ATHEROSCLEROSIS
AND
CARDIOVASCULAR
DISEASE

7TH INTERNATIONAL MEETING

ATHEROSCLEROSIS
AND
CARDIOVASCULAR
DISEASE

7TH INTERNATIONAL MEETING

EDITED BY

G.C. DESCOVICH, A. GADDI
G.L. MAGRI AND S. LENZI

Clinica Medica Generale e Terapia Medica I
Policlinico S. Orsola
via Massarenti, 9
40138 Bologna
Italy

KLUWER ACADEMIC PUBLISHERS
DORDRECHT / BOSTON / LONDON

Distributors

for the United States and Canada: Kluwer Academic Publishers, PO Box 358, Accord Station, Hingham, MA 02018-0358, USA
for all other countries: Kluwer Academic Publishers Group, Distribution Center, PO Box 322, 3300 AH Dordrecht, The Netherlands

British Library Cataloguing in Publication Data

Atherosclerosis and cardiovascular disease
1. Man. Cardiovascular system. Diseases
I. Descovich, G.C. (Giancarlo C.)
616.1
ISBN 0-7923-8938-7

Published in the United Kingdom by Kluwer Academic Publishers, PO Box 55, Lancaster, UK.

Kluwer Academic Publishers BV incorporates the publishing programmes of D. Reidel, Martinus Nijhoff, Dr W. Junk and MTP Press.

Printed in Great Britain by Butler & Tanner Limited, Frome and London

Contents

Contents

THE VEGETATIVE NERVOUS SYSTEM AND CARDIOVASCULAR DISEASE

NOSOLOGY OF HYPERLIPOPROTEINEMIAS

NUTRITION: POPULATION STUDIES

NUTRITION: SPECIAL DIETS AND METABOLIC EFFECTS OF FATS AND PROTEINS

RATIONALE FOR PREVENTION IN HIGH RISK SUBJECTS

HYPERLIPOPROTEINEMIA THERAPY: WHEN TO OPT FOR DRUG COMBINATIONS

HYPERTENSION AS A RISK FACTOR

INVASIVE THERAPY OF CORONARY AND CEREBROVASCULAR DISEASES

Preface

The advances in the field of atherosclerosis and cardiovascular disease continue at an increasingly rapid pace and it is an arduous task for those not directly involved to keep up with the latest developments.

The papers presented at the 7th Meeting on Atherosclerosis and Cardiovascular Disease, held in Bologna, as part of the Ninth Centenary of the foundation of the University of Bologna, have been collected together here with the aim of providing all the latest information for doctors and research workers concerned with this important branch of medicine.

We are pleased to be able to thank all those who joined us in celebrating the oldest university in the world.

The scientific contributions, of the highest level, are valid proof of the tradition of exchanging experiences and of the continual up-dating of knowledge in the different sectors of lipid metabolism, genetics, physiopathology, pathological anatomy, biochemical and clinical diagnosis, diet, pharmacological and non-pharmacological therapy. The numerous contributions made by authors in the field of epidemiology and the prevention of atherosclerosis were also fundamental since not only research centres but also doctors all over the world are engaged in the battle which was defined by the WHO, twenty-five years ago, as the most important epidemic of the modern age. The crucial importance of this sector of medicine cannot be overemphasized, since the awaited results concern entire communities or nations, and also because of the social, behavioural, ethical and economic implications which derive from the different strategic and/or working choices made in the health sector.

It is impossible to single out the most important papers: each one contributes to making this volume worthy of a place in the most highly specialized libraries of research workers, scholars, students and, in general, all those who recognize the urgency of the hyperlipoproteinaemia problem and the diseases linked to it.

All these readers will find appropriate and up-to-date answers to their questions in the various sections making up this book, which also provides a clear picture of the direction in which research in the field of atherosclerosis is moving.

The editors would like to express their gratitude to all the authors, and to the publishers who made it possible to publish this volume so rapidly.

Giancarlo Descovich
Antonio Gaddi
Gianluigi Magri
Sergio Lenzi

List of Contributors

G. Abate
Istituto di Gerontologia e Geriatria
via Nicolini 2
66100 Chieti CH
Italy

S. Alati
Department of Preventive Pediatrics and Neonatology
Università di Bologna
via Massarenti 11
40138 Bologna
Italy

R. Alessandroni
Department of Preventive Pediatrics and Neonatology
Università di Bologna
via Massarenti 11
40138 Bologna
Italy

M. Alle
Divisions of Cardiology and Cardiothoracic Surgery
Johann W. Goethe-University
Theodor-Stern-Kai 7
6000 Frankfurt a.M.
Federal Republic of Germany

P. Altieri
Divisione di Nefrologia e Dialisi
Ospedale "G. Brotzu"
via Peretti
09134 Cagliari
Italy

S. Amato
Internal Medicine and Geriatrics Institute
Department of Pathological Medicine
via del Vespro 143
University of Palermo
90127 Palermo
Italy

K.M. Anderson
Framingham Heart Study
118 Lincoln Street
Framingham, MA 02167
USA

F. Angelico
Institute of Systematic Medical Therapeutics
University of Rome "La Sapienza"
Policlinico Umberto I
viale del Policlinico
00161 Roma
Italy

G. Angelini
Department of Geriatrics
Institute of Clinical Medicine
University of Bari Medical School
Policlinico
70124 Bari
Italy

R. Antonini
Istituto di Scienze Farmacologiche
Facoltà di Farmacia
Università di Milano
via Balzaretti 9
20133 Milano
Italy

M. Arca
Department of Gerontology and Atherosclerosis Centre
University of Bologna
via Massarenti 9
40138 Bologna
Italy

P. Arrichiello
Institute of Internal Medicine
2nd School of Medicine
via S. Pansini 5
80135 Naples
Italy

G. Avellone
Istituto di Scienze Farmacologiche
Facoltà di Farmacia
Università di Milano
via Balzaretti 9
20133 Milano
Italy

M.R. Averna
Internal Medicine and Geriatrics Institute
Department of Pathological Medicine
via del Vespro 143
University of Palermo
90127 Palermo
Italy

P. Avogaro
Ospedale Regionale Generale
Divisione Medica II
30122 Venezia VE
Italy

M.R. Baiocchi
Istituto di Scienze Farmacologiche
Facoltà di Farmacia
Università di Milano
via Balzaretti 9
20133 Milano
Italy

R. Balestreri
Atherosclerosis Prevention Centre
Department of Internal Medicine
University of Genoa
viale Benedetto XV 6
16132 Genova GE
Italy

C.M. Barbagallo
Internal Medicine and Geriatrics Institute
Department of Pathological Medicine
via del Vespro 143
University of Palermo
90127 Palermo
Italy

J.M. Bard
Institut Pasteur
SERLIA et U. Inserm 325
1 rue Calmette
59019 Lille Cédex
France

G. Barozzi
Department of Gerontology and Atherosclerosis Centre
University of Bologna
via Massarenti 9
40138 Bologna
Italy

A. Barracca
Divisione di Nefrologia e Dialisi
Ospedale "G. Brotzu"
via Peretti
09134 Cagliari CA
Italy

J. Beitz
Department of Pharmacology and Toxicology
Martin Luther University
Halle-Wittenberg
German Democratic Republic

S. Bellosta
Institute of Pharmacological Sciences
University of Milan
via del Sarto 21
20129 Milano MI
Italy

M.S. Benassi
Istituto Patologia Speciale Medica e Metodologia Clinica
Università degli Studi di Bologna
via Massarenti 9
40138 Bologna BO
Italy

K. Berg
Institute of Medical Genetics
University of Oslo
PO Box 1036 Blindern
0315 Oslo 3
Norway

P. Bernardi
Istituto di Patologia Medica
Università di Bologna
Policlinico S. Orsola
via Massarenti 9
40138 Bologna
Italy

F. Bernini
Institute of Pharmacological Sciences
University of Milan
via del Sarto 21
20129 Milano MI
Italy

S. Bertolini
Atherosclerosis Prevention Centre
Department of Internal Medicine
University of Genoa
viale Benedetto XV 6
16132 Genova GE
Italy

A.C. Beynen
Department of Laboratory Animal Science
Veterinary Faculty
University of Utrecht
PO Box 80.166
3508 TD Utrecht
The Netherlands

V. Bianchi
Institute of Internal Medicine
2nd School of Medicine
via S. Pansini 5
80135 Naples
Italy

G. Bianciardi
Istituto di Anatomia e Istologia Patologica
Centro di Ricerche Arteriosclerosi
via delle Scotte 6
53100 Siena SI
Italy

M. Bihari-Varga
Semmelweis Medical University
II Department of Pathology
Biochemistry Division
Üllöi ut 93
H-1091 Budapest
Hungary

G. Bittolo Bon
Ospedale Regionale Generale
Divisione Medica II
30122 Venezia VE
Italy

G.F. Blane
Laboratoires Fournier SA
Centre de Recherche de Daix
50 Rue de Dijon
21121 Fontaine-les-Dijon
France

T. Bombardini
Cardiac Surgery Department
Policlinico S. Orsola
via Massarenti 9
40138 Bologna BO
Italy

D. Bonfiglioli
Second Department of Medicine
L. Sacco Hospital
University of Milan
via G.B. Grassi 74
20157 Milan
Italy

D. Bonaduce
Institute of Internal Medicine
2nd School of Medicine
via S. Pansini 5
80135 Naples
Italy

A. Bonanome
Clinica Medica I
University of Padova
Padova
Italy

G. Bondjers
Wallenburg Laboratory for Cardiovascular Research
Sahlgren's Hospital
University of Gothenburg
413 45 Gothenburg
Sweden

D. Bonfiglioli
Second Department of Medicine
L. Sacco Hospital
University of Milan
via G.B. Grassi 74
20157 Milan
Italy

M. Bonvicini
Department of Cardiology
University of Bologna
via Massarenti 9
40138 Bologna
Italy

A. Borghi
Institute of Pathological Medicine and CCU
Policlinico S. Orsola
University of Bologna
via Massarenti 9
40138 Bologna BO
Italy

M.L. Borlotti
Department of Geriatrics and Lipid Clinic
University of Bologna
40138 Bologna
Italy

C. Bozzoli
Instituto di Patologia Speciale Medica e Metodologia Clinica
Università di Bologna
S. Orsola Hospital
via Massarenti 9
40138 Bologna
Italy

A. Branchi
Institute of Internal Medicine and Medical Physiopathology
University of Milan
via G.B. Grassi 74
20157 Milan
Italy

A. Branzi
Institute of Cardiovascular Diseases
University of Bologna
Policlinico S. Orsola
via Massarenti 9
40138 Bologna BO
Italy

H. Braunsteiner
Department of Medicine
University of Innsbruck
Anichstrasse 35
6020 Innsbruck
Austria

E. Bruckert
Service d'Endocrinologie-Métabolisme
Hôpital de la Pitié
83 bv. de l'Hôpital
75013 Paris Cédex 13
France

G. Brunetti
2nd Department of Internal Medicine
University of Perugia
Policlinico Monteluce
06100 Perugia PG
Italy

T. Brüning
Institut für Klinische Chemie und Laboratoriumsmedizin
Arterioskleroseforsch. Institut
Westfälische Wilhelms-Univ.
Albert-Schweitzer-Strasse 33
D-4400 Münster
Federal Republic of Germany

A. Bucci
Istituto di Terapia Medica Sistemica
Cattedra di Ematologia
Università di Roma "La Sapienza"
Policlinico Umberto I
00161 Roma RM
Italy

H. Buchwald
Department of Surgery
University of Minnesota
420 Delaware Street
Minneapolis, MN 55455
USA

R. Bugiardini
Institute of Pathological Medicine and CCU
Policlinico S. Orsola
University of Bologna
via Massarenti 9
40138 Bologna BO
Italy

G. Busnach
Center E. Grossi Paoletti
Institute of Pharmacological Sciences
University of Milan
Niguarda Cà Granda Hospital
Milano
Italy

L. Calabresi
Center E. Grossi Paoletti
Inst. of Pharmacological Science
Department of Nephrology
University of Milano
Niguarda Cà Granda Hospital
Milano
Italy

S. Calandra
Institute of General Pathology
University of Modena
via Campi 287
41100 Modena
Italy

G. Camejo
Wallenburg Laboratory for Cardiovascular Research
Sahlgren's Hospital
University of Gothenburg
413 45 Gothenburg
Sweden

W. Campora
Atherosclerosis Prevention Centre
Department of Internal Medicine
University of Genoa
viale Benedetto XV 6
16132 Genova GE
Italy

C.T. Campos
Department of Surgery
Box 290
University of Minnesota
420 Delaware Street
Minneapolis, MN 55455
USA

A. Capurso
Department of Geriatrics
Institute of Clinical Medicine
University of Bari Medical School
Policlinico
70124 Bari
Italy

R. Carmena
Departmnt of Internal Medicine
Hospital Clinico Universitario
46010 Valencia
Spain

K.K. Carroll
Department of Biochemistry
University of Western Ontario
London
Ontario N6A 5C1
Canada

G. Castellani
Department of Physics
Università di Bologna
via Irnerio 46
40126 Bologna
Italy

M.A. Cavina
Department of Geriatrics and Lipid Clinic
University of Bologna
40138 Bologna
Italy

A.L. Catapano
Istituto di Scienze Farmacologiche
Facoltà di Farmacia
Università di Milano
via Balzaretti 9
20133 Milano
Italy

M.A. Cavina
Department of Geriatrics
University of Bologna
via Massarenti 9
40138 Bologna
Italy

M.A. Cavoni
Istituto di Gerontologia e Geriatria
via Nicolini 2
66100 Chieti CH
Italy

M. Cazzato
Cardiac Surgery Department
Policlinico S. Orsola
via Massarenti 9
40138 Bologna BO
Italy

G. Cazzolato
Ospedale Regionale Generale
Divisione Medica II
30122 Venezia VE
Italy

E. Celentano
Institute of Internal Medicine and Metabolic Disease
2nd Medical School
via Sergio Pansini 5
80131 Naples
Italy

L. Centi
Istituto di Anatomia e Istologia Patologica
Centro di Ricerche Arteriosclerosi
via delle Scotte 6
53100 Siena SI
Italy

A.M. Cerbone
Istituto di Medicina Interna e Malattie Dismetaboliche
Cattedra di Immunoematologia
II. Policlinico
Università degli Studi di Napoli
Napoli
Italy

C. Ceredi
Department of Geriatrics and Lipid Clinic
University of Bologna
40138 Bologna
Italy

S. Cerutti
Istituto Ricerche Cardiovascolari CNR
Patologia Medica
Ospedale "L. Sacco"
Università di Milano
via Bonfadini 214
20138 Milano
Italy

G. Chiesa
Center E. Grossi Paoletti
Institute of Pharmacological Sciences
Department of Nephrology
University of Milano
Niguarda Cà Granda Hospital
Milano
Italy

D. Ciancia
Department of Geriatrics
Institute of Clinical Medicine
University of Bari Medical School
Policlinico
70124 Bari
Italy

A. Ciarrocchi
Department of Gerontology
Atherosclerosis Centre
University of Bologna
via Massarenti 9
40138 Bologna
Italy

A. Cicognani
Istituto di Medicina Legale
Università di Bologna
40138 Bologna
Italy

M.R. Cingi
Institute of General Pathology
University of Modena
via Campi 287
41100 Modena
Italy

F. Cirillo
Istituto di Medicina Interna e Malattie Dismetaboliche
Cattedra di Immunoematologia
Università degli Studi di Napoli
Napoli
Italy

V. Clavey
Institut Pasteur
SERLIA et U. Inserm 325
1 rue Calmette
59019 Lille Cédex
France

D. Colombo
Department of Chemistry and Biochemistry
School of Medicine
Università di Milano
via Balzaretti 9
20133 Milano MI
Italy

C. Colucci
Department of Preventive Pediatrics and Neonatology
Università di Bologna
via Massarenti 11
40138 Bologna
Italy

G. Conforti
Institute of Internal Medicine
2nd School of Medicine
via S. Pansini 5
80135 Naples
Italy

A. Corsini
Institute of Pharmacological Sciences
University of Milan
via del Sarto 21
20129 Milano MI
Italy

F. Cuccurullo
Istituto di Patologia Speciale Medica
Università G. D'Annunzio
via dei Vestini
66013 Chieti CH
Italy

M. D'Addato
Department of Vascular Surgery
University of Bologna
via Massarenti 9
40138 Bologna BO
Italy

S. D'Addato
Department of Geriatrics
University of Bologna
via Massarenti 9
40138 Bologna BO
Italy

F. Dairou
Service d'Endocrinologie-Métabolisme
Hôpital de la Pitié
83 bv. de l'Hôpital
75013 Paris Cédex 13
France

C. Dal Palu'
Clinica Medica I
Università di Padova
via Giustiniani 2
35100 Padova PD
Italy

G. Davì
Ematologia
Università di Chieti
Italy

J. Davignon
Hyperlipidemia & Artherosclerosis Research Group
Clinical Research Institute of Montreal
110 Pine Avenue West
Montreal
Quebec H2W. IR7
Canada

C. De Collibus
Istituto Patologia Speciale Medica e Metodologia Clinica
Università degli Studi di Bologna
via Massarenti 9
40138 Bologna BO
Italy

J.L. De Gennes
Service d'Endocrinologie-Métaboiisme
Hôpital de la Pitié
83 bv. de l'Hôpital
75013 Paris Cédex 13
France

M. Del Ben
Institute of Systematic Medical Therapeutics
University of Rome "La Sapienza"
Policlinico Umberto I
00161 Roma
Italy

G. Del Boccio
Istituto di Scienze Biochimiche
Università G. D'Annunzio
via dei Vestini
66013 Chieti CH
Italy

D. De Nardo
Department of Internal Medicine
Institute of Clinical Medicine
II University of Rome "Tor Vergata"
Rome
Italy

G.C. Descovich
Department of Gerontology and Atherosclerosis Centre
University of Bologna
via Massarenti 9
40138 Bologna
Italy

G. De Simone
Department of Geriatrics and Lipid Clinic
University of Bologna
40138 Bologna
Italy

G. Di Minno
Istituto di Medicina Interna e Malattie Dismetaboliche
Cattedra di Immunoematologia
Università degli Studi di Napoli
Napoli
Italy

U. Dimita
Internal Medicine and Geriatrics Institute
Department of Pathological Medicine
via del Vespro 143
University of Palermo
90127 Palermo
Italy

G. Di Paola
Internal Medicine and Geriatrics Institute
Department of Pathological Medicine
via del Vespro 143
University of Palermo
90127 Palermo
Italy

M. Di Tommaso
Department of Geriatrics
Institute of Clinical Medicine
University of Bari Medical School
Policlinico
70124 Bari
Italy

A. Dormi
Department of Geriatrics and Lipid Clinic
University of Bologna
40138 Bologna
Italy

H. Drexel
Department of Medicine
University of Innsbruck
Anichstrasse 35
6020 Innsbruck
Austria

C.A. Dujovne
Lipid and Arteriosclerosis Prevention Clinic
Division of Clinical Pharmacology
University of Kansas Medical Center
1348 Bell 39th and Rainbow
Kansas City, KS 66103
USA

S. Eisenberg
Hadassah University Hospital
Department of Internal Medicine B
POB 12000
il-91120 Jerusalem
Israel

N. Elicio
Atherosclerosis Prevention Centre
Department of Internal Medicine
University of Genoa
viale Benedetto XV 6
16132 Genova GE
Italy

F.H. Epstein
Institute of Social and Preventive Medicine
University of Zürich
Sumatrastrasse 30
CH 8006 Zürich
Switzerland

G. Fager
Wallenburg Laboratory for Cardiovascular Research
Sahlgren's Hospital
University of Gothenburg
413 45 Gothenburg
Sweden

E. Faggioli
Department of Geriatrics and Lipid Clinic
University of Bologna
40138 Bologna
Italy

C. Falco
Istituto di Medicina Interna e Malattie Dismetaboliche
Cattedra di Immunoematologia
II Policlinico
Università degli Studi di Napoli
Napoli
Italy

G. Faldella
Department of Preventive Pediatrics and Neonatology
Università di Bologna
via Massarenti 11
40138 Bologna
Italy

M. Fallani
Istituto di Medicina Legale
Università di Bologna
40138 Bologna
Italy

S. Fantappie
Istituto di Scienze Farmacologiche
Facoltà di Farmacia
Università di Milano
via Balzaretti 9
20133 Milano
Italy

E. Farinaro
Institute of Internal Medicine and Metabolic Disease
2nd Medical School
via Sergio Pansini 5
80131 Naples
Italy

A. Fasoli
Institute of Internal Medicine and Medical Physiopathology
University of Milan
via G.B. Grassi 74
20157 Milan
Italy

R. Fattori
Institute of Cardiovascular Diseases
University of Bologna
Policlinico S. Orsola
via Massarenti 9
40138 Bologna BO
Italy

R. Fellin
Istituto di Scienze Farmacologiche
Facoltà di Farmacia
Università di Milano
via Balzaretti 9
20133 Milano
Italy

C. Fieschi
Department of Neurosciences
University of Rome "La Sapienza"
viale dell'Università 30
00185 Roma RM
Italy

L. Finazzo
Gerontology & Atherosclerosis Centre
University of Bologna
via Massarenti 9
40138 Bologna
Italy

F. Fontana
Istituto di Patologia Medica
Università di Bologna
Policlinico S. Orsola
via Massarenti 9
40138 Bologna
Italy

G. Fortuni
Istituto di Medicina Legale
Università di Bologna
40138 Bologna
Italy

G. Franceschini
Center E. Grossi Paoletti
Inst. of Pharmacological Sci.
University of Milano
Niguarda Cà Granda Hospital
Milano
Italy

M. Frontoni
Department of Neurosciences
University of Rome "La Sapienza"
viale dell'Università 30
00185 Roma RM
Italy

J.C. Fruchart
Institut Pasteur
SERLIA et U. Inserm 325
1 rue Calmette
59019 Lille Cédex
France

H. Fujita
The Second Department of Internal Medicine
Kanazawa University School of Medicine
Takara-machi 13-1
Kanazawa 920
Japan

R. Fumagalli
Institute of Pharmacological Sciences
University of Milan
via del Sarto 21
20129 Milano MI
Italy

G. Fusco
Institute of Internal Medicine and Metabolic Disease
2nd Medical School
via Sergio Pansini 5
80131 Naples
Italy

A. Gaddi
Department of Gerontology and Atherosclerosis Centre
University of Bologna
via Massarenti 9
40138 Bologna
Italy

R. Galasso
Institute of Internal Medicine and Metabolic Disease
2nd Medical School
via Sergio Pansini 5
80131 Naples
Italy

G. Galli
Institute of Pharmacological Sciences
School of Pharmacy
Università di Milano
via Balzaretti 9
20133 Milano MI
Italy

I. Galligani
Department of Mathematics
University of Bologna
40125 Bologna BO
Italy

E. Ganga
Centro Regionale per le Malattie Dismetaboliche e l'Arteriosclerosi
Ospedale S. Michele
USL 21 via Peretti
09100 Cagliari CA
Italy

C. Gaudio
II Department of Cardiology
University of Rome "La Sapienza"
00161 Rome
Italy

G. Ghiselli
Baylor College of Medicine
6565 Fannin Street
Houston, TX 77030
USA

M. Giacchi
Istituto di Scienze Farmacologiche
Facoltà di Farmacia
Università di Milano
via Balzaretti 9
20133 Milano
Italy

D. Giumetti
Institute of Internal Medicine and Metabolic Disease
2nd Medical School
via Sergio Pansini 5
80131 Naples
Italy

A. Gnasso
Istituto di Medicina Interna e Malattie Dismetaboliche
Cattedra di Immunoematologia
II. Policlinico
Università degli Studi di Napoli
Napoli
Italy

N. Gorder
Baylor College of Medicine
6565 Fannin Street
Houston, TX 77030
USA

A.M. Gotto Jr
Department of Medicine
The Methodist Hospital
6565 Fannin Street
Houston, TX 77030
USA

M. Gozzer
Istituto di Terapia Medica Sistemica
Cattedra di Ematologia
Università di Roma "La Sapienza"
Policlinico Umberto I
00161 Roma RM
Italy

M.J. Halpern
Centre for Lipid Research
Department of Biochemistry
Faculty of Medical Science of UNL
Campo Santana 130
1100 Lisbon
Portugal

W.S. Harris
Lipid and Arteriosclerosis Prevention Clinic
Division of Clinical Pharmacology
University of Kansas Medical Center
1348 Bell 39th and Rainbow
Kansas City, KS 66103
USA

R. Homan
Division of Atherosclerosis and Lipoprotein Research
Baylor College of Medicine
The Methodist Hospital
6565 Fannin Street
Houston, TX 77030
USA

Th. Hopferwieser
Department of Medicine
University of Innsbruck
Anichstrasse 35
6020 Innsbruck
Austria

E. Hurt-Camejo
Wallenburg Laboratory for Cardiovascular Research
Sahlgren's Hospital
University of Gothenburg
413 45 Gothenburg
Sweden

T.L. Innerarity
Galdstone Foundation Laboratories for Cardiovascular Disease
Cardiovascular Research Institute
University of California
San Francisco, CA 94140-0608
USA

G.C. Isacchi
Istituto di Terapia Medica Sistemica
Cattedra di Ematologia
Università di Roma "La Sapienza"
Policlinico Umberto I
00161 Roma RM
Italy

Z. Jericevic
The Methodist Hospital
Department of Cell Biology
6565 Fannin Street
Houston, TX 77030
USA

F. Jossa
Institute of Internal Medicine and Metabolic Disease
2nd Medical School
via Sergio Pansini 5
80131 Naples
Italy

I. Juhan-Vague
Institut Pasteur
SERLIA et U. Inserm 325
1 rue Calmette
59019 Lille Cédex
France

K. Kajinami
The Second Department of Internal Medicine
Kanazawa University School of Medicine
Takara-machi 13-1
Kanazawa 920
Japan

M. Kaltenbach
Divisions of Cardiology and Cardiothoracic Surgery
Johann W. Goethe-University
Theodor-Stern-Kai 7
6000 Frankfurt a.M.
Federal Republic of Germany

W.B. Kannel
Section of Preventive Medicine & Epidemiology
Boston University School of Medicine
720 Harrison Avenue
Boston, MA 02118
USA

M.B. Katan
Department of Human Nutrition
Agricultural University
PO Box 8129
6700 EV. Wageningen
The Netherlands

P. Khosla
Department of Biochemistry
University of Western Ontario
London
Ontario N6A 5C1
Canada

E. Knapp
Department of Medicine
University of Innsbruck
Anichstrasse 35
6020 Innsbruck
Austria

G. Kober
Divisions of Cardiology and Cardiothoracic Surgery
Johann W. Goethe-University
Theodor-Stern-Kai 7
6000 Frankfurt a.M.
Federal Republic of Germany

J. Koizumi
2nd Department of Internal Medicine
Kanazawa University School of Medicine
Takara-machi 13-1
Kanazawa 920
Japan

G.M. Kostner
Institute of Medical Biochemistry
University of Graz
Harrachgasse 21/III
A-8010 Graz
Austria

S.G. Kozlov
USSR Cardiology Research Center
Academy of Medical Sciences
Moscow 121552
USSR

D. Kritchevsky
Wistar Institute of Anatomy & Biology
3601 Spruce Street
Philadelphia, PA 19104
USA

M. Labisi
Internal Medicine and Geriatrics Institute
Department of Pathological Medicine
via del Vespro 143
University of Palermo
90127 Palermo
Italy

G. Lamm
Institute for Clinical Social Medicine
University Medical Clinic Heidelberg
Bergheimer Strasse 58
6900 Heidelberg 1
Federal Republic of Germany

M. Lanari
Department of Preventive Pediatrics and Neonatology
Università di Bologna
via Massarenti 11
40138 Bologna
Italy

T. Lanzillo
Institute of Internal Medicine
2nd School of Medicine
via S. Pansini 5
80135 Naples
Italy

D. Lapenna
Istituto di Patologia Speciale Medica
Università G. D'Annunzio
via dei Vestini
66013 Chieti CH
Italy

R. Laschi
Institute of Clinical Electron Microscopy
University of Bologna
S. Orsola Hospital
via Massarenti 9
40138 Bologna BO
Italy

Y.C. Lin-Lee
Baylor College of Medicine
6565 Fannin Street
Houston, TX 77030
USA

F. Lombardi
Istituto Ricerche Cardiovascolari CNR
Ospedale "L. Sacco"
Università di Milano
via Bonfadini 214
20138 Milano
Italy

G. Lupattelli
2nd Department of Internal Medicine
University of Perugia
Policlinico Monteluce
06100 Perugia PG
Italy

A.A. Lyakishev
USSR. Cardiology Research Center
Academy of Medical Sciences
Moscow 12 1552
USSR

H. Mabuchi
The Second Department of Internal Medicine
Kanazawa University School of Medicine
Takara-machi 13-1
Kanazawa 920
Japan

G.L. Magri
Department of Geriatrics and Lipid Clinic
University of Bologna
40138 Bologna
Italy

R.W. Mahley
Galdstone Foundation Laboratories for Cardiovascular Disease
Cardiovascular Research Institute
University of California
San Francisco, CA 94140-0608
USA

B. Malavasi
Institute of Pharmacological Sciences
School of Pharmacy
Università di Milano
via Balzaretti 9
20133 Milano MI
Italy

A. Malliani
Istituto Ricerche Cardiovascolari
Centro Ricerche Cardiovascolari CNR
Ospedale "L. Sacco"
Università Milano
via Bonfadini 214
20138 Milano MI
Italy

M. Mancini
Institute of Internal Medicine and Metabolic Disease
2nd Medical School
via Sergio Pansini 5
80131 Naples
Italy

C.F. Manetti
Istituto Patologia Speciale Medica e Metodologia Clinica
Università degli Studi di Bologna
via Massarenti 9
40138 Bologna BO
Italy

G. Mannino
Department of Mathematics
Department of Numerical Analysis
University of Modena
Modena
Italy

P.M. Mannucci
Institute of Internal Medicine
A. Bianchi Bonomi Hemophilia and Thrombosis Center
University of Milan
20122 Milano MI
Italy

A. Marcenaro
Atherosclerosis Prevention Centre
Department of Internal Medicine
University of Genoa
viale Benedetto XV 6
16132 Genova GE
Italy

M. Margaglione
Istituto di Medicina Interna e Malattie Dismetaboliche
Cattedra di Immunoematologia
II. Policlinico
Università degli Studi di Napoli
Napoli
Italy

D. Mari
Institute of Internal Medicine
A. Bianchi Bonomi Hemophilia and Thrombosis Center
University of Milan
20122 Milano MI
Italy

G. Marinelli
Cardiac Surgery Department
Policlinico S. Orsola
via Massarenti 9
40138 Bologna BO
Italy

G. Marino
Internal Medicine and Geriatrics Institute
Department of Pathological Medicine
via del Vespro 143
University of Palermo
90127 Palermo
Italy

G. Marra
Department of Gerontology and Atherosclerosis Centre
University of Bologna
via Massarenti 9
40138 Bologna
Italy

C. Marrozzini
Institute of Cardiovascular Diseases
University of Bologna
Policlinico S. Orsola
via Massarenti 9
40138 Bologna BO
Italy

A. Marzocchi
Institute of Cardiovascular Diseases
University of Bologna
Policlinico S. Orsola
via Massarenti 9
40138 Bologna BO
Italy

M. Masci
Istituto di Terapia Medica Sistemica
Cattedra di Ematologia
Università di Roma "La Sapienza"
Policlinico Umberto I
00161 Roma RM
Italy

P. Mascia
Centro Regionale per le Malattie Dismetaboliche e l'Arteriosclerosi
Ospedale S. Michele
USL 21 via Peretti
09100 Cagliari CA
Italy

J.B. Massey
Division of Atherosclerosis and Lipoprotein Research
Baylor College of Medicine
6565 Fannin Street
Houston, TX 77030
USA

B. Mazzarella
Istituto di Terapia Medica Sistemica
Cattedra di Ematologia
Università di Roma "La Sapienza"
Policlinico Umberto I
00161 Roma RM
Italy

G. Melandri
Institute of Cardiovascular Diseases
University of Bologna
Policlinico S. Orsola
via Massarenti 9
40138 Bologna BO
Italy

R.P. Mensink
Department of Human Nutrition
Agricultural University
PO Box 8129
6700 EV. Wageningen
The Netherlands

M. Mercuri
2nd Department of Internal Medicine
University of Perugia
Policlinico Monteluce
06100 Perugia PG
Italy

M.F. Mesquita
Centre for Lipid Research
Department of Biochemistry
Faculty of Medical Science of UNL
Campo Santana 130
1100 Lisbon
Portugal

H.J. Mest
Department of Pharmacology and Toxicology
Martin Luther University
Halle-Wittenberg
East Germany

E. Millefiorini
Department of Neurosciences
University of Rome "La Sapienza"
viale dell'Università 30
00185 Roma RM
Italy

A. Minardi
Department of Geriatrics
University of Bologna
via Massarenti 9
40138 Bologna
Italy

A.M. Mogavero
Department of Geriatrics
Institute of Clinical Medicine
University of Bari Medical School
Policlinico
70124 Bari
Italy

M.V. Montemurro
Institute of Internal Medicine
2nd School of Medicine
via S. Pansini 5
80135 Naples
Italy

G. Morgagni
Institute of Pathological Medicine and CCU
Policlinico S. Orsola
University of Bologna
via Massarenti 9
40138 Bologna BO
Italy

G. Morgano
Institute of Internal Medicine
2nd School of Medicine
via S. Pansini 5
80135 Naples
Italy

M. Mosca
Istituto Patologia Speciale Medica e Metodologia Clinica
Università degli Studi di Bologna
via Massarenti 9
40138 Bologna BO
Italy

V. Mühlberger
Department of Medicine
University of Innsbruck
Anichstrasse 35
6020 Innsbruck
Austria

S. Muntoni
Centre for Metabolic Diseases and Atherosclerosis
Ospedale "G. Brotzu"
via Peretti
09134 Cagliari
Italy

R. Musanti
Baylor College of Medicine
6565 Fannin Street
Houston, TX 77030
USA

A. Muscari
Istituto di Patologia Speciale Medica e Metodologia Clinica
Università di Bologna
S. Orsola Hospital
via Massarenti 9
40138 Bologna
Italy

P.G. Nanni
Department of Physics
Università di Bologna
via Irnerio 46
40126 Bologna
Italy

G. Negro
Department of Geriatrics and Lipid Clinic
University of Bologna
40138 Bologna
Italy

M. Nichelatti
Pierrel Farmaceutici
via Bisceglie 96
20152 Milano
Italy

F. Nobili
Institute of Neurophysiopathology
Università di Genova
viale Benedetto XV 6
16132 Genova GE
Italy

A. Notarbartolo
Internal Medicine and Geriatrics Institute
Department of Pathological Medicine
via del Vespro 143
University of Palermo
90127 Palermo
Italy

S. Nucci
Immunohematology and Transfusional Centre
University of Bologna
S. Orsola Hospital
via Massarenti 9
40138 Bologna BO
Italy

M.F. Oliver
Wynn Institute for Metabolic Research
London NW8 9SQ
United Kingdom

A.N. Orekhov
USSR. Cardiology Research Center
Academy of Medical Sciences
Moscow 12 1552
USSR

P. Oriente
Istituto di Scienze Farmacologiche
Facoltà di Farmacia
Università di Milano
via Balzaretti 9
20133 Milano
Italy

F. Ottani
Institute of Pathological Medicine and CCU
Policlinico S. Orsola
University of Bologna
via Massarenti 9
40138 Bologna BO
Italy

A. Pagnan
Patologia Speciale Medica
University of Padova
35139 Padova PD
Italy

C. Pallotti
Department of Physics
Università di Bologna
via Irnerio 46
40126 Bologna
Italy

G. Pallotti
Department of Physics
Università di Bologna
via Irnerio 46
40126 Bologna
Italy

S. Palmisano
Department of Geriatrics
Institute of Clinical Medicine
University of Bari Medical School
Policlinico
70124 Bari
Italy

S. Panico
Institute of Internal Medicine and Metabolic Disease
2nd Medical School
via Sergio Pansini 5
80131 Naples
Italy

P. Pantano
Department of Neurosciences
University of Rome "La Sapienza"
viale dell'Università 30
00185 Roma RM
Italy

R. Paoletti
Institute of Pharmacological Sciences
University of Milan
via del Sarto 21
20129 Milano MI
Italy

H.J. Parra
Institut Pasteur
SERLIA et U. Inserm 325
1 rue Calmette
59019 Lille Cédex
France

G. Pasquinelli
Institute of Clinical Electron Microscopy
University of Bologna
S. Orsola Hospital
via Massarenti 9
40138 Bologna BO
Italy

J.R. Patsch
Department of Medicine
Baylor College of Medicine
The Methodist Hospital
6565 Fannin Street
Houston, TX 77030
USA

W. Patsch
Baylor College of Medicine
6565 Fannin Street
Houston, TX 77030
USA

P. Pauletto
Clinica Medica I
Università di Padova
via Giustiniani 2
35100 Padova PD
Italy

A. Pennelli
Istituto di Scienze Biochimiche
Università G. D'Annunzio
via dei Vestini
66013 Chieti CH
Italy

M. Petretta
Institute of Internal Medicine
2nd School of Medicine
via S. Pansini 5
80135 Naples
Italy

P. Pettazzoni
Department of Physics
Università di Bologna
via Irnerio 46
40126 Bologna
Italy

F.M. Picchio
Department of Cardiology
University of Bologna
via Massarenti 9
40138 Bologna
Italy

A. Pierangeli
Cardiac Surgery Department
Policlinico S. Orsola
via Massarenti 9
40138 Bologna BO
Italy

C. Pini
Institute of Internal Medicine
and Medical Physiopathology
University of Milan
via G.B. Grassi 74
20157 Milan
Italy

F. Pintus
Centro Regionale Malattie
Dismetaboliche e
l'Arteriosclerosi
Ospedale S. Michele
USL 21 via Peretti
09100 Cagliari CA
Italy

G. Piovaccari
Institute of Cardiovascular
Diseases
University of Bologna
Policlinico S. Orsola
via Massarenti 9
40138 Bologna BO
Italy

E.M. Pivovarova
USSR. Cardiology Research
Center
Academy of Medical Sciences
Moscow 12 1552
USSR

R. Pizzorno
Atherosclerosis Prevention
Centre
Department of Internal
Medicine
University of Genoa
viale Benedetto XV 6
16132 Genova GE
Italy

E. Porreca
Istituto di Patologia Speciale
Medica
Università G. D'Annunzio
via dei Vestini
66013 Chieti CH
Italy

A. Postiglione
Istituto di Medicina Interna e
Malattie Dismetaboliche
Cattedra di Immunoematologia
II. Policlinico
Università degli Studi di Napoli
Napoli
Italy

L. Postiglione
Istituto di Scienze
Farmacologiche
Facoltà di Farmacia
Università di Milano
via Balzaretti 9
20133 Milano
Italy

H.J. Pownall
Division of Atherosclerosis and
Lipoprotein Research
Baylor College of Medicine
The Methodist Hospital
6565 Fannin Street
Houston, TX 77030
USA

A. Pozzati
Institute of Pathological
Medicine and CCU
Policlinico S. Orsola
University of Bologna
via Massarenti 9
40138 Bologna BO
Italy

F. Prati
Institute of Cardiovascular
Diseases
University of Bologna
Policlinico S. Orsola
via Massarenti 9
40138 Bologna BO
Italy

G.M. Puddu
Istituto Patologia Speciale Medica e Metodologia Clinica
Università di Bologna
S. Orsola Hospital
via Massarenti 9
40138 Bologna BO
Italy

P. Puddu
Istituto Patologia Speciale Medica e Metodologia Clinica
Università di Bologna
S. Orsola Hospital
via Massarenti 9
40138 Bologna BO
Italy

S.C. Rall Jr.
Galdstone Foundation Laboratories for Cardiovascular Disease
Cardiovascular Research Institute
University of California
San Francisco, CA 94140-0608
USA

D. Reggiani
Institute of General Pathology
University of Modena
via Campi 287
41100 Modena
Italy

N. Reifart
Divisions of Cardiology and Cardiothoracic Surgery
Johann W. Goethe-University
Theodor-Stern-Kai 7
6000 Frankfurt a.M.
Federal Republic of Germany

F. Resta
Department of Geriatrics
Institute of Clinical Medicine
University of Bari Medical School
Policlinico
70124 Bari
Italy

G. Ricci
Istituto di Scienze Biochimiche
Università L'Annunzio
via dei Vestini
66013 Chieti CH
Italy

G. Ricci
Institute of Systematic Medical Therapeutics
University of Rome "La Sapienza"
Policlinico Umberto I
00161 Roma
Italy

I. Richichi
Cardiovascular Prevention Center
Policlinico S. Matteo
P. le Golgi 2
27100 Pavia PV
Italy

S. Rimondi
Department of Gerontology and Atherosclerosis Centre
University of Bologna
via Massarenti 9
40138 Bologna
Italy

G. Rodriguez
Institute of Neurophysiopathology
Università di Genova
via le Benedetto XV 6
16132 Genova GE
Italy

P. Roebruck
Divisions of Cardiology and Cardiothoracic Surgery
Johann W. Goethe-University
Theodor-Stern-Kai 7
6000 Frankfurt a.M.
Federal Republic of Germany

P. Roma
Istituto di Scienze Farmacologiche
Facoltà di Farmacia
Università di Milano
via Balzaretti 9
20133 Milano
Italy

A. Romagnoli
Department of Geriatrics and Lipid Clinic
University of Bologna
40138 Bologna
Italy

R. Rossini
Department of Preventive Pediatrics and Neonatology
Università di Bologna
via Massarenti 11
40138 Bologna
Italy

C. Rotella
Atherosclerosis Prevention Centre
Department of Internal Medicine
University of Genoa
viale Benedetto XV 6
16132 Genova GE
Italy

A. Rovellini
Institute of Internal Medicine and Medical Physiopathology
University of Milan
via G.B. Grassi 74
20157 Milan
Italy

D. Rovinetti
Istituto Patologia Speciale Medica e Metodologia Clinica
Università degli Studi di Bologna
via Massarenti 9
40138 Bologna BO

M. Ya. Ruda
USSR. Cardiology Research Center
Academy of Medical Sciences
Moscow 12 1552
USSR

O. Russo
Istituto di Medicina Interna e Malattie Dismetaboliche
Cattedra di Immunoematologia
II. Policlinico
Università degli Studi di Napoli
Napoli
Italy

M. Sacchetti
Department of Neurosciences
University of Rome "La Sapienza"
viale dell'Università 30
00185 Roma RM
Italy

R. Sala
Istituto Ricerche Cardiovascolari CNR
Patologia Medica
Ospedale "L. Sacco"
Università di Milano
via Bonfadini 214
20138 Milano
Italy

M. Salvi
Istituto di Anatomia e Istologia Patologica
Centro di Ricerche Arteriosclerosi
via delle Scotte 6
53100 Siena SI
Italy

G.P. Salvioli
Department of Preventive Pediatrics and Neonatology
Università di Bologna
via Massarenti 11
40138 Bologna
Italy

S. Samman
Department of Biochemistry
University of Western Ontario
London
Ontario N6A 5C1
Canada

G. Sandrone
Istituto Ricerche Cardiovascolari CNR
Patologia Medica
Ospedale "L. Sacco"
Università di Milano
via Bonfadini 214
20138 Milano
Italy

M. Sangiorgi
Cattedra di Clinica Medica Generale e Terapia Medica
Departimento di Medicina Interna
II Università degli Studi di Roma
00144 Roma
Italy

Z. Sangiorgi
Department of Gerontology and Atherosclerosis Centre
University of Bologna
via Massarenti 9
40138 Bologna
Italy

M. Santarella
Brisighella Hospital
Brisighella
Italy

P. Satter
Divisions of Cardiology and Cardiothoracic Surgery
Johann W. Goethe-University
Theodor-Stern-Kai 7
6000 Frankfurt a.M.
Federal Republic of Germany

V. Sau
Divisione di Nefrologia e Dialisi
Ospedale "G. Brotzu"
via Peretti
09134 Cagliari CA
Italy

G. Scannapieco
Clinica Medica I
Università di Padova
via Giustiniani 2
35100 Padova PD
Italy

L. Scandiani
Institute of Internal Medicine and Medical Physiopathology
University of Milan
via G.B. Grassi 74
20157 Milan
Italy

A.M. Scanu
Department of Medicine, Biochemistry & Molecular Biology
University of Chicago
Pritzker School of Medicine
5841 South Maryland Avenue
Chicago, IL 60637
USA

N. Scarpato
Istituto di Medicina Interna e Malattie Dismetaboliche
Cattedra di Immunoematologia
II. Policlinico
Università degli Studi di Napoli
Napoli
Italy

W. Scheuermann
Institute for Clinical Social Medicine
University Medical Clinic Heidelberg
Bergheimer Strasse 58
6900 Heidelberg
Federal Republic of Germany

G. Schmitz
Institut für Klinische Chemie und Laboratoriumsmedizin
Wilhelms-Universität
Albert-Schweitzer-Strasse 33
D-4400 Münster
Federal Republic of Germany

W. Schneider
Divisions of Cardiology and Cardiothoracic Surgery
Johann W. Goethe-University
Theodor-Stern-Kai 7
6000 Frankfurt a.M.
Federal Republic of Germany

E. Sehayek
Hadassah University Hospital
Department of Internal Medicine B
POB 12000
il-91120 Jerusalem
Israel

U. Senin
2nd Department of Internal Medicine
University of Perugia
Policlinico Monteluce
06100 Perugia PG
Italy

G. Sermasi
Immunohematology and Transfusional Centre
University of Bologna
S. Orsola Hospital
via Massarenti 9
40138 Bologna BO
Italy

M. Shimizu
2nd Department of Internal Medicine
Kanazawa University School of Medicine
Takara-machi 13-1
Kanazawa 920
Japan

G.B. Sisca
Department of Geriatrics and Lipid Clinic
University of Bologna
40138 Bologna
Italy

M.R. Slawomirski
Department of Mathematical Modelling
Polish Petroleum Institute
PL 31-935 Krakow
Poland

L.C. Smith
Baylor College of Medicine
Department of Medicine
6565 Fannin Street
Houston, TX 77030
USA

D. Sommariva
Second Department of Medicine
L. Sacco Hospital
University of Milan
via G.B. Grassi 74
20157 Milan
Italy

L. Sottocornola
Istituto di Scienze Farmacologiche
Facoltà di Farmacia
Università di Milano
via Balzaretti 9
20133 Milano
Italy

H.F. Spies
Divisions of Cardiology and Cardiothoracic Surgery
Johann W. Goethe-University
Theodor-Stern-Kai 7
6000 Frankfurt a.M.
Federal Republic of Germany

L. Steffanon
Istituto Patologia Speciale Medica e Metodologia Clinica
Università degli Studi di Bologna
via Massarenti 9
40138 Bologna BO

C. Stefanutti
Istituto di Terapia Medica Sistemica
Cattedra di Ematologia
Università di Roma "La Sapienza"
Policlinico Umberto I
00161 Roma RM
Italy

A. Strano
Patologia Medica
II Università di Roma
via di Vigna Stelluta 40
00191 Roma RM
Italy

W. Strobl
Baylor College of Medicine
6565 Fannin Street
Houston, TX 77030
USA

A. Susta
2nd Department of Internal Medicine
University of Perugia
Policlinico Monteluce
06100 Perugia PG
Italy

M.I. Sztern
Lipid and Arteriosclerosis Prevention Clinic
Division of Clinical Pharmacology
University of Kansas
1348 Bell 39th and Rainbow
Kansas City, KS 66103
USA

R. Takeda
2nd Department of Internal Medicine
Kanazawa University School of Medicine
Takara-machi 13-1
Kanazawa 920
Japan

P. Tanganelli
Istituto di Anatomia e Istologia Patologica
Centro di Ricerche Arteriosclerosi
via delle Scotte 6
53100 Siena SI
Italy

R. Taverniti
Department of Geriatrics
Institute of Clinical Medicine
University of Bari Medical School
Policlinico
70124 Bari
Italy

M.T. Tenconi
Istituto di Scienze Farmacologiche
Facoltà di Farmacia
Università di Milano
via Balzaretti 9
20133 Milano
Italy

V.V. Tertov
USSR. Cardiology Research Center
Academy of Medical Sciences
Moscow 12 1552
USSR

R. Tiozzo
Institute of General Pathology
University of Modena
via Campi 287
41100 Modena
Italy

M. Tirrito
Second Department of Medicine
L. Sacco Hospital
University of Milan
via G.B. Grassi 74
20157 Milan
Italy

D. Toni
Department of Neurosciences
University of Rome "La Sapienza"
viale dell'Università 30
00185 Roma RM
Italy

U. Tortorolo
Atherosclerosis Prevention Centre
Department of Internal Medicine
University of Genoa
viale Benedetto XV 6
16132 Genova GE
Italy

J. Truffert
Service d'Endocrinologie-Métabolisme
Hôpital de la Pitié
83 bv. de l'Hôpital
75013 Paris Cédex 13
France

C. Turchi
Department of Agriculture and Nutrition
Emilia-Romagna Region
Italy

B. Turinetto
Cardiac Surgery Department
Policlinico S. Orsola
via Massarenti 9
40138 Bologna BO
Italy

Y. Uno
2nd Department of Internal Medicine
Kanazawa University School of Medicine
Takara-machi 13-1
Kanazawa 920
Japan

G.C. Urbinati
Institute of Systematic Medical Therapeutics
University of Rome "La Sapienze"
Policlinico Umberto I
00161 Roma
Italy

G. Vecchione
Istituto di Medicina Interna e Malattie Dismetaboliche
Cattedra di Immunoematologia
II. Policlinico
Università degli Studi di Napoli
Napoli
Italy

M.G. Vedovelli
2nd Department of Internal Medicine
University of Perugia
Policlinico Monteluce
06100 Perugia PG
Italy

A. Ventura
2nd Department of Internal Medicine
University of Perugia
Policlinico Monteluce
06100 Perugia PG
Italy

D. Vesselinovitch
Department of Pathology
University of Chicago
5841 South Maryland Avenue
Chicago, IL 60637
USA

P. Viale
Atherosclerosis Prevention Centre
Department of Internal Medicine
University of Genoa
viale Benedetto XV 6
16132 Genova GE
Italy

M. Vigna
Department of Geriatrics and Lipid Clinic
University of Bologna
40138 Bologna
Italy

A. Vivenzio
Istituto di Terapia Medica Sistemica
Cattedra di Ematologia
Università di Roma "La Sapienza"
Policlinico Umberto I
00161 Roma RM
Italy

M.R. Wardell
Galdstone Foundation Laboratories for Cardiovascular Disease
Cardiovascular Research Institute
University of California
San Francisco, CA 94140-0608
USA

G. Weber
Istituto di Anatomia e Istologia Patologica
Centro di Ricerche Arteriosclerosi
via delle Scotte 6
53100 Siena SI
Italy

K.H. Weisgraber
Galdstone Foundation Laboratories for Cardiovascular Disease
Cardiovascular Research Institute
University of California
San Francisco, CA 94140-0608
USA

O. Wiklund
Wallenburg Laboratory for Cardiovascular Research
Sahlgren's Hospital
University of Gothenburg
413 45 Gothenburg
Sweden

E. Williamson
Institut für Klinische Chemie und Laboratoriumsmedizin
Wilhelms-Universität
Albert-Schweitzer-Strasse 33
D-4400 Münster
Federal Republic of Germany

P.W.F. Wilson
Framingham Heart Study
118 Lincoln Street
Framingham, MA 02167
USA

R.W. Wissler
Department of Pathology
University of Chicago
5841 South Maryland Avenue
Chicago, IL 60637
USA

T. Yasugi
Nihon University
School of Medicine
2nd Department of Internal Medicine
30–1 Ohotanighuchi
Uenachi Itabashiku
Tokyo
Japan

F. Zaca'
Istituto Patologia Speciale Medica e Metodologia Clinica
Università degli Studi di Bologna
via Massarenti 9
40138 Bologna BO

M. Zito
Istituto di Gerontologia e Geriatria
via Nicolini 2
66100 Chieti CH
Italy

P. Zucchelli
Immunohematology and Transfusional Centre
University of Bologna
S. Orsola Hospital
via Massarenti 9
40138 Bologna BO
Italy

1
Cholesterol–CHD connection: evidence for the benefit of lipoprotein modification

A.M. GOTTO, Jr.

Department of Medicine, Chief, Internal Medicine Service, The Methodist Hospital, 6565 Fannin, M.S. A-601, Houston, TX 77030, USA

Several clinical studies using lipid-lowering diets or agents have shown that lowering total cholesterol and low density lipoprotein (LDL) -cholesterol can help prevent coronary heart disease (CHD) death and non-fatal myocardial infarction [1,2]. In addition, two recent studies have shown that elevated levels of high density lipoprotein (HDL) -cholesterol also prevent CHD events [3,4].

Together, these studies have lent credence to the cholesterol hypothesis: CHD risk increases with elevated levels of total cholesterol and LDL-cholesterol, but decreases with elevated levels of HDL-cholesterol.

The strongest support for the hypothesis comes from the Lipid Research Clinics' Coronary Primary Prevention Trial (CPPT) [1]. More than 3800 asymptomatic hypercholesterolemic men, ages 35 to 59, participated in this double blind trial. The men were placed on low-fat diets, and were then randomized and treated with either the bile-acid sequestrant, cholestyramine, or placebo.

Over the 7-year trial, the cholestyramine group reduced total cholesterol and LDL-cholesterol levels by averages of 9% and 12%, respectively, when compared to the placebo group.

In turn, the rates of definite CHD death and nonfatal myocardial infarction were, respectively, 24% and 29% lower in the cholestyramine group than in the placebo group. The incidence of CHD events between the two groups differed significantly after the study's second year, indicating a lag period between lipid modification and reduced CHD risk. The CPPT also indicated a 1:2 ratio between the degree of total cholesterol lowering and CHD reduction.

The more than 4000 subjects in the 5-year Helsinki Study [3], a double-blind randomized trial, were also asymptomatic, middle-aged men with hypercholesterolemia. Overall, 63% of the men had Fredrickson type IIa hyperlipoproteinemia, 28% type IIb, and 9% type IV. Compared with the placebo group, the men treated with the fibric acid derivative, gemfibrozil, lowered their total cholesterol by 10%, LDL-cholesterol by 11%, triglycerides by 35%, and increased their HDL-cholesterol by 11%.

While changes in HDL-cholesterol were similar in all of the treated men, the largest drops in total cholesterol and LDL-cholesterol were seen in the type IIa and the smallest change of LDL in the type IV. Based on the 1:2 ratio of the CPPT, the men in the Helsinki gemfibrozil group were expected to have 20% fewer CHD events than the placebo group since their total cholesterol fell by 10% more than that of others.

Instead, they experienced 34% fewer cardiac deaths and non-fatal myocardial infarctions. The reduction of CHD incidence over placebo was largest in type IIb and smallest in type IIa.

The results suggest that a combination therapy of lowering total and LDL-cholesterol, while raising HDL-cholesterol, exerts a stronger effect on CHD incidence than lowering LDL-cholesterol alone. As with the CPPT, there was an indicted lag of about two years between lipid modification and CHD reduction.

As part of the NHLBI's Coronary Drug Project, 1119 male survivors of myocardial infarction were treated with niacin (nicotinic acid), and 2789 male survivors with placebo [3]. At the conclusion of the 6-year trial, the niacin group had reduced total cholesterol levels by 10% over the placebo group. While the lipid reductions were credited with a slightly lower rate of reinfarction in the niacin group, no difference in total mortality was observed. However, in a 15-year follow-up, almost 9 years after the trial's completion, mortality in the niacin group was 11% lower than in the placebo group. This difference was linked to the earlier effect of niacin on reducing reinfarction and/or the cholesterol-lowering effect of the drug.

Over 1200 middle-aged, hypercholesterolemic men in the Oslo Study Diet and Antismoking Trial were randomized either to a control or intervention group [5]. At the end of this 5-year trial, total cholesterol levels for the intervention group had been reduced by an average of 13%, compared to only 3% in the control counterpart, which included fatal and non-fatal mayocardial infarction and sudden death, was 47% lower in the intervention than in the control group.

A follow-up some 3 to 4 years after the trial's completion, showed that these trends had continued: The intervention group had 45% fewer coronary events than did the placebo group. Moreover, the difference between the group's total mortality rate had widen by the follow-up survey: at the 5-year mark, there was a 33% lower incidence of mortality in the intervention group; at the 8 to 9 year mark, the difference was 40%.

The beneficial effect of lipid modification on lower mortality rates was also observed in the 5-year Stockholm Ischemic Heart Study of myocardial infarction survivors [6]. The more than 560 participants, half of whom had hypertriglyceridemia, were randomized into a control group or a group given a combined treatment of clofibrate and niacin. The treatment group lowered its total cholesterol and triglycerides by 13% and 10%, compared to the control group. The treated group also experienced 26% fewer deaths than did the control group, with 36% fewer deaths due to ischemic heart disease.

Finally, the Cholesterol Lowering Atherosclerosis Study (CLAS) - of 162 patients who had coronary artery bypass surgery - showed that lipid modification could also benefit patients with established coronary disease [4]. The daily therapy of 29.5g of colestipol plus 4.5g of niacin reduced LDL-cholesterol by 43% and raised HDL by 37% over two years. Based on global coronary artery scores, 16% of the patients receiving therapy had evidence of atherosclerotic regression, compared to 3.5% of the patients taking placebo.

Thus, evidence is accumulating that pharmacologic intervention with cholesterol-lowering drugs can reduce the incidence of CHD within a few years. It is also becoming apparent that the greater the magnitude and duration of the decrease in LDL-cholesterol and the increase in the HDL-cholesterol, the greater is the reduction of CHD risk.

Acknowledgement:

This manuscript was prepared with the editorial assistance of Anita Cecchin.

References:

1. Lipid Research Clinics Program: The Lipid Research Clinics' Coronary Primary Prevention Trial (CPPT) Results. I and II. JAMA 1984;251:351-374.

2. Canner PL, Berge KG, Wenger NK, et al: Fifteen year

mortality in Coronary Drug Project patients: long-term benefit with niacin. J Am Coll Cardiol 1986;8:1245-1255.

3. Manninen V, Elo MO, Frick MH, et al: Lipid alterations and decline in the incidence of coronary heart disease in the Helsinki Heart Study. JAMA 1988;260:641-651.

4. Blankenhorn DH, Nessim SA, Johnson RL, et al: Beneficial effects of combined colestipol-niacin therapy on coronary atherosclerosis and coronary venous bypass graphs. JAMA 1987;257:3233-3240.

5. Hjermann I, Holme I, Leren P: Oslo Study Diet and Antismoking Trial. Results after 102 months. Am J of Med 1986;80(2A):7-11.

6. Carlson LA, Rosenhamer G: Reduction of mortality in the Stockholm Ischemic Heart Disease Secondary Prevention Study by combined treatment with clofibrate and nicotinic acid. Acta Med Scand 1988;223:405-418.

EPIDEMIOLOGICAL STUDIES ON ATHEROSCLEROSIS AND CORONARY HEART DISEASE

2
The effect of coronary heart disease prevention on the prevention of non-cardiovascular diseases

F.H. EPSTEIN

Institute of Social and Preventive Medicine, University of Zürich, Sumatrastrasse 30, CH 8006 Zürich, Switzerland

At the preceding Bologna meeting, evidence was presented that measures to prevent coronary heart disease (CHD) are likely to provide protection against some of the other, major chronic diseases as well [1]. Of the latter, the most important is cancer in its different manifestations. During the last few years, a high level of consensus has been reached that CHD is, indeed, preventable through risk factor control and that both a population and a high-risk strategy are needed to make prevention optimally effective on the population level [2-6]. However, there is still opposition to these recommendations, even though they become more and more accepted by the scientific and medical community.The most serious of these objections is the allegation that the reduction in CHD risk resulting from lowering one of the three main risk factors, serum cholesterol, would be counterbalanced by an increase in cancer risk, leaving total mortality unchanged [7]. It is the present purpose to show that these concerns are unfounded, based on a comprehensive review of available data, bearing both on cancer and total mortality.

1. Serum cholesterol and cancer risk

1.1. EVIDENCE FROM PROSPECTIVE EPIDEMIOLOGICAL STUDIES

The question whether serum cholesterol lowering might lead to an increase of cancer risk arose from the results of CHD risk reduction trials in the late 1960ies. However, Ederer and colleagues, reviewing the experience of 5 such trials, concluded in 1971 that there was no evidence for a connection between serum cholesterol reduction and cancer risk [8]. Nevertheless, the matter did not come to rest because the data from some prospective epidemiological observational studies, as opposed to intervention studies, suggested an inverse relationship between serum cholesterol level and cancer incidence or mortality. The problem was considered sufficiently serious to convene a Workshop, sponsored by the National Heart, Lung and Blood Institute, National Institutes of Health in Bethesda in 1981, to review all the available epidemiological data [9, 10]. It was concluded that there was no cause for concern but, at the same time, there was a need to keep an eye on the situation and to collect further information. Now, 8 years later, it is time to take stock again.

In assessing the findings from prospective epidemiological studies, it is essential to take into account the 'preclinical cancer effect', reflecting that serum cholesterol levels may be low prior to death or onset of manifest disease because latent cancer is already present. In the analysis of results, it is usually assumed that this effect covers 2-3 years so that data are analysed in terms of the total experience and, if an inverse relationship between cancer and low serum cholesterol levels exists, a re-analysis after excluding all deaths or incident cases occurring within a few years after the serum cholesterol determination is done.

Among men, there are 22 studies in which an inverse relationship between serum cholesterol level and total cancer risk was found. In 8 of these studies, the relationship disappeared when the preclinical cancer effect was excluded, [10 (WHO Clofibrate Trial reference group) 11-16, 17 (non-smokers)], in a further 10 studies, the relationship persisted after testing for this effect [18-27], in 4 studies, the preclinical effect was not tested [28, 29, 10 (Minnesota business men), 10 (Hiroshima-Nagasaki Study)], while 16 studies failed to show a relationship[10 (Oslo Study 1972-1978), 10 (Western Collaborative Study), 10 (Tecumseh Study), 10 (Lipid Research Clinics Study, USA), 10 (Kiryat Yovel Study, Jerusalem), 17 (smokers), 30-35, 29 (Southern Europe), 29 (US Railroad)]. In one additional study in which men and women were combined in the analysis, the inverse relationship became non-significant after a preclinical cancer effect was taken into consideration [36].

Among women, there exist altogether 17 studies, 9 of which show no relationship between serum cholesterol and cancer risk [10 (Tecumseh, Michigan), 10 (Hiroshima-Nagasaki Study), 10 (Lipid Research Clinics Study, USA), 13, 17 (smokers), 22, 27, 31, 34], three studies show an inverse relationship which disappears after excluding early cancer events or deaths [15, 17 (non-smokers), 25], while, in 5 further studies, an inverse relationship persists after testing for a preclinical cancer effect [10 (Kiryat Yovel Study, Jerusalem), 18, 19, 23, 26]; in tow of these [18, 23], the trend is non-significant and in one [26], the inverse relationship is limited to diseases associated with smoking.

The data relating to colon cancer are of particular importance because cholesterol has been considered a co-carcinogen. It is conceivable that people have low serum cholesterol levels because they excrete more cholesterol from the gut which, in turn, makes them more susceptible to colon cancer. For men, there are 22 studies with data on colon cancer risk and serum cholesterol levels. In 11 of them, there ist no relationship [13, 15, 17, 27, 32, 34, 35, 37, 38], in 3 studies, an inverse relationship disappears after excluding early cancers [14, 16, 25], in another three, the relationship is inverse without a preclinical cancer effect [39, 40, 41], while in the remaining five, no test was made for such an effect [10 (Hiroshima-Nagasaki Study), 18, 23, 26, 28]. In 13 studies among women, there was no relationship in 12 [10 (Hiroshima-Nagasaki Study), 13, 15, 26, 27, 32, 34, 37, 38, 41], and only one study in which there was a persistent, inverse relationship [17].

The entire evidence on serum cholesterol and cancer risk may now be summarized (Table 1).

Table 1. Serum cholesterol and cancer risk - summary of studies

	ALL CANCERS		COLON CANCER	
	Men	Women	Men	Women
Total studies	34*	17	17**	13
No relationship	16	9	11	12
Inverse relationship - preclinical cancer effect present	8+	3	3+	-
Inverse relationship - no preclinical cancer effect	10	5	3	1

* excluding 4 studies in which preclinical cancer effect was not tested.
** excluding 5 studies in which preclinical cancer effect was not tested.
\+ excluding one additional study [36] in which the analysis was carried out for men and women combined.

As regards all cancers, only 10 out of 34 studies among men (29 %) and 5 out of 17 studies among women (29 %) show an inverse relationship which persists after allowing for a preclinical cancer effect. Thus, a little over two-thirds of the studies show either no relationship or a relationship which is accounted for by a preclinical cancer effect, the majority showing no relationship at all. For colon cancer, the vast majority show no or even a positive relationship. In the face of such weak evidence, it would be hard to maintain that there is a cause-and-effect connection between low serum cholesterol levels and cancer risk. Possibly, the association is even weaker than indicated because, based on the Framingham experience, a preclinical cancer effect may be present for a good deal longer than around 4 years [41] so that the proportion of studies without a preclinical cancer effect may be even smaller. Some kind of biological relationship between cancer risk and sterol metabolism may well exist but it would, in all likelihood, be much more complex than could be expressed by the simplistic formula 'low serum cholesterol-high cancer risk'. As an example, both in the Scottish [27] and the Evans County Studies [42], the relationship between serum cholesterol level and, respectively, colon and total cancer risk is U-shaped. It would be difficult to find a single explanation for the finding that both low and high levels carry increased cancer risk!

1.2. EVIDENCE FROM CROSS-CULTURAL STUDIES

On the basis of cross-cultural studies, there is no question that populations with habitual dietary patterns associated with low serum cholesterol levels are characterized not only by low mortality and morbidity for coronary heart disease but show cancer mortality rates which are either not increased or are even relatively low. Total cancer mortality, based on data from 20 countries, is strongly correlated with total calories, total and saturated fat intake, the daily intake of cholesterol and, inversely, with the polyunsaturated/saturated dietary fat ratio [43]. Similar correlations exist for colorectal cancer and there is a strong relationship between CHD and colorectal cancer mortality [43]. Serum cholesterol levels and cancer mortality show a linear relationship in the Seven Countries Study [43, 44].

In discussions concerning serum cholesterol and cancer, those who warn against the possible dangers of cholesterol reduction emphasize the data from prospective epidemiological studies, some of which, as already described, do show an inverse relationship which is apparently not accounted for by a preclinical cancer effect. Actually, the cross-cultural data which are, taken as a whole, unequivocal, are in a way more telling because they reflect the lifetime exposure to a pattern of lifestyles, especially diet, rather than the experience of a cohort of middle-aged individuals over a limited period of time. The individual experience always reflects the interaction between genetic predisposition and environmental influences. Within the same population, different individuals are, on the whole, under similar environmental exposures so that so that it will be largely a matter of genetics whether a person will develop heart disease or cancer. However, this same person, given her or his genetic make-up, can modify this risk of heart disease or cancer by lifestyle changes. In fact, heart disease and some types of cancer are likely under the influence of the same lifestyles [1].

1.3. EVIDENCE FROM INTERVENTION STUDIES

The claim that intervention studies conducted to lower the risk of CHD through serum cholesterol reduction have indicated an increase in cancer risk is unsupported. It was already mentioned in the beginning that the whole subject under discussion came to attention on account of such a claim which could be discounted [8]. In a review published in 1983 [43], it was concluded that only one of eight clinical trials showed an increase in cancer risk; this was the W.H.O. Clofibrate trial in which there was also an increased risk of death from other major causes. The evidence has been brought up to date by R. Peto in a careful analysis of 20 trials concerned with reduction of serum cholesterol to lower CHD risk (unpublished information). These trials included over 30,000 persons of whom about 1,200 died of non-cardiac, non-gallstone related causes. In this group, there were only 34 more deaths than would have been expected by chance alone; 13 of those were due to cancer. A detailed analysis of these 13 deaths due to neoplasms showed that most came from the W.H.O. Clofibrate trial; all dietary trials except one showed a reduction of cancer deaths in the treated group. None of these differences relating to neoplasms were statistically significant. A causal relationship between reduction in serum cholesterol and cancer risk is not only unlikely on statistical grounds but because excessive deaths, equally very small in number, were also observed for other non-cardiac, non-neoplastic deaths.

Thus, data from intervention studies provide no ground for any claim that a reduction of CHD risk through serum cholesterol lowering ist counterbalanced by an increase in cancer risk. It must not be forgotten that all of these trials were designed to have adequate numers to test a preventive effect on CHD but not on cancer which is less frequent. Therefore, a future single trial with larger numbers may yet yield sufficient numbers of cancer deaths to test any effect on cancer mortality with adequate statistical power. However, the results of the metaanalysis of extant trials quoted above, based on very large numbers, make it improbable that the conclusions would be different.

2. The influence of serum cholesterol reduction on total mortality

Having concluded from three lines of evidence that reduction of serum cholesterol does not increase cancer risk and accepting that it will decrease the risk of CHD, cancer and CHD accounting together for most deaths, it should not be necessary to discuss any possible effect on total mortality. However, the matter is raised again and again in order to caution against the current, concerted efforts to promote CHD prevention in the population through dietary measures which would reduce serum cholesterol levels not only in high-risk persons but the population as a whole. In this connection, there is frequent reference to a publication which is said to indicate that the results of intervention studies show an excess of non-cardiac deaths in the face of a reduction in CHD deaths, implying failure to affect total mortality [45]. In fact, the first author of this publication has stated that '... the observed increase in non-CHD is consistent with chance ' [46].

The same group of authors have asked the question how many events, in this case deaths, would be required in the control group of an intervention study to provide statistically significant evidence of risk reductions of a given degree [47]. In a primary prevention trial, it could not be expected to lower mortality from all causes through serum cholesterol lowering by much more than 10 %, considering that a number of non-cardiovascular causes of death are unrelated to serum cholesterol level. Given a risk reduction of 10 %, 1,800 total deaths would be required in the control group to indicate at a significance level of 5 % that the intervention was effective [47]. It can now be asked whether the main primary prevention studies published so far had adequate numbers to yield the total number of deaths required to test an effect not only on CHD but also on total mortality. Ten such trials are summarized in Table 2. The method of intervention was diet in the first 3 trials, cholesterol-lowering drugs in the second 3 trials while the last 4 trials involved multifactorial intervention; in the latter group, serum cholesterol lowering was only one of the targets of intervention. It will be seen that 8 of the 10 trials fall far short of the needed number of 1,800 deaths, the Göteborg trial is non-contributary because, for several reasons, it was largely ineffective as far as CHD reduction was concerned but the WHO European trial, even though it accumulated about 600 fewer deaths than required, did show a significant reduction in total mortality [58]. It is concluded that trials to date did not have the statistical power to permit <u>any</u> statement regarding the effect of intervention on total mortality. It ist unjustified, therefore, to claim that serum cholesterol reduction has no effect on total mortality.

Table 2 Is statistical power of completed intervention studies sufficient to test their effect on total mortality?

Study	Size of Control Group (N)	Total Deaths* (N)	Reference
1. Veterans Administration (Dayton)	422	177	48
2. Minnesota (Frantz)	4,738	248	49
3. Oslo (Hjerman)	628	24	50
4. WHO Clofibrate	5,296	317	51
5. Lipid Research Clinics-CPPT	1,900	68	52
6. Helsinki (Gemfibrozil)	2,030	42	53
7. MRFIT	6,438	260	54
8. WHO European Trial	26,971	1,186	55
9. Göteborg (Wilhelmsen)	10,011	1,304	56
10. Helsinki (T.A. Miettinen)	1,203	8	57

* In control group
For interpretation, see text.

3. Summary and conclusions

This review addressed the question whether reduction of serum cholesterol to reduce coronary heart disease risk might carry with it the danger of increasing the risk of cancer, thus making no dent in total mortality. A scrutiny of the evidence provides no grounds for such concerns. The majority of prospective epidemiological studies show no inverse relationship between serum cholesterol level and total or colon cancer risk, taking into account a preclinical cancer effect, and there is, likewise, no significant increase in cancer risk in intervention studies to lower CHD risk. Cross-cultural studies, reflecting life-long habits, suggest on the contrary that lifestyles associated with a lower CHD risk carry with it a protection against cancer. The claim that trials conducted to test the effect of serum cholesterol lowering on CHD risk leave total mortality unchanged cannot be supported because these trials fell far short of the statistical power needed to test an effect on total mortality. Thus, there appear to be no valid scientific reasons to caution against treatment of hypercholesterolemia, a need also stressed in a recent editorial [59], on the high-risk strategy level of CHD prevention, or against the population strategy aimed at lowering serum cholesterol levels through dietary modifications in the population at large.

References

1. Epstein, F.H. (1986) 'Prevention of coronary heart disease - links with other chronic disorders', in S. Lenzi and G.C. Descovich eds., Atherosclerosis and Cardiovascular Diseases, MTP Press Ltd. Lancaster, Boston, The Hague, Dordrecht, pp. 157-162.
2. 'Prevention of coronary heart disease' (1982) Report of a W.H.O. Expert Committee, Technical Report Series 678, World Health Organization, Geneva, Switzerland.
3. Study Group, European Atherosclerosis Society (1987) 'Strategies for the prevention of coronary heart disease', Europ.Heart J. 8, 77-88.
4. Study Group, European Atherosclerosis Society (1988) 'The recognition and management of hyperlipidaemia in adults: a policy statement of the European Atherosclerosis Society', Europ.Heart J. 9, 571-600.
5. The Expert Panel (1988) 'Report of the National Cholesterol Education Program Expert Panel on Detection, Evaluation, and Treatment of High Blood Cholesterol in Adults', Arch.Int.Med. 148, 36-69.
6. Havel,R.J. (1988) 'Lowering cholesterol, 1988, rationale, mechanisms and means', J.Clin.Invest. 81, 1653-1660.
7. Oliver,M.F. (1988) 'Reducing cholesterol does not reduce mortality', J.Am.Coll.Cardiol. 12, 814-817.
8. Ederer,F. et al. (1971) 'Cancer among men on cholesterol-lowering diets. Experience from clinical trials', Lancet 2, 203-206.
9. Anon (1981) 'Cholesterol and non-cardiovascular mortality', J.Am.Med.Ass. 246, 731.
10. 'Workshop on cholesterol, and non-cardiovascular disease mortality', National Heart, Lung and Blood Institute and National Cancer Institute, National Institutes of Health, Bethesda, Maryland, U.S.A., May 11-12, 1981.
11. Cambien,F., Ducimetière,P. and Richard,J. (1980) 'Total serum cholesterol and cancer mortality in a middle-aged male population', Am.J.Epidemiol. 112, 388-394.
12. Rose,G. and Shipley,M.J. (1980) 'Plasma lipids and mortality: a source of error', Lancet 1, 523-525.
13. Wallace,R.B. et al. (1982) 'Cancer incidence in humans: relationships to plasma lipids and relative weight', J.Nat.Cancer Inst. 68, 915-918.
14. International Collaborative Group (1982) 'Circulating cholesterol level and risk of death from cancer in men aged 40 to 69 years', J.Am.Med.Ass. 248, 2853-2859.
15. Hiatt,R.A. and Firemen,B.H. (1986) 'Serum cholesterol and the incidence of cancer in a large cohort', J.Chronic Dis. 39, 861-870.
16. Sherwin,R.W. et al. (1987) 'Serum cholesterol levels and cancer mortality in 361 662 men screened for the multiple risk factor intervention trial', J.Am.Med.Ass. 257, 943-948.
17. Knekt,P. et al. (1988) 'Serum cholesterol and risk of cancer in a cohort of 39,000 men and women', J.Clin.Epidemiol. 41, 519-530.
18. Kark,J.D., Smith,A.H. and Hames,C.G. (1980) 'The relationship of serum cholesterol to the incidence of cancer in Evans County, Georgia', J.Chronic Dis. 33, 311-322.
19. Beaglehole,R. et al. (1980) 'Cholesterol and mortality in New Zealand Maoris', Brit.Med.J. 1, 285-287.
20. Garcia-Palmieri,M.R. (1981) 'An apparent inverse relationship between serum cholesterol an cancer mortality in Puerto Rico', Am.J.Epidemiol. 114, 29-40.
21. Kagan,A. et al (1981) 'Serum cholesterol and mortality in a Japanese-American population', Am.J.Epidemiol. 114, 11-20.

22. Williams,R.R. et al. (1981) 'Cancer incidence by level of cholesterol' (Framingham Study), J.Am.Med.Ass. 245, 247-252.
23. Böttiger,L.E. and Carlson,L.A. (1982) 'Risk factors for death for males and females', Acta Med.Scand. 211, 437-442.
24. Petersen,B., Trell,E. and Sternby,N.H. (1981) 'Low cholesterol level as risk factor for noncoronary death in middle-aged men', J.Am.Med.Ass. 245, 2056-2057.
25. Gerhardsson,M. et al. (1986) 'Serum cholesterol and cancer - a retrospective case-control study', Int.J.Epidemiol. 15, 155-159.
26. Schatzkin,A. et al. (1988) 'Site-specific analysis of total serum cholesterol and incident cancer in the National Health and Nutrition Examination Survey I Epidemiologic Follow-up Study', Cancer Research 48, 452-458.
27. Isles,C.G. et al. (1989) 'Plasma cholesterol, coronary heart disease, and cancer in the Renfrew and Paisley survey', Brit.Med.J. 298, 920-924.
28. Kozarevic,D. et al. (1981) 'Serum cholesterol and mortality. The Yugoslavia Cardiovascular Disease Study', Am.J.Epidemiol. 114, 21-28.
29. Keys,A. et al. (1985) 'Serum cholesterol and cancer mortality in the Seven Countries Study', Am.J.Epidemiol. 121, 870-883.
30. Westlund,K. and Nicolaysen,R. (1972) 'Ten-year mortality and morbidity related to serum cholesterol', Scand.J.Clin.Labor.Invest. 30, Suppl. 127, 3-24.
31. Salonen,J. (1982) 'Risk of cancer and death in relation to serum cholesterol', Am.J.Epidemiol. 116, 622-630.
32. Dyer,A.R. et al. (1981) 'Serum cholesterol and risk of death from cancer and other causes in three Chicago epidemiological studies', J.Chronic Dis. 34, 249-620.
33. Thomas,C.B., Duszynski,K.R. and Schaffer,J.W. (1982) 'Cholesterol levels in young adulthood and subsequent cancer: a preliminary note', Johns Hopkins Med.J. 150, 89-94.
34. Wingard,D.L. et al. (1984) 'Plasma cholesterol and cancer morbidity and mortality in an adult community', J.Chronic Dis. 37, 401-406.
35. Yaari,S. et al. (1981) 'Associations of high density lipoprotein and total cholesterol with total cardiovascular, and cancer mortality in a 7-year prospective study of 10,000 men', Lancet 1, 1013-1015.
36. Morris,D.L. et al. (1983) 'Serum cholesterol an cancer in the Hypertension Detection and Follow-up Program', Cancer 52, 1754-1759.
37. Törnberg,S.A. et al. (1986) 'Risk of cancer of the colon and rectum in relation to serum cholesterol and betalipoprotein', New Eng.J.Med. 315, 1629-1633.
38. Mannes,G.A. et al. (1986) 'Relation between the frequency of colorectal adenoma and the serum cholesterol level', New Eng.J.Med. 315, 1634-1638.
39. Rose,G. et al. (1974) 'Colon cancer and blood-cholesterol', Lancet 1, 181-183.
40. Stemmermann,G.N. et al. (1981) 'Serum cholesterol and colon cancer incidence in Hawaian Japanese men', J.Nat.Cancer Inst. 67, 1179-1182.
41. Sorlie,P.D. and Feinleib,M. (1982) 'The serum cholesterol-cancer relationship: an analysis of time trends in the Framingham Study', J.Nat.Cancer Inst. 69, 989-996.
42. Davis,C.E. et al (1983) 'Serum cholesterol and cancer mortality: Evans County 20-year follow-up study', in: E.G.Perkins, W.J.Visek, eds., Dietary Fats and Health, Am. Oil Chemists Soc., Champaign, Illinois, pp. 892-900.
43. Sydney,S. and Farquhar,J.W. (1983) 'Cholesterol, cancer, and public health policy', Am.J.Med. 75, 494-508.

44. Keys,A. (1980) Seven Countries - A Multivariate Analysis of Death and Coronary Heart Disease, Harvard University Press, Cambridge, Mass. and London.
45. Yusuf,S. and Furberg,C.D. (1987) 'Single factor trials', in: A.G.Olsson,ed.,Atherosclerosis - Biology and Clinical Science, Churchill Livingstone, Edinburgh, London, Melbourne and New York, pp. 389-398.
46. Yusuf,S., Wittes,J. and Friedman,L. (1989) 'Randomized clinical trials in heart disease', J.Am.Med.Ass., 261, 2953-2954 (letter to the Editor).
47. Yusuf,S., Wittes,J. and Friedman,L. (1988) 'Overview of results of randomized clinical trials in heart disease, II' J.Am.Med.Ass. 260, 2259-2263.
48. Dayton,S. et al. (1969) 'A controlled trial of a diet high in unsaturated fat', Circulation 40 (Suppl.II) 1-62.
49. Frantz,I.D., Jr. et al. (1989) 'Test of effect of lipid lowering by diet on cardiovascular risk', Arteriosclerosis 9, 129-135.
50. Hjerman,I. et al. (1981) 'Effect of diet and smoking intervention on the incidence of coronary heart disease', Lancet 2, 1303-1310.
51. Committee of Principal Investigators (1980) 'WHO Cooperative Trial on primary prevention of ischaemic heart disease using clofibrate to lower serum cholesterol: mortality follow-up', Lancet 2, 379-385.
52. Lipid Research Clinics Program (1984) 'The Lipid Research Clinics Coronary Primary Prevention Trial results', J.Am.Med.Ass. 251, 351-364.
53. Frick,M.H. (1987) 'Helsinki Heart Study: primary prevention trial with gemfibrozil in middle-aged men with dyslipidemia', New Eng.J.Med. 317, 1237-1245.
54. Multiple Risk Factor Intervention Trial Research Group (1982) 'Multiple risk factor intervention trial. Risk factor changes and mortality results', J.Am.Med.Ass. 284, 1465-1477.
55. WHO European Collaborative Group (1986) 'European Collaborative Trial of multifactorial prevention of coronary heart disease: final report on the 6-year results', Lancet 1, 869-872.
56. Wilhelmsen,L. et al. (1986) 'The multifactor primary prevention trial in Göteborg, Sweden', Europ.Heart J. 7, 279-288.
57. Miettinen,T.A. et al. (1985) 'Multifactorial primary prevention of cardiovascular diseases in middle-aged men', J.Am.Med.Ass. 254, 2097-2102.
58. Rose,G. (1987) 'European Collaborative Trial of multifactorial prevention of coronary heart disease', Lancet 1, 685 (letter to the Editor).
59. Anon (1989) 'Low cholesterol and increased risk', Lancet 1, 1423-1425.

3
The meaning and relevance of intervention trials in prevention

G. LAMM and W. SCHEUERMANN

Institute for Clinical Social Medicine, University Medical Clinic Heidelberg, Bergheimer Strasse 58, 6900 Heidelberg, Federal Republic of Germany

ABSTRACT. A disease can be prevented theoretically in three different ways: by eradication, by avoiding the risk of acquiring and finally by managing, manipulating already established risk factors. In the case of atherosclerotic diseases only the third, least satisfactory approach is amenable to test the hypothesis of preventability by means of intervention trials. Prevention through correction of already established high risk is a fringe benefit of the purely medical approach to test the risk factor theory. The original postulate was simply: low risk profile goes with low incidence of the disease. Intervention trials contributed substantially to the broader acceptance of the preventability of atherosclerosis. The internal validity of the trial results is only one aspect of this problem, although this is the most often debated. The inference from or generalisability of positive and of course also of the negative trials poses problems only recently delt with in the literature. Issues of the sampling frame, exclusions, subjects eligible but not randomized, subgroup results, etc. and their influence on inference will be discussed, with the aim to redress the balance between randomised trials and good observational studies in prevention.

An argument often used in the still not fully resolved debate between the so called population and high risk strategy in cardiovascular disease (CVD) prevention is, that the former has never been tested properly, i.e. in a controlled intervention trial. Within the limitations of this short paper I will try to address this statement from three different angles. First the inherent scientific validity of randomised controlled clinical trials (RCCTs). Second, the differences between therapeutic and preventive trials and finally the public health relevance of such trials. To illustrate my views I shall use selected examples from trials well known to all of you.

According to Peter Armitage (1) the first randomised controlled trial was conducted by the Medical Resarch Council (MRC) on streptomyicin in 1948. Thanks to the uncontested authority and fame of such men like Sir Bradford-Hill (2) and A. Cochrane (3) RCCTs became quickly the yardstick of good medical practice. The salubrious substitution of belief, impression and conviction for trial evidence heralded a new era in clinical medicine although up to this day only a tiny proportion of our judgements are based on such firm grounds. Table 1 shows some of the most important benefits of RCCTs. They are free from the subjectivity of choice, be it exerted from the physician or from the patient. In its double-blind form RCCT does take proper care of the placebo effect, while not abolishing important features such as "tender loving care", belief in the doctor, hope for getting better, etc. They are eminently suited for testing hypothesis – like treatment A is better than treatment B –. In case of early collaboration with the proper expert a well planned RCCT is always amenable to statistical evulation.

Table 1:

Randomised Controlled Trial

Advantages

Freedom from subjective choice

Freedom from self selection

Avoidance of placebo effect (especially in double blind)

Testing of preformulated hypothesis

Amenability to statistical evaluation

The traditional development from resistance through acceptance to overenthusiasm finally ended up by acclaiming RCCTs as guardians of the ultimate truth in medicine. However, like any good medicine, RCCTs are working only when they are applied to the proper patient, after correct diagnosis and in the appropriate dosage. They are no panacea: a selection of their limitations is shown on table 2.

Table 2:

Randomised Controlled Trials

Limitations

Sampling frame

Selection bias

Eligible but not randomized

Randomized but switched

Compliance

One of the most neglected but very often misused criteria for the validity of the findings of a RCCT is the sampling frame or in other words the basic population from which the trial participants are finally selected by randomisation. Let this be demonstrated on a practical example. In the well known and widely publicized trial on hospital versus home treatment of acute myocardial infarction (AMI), Mather et al. (4) "considered" 1,895 AMI-patients (table 3). As it clearly emerges from their summary table only 24% of the "considered" nearly 2,000 patients entered the randomisation phase, the rest (68%) went to hospital by "force" (own or of the physician) and only a small proportion – 8% – remained at home on their own volition. The sampling frame thus was not the 1,895 patients with AMI, but 450 such patients, who after elimination of the most severe cases (24%), were ready to resign the decision about home versus hospital treatment in favour of chance.

Table 3:

Randomized trial of home versus hospital

care of AMI patients (Mather et al. 1976)

1895 patients considered, 450 randomized

	Random home	Random hospital	Elective home	Elective hospital	Mandatory hospital	Total
Number (%) of patients	226 (12)	224 (12)	151 (8)	837 (44)	457 (24)	1895

The next example is about the sampling bias. Some two years after the mentioned trial, another one was published on the same issue by Hill et al. (5). In order to overcome a number of medical and ethical difficulties, they used mobile teams to observe – and in case of need assist – the AMI patients in their home. Then, 4 hours after the onset of symptoms volunteering patients were randomly allocated to home and hospital treatment groups, and their survival was evaluated. Table 4 makes it evident on the basis of the WHO AMI Register Study results, that randomisation at 4 hours introduces a severe selection bias: Almost half of the patients to be dead within one month died already during these first hours. Thus, sudden death due to electric instability against which CCUs are eminently suited, has already taken its toll. The two examples were taken from a field where the present consensus is distinctly against the conclusions derived from these RCCTs.

Table 4:

	AMI mortality (%) in the first 28 days (100%)	Randomised study of home versus hospital care	
< 1/2 h	32		
1/2 - 1 h	6		
1 - 2 h	5	Home observation	
2 - 3 h	3		
3 - 4 h	2		
0 - 4 h	48	Randomisation	
		home	hospital
(WHO AMI Register, 1979)			(Hill et al., 1978)

In his oration at the acceptance of the J.A. Taylor prize Feinstein (6) calls the attention to the limitations of RCCTs and asserts that with the advent of modern calculators other methods based entirely on observed data might be used successfully to deal with the problems of probability.

In summary: even in their original, well defined territory, randomised controlled clinical trials constitute only partial "proof" and even then only with the observance of quality requirements.

How do then RCCTs perform in prevention? Table 5 lists some of the differences between therapeutic and preventive trials.

Table 5:

Difference between therapeutic and preventive trials

Goal	Treatment A better than Treatment B	Action is better than non-action
Intervention	Medical	Public health
Compliance	Usually good	Usually poor
Sample size	Modest	Enormous
Ethical considerations	Easy to resolve	Difficult
Latency	Little effect	Large effect
Duration	Short-medium	Long - very long

A therapeutic trial assesses the value of one treatment over another. In contrast the essential question in prevention is whether action is better than non-action. For instance: Should nutrition be changed for better health or should it be left to its natural (or unnatural) changing trend. One can of course substitute nutrition for smoking, physical activity or environment. The conceptual, ethical, and methodological problems arising from this first difference are tremendous. Intervention in therapeutic trials is in general a well defined medical or surgical activity aimed to correct something in the body: blood pressure, flow, biochemistry, etc. Preventive trials must deal with problems of behaviour using intervention measures much less developed and tested. Partly as a consequence, medical interventions are usually well accepted and adhered to whereas public health measures are difficult to introduce. The rest of the listed differences are mainly of technical character in contrast to the first three essential ones.

Some of the limitations ensuing from these differences are listed in table 6. Point one is self-evident and does not need elaboration. How far even the largest preventive trials lag behind the ideal stated in item two will be exemplified on hand of the Lipid Research Clinic Primary Prevention Trial (7), summarized in table 7.

Table 6:

Limitations ensuing from these differences

Preventive trials are:

Difficult to organize

Should ideally include everybody

Their optimal duration exceeds

- **interest of investigators**
- **patience of participants**
- **willingness of granting bodies**

Are prone to β-type of error

Table 7:

LRC Primary Prevention Trial

Screened:	**480,000 men**	
Randomised:	**3,810 men**	
Selection criteria:	**Cholesterol > 265 mg%**	
Exclusion criteria:	**CVD**	**Hyperuricaemia**
	Diabetes	**Gross obesity**
	Hypothyroidism	**Hypertension**
	Nephrotic syndrom	**Cancer**
	Liver disease	**Long term medication**
	Female sex	

The fact that from almost 1/2 million screened men only a meagre four thousand entered the trial, depicts only the quantitative dimensions. The conceptual consequence behind these shrinking numbers is what really matters. Subjects with cholesterol levels below the predefined level are excluded. But even the group above 265 mg% is further trunkated through omission of all those carrying one or another exclusion criteria although these people are all part of the general population. One could argue, that these exclusions limit only the possibility of inference from and not the internal validity of such trials. However, if one recalls the multiple risk concept and ponders on the still poorly understood interrelation between various chronic diseases some doubts about the internal validity may appear to be justified.

The latency period of risk accumulation and disease evolution is poorly known, not to speak about the latency between risk reversal and disease decline. The magic 5-6 year duration of the major preventive trials is much more a compromise between the endurance of the investigators, the patience of the participants and the toleration of granting bodies, than a sound biological estimate. In the latter case 10-20 year long trials would be closer to reality.

My last argument on the limitations of preventive trials refers to their increased vulnerability to type-β errors. In other words, they are much more prone to miss a response when it is there, rather than to demonstrate an effect when in fact there is none.

The danger of a false negativ conclusion in preventive trials originates from two main sources. The first is bound to the difficulty of proper planning in such trials. Table 8 taken from the MRFIT-trial (8) will help to demonstrate this.

Table 8:

M R F I T

Screened: 361,662 men

Randomised: 12,866 men into

usual care (UC) and special intervention (SI) groups

Results

	Expected		Observed	
	UC	**SI**	**UC**	**SI**
CHD mortality/1,000	**29,0**	**21,3**	**19,3**	**17,9**

The trial was planned in the early seventies on the ground of experience coming from the Framingham Study. The use of old numerical data from Framingham proved itself as detrimental as shown in the discrepancy between expected (planned) and observed results. When MRFIT ended in 1982 the observed mortality in the control-group (UC) was 1/3 lower than predicted and the similarly smaller than projected effect of intervention (SI) became nonsignificant. After the turning point in 1967 CHD mortality declined steadily in the USA making the Framingham estimates though qualitatively valid, quantitatively obsolate.

In summary the pre-test probability of the Bayes theorem is much more shaky in a preventive -, than in a therapeutic trial.

The second main reason for a tendency to type-β error is bound to the so called "drop in" phenomenon in preventive trials. The two columns on the left on table 9 show the main risk factor levels at the end of the MRFIT trial according to expectation. On the right the effectively observed levels in the two groups are shown. The largest discrepancy between expectation and reality is seen in UC control group. The basic assumption that cholesterol and diastolic blood pressure will remain unchanged in the UC group turned out to be false. These values diminished substantially even in the controls, obfuscating the effects of intervention.

Table 9:

M R F I T Risk factor changes

	Expected		**Observed**	
	UC	**SI**	**UC**	**S I**
Cholesterol, mg%	**2 5 3**	**2 2 8**	**2 4 0**	**2 3 5**
Diastolic, BP Hgmm	**9 1**	**8 2**	**83,6**	**80,5**
Cigarettes, No/d	**38-22-17**	**30-15-9**	**?**	**?**
quit rate, %	**?**	**?**	**2 9**	**4 6**

Preventive trials are testing the value of action against non-action and as shown in this example, it is almost impossible to predict the consequences of this non-action. While the research team is not acting on the control group, many other biological and social forces do. Pantha rei!

Finally, I should like to make a few comments on the public health relevance of preventive trials. The most fundamental limitation of the hitherto known trials lies in their character: they are set out to test the effect of reversal of high risk, whether in subjects or in populations. This is a fundamental medical approach. The public health issue, however, is, whether avoidance of risk elevation brings reasonable benefit to the whole population, or not.

Two more technical aspects should be added. One is trivial and refers to the tremendous size, difficulties, duration and costs of such trials. More serious is the second about the dangers of inference from successfully completed trials. If the outcome is as expected, like in the case of LRC Primary Prevention Trial, it is difficult to resist the temptation to expand the results to those never tested: i.e. to women, people younger, at lesser risk, etc.

In cases like MRFIT where the indications for a type-β error are overwhelming the public health consequence might be even more detrimental. By failing to detect an effect when in fact there has been one, the whole idea of cardiovascular disease prevention becomes jeopardized and may be abandoned for who knows how long.

Summary and conclusion:

RCCTs when properly conducted are excellent tools in promoting medical science. New knowledge is, however, never established by one single approach but from a complexity of basic, laboratory, observational and experimental evidence. Last but not least: good science is not by necessity good public health – let us remember the Manhattan Project!

References

Armitage, P. (1989) 'Inference and dicision in clinical trials', J. Clin. Epidemiol. 42, 293-299.

Bradford Hill, A. (1962) Statistical methods in Clinical and Preventive Medicine, Livingstone, Edinburgh

Cochrane, A.L. (1972) Effectiveness and efficiency, The Nuffield Provincial Hospital Trust, London.

Mather, H.G., Morgan D.C., Pearson N.G. et al. (1976) 'Myocardial infarction: a comparison between home and hospital care for patients', Br. Med. J. i, 925-929.

Hill, J.D., Hampton J.R., Mitchell J.R.A. (1978) 'A randomised trial of home-versus-hospital management for patients with suspected myocardial infarction' Lancet i, 837-841.

Feinstein, A.R. (1989) 'Models, methods and goals', J. Clin. Epidemiol. 42, 301-308.

LRC Programm (1984) 'The Lipid Research Clinics Coronary Primary Prevention Trial Results', J.A.M.A. 251, 351-364.

MRFIT Research Group (1982) 'Multiple Risk Factor Intervention Trial', J.A.M.A. 248, 1465-77.

4
Prospects for primary prevention of coronary heart disease

W.B. KANNEL

Boston University School of Medicine, Section of Preventive Medicine and Epidemiology, 720 Harrison Avenue, Suite 1105, Boston, MA 02118, USA

ABSTRACT. Major contributors to coronary heart disease have been identified through epidemiologic research. These risk factors fall into a number of interdependent categories including: atherogenic personal attributes, living habits which promote them, signs of a compromised circulation and host susceptibility to these risk factors. Modifiable atherogenic risk attributes include blood lipids, blood pressure, glucose tolerance and fibrinogen. The risk associated with each is markedly affected by those others which coexist. Modifiable living habits exist which promote these atherogenic traits including overeating, unrestrained weight gain, faulty diet, cigarette smoking, and lack of exercise. Innate susceptibility is signified by a family history of premature vascular disease, identifying persons in particular need of risk factor control. At a given level of serum total cholesterol risk varies widely depending on total/HDL-cholesterol ratio providing an efficient and practical means for assessing the joint effect of the two-way traffic of total cholesterol. Optimal treatment must improve this lipid profile. Diabetes on average doubles CHD mortality imparting greater risk in women than men and exerting an independent effect. Risk in diabetics varies widely depending on coexistent risk factors providing a means for reducing the risk. The same applies for hypertension and dyslipidemia. Preclinical indicators of a compromised coronary circulation and ischemic myocardial involvement include ECG evidence of left ventricular hypertrophy, blocked intraventricular function, repolarization abnormality and abnormal response to exercise. Such persons are in dire need of correction of modifiable risk factors. Optimal risk predictions require a quantitative synthesis of risk factors into a composite estimate. Handbooks, hand calculators and P.C. software, based on multiple logistic risk formulations have been devised for office use requiring only ordinary office procedures and simple laboratory tests to measure the risk factor ingredients. Preventive management as well as risk estimation should be multifactorial if good results are to be acheived. Preventive strategies should include public health measures to alter the ecology so as to shift the whole distribution of risk factors to a more favorable level, health education to enable people to protect their own health and preventive medicine for high risk candidates. Greater skill at modifying behavior must be developed to carry out such risk factor interventions.

Introduction

Chances of a major cardiovascular catastrophe before age 60 are one in three in most affluent countries and one in five men will have a coronary attack before that age. Women lag men in incidence by ten years, but cardiovascular disease is also their chief cause of death. Coronary disease must be anticipated and prevented because one in five attacks present with sudden death as the first, last and only symptom and half of all coronary deaths are sudden deaths (1).

Fortunately, vulnerability can be readily assessed from a risk profile comprised of blood lipids, blood pressure, fibrinogen, glucose, cigarette habit and ECG findings using only ordinary office procedures and simple laboratory tests (2). These modifiable atherogenic risk attributes are promoted by a faulty life-style typified by a diet too rich in calories, saturated fat, and salt; and too low in fiber, vegetable content, calcium and magnesium. Fish in the diet, by providing omega-3 fatty acids in abundance, and by substituting for red meat, has been found to be protective against coronary mortality in three major epidemiologic studies. Sedentary habits, unrestrained weight gain and cigarettes also predispose.

Risk Factor Analysis

Coronary heart disease (CHD) is the leading cause of mortality and a major determinant of morbidity in the industrialized countries. Epidemiologic investigation has been instrumental in identifying risk factors for CHD. Many studies have shown a strong and consistent relationship of subsequent rates of development of CHD to antecedent serum total cholesterol and its low-density lipoprotein fraction. High levels of the high-density lipoprotein (HDL) fraction have been found to be protective (3). Triglycerides appear not be an independent risk factor for CHD in men, but may be in women. The weight of evidence indicates that a high-fat diet is related to coronary disease through its influence on blood lipid precursors (4). Hypertension is a powerful contributor to coronary disease (5,6,7). At any age, in either sex, risk of coronary events is proportional to the height of the blood pressure, systolic or diastolic, casual or basal. Systolic hypertension in the elderly is not innocuouc, being associated with an increased risk of CHD and stroke. Cigarette smoking is another important independent predictor of coronary disease; the risk of myocardial infarction increases in relation to the number of cigarettes smoked daily (8). Diabetes is a cardiovascular risk factor for both men and women, with the incidence in diabetic men and women being, respectively, two and three times that in nondiabetics (9). Although obesity is often found not to be an independent predictor of coronary disease, obesity is important because of its promotion of other risk factors like hypercholesterolemia, hypertension and diabetes (4). Left ventricular hypertrophy on ECG is an ominous accompaniment of hypertension and cardiovascular disease, and is a powerful predictor of subsequent coronary events in its own right (10,11).

Physical activity has been shown to be protective for CHD, but the data are not entirely consistent, and the precise type and amount of protective physical activity is unclear (12). Coffee consumption has not been shown to be a consistent risk factor for coronary disease (4). Heavy alcohol consumption clearly damages hear muscle and predisposes to hypertension, but there has been a suggestion tha tmoderate intake may actually reduce coronary risk (4). Type A behavior has been shown in some--but not all--studies to be an independent predictor of CHD. Evidence on the role of social supports and the acculturation is inconsistent (13). Pre-menopausal status seems to confer protection on women, and there is a definite narrowing of the gap in incidence between the sexes with advancing age. However, the precise hormonal substrates of atherogenesis are not well understood (14,15).

Because a constellation of risk factors provides substantially better risk predictions than any single factor, efficient multivariate risk assessment methods have been developed (2). Risk factor analysis enables clinicians to identify persons at high risk of developing CHD. The dramatic and gratifying decline in cardiovascular mortality in the USA, Australia, Canada and New Zealand since 1968, which coincides with reductions in cholesterol levels, cigarette smoking, and uncontrolled hypertension in the populations, suggests that the modern coronary epidemic is indeed amenable to primary prevention (16).

The rise and fall in coronary mortality in the USA over the past three decades indicates the existence of powerful correctable environmental influences making coronary heart disease avoidable by changes in lifestyles. Recent declines in coronary heart disease mortality in the USA and in the Framingham cohort have coincided with improved risk factor levels and changes in relevant living habits (16).

Through epidemiologic research over the last three decades at the Framingham Study a number of major predictors of coronary attacks have been delineated which have allowed identification of high risk coronary candidates. Markers of increased vulnerability were documented and quantified. Indicators of accelerated atherogenesis identified include blood lipids, blood pressure, glucose tolerance and fibrinogen values. Predisposing living habits include cigarette smoking, physical inactivity, unrestrained weight gain and faulty diet. Preclinical signs of a compromised circulation have been discerned which include ECG abnormalities on exercise and at rest. Evidence of innate susceptibility is indicated by a family history of premature cardiovascular disease in parents and siblings.

These epidemiologic studies have clarified in what particulars those who fall victim to cardiovascular disease differ from those who avoid it, providing insight into the risk factors. Information has accumulated on the incidence of cardiovascular disease; the undistorted, full clinical spectrum in all sho have it, its importance as a force of morbidity and mortality, clues to pathogenesis and the chain of circumstances leading to its occurrence. The common occurrence of silent myocardial infarction, accounting for a third of all MI's, and its serious prognosis has been documented (17).

The risk factor concept derived from epidemiologic investigations relating suspected predisposing factors to the subsequent development of disease. As the risks associated with these promoters of cardiovascular disease were quantified, concepts of normality changed from usual to optimal values more conducive to long-term freedom from disease.

The lipid profile promoting accelerated atherogenesis has been refined from a preoccupation with cholesterol to a consideration of cholesterol-lipoprotein subfractions (3). High LDL-cholesterol was shown to be positively related to incidence of coronary heart disease and elevated HDL-cholesterol to be inversely related to occurrence of coronary heart disease (3). The Total/HDL-cholesterol ratio has been shown to be an efficient profile for estimating the joint effect of the two-way traffic of cholesterol.

The association of the serum total cholesterol with coronary disease derives from the atherogenic LDL component and there is also a protective HDL component inversely related to coronary disease risk. At a given level of total cholesterol, including seemingly optimal values around 200 mg/dl, HDL strongly influences coronary risk (Figure 1).

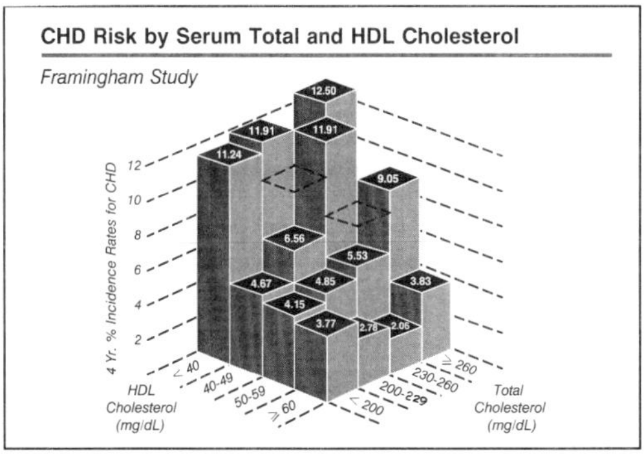

The Total/HDL-cholesterol ratio is a practical clinical indicator of the joint effect of the two-way traffic of LDL and HDL-cholesterol entering and leaving the arteries. A ratio of 3.5, corresponding to half the high average American risk, is optimal. Elevations of blood pressure, glucose and fibrinogen markedly increase the risk associated with dyslipidemia and cigarette smoking can precipitate attacks in those so predisposed and can also lower HDL. These associated risk factors must be taken into account in evaluating the urgency to treat an elevated serum cholesterol (Figure 2).

Misconceptions about hypertension were discerned. Systolic pressure in general and isolated systolic hypertension in particular have been shown to be major contributors to cardiovascular disease

(Figure 3).

Fig. 2. Risk of cardiovascular disease according to serum cholesterol at specified levels of other risk factors

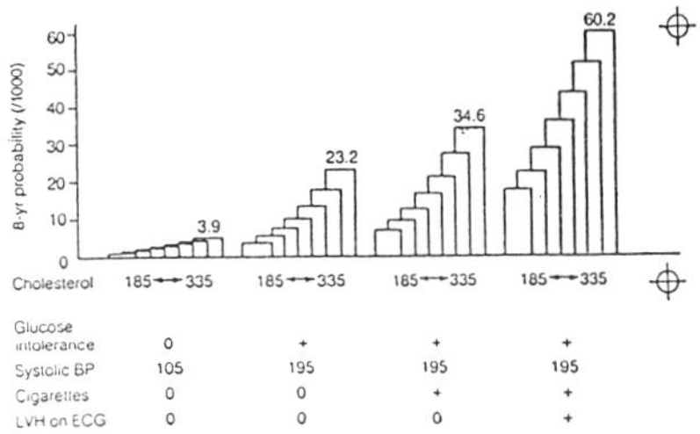

Framingnam Study, 18-yr follow-up, men aged 35

Source: Kannel, *Am J Cardiol* 1983*

Risk of Cardiovascular Disease According to
Systolic Blood Pressure. Persons With
Diastolic Blood Pressure ≤ 95
Men and Women 50-79
Framingham Study, 20 Year Follow-Up

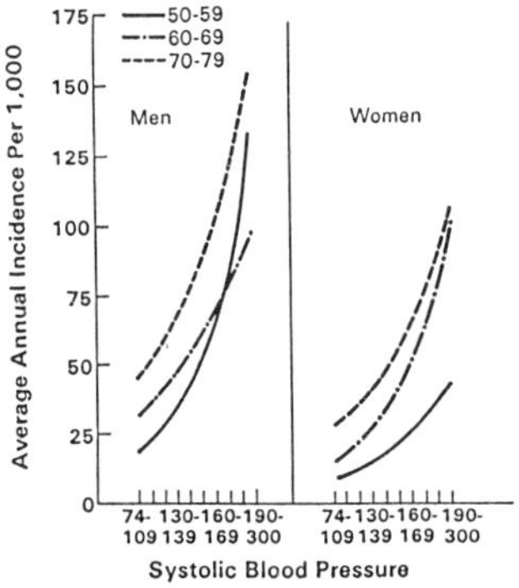

Lability was shown to be a faulty concept. Women and the elderly were found to tolerate hypertension no better than the middle-aged candidate or men. No critical blood pressure value was found and even modest elevations were shown to be hazardous. More than the nature of the blood pressure elevation, the associated cardiovascular risk profile has been shown to determine the outlook for any degree of hypertension.

Diabetes was shown to be a major, unique contributor, which in women, eliminated their advantage over men in coronary heart disease incidence. Fibrinogen, within the usual range was found to be independently associated with rate of occurrence of coronary heart disease and stroke, taking coexistent correlated risk factors into account (18).

Elements of lifestyle have been shown to promote risk factors and influence the incidence of coronary heart disease. This lifestyle is typified by a diet excessive in calories, fat and salt, a sedentary lifestyle, unrestrained weight gain and the cigarette habit. Alcohol, when used in moderation, was found to be associated with a reduced risk of coronary heart disease events. Coffee intake was unrelated to coronary heart disease incidence when highly correlated cigarette smoking was taken into account. In the sedentary Framingham cohort, cardiovascular and coronary heart disease mortality were found to be inversely related to level of physical activity in men but not women (12). A moderate level of activity was shown to be protective. Obese persons were found to be vulnerable to coronary disease and angina and sudden death in particular (10). This effect was only partly due to the associated cardiovascular risk factors which weight gain promotes (Table 1).

TABLE 1. Weight Fluctuations and Cardiovascular Risk Factors on Biennial Exams. The Framingham Study.

C.V. Risk Factors	Influence of 10 lb. Weight Change on C.V. Risk Factors: Men	Women
Serum Cholesterol	7.5 mg/dl.	5.8 mg/dl.
Systolic Blood Pressure	4.4 mmHg.	4.2 mmHg.
Blood Glucose	0.6 mg/dl.	1.2 mg/dl.
Uric Acid	0.2 mg/dl.	0.1 mg/dl.

Cigarette smoking was consistently shown to be a powerful independent risk factor for coronary heart disease which is particularly hazardous in those with a poor cardiovascular risk profile and in women taking estrogen (8). The effect appears to be non-cumulative and transient increasing with daily exposure. Those who quit smoking were found to have only half the risk of those who continue to smoke regardless of how long they formerly smoked. Substitution of filter cigarettes did not reduce coronary heart disease risk (8).

Type A behavior conferred a two-fold excess of coronary heart disease in the Framingham Study, confirming some, but not all epidemiologic studies (13). In women, the association was noted both in housewives and in those working outside the home. In men, the association was confined to white collar workers. Suppressed hostility was also associated with an increased risk. Men with highly educated wives were at increased risk of coronary heart disease, but only if their spouse worked outside the home (13).

Preclinical signs of ischemic myocardial involvement can be detected in subjects with a poor cardiovascular risk profile by ECG examination for silent myocardial infarction, ECG-LVH, blocked intraventricular conduction and repolarization abnormalities (10,11). Such persons were shown to have a clinical course much like persons with clinically overt coronary heart disease (Figure 4).

The incidence of myocardial infarction in the Framingham Study was significantly related to the myocardial infarction experience of male siblings. There was a 2-fold excess risk in those with a positive family member even controlling for a shared tendency to hypertension, hypercholesterolemia and the cigarette habit (19).

An abrupt rise of coronary heart disease incidence occurred in women undergoing the menopause, doubling their risk and the severity of the clinical manifestations of the disease. Estrogen administration did not eliminate this excess risk in cigarette smokers (15).

RISK OF CHD BY ECG ABNORMALITY IN MEN AND WOMEN AGED 35-64 YEARS
(FRAMINGHAM 30 YR FOLLOW-UP)

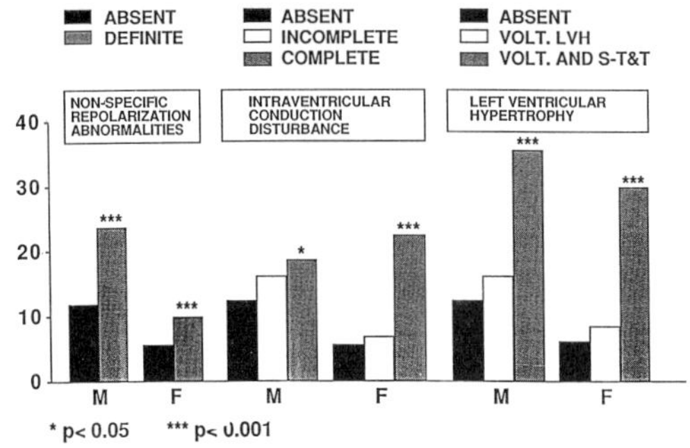

Optimal risk prediction was shown to require a quantitative synthesis of risk factors into a composite risk profile. Only by such multivariate combination of risk factors is it possible to avoid overlooking coronary candidates with multiple marginal risk factor values who are often missed by categorical evaluations of arbitrarily defined "risk factors". Handbooks and computer applications have been produced to facilitate multivariate assessments of risk (Table 2).

PROBABILITY OF DEVELOPING CORONARY HEART DISEASE
IN 6 YEARS: MEN (AGED 35-70)

Points	0	1	2	3	4	5	6	7	8	9	10
SBP	100	110	120	130	140	150	160	170	180	190	200
Cig	No				Yes						
LVH	No						Yes				
Glu	No		Yes								

HDL-C
Age/chol
multiplier

HDL-C (mg/dL)	*Factor*
30	1.82
35	1.49
40	1.22
45	*1.00*
50	0.82
55	0.67
60	0.55
65	0.45

Chol \ Age	36	38	40	42	44	46	48	50	55	60	65	70
165	3	6	9	11	14	16	18	19	23	26	27	27
180	5	8	10	13	15	17	19	20	24	26	27	27
195	7	9	12	14	16	18	20	21	24	26	27	27
210	8	11	13	15	17	19	21	22	25	27	27	27
225	10	12	15	17	19	20	22	23	26	27	28	27
240	11	14	16	18	20	21	23	24	27	28	28	27
255	13	15	17	19	21	23	24	25	27	28	28	27
270	15	17	19	21	22	24	25	26	28	29	28	26
285	16	18	20	22	24	25	26	27	29	29	28	26
300	18	20	22	23	25	26	27	28	29	29	28	26
315	20	22	23	25	26	27	28	29	30	30	29	26

Calculation of probability

Enter points (in red) for

______ Systolic blood pressure
\+ ______ Cigarette smoking
\+ ______ Left ventricular hypertrophy
\+ ______ Glucose intolerance
\+ ______ Age/serum cholesterol
= ______ Total points → probability

TP	Prob	TP	Prob	TP	Prob
5	.003	20	.021	35	.13
6	.004	21	.024	36	.14
7	.004	22	.028	37	.16
8	.005	23	.031	38	.17
9	.006	24	.035	39	.19
10	.006	25	.040	40	.21
11	.007	26	.045	41	.23
12	.008	27	.050	42	.25
13	.009	28	.057	43	.28
14	.010	29	.064	44	.30
15	.012	30	.071	45	.33
16	.013	31	.080	46	.36
17	.015	32	.090	47	.39
18	.017	33	.100	48	.42
19	.019	34	.110	49	.45

Left ventricular hypertrophy — as evaluated by ECG
Glucose intolerance — as manifested by diabetes, or a trace or more of sugar in the urine, or a non-fasting whole blood glucose level of 120 mg% or greater

Compiled by Erica Brittain at Stanford University, 1979, from multiple logistic functions in The Framingham Study, U.S. Government Printing Office.

From "Hospital Medicine", February, 1985, Pages 153 & 157.

These Framingham risk formulations have been tested and found to accurately predict disease in a variety of American population samples and in the elderly as well as younger coronary candidates.

The coronary risk profile can be done quickly, easily and inexpensively in any physician's office. However, efforts to prevent coronary heart disease are not as simple, requiring behavior modification and a sustained effort on the part of the physician and patient and involvement of the whole family. The rationale for prevention is sound, favorable evidence of efficacy is growing and the preventive measures advocated are safe and hygienic. Health agencies should attempt to improve the population levels of the major risk factors through health education, alteration of the ecology by government regulations and preventive medicine for high risk candidates.

There is reason for optimism about combatting the epidemic of coronary disease as this has taken a dramatic downturn in the United States, Canada, Australia and New Zealand, coincident with improvements in diet and risk factors. Major changes in all the atherogenic risk factors can be acheived by palatable alterations in diet along with weight control, exercise and avoidance of cigarettes. Behavior modification skills of prevention-minded physicians need to be improved and changes in the national diet promoted.

REFERENCES

[1] Gordon, T., Kannel, W.B. (1971) 'Premature mortality from coronary heart disease. The Framingham Study', JAMA 215,1617-1625.

[2] Kannel, W.B., McGee, D.L. (1976) 'A general cardiovascular risk profile: The Framingham Study', Am J Cardiol 38,46-51.

[3] Kannel, W.B. (1983) 'High density lipoproteins: Epidemiologic profile and risks of coronary artery disease', Am J Cardiol 52,9B-12B.

[4] Report of Intersociety Commission for Heart Disease Resources. (1984) 'Optimal resources for primary prevention of atherosclerotic disease', Circ 70,155A-205A.

[5] Kannel, W.B., Sorlie, P., Gordon, T. (1980) 'Labile hypertension: A faulty concept?' Circ 61,1183-1187.

[6] Kannel, W.B., Dawber, T.R., McGee, D.L. (1980) 'Perspectives on systolic hypertension: The Framingham Study', Circ 61,1179-1182.

[7] Kannel, W.B., Wolf, P.A., McGee, D.L. (1981) 'Systolic blood pressure, arterial rigidity and risk of stroke: The Framingham Study', JAMA 245,1442-1448.

[8] Kannel, W.B., McGee, D.L., Castelli, W.P. (1984) 'Latest perspective on cigarette smoking and cardiovascular disease: The Framingham Study', J Cardiac Rehav 4,267-277.

[9] Kannel, W.B., McGee, D.L. (1979) 'Diabetes and cardiovascular disease: The Framingham Study', JAMA 241,2035-2038.

[10] Kannel, William B., Gordon, Tavia (1974) 'The Framingham Study: An epidemiologic investigation of cardiovascular disease. Section 30, Monograph. Some characteristics related to the incidence of cardiovascular disease and death. 18 year foolow-up. U.S. Dept., HEW, PHS, NIH, DHEW, Publication No. (NIH)74-599.

[11] Kannel, W.B., Sorlie, W.P. (1981) 'Left ventricular hypertrophy in hypertension. Prognostic and pathogenetic implications. The Framingham Study', In, The Heart in Hypertension. Ed., B. E. Strauer, Springer-Verlag Publishing, Berlin pp. 223-242.

[12] Kannel, W.B., Belanger, A.J., D'Agostino, R.B., Israel, I. (1986) 'Physical activity and physical demand on the job and risk of cardiovascular disease and death. The Framingham Study', Am Heart J 112,820-825.

[13] Kannel, W.B., Eaker, E.D. (1986) 'Psychosocial and other features of coronary heart disease: Insights from the Framingham Study', Am Heart J, 112,5,1066-1073.

[14] Kannel, W.B., Hjortland, M.C., McNamara, P.M. (1976) 'Menopause and risk of cardiovascular disease: The Framingham Study', Ann Intern Med 85,447.

[15] Wilson, P.W.F., Garrison, R.J., Castelli, W.P. (1985) 'Post-menopausal estrogen use, cigarette smoking and cardiovascular morbidity in women over 50. The Framingham Study', N Engl J Med, 313,1038-1043.

[16] Thom, T., Kannel W.B. (1981) 'Downward trend in cardiovascular mortality', Annual Rev Med 32,427-434.

[17] Kannel, W.B., Abbott, R.D. (1984) 'Incidence and prognosis of unrecognized myocardial infarction: An update on the Framingham Study', N Engl J Med 311,1144.

[18] Wilhelmsen, L., Svansudd, M.D., Korson-Bengtsenk. (1984) 'Fibrinogen as a risk factor for stroke and myocardial infarction', N Engl J Med 311,501-505.

[19] Snowden, C.B., McNamara, P.M., Garrison, R.J. (1980) 'Predicting CHD in siblings. A multivariate assessment. The Framingham Study', Am J Epidemiol 115,217-222.

5
Dyslipemia in Portugal

M.J. HALPERN and M.F. MESQUITA

Center for Lipid Research, Department of Biochemistry, Faculty of Medical Sciences of UNL, Campo Santana, 130, 1100 Lisbon, Portugal

ABSTRACT. The Authors found a great prevalence of hypertriglyceridemia in the general population. In coronary disease the most important risk factors are, smoking, hypertension, obesity, hypercholesterolemia. hypertriglyceridemia and hypoHDLemia. In newborns they described 10 cases of hypertriglyceridemia in 188 newborns. In a study did in 600 subjects of a health center they found a great prevalence of increased Lp(a).

1. DEATH RATES IN PORTUGAL

The distribution of death rate for atherosclerosis in Portugal is diferent from EEC mean (table 1) - much lower for coronary disease and much

Table 1. Death rate for atherosclerosis

	Portugal	EEC
Coronary disease	80,4	144,6
Cerebrovascular disease	237,6	110,6

higher for cerebrovascular disease (1).

2.DYSLIPEMIA IN GENERAL POPULATION

In 1973 we described for the first time the prevalence of hypertriglyceridemia in two samples of the Portuguese population (2).

Table 2. Hyperlipemia in 2 samples of Portuguese population

Type	Urban population	Rural population
Normal	71,9	59,9
IIa	32	4
IIb	2,2	5,3
IV	23,7	30,9

Serra e Silva (3) confirmed these results in Coimbra but described a higher prevalence of hypercholesterolemia in medical doctor as compared against general population.

3. DYSLIPEMIA AND RISK FACTORS IN CORONARY DISEASE

In a study did in infarction patients 3 and 6 months after infarction (4) we observed also the higher prevalence of hypertriglyceridemia (table III).

Table 3. Dyslipemia in infarction (%)

Type	3 months	6 months
Normal	35,5	29,6
IV	38,4	46,6
Latent IV	7,3	11,1
IIa	13,3	10,3
IIb	3,4	7,3

In cerebrovascular diseases the hypertrigliceridemia prevalence is more important (5).

Pedro et all (6) did a retrospective study in 666 coronary patients with coronography. The most important risk factors are shown in table 4.

Table 4. % of found risk factors

Factor	Man	Women
Smoking	47,8	21,6
Hypertension	36,6	61
Obesity	14	16,7
Cholesterol	64	72
Triglycerides	40	32,6
HDL	28	58

They found also a direct relationship between the number of observed risk factors and the coronary score or the numbers of stenosated vessels.

4. NEWBORNS

In 1972 Glueck (7) described hypercholesterolemia in cord blood. In 1973 we described for the first time hypertriglyceridemia in the newborn - 4 cases in 60 newborns (8, 9). Recently (10, 11) we described 10 hypertriglyceridemia in 188 newborns (table 5).

In 6 cases we determined triglycerides also at 5 months of age (table 6). In table 7 we show the mother and newborn principal characteristics in order to excluse fetal distress as cause of hypertriglyceridemia.

Table 5. Newborn hyperlipemia

Case	Chol	TG	HDL
A	84	160	21
B	113	208	18
C	126	151	33
D	76	126	28
E	151	154	38
F	97	206	23
G	131	150	42
H	98	126	24
I	63	128	18
J	92	164	24

Table 6. Lipides after 5 months

Case	Chol.		TG		HDL	
	0 month	5 m.	0	5	0	5
A	84	118	166	154	21	35
B	113	136	208	177	18	28
D	76	163	126	280	28	29
F	97	113	206	212	23	22
H	98	120	126	160	24	30
J	92	140	164	144	25	31

Table 7. Newborn and mother characteristics

Case	Gestacional age	Delivery	Apgar Index	Weight for gest. age
A	40	C	8-10	AIG
B	40	V	10-10	AIG
C	40	V	9-10	AIG
D	38	V	9-10	AIF
E	39	F	5-9	GIG
F	38	C	3-8	LIG
G	36	F	6-9	LIG
H	35	V	9-10	AIG
I	35	C	9-10	AIG
J	39	V	9-10	LIG

C-Cesarean V-Vaginal F-Forceps
AIG - Adequate for gestational age
L-light G-Great

5. AIFRA PROJECT

In order to assure a strategy for prevention and treatment of atherosclerosis we organized an intervention trial, the AIFRA project (from the initials of the portuguese words Avaliação e Intervenção sobre os Factores de Risco da Ateroesclerose). The project consists in (1) Inquiry on risk factors (2). Analysis of chol., TG, HDL, HDL2, apo AI, apo B and Lp(a) (3), computerized evaluation of the results (4) lipid clinics.

We shall do oportunistic screening (health centers) and generalized screenings (companies, army, schools). We shall present data from 600 subjects of a Health Center.

5.1. Life style

The most striking data were the consumption of saturated fatty acids (85% of sample). 90% consume olive oil but 90% of them associated to saturated fatty acids. Other interesting findings were increased salt consumption (31%), obesity (24%) and hypertension (88%). 55% eated fish at least 4 times a week. Smoking and alcoholism were not important in this group (12 and 16%).

5.2. Lipids and apoproteins

We found 30,3% of borderline cholesterol (200-240 mg) and 35% of hypercholesterolemia (>240) but only 8% with cholesterol levels superior to 300.

We found hypertriglyceridemia (>200 mg%) in 9,7%, hypo HDL

(<35 mg% in men and 45 in women) in 15%, hypo HDL2 (<15) in 50% hyper apo B (>105) in 22%, hypo apo A1 (<95) in 20,3% . Concerning Lp(a) we observed a great prevalence of increased values 58% superior to 20mg% and 43% superior to 30.

6. REFERENCES

1. Cruz, A.(1987). Rev. Centro de Estudos de Nutrição 11(3) 3-22
2. Miguel J.P. and Halpern M.J. (1973) Ann. Biol. Clin. 3:145-147
3. Serra e Silva P. et al (1986) in M.J. Halpern (ed) " Lipid metabolism and its Pathology". Elsevier, Amsterdam,pp 175-184
4. França A. et al (1986) in M.J. Halpern "Lipid metabolism and its Pathology". Elsevier, Amsterdam, pp 119-126.
5. Ribeiro H.M. et al. (1986) in M.J. Halpern (ed) "Lipid metabolism and its Pathology". Elsevier, Amsterdam, pp127-131.
6. Pedro E. et al. (1989) Com. Congresso Sociedade Portuguesa de Cardiologia.
7. Glueck C.J. and Tsang R.C. (1972) Am. J. Clin. Nutr, 25:224-230.
8. Maymone Martins et al (1973) Brit. Med. J. I 544-545.
9. Maymone Martins et al (1973) Rev. Port. Ped. 4 (4) 1-10.
10. Amaral J.M. et al (1987) Ateroma, 5:30-32.
11. Pedro E. "Dislipemias dos recemnascidos (Author Edition).

6
The Brisighella study: plasma lipid trend in the elderly observed over a twelve year period

G.C. DESCOVICH, C. CEREDI, G. DE SIMONE, A. DORMI, G.L. MAGRI, A. MINARDI, M. SANTARELLA[1], G.B.SISCA, Z.SANGIORGI, M. VIGNA and G. MANNINO[2]

Department of Geriatrics and Lipid Clinic, University of Bologna. [1]Head, Brisighella Hospital; [2]Department of Mathematics and Chair of Numerical Analysis, University of Modena, Italy

ABSTRACT. Several intervention trials have shown the efficacy of a preventive strategy against cardiovascular risk factors, but in elderly the problem still remains open. In the Brisighella population, between 1972 and 1984 there was a marked increase in mean total cholesterol levels although the phenomenon was less marked amongst the elderly. The application of Multiple Logistic Function underlines the predictive role of total plasma cholesterol and systolic blood pressure. This study emphasizes the role of total plasma cholesterol in the development of coronary heart disease even in men over the age of 64. This observation strengthens the indications for preventive or therapeutic intervention, against the causal risk factor "cholesterol", at least up to the age of 70.

Introduction

The clear role of "risk factor(s)" in chronic cardiovascular disease has emerged from large epidemiological studies, namely from the observational longitudinal ones, but also from clinical trials.

Total plasma cholesterol, as a predictive or better as a "causal" factor for coronary heart disease (CHD) suggested by the Framingham Heart Study [1] and by the Seven Countries Study [2], was found to be crucial also from an etiopathological point of view by means of the more recent metabolic and clinical studies [3, 4, 5].

In the elderly, however, the role of cholesterol is less documented. The rare epidemiological and clinical studies are confusing, considering that the ageing physiology, the age-related functional modifications and the natural selection caused by diseases makes it difficult to evaluate whether the elderly have the same sensitivity to nutritional stimulation and/or modification as younger subjects.

The United States Senate Special Committee on Aging [6] in 1986 provided morbidity data for the American population over 65 years: chronic arthritis 44%, hypertension 38%, cardiovascular disease 27%, hearing (28%) and sight (12%) problems.

In a cohort of the Gubbio Study [7] people over 59 years had total cholesterol over 250 mg/dL (30% in women and 20% in men).

In the Framingham Heart Study [8] in the age group 65-74 blood pressure and smoking habits, but not total cholesterol, positively correlated with mortality from all causes and cardiovascular death. In women aged 65-94, total cholesterol was a risk factor for CHD; for the same age group and in both sexes, high LDL cholesterol and low HDL cholesterol levels were risk factors for CHD.

In the Lipid Research Clinic Program follow-up Study [9] of a population sample aged over 65, multivariated analysis showed a significant positive correlation between total and LDL cholesterol and CHD mortality in both sexes, while the protective role of HDL cholesterol was found only in women.

In the Los Angeles Veterans Administration Domiciliary Facility Study [10] the efficacy of dietary modification was tested on a sample of men, (mean age 65.5 years): the effect was more pronounced in men under 65.5 with the highest total cholesterol levels, but was also present in men over 65.5 years. Moreover, in all treated subjects the incidence of new cardiovascular events fell by 31% during a 8.5 year follow-up.

The Brisighella Study.

The Brisighella study started in 1972 with the aim [11] of analyzing every four years the levels of the main atherosclerosis risk factors and their correlation with cardiovascular disease, as well as of recording all fatal and nonfatal new events[12].

The population consisted of 1,491 men and 1,448 women, aged from 14 to 84 years and the geriatric sample was composed of 672 (357 men and 315 women) citizens.

From 1972 to 1984 in the whole population, mean total cholesterol values for men ranged from 222.6 mg/dL to 247.2 mg/dL, with an average increase of 2 mg/dL a year. Corresponding values for women ranged from 226.2 mg/dL to 259.6 mg/dL, with an average annual increase of 3 mg/dL. Plasma triglyceride levels also increased during this period, from 152.9 mg/dL to 174.1 mg/dL for men and from 129.1 mg/dL to 155.8 mg/dL for women. When these cholesterol values are seen in the context of the classification established by the National Cholesterol Education Program [13], it becomes clear that the Brisighella populations falls within the borderline-high (200-239 mg/dL) and high-risk (240 mg/dL or above) categories.

In subjects aged over 60 years the total cholesterol increase was less marked than in middle-aged and in younger subjects of both sexes (fig.1, 2).

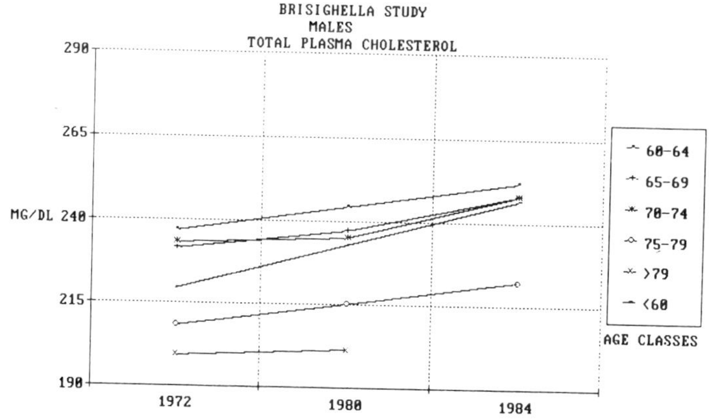

Figure 1

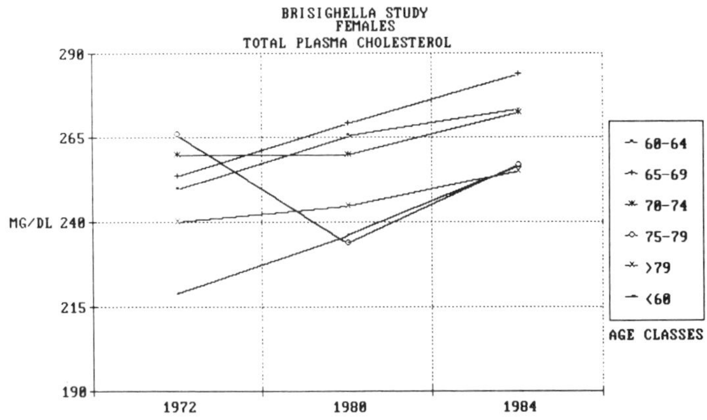

Figure 2

Fasting blood sugar (FBS) and serum uric acid (SUA) did not change during the twelve year observation period (fig.3, 4).

Systolic blood pressure (SBP) and diastolic blood pressure (DBP) showed an irregular trend, but always towards a decrease (fig.5); and the prevalence of hypertensives in 1984 showed a marked decrease (-6.8% in men and -18.3% in women). The analysis of drug consumption demonstrated a very frequent use of antihypertensive drugs both in 1980 and in 1984 in the two sexes, while the hypolipidemic agents were rarely used (6-7% in men and 13-14% in women) (fig.6). This may explain the decrease in SBP and DBP even in the elderly between 1972 to 1984 and the increase in total cholesterol in the same period.

To verify whether some risk factors maintained their predictive power for all cardiovascular deaths and in particular coronary deaths, solutions of the Multiple Logistic Function (MLF) were applied to all subjects enrolled in 1972. The parameters considered for the calculation of individual risk were age (A), physical activity (PA), cigarette consumption (CC), SBP and total plasma cholesterol (TC). This procedure was applied for the whole population, and in age classes 35-59, >59, >64 and >69 years (fig.7, 8).

In the whole male population a very good correlation was obtained for all the parameters considered versus CHD and all fatal cardiovascular new events.

Obviously in the oldest subjects, only age was highly statistically significant for the prediction of all cardiovascular diseases. PA and CC lost their predictive power in the population over 60; SBP and TC maintained the predictive power only in subjects under 65 years. On the contrary, the predictive power of TC was maintained in the subjects over 64 for CHD.

This means that cholesterol exerts its atherogenic activity also during the last years of life and for this reason all the intervention programmes aimed at reducing total plasma cholesterol levels are justified.

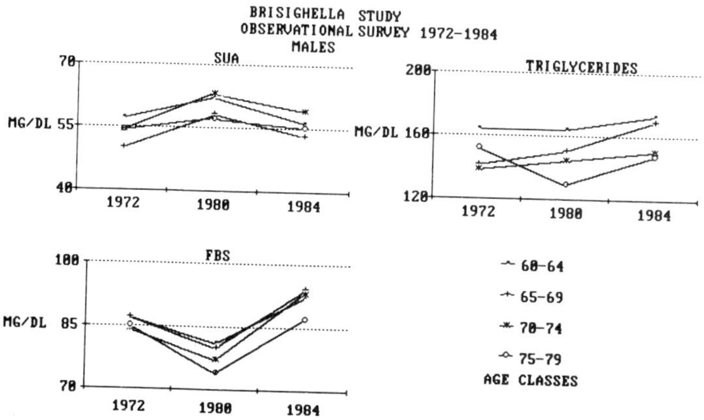

Figure 3

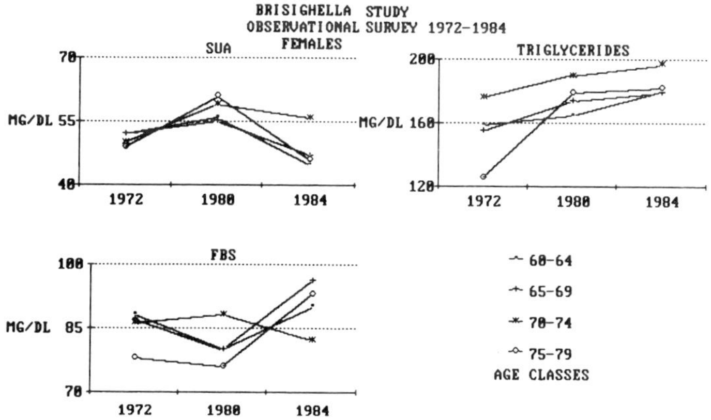

Figure 4

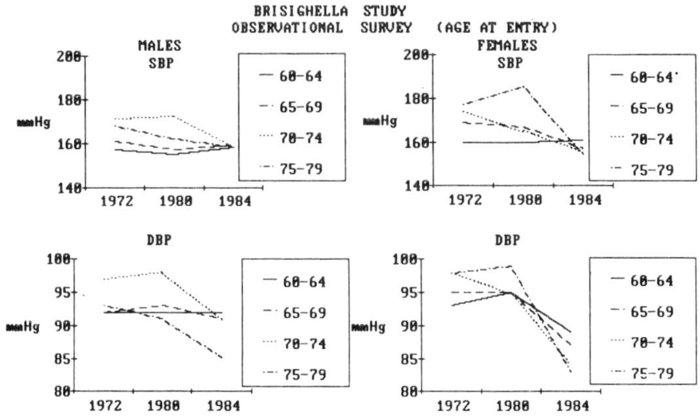

Figure 5

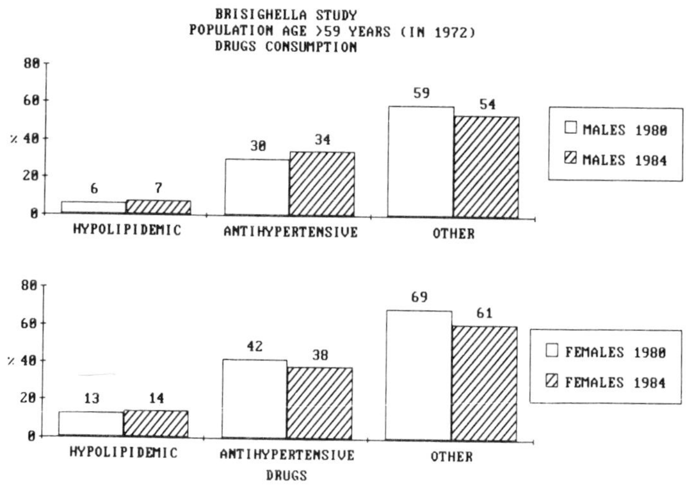

Figure 6

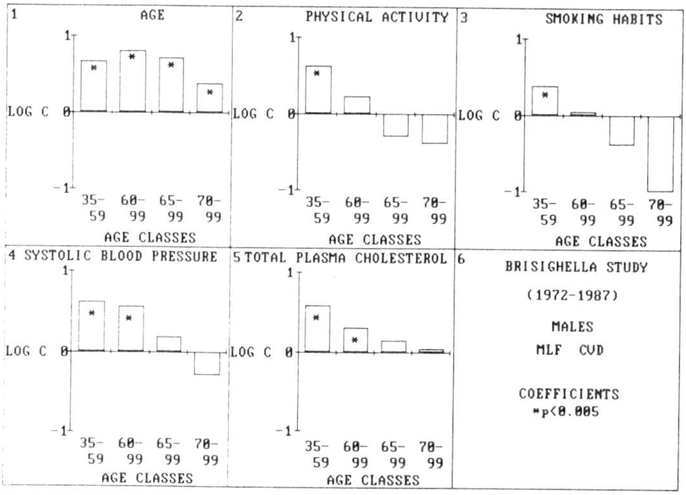

Figure 7

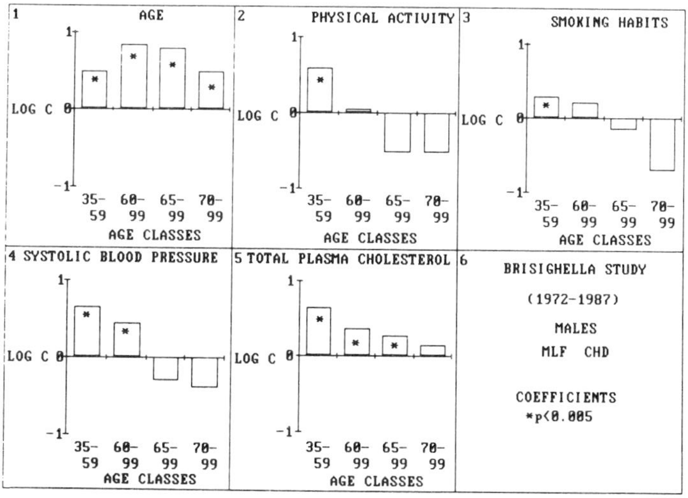

Figure 8

Furthermore, subdividing the population into cholesterol quintiles and considering fatal cardiovascular new events,the "case" distribution for each one appears to be "J" shaped, with higher numbers of deaths in the fifth quintile. It is worth underlining that the age of death is ten years less in the fifth quintile compared to the first one (fig.9, 10).

Moreover, constructing life tables for males over 60 subdivided into TC classes according to the US Consensus Conference [14] it appears that citizens with high TC survive less than people in borderline or low-risk cholesterol categories (fig.11).

Several intervention studies demonstrate the efficacy of a preventive strategy in pregeriatric subjects on cardiovascular mortality, but observational epidemiological studies supply insufficient data on geriatric subjects.

Through the application of MLF, the Brisighella Study confirms the importance of TC as a risk factor also in men aged over 64, thus strongly supporting the validity of a preventive strategy mainly oriented towards modifications in dietary habits. All data derived from the Brisighella Study support the hypothesis that it is never too early, but also never too late, to start an intervention program.

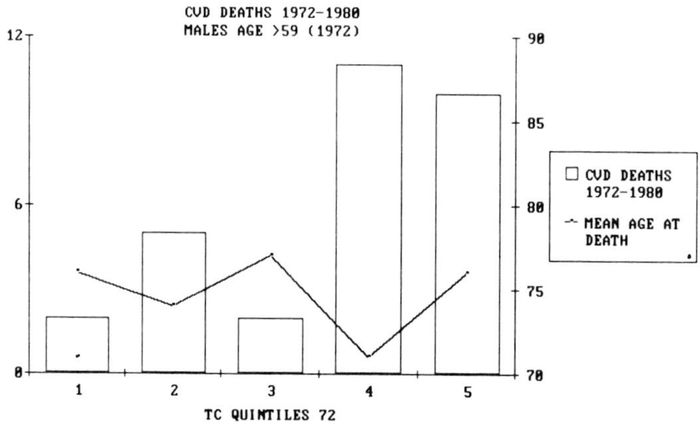

Figure 9

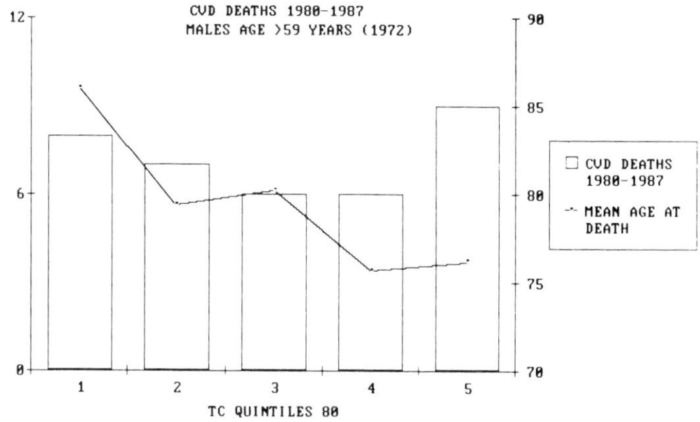

Figure 10

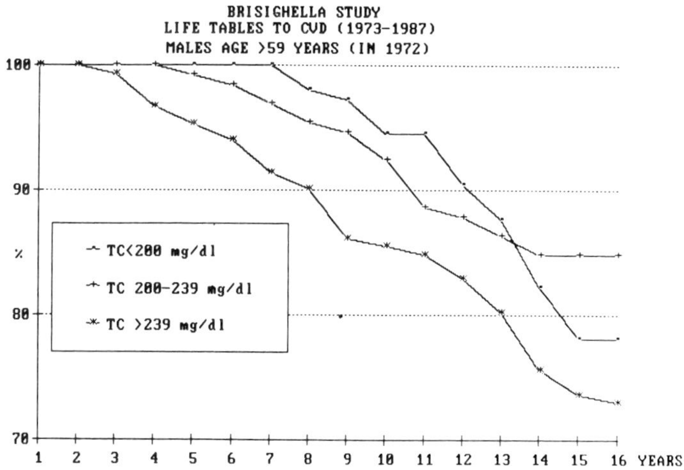

Figure 11

BRISIGHELLA HEART STUDY MEMBERS	(All Researchers listed in the appendix must be considered "Authors" of the present papers)
Coordinator:	G.C. Descovich - Bologna
Cholelithiasis Staff:	Chairman E. Roda
Bologna Medical Staff:	G.C. Descovich, G. Barozzi, A. Cavina, C. Ceredi, M. Colletta, A. Ciarrocchi, G. De Simone, A. Gaddi, A. Minardi, C. Naldoni, S. Paci, A.Romagnoli, M. Vigna
Bologna Biochemical Laboratory Staff:	Dir. Z. Sangiorgi, G. Copparoni, I. Faenza, G. Gamberi, G. La Regina, C. Meotti
Bologna Nutritional Laboratory Staff:	M.L. Borlotti, F. Brini, E. Faggioli, G. Negro, E. Tabanelli, G. Tarrini
Bologna Biometrics Laboratory Staff:	Dir. G. Mannino, A. Dormi, A. Braiato
Bologna ECG Reading and Coding Staff:	Dir. S. Rimondi, L. Finazzo
Bologna Echographic Reading and Coding Staff:	S. D'Addato, D. Festi, G.L. Magri, G. Manganaro, A. Matteucci
Bologna Rheumatism Staff:	S. Ferri
Medical Students Field Operators:	M. Ceccardi, G. Sisca, B. Descovich, C. Descovich B. Benassi
General Secretariat:	C. Maurizzi, M. Nanni
Brisighella Gen. Practitional Staff:	J. Drei, I. Gamberi, A. Naldi, F. Onofri, C. Samore' L. Savorani, G. Trere', F.M. Valpondi, P. Viozzi
Brisighella Hospital Staff:	Dir. M. Santarella, A. Callea, D. Casadei-Giunchi, C. Colombi, M. Gualdrini, S. Milletti, F.M. Montanari, G. Pagano, O. Quercia, R. Ramponi, A. Sarti, F. Tavoni, A. Zambon, A. Zamboni, R. Zucchini
Brisighella Biochemical Laboratory Staff:	E. Folco-Zambelli
Brisighella Coordination Staff:	E. Pelliconi, R. Bandini, B. Alboreti, F. Silvestrini
Brisighella Anagraphic Staff:	L. Sbarzaglia
Emilia-Romagna Region:	
Assessorato all'Agricoltura e all' Alimentazione:	G. Ceredi, M.C. Turchi
Press Office:	F. Gencarelli, I. Cattania
U.S.L. 37 Faenza:	F. Laghi, R. Bertoni, P. Fabbri
Mass media Staff: E. Marino	Pedagogic Staff: R. Bianco Finocchiaro

References

1) Truett, J., Cornfield, J., Kannel, W. (1967) 'A multivariate analysis of the risk of coronary heart disease in Framingham'. J. Chron. Dis. 20, 511-524
2) Keys, A. (ed.) (1970) 'Coronary heart disease in seven countries'. Circulation 41 suppl., 1-211
3) Stamler, J., Wentworth, D., Neaton, J.D. for the MRFIT Research Group (1986): 'Is relationship between serum cholesterol and risk of premature death from coronary heart disease continuous and graded? Findings in 356222 primary screenings of the Multiple Risk Factor Intervention Trial (MRFIT)'. JAMA, 256, 2823
4) Brensike, J.F., Levy, R.I., Kelsey, S.F. et al. (1984) 'Effects of therapy with cholestyramine on progression of coronary arteriosclerosis: results of the NHLBI Type II coronary intervention study'. Circulation 69, 313-324
5) Artzenius, A.C., Kromhout, D., Barth, J.D. et al. (1985) 'Diet, lipoproteins, and progression of coronary atherosclerosis. The Leiden Intervention Trial'. N. Engl. J. Med. 312, 805-811
6) United States Senate Special Committee on Aging (1986) 'Developments in Aging: 1985'. Government Printing Office
7) Laurenzi, M., Mancini, M. (1988) 'Plasma lipids in elderly men and women'. Eur. Heart J., 9 suppl.D, 69-74
8) Kannel, W.B., Vokonas, P.S. (1986) 'Primary risk factors for coronary heart disease in the elderly: The Framingham study', in N.K. Wenger, C.D. Furberg and E. Pitt (eds.), Coronary Heart Disease in the Elderly, Elsevier Science Publ., 60-92
9) Bush, T. (1989) 'Risk Factors for Atherosclerosis in the Elderly'. Communication at XIV International Congress of Gerontology, Acapulco, SY-CM10, 46
10) Dayton, S., Pearce, M.L., Hashimoto, S., Dixon, W.J., Tomiyasu, U. (1969) 'A controlled clinical trial of a diet high in unsaturated fat in preventing complications of atherosclerosis'. Circulation, 39-40 suppl.2, 1-63
11) Descovich, G.C., Dalmonte, G., Dormi, A. et al. (1984) 'The Brisighella Study: a community survey', in S. Lenzi and G.C. Descovich (eds.), Atherosclerosis and Cardiovascular Disease, MTP Press Limited, Lancaster, 467-477
12) Descovich, G.C., Dormi, A., Gaddi, A. et al. (1987) 'From observational to intervention programmes. The Brisighella study', in S. Lenzi and G.C. Descovich (eds.), Atherosclerosis and Cardiovascular Diseases, MTP Press Limited, Lancaster, 215-222
13) Poli A. (1989) Italian National Cholesterol Education Programme, in this book
14) Consensus Conference (1985): 'Lowering blood cholesterol to prevent heart disease'. JAMA 253, 2080-2086

GENETICS OF CORONARY HEART DISEASE AND ATHEROSCLEROSIS: CLINICAL AND EPIDEMIOLOGICAL IMPLICATIONS

7
FH gene phenotypic expression: insight for therapeutic strategy

A. GADDI, A. CIARROCCHI, G. BAROZZI, M. ARCA, G. MARRA, G. SERMASI, P. ZUCCHELLI, Z. SANGIORGI, A. DORMI, L. FINAZZO, S. RIMONDI and G.C. DESCOVICH

Chair of Gerontology and Atherosclerosis Centre, University of Bologna, via Masserenti 9, 40138 Bologna, Italy

ABSTRACT. For the last few years an Official Health Research Project of the Emilia Romagna Region has been underway to define the best diagnostic and therapeutic strategy for familial hypercholesterolemia. The data collected to date, referring to a survey of more than 500 subjects, indicate the severity and early type of coronary and carotid atheromatous lesions in Italian heterozygotes but also report, unlike surveys in other countries, the low prevalence of xanthomata and of xanthelasmas. The aim of this paper is to discuss the current diagnostic possibilities in relation to the clinical-laboratory picture and to the therapeutic needs and cardiovascular instrumental diagnosis of the FH patient.

Introduction

The patients with heterozygote familial hypercholesterolemia (FH) have a myocardial infarction risk 11 times (males) and 5 times (females) higher than that of the general population. Moreover, the mean age of the non-fatal infarction is, in males, 22 years less than that of the general population (1). There is no evidence, amongst heterozygote FHs, that this risk depends on the presence of xanthomata or xanthelasmas or other phenotypical expressions of the FH gene.

Treatment (drugs and/or LDL-apheresis) can, at least partially, correct the metabolic defect and perhaps prevent coronary events and/or prevent the extension of atheromatous lesions.

Immediate identification and treatment (always maximal) of FHs must therefore always be considered as imperative and inescapable objectives. This paper discusses the implications that diagnostic criteria may have on the decisions made in prescribing therapy (pharmacological, apheretic, para-pharmacological, surgical) and instrumental follow-ups (carotid echography, effort ECG, coronography, etc.) that the physician must face in the long-term treatment of heterozygote FH patients.

The main point of this discussion is the assumption that whereas on the one hand the heterozygote FH patient must be monitored from a cardiovascular point of view and given maximal treatment, on the other, it is not at present possible to assign these diagnostic resources and maximal treatments to all the secondary, sporadic, multigenic or hypercholesterolemic patients or in any case to all "suspect FHs".

Materials and Methods

A) DIAGNOSTIC CRITERIA

The following criteria all had to be satisfied for inclusion in the survey:

- presence of stable primary hypercholesterolemia with phenotype IIa in the propositus and in 50% of the first-degree relatives (approximation at 50% with the Robert test assuming X^2 values <2.6). Cut-off points: LDL-C > 230 mg/dl (» the median between the modes of the LDL-C distribution in FH families), VLDL-TG < 120 mg/dl, HDL-C between the 1st and 99th percentile of the control populations (2-4);
- presence of clear bimodal distribution of the LDL-C levels in the family;
- presence of clear vertical transmission of the trait;
- readiness of at least 8 members of the family to undergo repeated lipid profile check-ups;
- absence, for at least four consecutive check-ups over 6-10 months, of IIb phenotypes or at least of an increase in VLDL-TG in all the members of the family.

Great care was taken to avoid selection criteria based on other phenotypical signs of FH gene (xanthomata, xanthelasmas) or anamnestic criteria (history of angina or myocardial infarction).

The diagnoses were confirmed subsequently by assessing the B-E receptor activity on fibroplast explants (1-3 subjects per family).

FAMILIAL HYPERCHOLESTEROLEMIA STUDY

CASE REPORT #2 (August 1989): LIVING SUBJECTS

	N.	AGE: X	(SEM)	LOWER Q.	UPPER Q.
Parents (m) (*)	20	66.3	2.9	57	75
Parents (f) (*)	34	65.6	1.7	60	75
Propositi	48	42.9	1.7	33	52
Sibling (m)	57	50.4	1.8	41	60
Sibling (f)	65	52.6	1.9	46	64
Offspring I (m)	100	24.4	1.2	17	32
Offspring I (f)	80	24.5	1.2	17	33
Offspring II (m)	34	9.8	0.9	7	14
Offspring II (f)	26	11.5	1.3	6	16
Other (m) (*)	36	49.5	2.2	41	59
Other (f) (*)	45	41.7	1.4	35	47

(*) Excluded from lipoprotein-lipid data analysis

B) CASES SURVEYED

The data on the cases examined so far refer to 545 subjects (heterozygotes, +/Rbx, as well as "healthy" relatives, +/+) belonging to 48 families. The data on the causes of death were obtained from the analysis of more than 90 deceased subjects for whom reliable data was available on the cause of death and their lipidological conditions. The data referring to the incidence of new events were taken from a retrospective analysis of 27 families (enrolled from 1982 onwards) and refer to a three-year period during which the patients were not given any specific chronic therapy. Figure 1 shows the number, the average age (SEM, Upper and Lower Quartile) of the siblings and the offspring of the propositi (other = acquired relatives and/or uncertain relationship and/or homozygote subjects, all excluded during the data processing). Other features of the cases surveyed are reported in previous papers (5-7).

C) METHODS

All the lipidological analyses were carried out on venous blood samples collected after 12 hours of fasting.

Dosage of total plasma cholesterol (auto-analyzer Leitz Eppendorf, BBR reagent, Milan), triglyceridemia (idem), HDL-cholesterol (precipitation with dextran sulfate), Apo AI, Apo B, Apo CII, Apo CIII, Apo E (radial immunodiffusion), isoform apo E (IEF with Ampholine 4-6 and subsequent bidimensional electrophoreses on PAG) were carried out together with preparatory ultracentrifugation of the lipoproteins (UC Beckman L8-80, rotor 40.3, modified Havel method) and subsequent measurement of lipids and apoproteins.

All the methods were standardized and carried out following the directions of the Italian Lipid Clinics and the NHI (8-10); Quality Control of lipidic dosage was made in accordance with the WHO Lipid Reference Centre in Prague (Dir. Prof. D. Grafnetter).

Lipidological analyses were carried out approximately every 2 months. The LDL receptor activity was assessed as described elsewhere (11). Echographic investigations of the carotid district were made following the indications of the National Research Council (12). Clinical and instrumental cardiological examinations were carried out according to the general WHO directives (13).

Results

The prevailing causes of death in the cases examined were as follows: certain myocardial infarction (MI) (m=65.4%, f=23.3%); possible MI and/or sudden death (m=14.8%, f=19.3); stroke (m=7.4%, f=20.0%); neoplasms (M=1.2, f=20.0); other known causes (m=7.4%, f=16.7%); episodes (m=3.7%, f=0.0).

The estimate of the prevalence of new non-fatal events is almost identical to that of the causes of death: MI (m=63.8%, f=35.0%); effort angina (m=25.5%, f=35.0%); ac by-pass (m=6.4%, f= no case); stroke (m=2.1%, f=10.0%); TIA (m= no case, f=5.0%); others (m=2.1%, f=15%).

The data concerning the incidence of new fatal and non-fatal events, again in heterozygote FHs, are as follows: fatal MI (m=1300/100,000/y, f= no fatal case); non-fatal MI (m=800/100,000/y, f=480/100,000/y); typical effort angina with positive effort ECG for ischemia (m=400/100,000/y, f=445/100,000/y). The number of new stroke events or the new diagnoses of neoplasms (both found only in women) were too few for the calculation of a reliable indices.

Figures 2 and 3 show the average age (+95% CI) of the non-fatal (fig.2) and fatal (fig.3) cardiovascular events obtained from the prevalence data. It is clear that the data relative to certain myocardial infarction in males was concentrated in the decade 40-50 for the non-fatal events and 50-60 for the fatal ones.

Amongst the new non-fatal coronary events, 4 (effort angina n=1, ECG with positive effort n=2, positive coronography and subsequent angioplasty n=1; the first three are still being studied) were observed in subjects under the age of 25, all males. One woman, aged 34, had a myocardial infarction.

Figure 4 (*) shows the preliminary data for the prevalence of carotid atheromatous lesions in heterozygote FHs and the ages (+95% CI) of the respective groups. It can be seen that only 25% of the heterozygote FHs (with an average age of 30 (+7) show no sign of cholesterol deposition at a carotid level.

An analysis by sex and age of the data indicates a prevalence of echographic patterns indicating isolated or multiple maximal carotid stenoses in women over the age of 50 (84%).

FAMILIAL HYPERCHOLESTEROLEMIA STUDY
Mean age at Death of heterozygotes

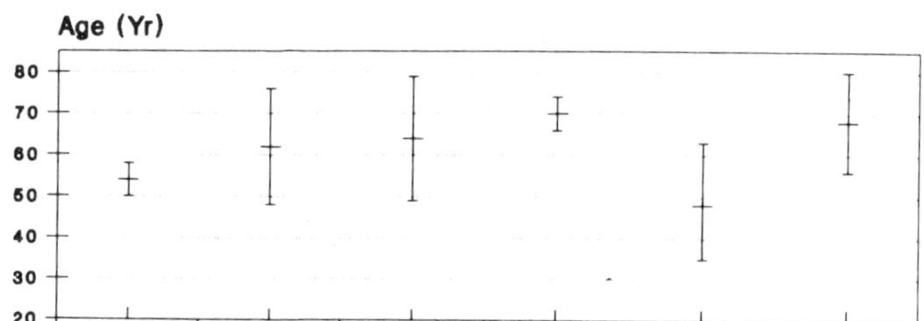

	MI (m)	MI (f)	CV (m)	CV (f)	D (m)	D (f)
95% CI	58	48	49	66	35	56
" "	50	76	79	74	63	80
Mean	54	62	64	70	48	68

I 95% CI ‡ Mean

MI - Myocardial Infarction
CV - Cerebrovascular Disease
D - Possible MI or Sudden Death

* The classification indicated (intimal lesion = IL, one stenosis = ST 1, two or more stenoses = ST>1) have a purely indicative value; analysis of the data in accordance with the previously standardized criteria (12) is still underway.

This brief summary of some of the clinical data relative to our survey tends to emphasize the severity of the coronary and carotid condition even in very young heterozygotes. An analysis of the results based on the presence of other risk factors, other symptoms or lipid levels, indicates at present slightly higher LDL-cholesterol levels (and slightly lower HDL-C) in subjects of both sexes with ischemic cardiopathy (as compared to the heterozygote relatives with no signs of CHD) and a higher number of smokers amongst the subjects with CHD (33%) as compared to the controls of the same age (heterozygote or non-heterozygote of the same families: 17%).

The prevalence of skin "signs" of hypercholesterolemia was as follows: xanthomata other than those on the Achilles' tendon = 3.5%; xanthelasmas = 20.8% (monolateral = 4.8%, bilateral = 16.0%); gerontoxon = 2.4%.

There was no difference in the prevalence or incidence indices of coronary conditions (MI, angina, coronography and/or positive effort ECG) or in the carotid patterns observed in relation to the presence or absence of xanthomata or xanthelasmas or both.

Discussion

The diagnostic "problem" presented by heterozygote familial hypercholesterolemia appears to be extremely complex and urgently requires a solution.

Simplified diagnostic criteria, easy for doctors to use on the entire population, could lead to an excessive number of false positives, with an enormous increase in costs for society (in terms of pharmaceutical and cardiovascular instrumental diagnostic costs) and excessive medical control of many young people or children.

On the other hand, the adoption of more selective, but also more sophisticated and complex criteria, besides increasing the initial diagnostic costs, would mean that diagnosis could only be made in specialized centres capable at least of measuring the LDL receptor activity. These centres would certainly not be able to cope with the load of all the Italian "possible FHs" (estimated heterozygote FHs in Italy: 130,000 subjects; indicative estimate of the number of subjects susceptible to differential diagnosis: > 500,000 subjects).

Moreover, the non-identification and the consequent lack of specific treatment of these subjects, besides being unacceptable from an ethical point of view, would lead to approximately 4,000 new events per year (MI, angina, by-pass, stroke, TIA, etc.) in the majority of cases in young working-age subjects, with a mortality which can be estimated at more than 20,000 in ten years.

On the other hand, diagnoses also based on the presence of clinical signs (e.g. xanthomata) are unthinkable, at least for Italian heterozygote FHs, given the low prevalence of these signs and given also the absence of reliable data which permit an assessment of the sensitivity, specificity and accuracy of diagnoses based on semeiotics (14). For example, in the case of the Italian heterozygotes, a diagnostic criterion based on the combination of the presence of LDL-C > 90th percentile (in the population from the same geographic area) and the presence of xanthomata and/or xanthelasmas would give a fair specificity (assuming that the problem of differential diagnosis as compared to severe II multigenics, combined familial forms and other non-FH monogenic hypercholesterolemias can be overcome with other criteria - still to be defined!), but, in any case, it would have a completely inacceptable sensitivity (<35%).

The use of FH gene markers (RFLP), of great scientific significance, does not however seem possible in clinical practice and, even where this might be possible in the future, the methods would need to be simplified.

LDL receptor measurement, besides the problems of overlapping between false

FAMILIAL HYPERCHOLESTEROLEMIA STUDY
Cardiovascular non fatal new events
(mean age)

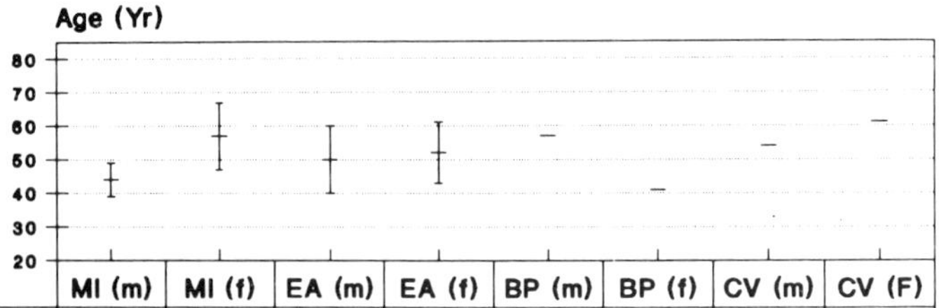

	MI (m)	MI (f)	EA (m)	EA (f)	BP (m)	BP (f)	CV (m)	CV (F)
95% CI	39	47	40	43				
" "	49	67	60	61				
Mean	44	57	50	52	57	41	54	61

MI = Myocardial Infarction
EA = Effort angina, BP = By pass a-c
CV = Cerebrovascular diseases

FAMILIAL HYPERCHOLESTEROLEMIA STUDY
CAROTID ATHEROSCLEROSIS IN HETEROZYGOTES

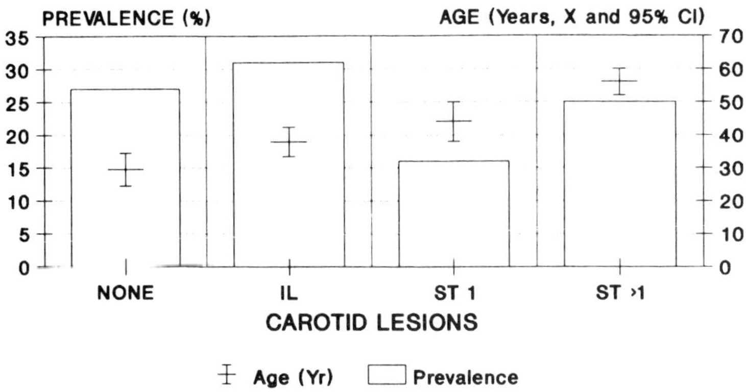

IL = lesion of intima
ST 1 = one stenosis
ST >1 = two or more stenoses

positive and false negative results, appears to be difficult to adopt on a large scale, as mentioned above.

The use of other clinical criteria (e.g. presence of early myocardial infarction), besides cancelling out the preventive purpose of treatment, would present new diagnostic problems, e.g. combined familial hyperlipidemia.

Finally mixed criteria (based on the measurement of lipids and/or apo B and/or preparatory UC of lipoprotein and/or type of E genotype and/or presence of clinical signs and/or analysis of geneological tree, etc.) would require, apart from high costs again, specialist expertise which could hardly be expected to fall within the normal routine of general practitioners.

All this at a time when the therapies available (in alphabetical order: cholesterol synthesis inhibitors, fibrates, ionic exchange resins, LDL-aphereses, nicotinic ac., probucol) promise encouraging results even in patients with heterozygote familial hypercholesterolemia and in whom early diagnosis and cardiovascular monitoring can permit surgical or parasurgical solutions which frequently resolve the problem and are not necessarily traumatic or costly (e.g. angioplasty).

On the basis of the data currently available, it would appear legitimate to suggest probabilistic solutions to the diagnostic problem, preferably using the total plasma cholesterol level, which can be used together with the more general indications of the Health Consensus Development Conference (15-17) (to avoid creating confusion among citizens and medical personnel), but which, together, offer sufficient diagnostic accuracy.

A working hypothesis may be that of resorting to the assessment of the final risk of heterozygosity, which, from preliminary data, appears to allow an acceptable probabilistic diagnosis (e.g. true negative for $p<0.05$, true positive for $p>0.95$) in most heterozygotes. Moreover, resorting to an assessment of all the cases available in a given family (through estimates of central tendencies and dispersion, easily used by anyone) may permit a very useful diagnostic specialization. Finally, not as a definite but a strongly convincing criteria, the presence of a hypercholestolemic child.

Acknowledgements

We thank Prof. S. Calandra and Prof. Tiozzo Costa (University of Modena, Italy) for their continued cooperation and for measuring the LDL receptor activity; Prof A.M. Gotto and Dr. G. Ghiselli (Baylor College of Medicine, Huston, USA) for their advice and for setting up the methods; Dr. H Mabuchi (Kanazawa, Japan) for critical discussion of some data; Dr. D. Grafnetter (WHO Lipid Reference Center, Prague) for the quality control of the lipidological analyses; S. West (Bologna) for translation of the text.

SUPPORTER: the study was partially financed by the Emilia Romagna Region (Official Health Research Programmes) and the University of Bologna.

References

1 Gaddi, A., Braiato, A., Marra, M., Magri, G. L., Mezzetti, M., Minardi, A., Sangiorgi, Z. and Descovich G. C. (1986) 'Familial hypercholesterolemias in Italy: plasma cholesterol evaluation and diagnostic insight', in S. Lenzi and G. C. Descovich (eds.), Atherosclerosis and Cardiovascular Diseases, MTP Press, Lancaster, pp. 279-88.

2 Descovich, G. C., Gaddi, A., Mannino, G. and Lenzi, S. (1981) 'L'indagine di Brisighella. I Fattori di Rischio Metabolici', Giorn. It. Cardiol. 11, 1591-603.

3 Descovich, G. C., Dormi, A., Gaddi, A., et al. (1987) 'From observational to Intervention Programmes. The Brisighella Study.', in S. Lenzi and G. C. Descovich (eds.), Atherosclerosis and Cardiovascular Diseases Prevention. Lancaster, MTP Press, pp. 346-51.

4 National Research Council Atherosclerosis Research Group. (1981) Atherosclerosis risk factors in nine Italian population samples. Am. J. Epidemiol. 113, 338-343.

5 Mezzetti, M., Gaddi, A. and Rimondi, S. et al. (1987) 'Familial Hypercholesterolemias in Emilia-Romagna Region.', in S. Lenzi and G. C. Descovich (eds.), Atherosclerosis and Cardiovascular Disease, Bologna, Ed. Compositori, pp. 1001-5.

6 Ciarrocchi, A., Gaddi, A., Barozzi, G., Marra, G., Colletta, M., Minardi, A., Nucci, S., La Regina, G., Sangiorgi, Z., Sermasi, G., Zucchelli, P. and Descovich, G. C. (1989) 'Ageing in familial hypercholesterolemic patients: clinical and metabolic implications' in G. C. Descovich, A. Gaddi and S. Lenzi (eds.), Atherosclerosis, Ed. Compositori, Bologna.

7 Ciarrocchi, A., Gaddi, A., Rimondi, S., Mezzetti, M. and Scaramuzzino, G. (1988) 'Ipercolesterolemia Familiare: aspetti clinici', Cardiologia 33 (11), 1055-60.

8 National Research Council. (1977) Laboratory Methods in Atherosclerosis Risk Factor Study. Ed. Dedalo, Bari, I, 1-76.

9 Manual of Laboratory Operations, (1974) Lipid Research Clinic Programme: Lipid and Lipoprotein Analysis. DHEW Publication no. (NHI) 75-628.

10 Lindgren, F. I., Jensen, L. C. and Hacth, F. T. (1972) 'The isolation and quantitative analysis of serum lipoproteins' in G. Wilson (eds.), Blood Lipids and Lipoproteins, Wiley & Sons Inc, pp. 181-207.

11 Ghisellini, M., Lelli, N., Cingi, M. R., Tiozzo, R., Calandra, S., Gaddi, A., Vergoni, W., Arca, M., Cortese, C., Pintus, F. and Bertolini, S. (1989) 'A survey of mutations of LDL-receptor gene in Italian patients with familial hypercholesterolemia', Atherosclerosis, in press.

12 Lenzi, S., Bucci, A., Crepaldi, G., Mancini, M., Menotti, A., Paoletti, R., Spagnoli, L. G., Ventura, A. and Weber, G. (1986) 'The CNR Program of Preventive Medicine - SP4 Ob. 44. Non-invasive techniques for the evaluation of atherosclerotic plaque progression or regression', in A. Ventura, G. Crepaldi, U. Senin (eds.), Extracoronary Atherosclerosis. Monograph on Atherosclerosis, Karger, pp 83-90.

13 Rose, G. A., and Blackburn, H. (1967) 'Cardiovascular survey methods', Geneva, Wld. Hlth. Org. Ed.

14 Crepaldi, G. (1986) 'Le Iperlipoproteinemie' Atti 87° Congresso Societa' Italiana Medicina Interna, Pozzi Editore, Roma, pp. 3-94.

15 National Institutes of Health Consensus Development Conference statement (1985) 'Lowering blood cholesterol to prevent heart disease', JAMA, 253, 2080-6.

16 Italian Consensus Conference, May 1986. 'Abbassare la colesterolemia per ridurre la cardiopatia ischemica'. National Research Council ed., Rome.

17 European Atherosclerosis Group, June 19-20th, 1986. 'A strategy for the prevention of coronary heart disease, a policy statement of the European Atherosclerosis Group', Naples.

8
Development of coronary heart disease in familial hypercholesterolemia

H. MABUCHI, H. FUJITA, K. KAJINAMI, Y. UNO, M. SHIMIZU, J. KOIZUMI and R. TAKEDA

The Second Department of Internal Medicine, Kanazawa University School of Medicine, Takara-machi 13-1, Kanazawa 920, Japan

ABSTRACT. We studied the development of coronary heart disease in 14 homozygous and 1043 heterozygous patients with familial hypercholesterolemia (FH). Forty-three (63%) out of the deceased 68 heterozygous patients died of coronary heart disease. The mean age at death was significantly less in male heterozygotes (56 years) than in female heterozygotes (68 years). Five homozygous and 105 male and 56 female heterozygous patients received coronary angiographic evaluation. The regression equations between age (X) and coronary stenosis index (Y) obtained by assigning score (0 to 4) to each of 15 coronary artery segments were Y=1.57X-20.43 in the homozygotes, Y=0.52X-9.1 in the male heterozygotes, and Y=0.47X-12.54 in the female heterozygotes. From these data, we can assume that coronary artery stenosis detectable by angiography will occur after 17 and 25 years of age in male and female heterozygotes, respectively, and the treatment of heterozygotes with lipid-lowering drugs can be delayed until late adolescence.

A new variant of low density lipoprotein (LDL) receptor gene (FH-Tonami-2) with 10kb deletion eliminating exons 2 and 3 deleted the first and second repeats of ligand binding domain of LDL receptor. Serum cholesterol levels in FH-Tonami-2 patients were lower than those of classical FH patients. All 4 true homozygotes with FH-Tonami-2 are presently alive at ages 62, 51, 48 and 33, and the heterozygotes have also survived longer than classical FH patients. From these results, we conclude that FH-Tonami-2, caused by a partially impaired LDL receptor with small deletion in its binding domain, produces a mild type of FH.

Introduction

FH is frequently associated with premature coronary heart disease (CHD), and the rate of death from CHD among heterozygotes is several times higher than that among the general population [1-4]. Homozygous patients does not survive to reach the age of 30 [1,5], whereas the mean age at death for male and female heterozygotes is 54 and 65 [4-7], respectively. There are no data, however, reporting when FH patients develop CHD documented by coronary angiography. Several authors [8], who have suggested that the earliest possible treatment of hypercholesterolemia can lead to the best results for FH patients, have treated children with FH. There are, however, no reports that indicate when CHD develops in FH and how rapidly it progresses. In the present study, we examined coronary angiographic findings to estimate the onset and progression of CHD in FH patients and to deduce when treatment of hypercholesterolemia can be initiated [9].

FH is a common autosomal dominant disorder resulting from a complete or partial defect of the gene for the low-density lipoprotein (LDL) receptor [1]. More than 30 different mutations in the LDL receptor gene have been reported [10], and thus, FH is a heterogenous disease at the molecular level. Here we studied if FH caused by the partially impaired LDL receptor may produce a mild type of FH and develop CHD slowly [11].

Materials and Methods

Consecutive 14 homozygous (7 men and 7 women) and 1043 heterozygous (515 men and 528 women) patients with FH from 560 families had been enrolled in this study since 1974. FH was diagnosed according to the following two criteria: 1) primary hypercholesterolemic patients (arbitrarily above 230 mg/dl in any age group) with tendon xanthomas [12], and 2) primary hypercholesterolemic patients with and without tendon xanthomas in a first-degree relative of FH patients. The diagnosis of homozygous FH was made on hypercholesterolemic patients with generalized xanthomas whose parents had been ascertained as heterozygous FH. Coronary angiography was performed with the Judkins technique before (first projection) and after (other projections) sublingual administration of 0.3 mg nitroglycerin. Coronary angiograms were interpreted by two or, in case of doubt, three investigators without knowledge of the patient's clinical history and serum lipid values. The extent and severity of stenotic changes were assessed by assigning scores to each of the 15 segments, according to the classification of the American Heart Association Grading Committee. The coronary stenosis index (CSI) was defined as the sum of these scores [13]. A normal coronary angiogram was graded 0, stenosis of less than 25% was graded 1, 25-50% stenosis was graded 2, 50-75% stenosis was graded 3, and more than 75% stenosis was graded 4. Thus, the highest possible CSI was graded 60. Coronary angiographic study was performed in 5 homozygotes, and 105 male and 56 female heterozygotes [9].

Blood samples, obtained in the morning after a 12-hour overnight fast, were allowed to clot at room temperature. Methods of lipoprotein fractions and lipid determinations were discussed in our previous study [15]. For statistical procedures, Student's t test and regression analysis were performed according to standard statistical methods with a computer system.

Results

Incidence of Myocardial Infarction

Myocardial infarction was diagnosed in 89 of 515 (17%) male patients and 39 of 529 (7%) female patients with heterozygous FH. Myocardial infarction was first noted in the men in the 3rd decade of life, with incidences gradually increasing by age (Figure 1). In the women the frequency of myocardial infarction rapidly increases after the menopause.

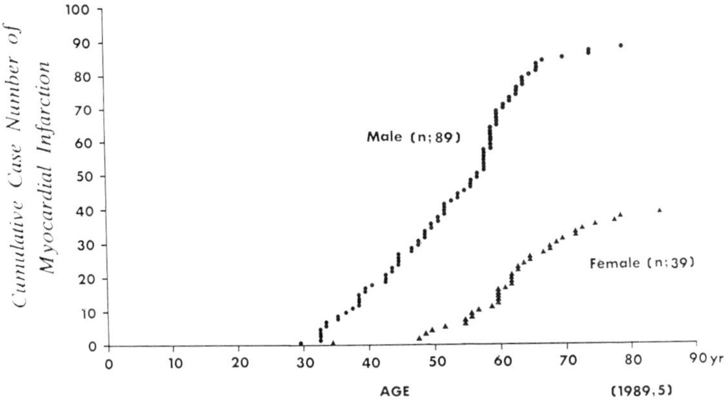

Figure 1. Cumulative case number of myocardial infarction by age in male and female heterozygotes with familial hypercholesterolemia.

Six of 14 homozygotes and 68 of 1043 heterozygotes have died. Sudden death or heart failure was the cause of death in all six deceased homozygotes (Table 1)[4]. Their average age at death was 26 years, with an average serum cholesterol level of 772 mg/dl. Forty-three (63%) out of the deceased 68 heterozygotes died of CHD. The mean age at death was significantly less in male heterozygotes (56 years) than in female heterozygotes (68 years)($p<0.001$)(Table 2). The mean serum cholesterol levels of deceased male and female heterozygotes were 369 and 354 mg/dl, respectively.

Coronary Angiographic Study

Five homozygous and 105 male and 56 female heterozygous patients received coronary angiographic evaluation. CSI and age of each patient are plotted in Figures 2A, 2B, and 2C. Their regression equations between age (X) and CSI (Y) are $Y=1.57X-20.43$ ($r=0.956$, $p<0.05$) in the homozygotes, $Y=0.52X-9.11$ ($r=0.438, p<0.001$) in the male heterozygotes, and $Y=0.47X-12.54$ ($r=0.343$, $p<0.01$) in the female heterozygotes (Figure 2D). As might be predicted from the regression equatons in Figure 2D, coronary stenosis should begin, on the average, at 13 years of age in the homozygotes and then at 17 and 25 years of age in the male and the female heterozygotes, respectively.

TABLE 1. Details of deceased homozygous patients with familial hypercholesterolemia

Patient	Age (yr)	Sex	Serum cholesterol (mg/dl)	Serum triglyceride (mg/dl)	Cause of death
Y.E.	16	M	900	300	Heart failure
M.I.	22	F	730	237	Sudden cardiac death
K.Y.	31	F	609	126	Sudden cardiac death
K.M.	42	F	610	180	Sudden cardiac death
S.T.	18	M	781	189	Heart failure
S.S.	29	F	1004	784	Sudden cardiac death
Mean	26		772	303	
SD	10		158	243	

TABLE 2. Causes of death, sex, age, serum cholesterol and triglyceride levels in 68 patients with heterozygous familial hypercholesterolemia (Values are given as means ± SD.)

Cause of death	Number of case		Age of death (yr)		Serum cholesterol (mg/dl)		Serum triglyceride (mg/dl)	
	M	F	M	F	M	F	M	F
Myocardial infarction	16	13	57±11	68±8	378±76	344±56	179±97	141±63
Sudden cardiac death	8	5	49±14	69±10	380±63	381±59	129±75	170±52
After CABG	1	0	58	-	376	-	146	-
Stroke	2	4	60±4	70±5	424±62	365±130	212	110±12
Cancer	8	3	59±9	59±14	299±125	349±19	217±96	187±35
Others	5	3	59±18	71±14	336±84	346±44	132±53	101±43
Total	40	28	56±12	68±9	369±72	354±65	173±81	142±55

The regression coefficient of the homozygotes was about three times that of male and female heterozygotes.

A New Variant of FH and Coronary Heart Disease

Four new variants of LDL receptor gene (FH-Tonami-1, FH-Tonami-2, FH-Kanazawa, FH-Okayama) were identified through analysis with Southern blotting of DNA samples from the members of 200 unrelated Japanese families[11,15,16]. FH-Tonami-2 has a variant of LDL receptor gene with 10 kb deletion eliminating exons 2 and 3 [11]. This mutant gene deleted the first and second repeats of ligand binding domain of LDL receptor, and serum cholesterol levels in FH-Tonami-2 patients were lower in both homozygotes and heterozygotes compared with those of "classical" FH patients. Development of coronary stenosis in FH-Tonami-2, determined by coronary angiography was slower than that of classical FH patients. All 4 true homozygotes with FH-Tonami-2

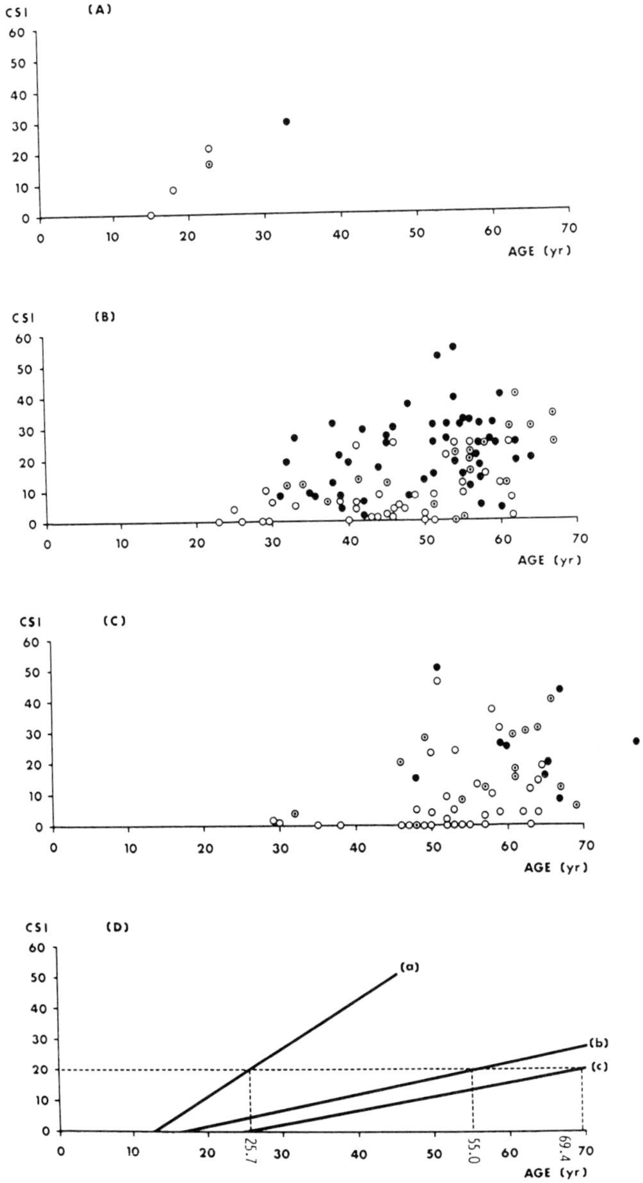

Figure 2. Plots of correlation between age (X) and coronary stenosis index (CSI;Y) in homozygous (A) and male (B) and female (C) heterozygotes. The regression equations in each patient group are shown (D). ●, Patients with myocardial infarction; ⊙, patients with angina pectoris or myocardial ischemia; O, asymptomatic patients. [9]

are presently alive at ages 62, 51, 48, and 33, and thus, we conclude that FH-Tonami-2, caused by a partially impaired LDL receptor with small deletion in its ligand binding domain, produces a mild type of FH.

Discussion

In the present study, coronary artery stenosis was documented in four of five homozygotes, and one male homozygote aged 15 years showed no coronary stenosis. Goldstein et al [1], who studied the prevalence of CHD in a group of 54 homozygotes, found that the prevalence of CHD in the age group 0-10 years was 60% in the receptor-negative homozygotes and 0% in the receptor-defective homozygotes. In the age group 10-20 years, the prevalence of CHD was 47% in the receptor-negative homozygotes and 36% in the receptor-defective homozygotes. Thus, homozygous patients should be treated as soon as the diagnosis is established, and plasma exchange [17], LDL-apheresis [18], or other drastic therapies such as liver transplantation [19] or portacaval shunt [20] rather than drug therapy have been applied.

About 70% of heterozygous patients died of CHD[4]. Heiberg [6] and Beaumont et al [7] reported that the incidence of CHD in FH was much higher in men than in women, and the mean age of onset was 9 years sooner in males. Kwiterowich et al [21] found that none of the 70 children with FH in his study had CHD in the 1st and 2nd decades, whereas half of their parents (mean age, 37.3 years) had CHD. The mean ages at which the affected men and women developed CHD was 39.7 and 41.3 years, respectively. Among the heterozygotes less than 30 years of age, the incidence was extremely low (about 5% for men and 0% for women). However, there are few papers reporting on CHD that have been documented by the coronary angiography of FH patients. Our study provides information about the course of CHD in FH [9].

FH is an autosomal dominant disease, which is completely expressed at birth and early in childhood [1]. The earlier the treatment of hypercholesterolemia is started, the better the outcome of CHD in FH. However, the view that treatment of hypercholesterolemia in childhood will reduce adult morbidity and mortality from CHD is necessarily based on extrapolation from controlled clinical trials in middle-aged, high-risk, hypercholesterolemic men, since such studies have not been done on children. The National Institutes of Health Consensus Conference has recommended special guidelines for management of children [22]. Strict dietary intervention is indicated, but treatment with a lipid-lowering agent in most children should be deferred until evidence is available about the safety and efficacy of drug therapy in children. Although no heterozygous patients less than 20 years of age underwent coronary angiography in the present study and the regression lines intercept at 17 and 25 years of age in male and female heterozygotes, respectively, there may in fact be a threshold at about age 20 in men and 30 in women before angiographic abnormalities are seen. As dietary modification will lower the plasma cholesterol levels in children and nutritional habits and other lifestyles develop early in life, dietary management should be started in childhood [22]. However, the possible adverse effects of a modified diet must always be carefully considered. Moreover, lipid-lowering drugs have been proved to be safe in general for adult patients, but no drugs have ever been proved safe for the long-term treatment of children. Because CHD does not usually develop until 30 years of age in male heterozygotes or until 40 years of age in female heterozygotes, treatment with lipid-lowering drugs or other drastic methods should not be required for the child heterozygotes and can instead be deferred until late adolescence.

Serum cholesterol levels in patients with FH-Tonami-2 were lower than those of classical FH patients [11]. The lower serum cholesterol levels and the slower development of coronary atherosclerosis in FH-Tonami-2 might be associated with their relative longevity [11]. This association was most prominent in the homozygotes. The LDL receptor activity was associated with the LDL cholesterol level and the age of onset of angina pectoris in classical homozygous patients, and the development of CHD in receptor-negative patients was faster than that in receptor-defective patients [1]. This indicates that residual receptor activity inversely correlated with the severity of the clinical picture. Therefore, FH-Tonami-2 patients, who possess high residual receptor activity, are likely to be the long-lived homozygotes.

References

1. Goldstein,J.L. and Brown,M.S.(1983)'Familial hypercholesterolemia', in J.B.Stunbury, J.B.Wyngaarden, D.S.Fredrickson, J.L.Goldstein and M.S.Brown (eds), The Metabolic Basis of Inherited Disease, ed 5, New York, McGraw-Hill Book Co, 1983, P672-712
2. Jensen,J., Blankenhorn,D.H. and Kornerup,V.(1967) 'Coronary disease in familial hypercholesterolemia', Circulation 36,77.
3. Stone,N.J., Levy,R.I., Fredrickson,D.S. and Verter,J.(1974) 'Coronary artery disease in 116 kindred with familial type II hyperlipoproteinemia', Circulation 49,476.
4. Mabuchi,H., Miyamoto,S., Ueda,K., Oota,M., Takegoshi,T., Wakasugi,T. and Takeda,R.(1986) 'Causes of death in patients with familial hypercholesterolemia', Atherosclerosis 61,1.
5. Mabuchi,H., Tatami,R., Haba,T., Ueda,K., Ueda,R., Kametani T., Itoh,S., Koizumi,J., Oota,S., Miyamoto,S., Takeda,R. and Takeshita,H. (1976) 'Homozygous familial hypercholesterolemia in Japan', Am J Med 65,290.
6. Heiberg,A.(1975)'The risk of atherosclerosis vascular disease in subjects with xanthomatosis', Acta Med Scand 198,249.
7. Beaumont,V., Jacotot,B. and Beaumont,J.L. (1976) 'Ischemic disease in men and women with familial hypercholesterolemia and xanthomatosis: A comparative study of genetic and environmental factors in 274

heterozygous cases', Atherosclerosis 24,441.
8. Kwiterowich,P.O.Jr., Bachorik,P.S., Franklin,F.A.Jr., Margolis,S., Georgopoulos,L., Teng,B. and Sniderman,A.D. (1985) 'Effect of dietary treatment and the plasma levels of lipids, lipoprotein cholesterol and LDL B protein in children with type II hyperlipoproteinemia: Detection and treatment of lipid and lipoprotein disorders in childhood', Prog Clin Biol Res 188,123.
9. Mabuchi,H., Koizumi,J., Shimizu,M., Takeda,R., and the Hokuriku FH-CHD Study Group (1989) 'Development of coronary heart disease in familial hypercholesterolemia', Circulation 79,225.
10. Russell,D.W., Esser, V. and Hobbs,H.H. (1989) 'Molecular basis of familial hypercholesterolemia' Arteriosclerosis Suppl I 9:I,8.
11. Kajinami,K., Fujita,H., Mabuchi,H., Uno,Y., Inazu,A., Itoh H., Koizumi,J., Takeda,R. and Oota M. 'Familial hypercholesterolemia with partial deletion in the ligand binding domain of low density lipoprotein receptor associated with mild hypercholesterolemia and normocholesterolemia: FH-Tonami-2, (Submitted for publication).
12. Mabuchi,H., Ito,S., Haba,T., Ueda,K., Ueda,R., Tatami,R., Kametani,T., Koizumi,J., Ohta,M., Miyamoto,S., Takeda,R. and Takegoshi,T. (1977) 'Discriminaton of familial hypercholesterolemia and secondary hypercholesterolemia by Achilles' tendon thickness',Atherosclerosis 28,61.
13. Tatami,R., Mabuchi,H., Ueda,K., Haba,T., Kametani,T., Ito,S., Koizumi,J., Ohta,M., Miyamoto,S., Nakayama,A., Kanaya,H., Oiwake,H., Genda,A. and Takeda,R. (1981) 'Intermediate-density lipoprotein and cholesterol-rich very low density lipoprotein in angiographically determined coronary artery disease',Circulation 64,1174.
14. Mabuchi,H., Kamon,N., Fujita,H., Michishita,I., Takeda,M., Kajinami,K., Itoh,H., Wakasugi,T. and Takeda,R. (1987) 'Effects of CS-514 on serum lipoprotein lipid and apolipoprotein levels in patients with familial hypercholesterolemia', Metabolism 36,475.
15. Kajinami,K., Mabuchi,H., Itoh,H., Michishita,I., Takeda,M., Wakasugi,T., Koizumi,J. and Takeda,R. (1988) 'New variant of low density lipoprotein receptor gene. FH-Tonami' Arteriosclerosis 8,187.
16. Kajinami K, Mabuchi,H., Inazu, A., Fujita,H., Koizumi,J., Takeda,R., Matsue,T. and Kibata,M (1989) 'Novel gene mutations at the low density lipoprotein receptor locus: FH-Kanazawa and FH-Okayama' J Internal Med (In press).
17. Thompson,G.R., Lowenthal,R, Myant,N.B. (1975) 'Plasma exchange in the management of homozygous familial hypercholesterolemia' Lancet 1,1208.
18. Mabuchi,H., Michishita,I., Takeda,M., Fujita,H., Koizumi,J., Takeda,R., Takada,S. and Oonishi,M. (1987) 'A new low density lipoprotein apheresis system using two dextran cellulose columns in an automated column regenerating unit (LDL continuous apheresis)' Atherosclerosis 68,19-25.
19. Bilheimer,D.W., Goldstein,J.L., Grundy,S.M., Starzl,T.E. and Brown,M.S. (1984) 'Liver transplantation to provide low-density lipoprotein receptors and lower plasma cholesterol in a child with homozygous familial hypercholesterolemia', N Engl J Med 311,1658.
20. Starzl,T.E., Chase,H.P., Ahrens,E.H.Jr., McNamara,D.J.,

Bilheimer,D.W., Schaefer,E.J., Rey,J., Porter,K.A., Stein,E., Francavilla,A. and Benson,L.N. (1983) ' Portacaval shunt in patients with familial hypercholesterolemia', Ann Surg 198,273.

21. Kwiterowich,P.O.Jr., Fredrickson,D.S. and Levy,R.I. (1974) 'Familial hypercholesterolemia (one form of familial type II hyperlipoproteinemia): A study of its biochemical, genetic, and clinical presentaton in childhood', J Clin Invest 53,1237.

22. Consensus conference: Lowering blood cholesterol to prevent heart disease', JAMA 253,2080.

9
Effect of genes on levels and variability of risk factors for coronary heart disease

K. BERG

Institute of Medical Genetics, University of Oslo, PO Box 1036 Blindern, 0315 Oslo 3, Norway

ABSTRACT. Present attempts to identify genes contributing to a person's predisposition or resistance to coronary heart disease (CHD) focus on "candidate genes" and traditional association tests have recently been supplemented with a more dynamic approach that takes risk factor variability into account. The new "variability gene" concept leads to the postulate that an individual's total genetic risk for CHD results from the person's combination of "level genes" and "variability genes".

Variability effects appear to be exerted on apolipoprotein B (apoB) and body mass index by the 3' part of the apoB gene. Recently discovered level gene as well as variability gene effects at the locus for cholesteryl ester transfer protein (CETP) suggest that more attention should be focused on "reverse cholesterol transport" in the study of CHD and its risk factors.

An important CHD risk factor that is not detected by traditional risk factor screening, is a high level of genetically determined Lp(a) lipoprotein. It should be analyzed in any diagnostic work-up in cases of CHD occurring prior to the age of 60-65 as well as in any risk factor screening of populations.

There is abundant evidence that specific genetic and environmental risk factors each contributes significantly to CHD risk and the study of interaction between genetic and environmental risk factors has started. Furthermore, the first example of gene - gene interaction influencing CHD risk factor levels has been uncovered: an interaction between normal genes at the low density lipoprotein receptor (LDLR) locus and genes at the apolipoprotein E (apoE) locus.

The already existing and forthcoming genetic knowledge should be utilized in risk profile assessment as a basis for a preventive strategy focusing on high risk individuals and families.

INTRODUCTION

It is well documented (for review, see Berg 1983, 1987a,b) that life style and nutritional factors as well as genetic factors contribute to the population variation in risk for coronary heart disease (CHD). Quantitative genetic analyses have shown that genes contribute significantly to the population variation in many risk or protective factors with respect to CHD, including total, low density lipoprotein (LDL), and high density lipoprotein (HDL) cholesterol, as well as apolipoproteins B (apoB), A-I (apoA-I), and A-II (apoA-II), and practically all the quantitative variation in the Lp(a) lipoprotein is genetically determined (Berg 1979; 1983; 1987a,b; 1989a,b).

Early attempts to identify genes responsible for risk factor variation made use of random genetic markers available at that time. Definite associations between genetic markers such as blood groups and serum types on the one hand, and overt disease or risk factor level on the other, were uncovered. These associations substantiated the findings in quantitative genetic studies of effects of genes on levels of risk factors or protective factors but in themselves provided little hope for a deeper insight into underlying molecular mechanisms.

CANDIDATE GENES FOR CORONARY HEART DISEASE

Present attempts to identify genes contributing to CHD risk focus on "candidate genes". With respect to CHD, a candidate gene could be any gene whose protein product is:

- involved in lipoprotein structure, lipoprotein metabolism or lipid metabolism
- involved in thrombogenesis, thrombolysis or fibrinolysis
- involved in regulation of blood flow in coronary arteries
- involved in regulation of blood pressure
- involved in reverse cholesterol transport
- present in atherosclerotic lesions
- involved in the regulation of growth of atherosclerotic lesions
- involved in the early development of coronary arteries.

Although the term "candidate gene" had not yet been coined, the candidate gene approach was in fact applied already in the early 1970ies. Direct association between the genetically determined Lp(a) lipoprotein (Berg 1963) and premature CHD was then demonstrated (Berg et al. 1974). This association has since been confirmed in many studies and a high Lp(a) lipoprotein level is today an established genetic risk factor for CHD.

In the mid-1970ies, association between lipid levels and the allotypic Ag variation of LDL was uncovered (Berg et al. 1976) and in the late 1970ies it was demonstrated that the apolipoprotein E (apoE) polymorphism is associated with cholesterol level in the general population (Utermann et al. 1979). Thus, lipid as well as disease associations were uncovered when the candidate gene approach was applied at the apolipoprotein level.

Lp(a) LIPOPROTEIN AND CORONARY HEART DISEASE

The association between overt CHD and genetically determined high level of Lp(a) lipoprotein which was discovered by workers in the Scandinavian countries (Berg et al. 1974, Dahlén et al. 1976, Frick et al. 1978) has been confirmed in a long series of studies (Brown and Goldstein 1987). The extensive study reported by Rhoads et al. (1986), in which quantity of Lp(a) lipoprotein was measured blindly in two different laboratories with excellent agreement between laboratories, is particularly informative. These workers calculated a population attributable risk of 28% for having myocardial infarction prior to age 60 in men with an Lp(a) lipoprotein level in the top quartile of the population distribution. The corresponding figure for males 60-69 years old was 13%. Durrington et al. (1988) in England reported that practically all familial clustering of early CHD cases in the absence of monogenic hyperlipidemia was attributable to a high level of this risk factor. Thus, a high Lp(a) lipoprotein level is an important risk factor for early CHD, in populations that are genetically and geographically well separated and that also have different life styles. Lp(a) lipoprotein does not exhibit strong association with any other relevant parameter and it must clearly be considered as an independent genetic risk factor for early CHD.

It was realized already in the very first studies that Lp(a) lipoprotein is a lipoprotein particle that very easily forms precipitates or aggregates, and Dahlén et al. (1978) showed that this will happen in vitro in the presence of glycosaminoglycans and also in the presence of calcium ions at near-physiological concentrations. This suggested that the reason for the association between Lp(a) lipoprotein and CHD is that this lipoprotein particle becomes easily trapped in the arterial wall. It was only after the recent cloning of cDNA representing the LPA gene (McLean et al. 1987) that alternative or additional mechanisms were suggested (Brown and Goldstein 1987). Total base sequence determination of cDNA representing the LPA gene revealed very extensive evolutionary homology with plasminogen, a much smaller protein of importance for thrombolysis/fibrinolysis in the body.

Harpel et al. (1989) observed affinity between Lp(a) lipoprotein and protease modified fibrinogen or fibrin. Hajjar et al. (1989) reported that Lp(a) lipoprotein modulates endothelial cell surface fibrinolysis. Miles et al. (1989) uncovered evidence of Lp(a) lipoprotein competition for plasminogen receptors by molecular mimicry. We found a correlation between Lp(a) lipoprotein level and fibrinogen concentration (Berg 1989a,b). It remains to be seen if these findings can help explain the association between Lp(a) lipoprotein and CHD.

We have conducted linkage analyses between the phenomenon that has been proven to be strongly associated with CHD: A high level of Lp(a) lipoprotein, and a restriction fragment length polymorphism (RFLP) in DNA at the plasminogen locus. For this purpose we selected families where a high level of Lp(a) lipoprotein segregated as a Mendelian trait from only one of the parents and where the same parent was heterozygous for the plasminogen RFLP (Berg 1989a,b). An update of our Lp(a) lipoprotein - plasminogen linkage data is given in Table 1.

TABLE 1. Lod scores for the Lp(a) lipoprotein - plasminogen relationship (adapted from Berg 1989b)

Segregation	Recombination fraction					
from	0.00	0.05	0.10	0.20	0.30	0.40
Males	2.71	2.34	1.97	1.25	0.62	0.17
Females	4.82	4.28	3.73	2.58	1.42	0.43
All	7.53	6.62	5.70	3.83	2.04	0.60

95% confidence limits of the recombination fraction, given linkage: 0.001-0.088

The lod score of 7.5 for recombination fraction zero is definite evidence of very close linkage between the LPA and plasminogen loci as well as for single-gene determination of Lp(a) lipoprotein levels. Although the two loci are close, the plasminogen polymorphism is not an adequate tool to study the genetics of Lp(a) lipoprotein because all genotypes within the plasminogen RFLP studied were found at all levels of genetically determined Lp(a) lipoprotein. The close linkage demonstrated is additional evidence for evolutionary relationship between plasminogen and Lp(a) lipoprotein. Others have examined this linkage relationship using either Lp(a) lipoprotein phenotypes as scored by double immunodiffusion (Weitkamp et al. 1988) or isoforms of the polypeptide chain carrying the Lp(a) antigen(s) (Drayna et al. 1988). Evidence of very close linkage between the two loci emerged also from these studies. The total body of evidence strongly suggests that all three phenomena, Lp(a) lipoprotein level, Lp(a) phenotype as scored by double immunodiffusion and isoforms of the polypeptide chain carrying the Lp(a) antigen(s), reflect variation at the same locus: the LPA locus. This must be on chromosome 6 (6q26-6q27), the area to which the plasminogen locus has been assigned.

The availability of DNA probes for the LPA gene makes it possible to search for DNA variation in this gene itself, although the extensive homology between plasminogen and Lp(a) lipoprotein causes difficulties. We have recently uncovered evidence for quantitative genetic variation at the LPA locus (Kondo and Berg 1989), which probably reflects varying numbers between individuals of kringle IV repeats. We have also evidence for a restriction site polymorphism at the LPA locus that appears to reside outside the kringle IV area, in the 3' part of the gene.

LEVEL GENES

Marker genes that exhibit a direct association with absolute risk factor levels may conveniently be referred to as "level genes". The Ag genes with their effect on cholesterol as well as triglyceride levels would belong to this category of genes. The same is the case with genes in the apoE polymorphism with their effect on total and LDL cholesterol levels.

The event of new DNA technology has significantly increased the possibilities for identifying level genes with respect to important CHD risk factors and interest has particularly focused on apolipoprotein genes. Law et al. (1986) found significantly lower cholesterol and triglyceride levels in people who lacked than in those who possessed a polymorphic XbaI restriction site at the apoB locus corresponding to residue 2,488 in the mature protein. This RFLP reflects a silent third base mutation which in itself could not cause structural differences between genetic types of the apolipoprotein. The effect of genes expressed as alleles in the XbaI polymorphism on absolute cholesterol and triglyceride levels has been confirmed (Berg 1986). This XbaI polymorphism is in strong allelic association (linkage disequilibrium) with the Ag(x) polymorphism, presence of the Ag(x) antigen being strongly associated with absence of the XbaI restriction site (Berg et al. 1986). Thus, the association between the Ag(x) and XbaI polymorphisms on one hand and between each polymorphism and lipid values on the other, are internally consistent. We have also found evidence of level gene effects at other candidate loci (Berg 1989c).

A word of caution is called for in the search for level gene effects. Some reported associations have proven to be difficult to reproduce. There are potentially many reasons for discrepancies. For example, type I errors have to be considered when many tests are conducted. More awareness of the potential sources of errors is needed (Berg 1989c,d).

VARIABILITY GENES

In addition to influencing absolute risk factor levels, genes could be of importance also by contributing to the frame within which nutritional, life style or other environmental factors can cause risk factor variation. Genes contributing to this frame may conveniently be referred to as "variability genes".

Several years ago, our group developed a method to detect variability genes, that does not require prolonged studies with environmental factors being controlled in a way that is very hard to achieve in man. This method is based on the fact that monozygotic (MZ) twins share all nuclear genes and that accordingly any difference in a quantitative parameter between the two members of an MZ pair must be caused by environmental factors. A restrictive variability gene would be expected to cause a lower mean within-pair difference in MZ twins having than in those lacking that gene, whereas a permissive variability gene should cause a greater within-pair difference (Berg 1981, 1984; Magnus et al. 1981). This method may be the best available to analyze gene - environment interactions.

Our early studies with a limited number of random markers were subsequently expanded to comprise 17 genetic marker systems and 5 quantitative lipid or apolipoprotein parameters (total cholesterol, fasting triglycerides, apoA-I level, apoA-II level and apoB level). Accordingly, a total of 85 analyses of variance were made and an outcome significant at the 5% level would therefore be expected to result from chance alone in approximately 4 of the analyses (or once if the level of significance was set at 1%). The total number of significant results was 10 (Berg 1984). This was more than expected by chance alone and it appeared likely that one or more of the results reflected true biological phenomena. We have recently reexamined the observation made in our first study of an effect of Kidd blood group genes on serum cholesterol variability. A new series of 142 MZ pairs, none of whom had been included in the first study, were examined. Again, we found a variability gene effect that was significant at the 2% level (Berg 1988). Our recent studies of DNA at apolipoprotein loci have uncovered evidence of variability gene effect on apoB at the apoB locus and also other suggestions of effects on risk factor variability, of candidate genes (Berg 1989c,d; Berg et al. 1989).

GENE - ENVIRONMENT INTERACTION

Early clinical studies suggested that variation in serum lipids may be even more significant than their absolute concentration in predicting the tendency to develop clinical evidence of CHD (Groover et al. 1960). It has been known for many years that strain differences in response to lipid intake exist in several animal species and such strain differences are almost certainly genetically determined (for review, see Berg 1979, 1989c). It has also been known that there are differences between humans in reaction to lipid intake but until recently this information was scarce. However, Katan and his coworkers have now convincingly demonstrated that hyporesponders and hyperresponders to lipid intake exist also in man and that these traits remain constant in an individual at least over several years (Beynen and Katan 1985, Katan et al. 1986, Katan and Beynen 1987). This makes it likely that hyporesponders and hyperresponders exist in man in a way similar to that in animals and that these phenotypes are genetically determined. This new knowledge underlines the need to develop more dynamic studies of CHD risk factors than traditional tests for association with absolute risk factor level.

In addition to the effect on apoB mentioned above, we have preliminary evidence of effect on body mass index variability of apoB genes probably caused by domains in the 3' part of the gene. This evidence agrees with the observation by Rajput-Williams et al. (1988) that certain haplotypes reflecting closely linked RFLPs at the apoB locus are associated with obesity and with findings in swine that LDL allotypes reflecting genetic apoB variation is associated with leanness or fatness (Dr. Jan Rapacz, personal communication).

If the variability gene concept is valid, it would follow that a person's total genetic risk to develop CHD most likely depends on his or her combination of level genes and variability genes (Table 2). This concept is eminently testable.

TABLE 2. Proposed, genetically determined, coronary heart disease risk resulting from the combination of genes affecting level and variability, respectively, of CHD risk factors (adapted from Berg 1989c)

Risk factor level specified by level genes	Total genetic risk if variability genes are permissive	restrictive
High	High, but reducible	Very high
Average	Average, but changeable	Average
Low	Low, but changeable	Very low

DNA VARIATION AT THE CHOLESTERYL ESTER TRANSFER PROTEIN (CETP) LOCUS AND CORONARY HEART DISEASE RISK FACTORS

Reverse cholesterol transport (Fielding and Fielding 1982) is the least understood part of lipid metabolism, but cholesteryl ester transfer protein (CETP) is believed to be a most important component of this lipid transport system. cDNA representing its locus has been cloned and RFLPs have been detected at the CETP locus (Drayna and Lawn 1987). This made it possible for us to examine DNA variants at the CETP locus with respect to level gene as well as variability gene effects. These studies uncovered a definite level gene effect on apoA-I as well as HDL cholesterol (Kondo et al. 1989) and also variability gene effect on total and LDL cholesterol (Berg et al. 1989). Although we can as yet not propose a mechanism by which one and the same gene (expressed as the 2-allele in this TaqI"B" RFLP) can at the same time cause high levels of apoA-I and HDL cholesterol and exert a restrictive effect on total and LDL cholesterol variability, the findings suggest the need to pay much more attention to genetic variation in components involved in reverse cholesterol transport, in the study of CHD risk factors.

GENE - GENE INTERACTION AND CORONARY HEART DISEASE RISK FACTORS

In the attempts to uncover the complex etiology of CHD, attention must also be paid to possible gene - gene interaction, in addition to effects of genes alone, environmental factors alone, or their interaction. Recent studies in our group have uncovered both an effect of normal genes at the LDLR locus on total and LDL cholesterol levels and an interaction between LDLR genes and apoE genes (Pedersen and Berg 1988; 1989). The first observation confirmed suggestions from our group made several years ago that normal alleles at the LDLR locus may contribute to the population variation in cholesterol (Maartmann-Moe et al. 1981).

When the people examined were grouped both according to genotype in the LDLR RFLP and with respect to presence or absence of the apoE4 gene (which is known to increase cholesterol level) it turned out that the well established effect of apoE4 was present only in homozygotes for absence of the polymorphic PvuII restriction site at the LDLR locus (Pedersen and Berg 1989). The effect of LDLR genes on cholesterol was only present in people possessing the apoE4 allele (Table 3). Apparently, presence of a normal gene, identified by

TABLE 3. Interaction between apolipoprotein E (apoE) alleles and normal alleles at the low density lipoprotein receptor (LDLR) locus expressed as a PvuII restriction site polymorphism, in determining age and sex adjusted total cholesterol (adapted from Pedersen & Berg 1989)

ApoE4 allele	Mean total cholesterol (mmol/l) In people with LDLR genotype A2A2	A1A1 or A1A2	In total series
Present	7.06* (n=31)	5.87 (n=15)	6.67 (n=46)
Absent	6.08* (n=69)	5.84 (n=41)	5.99 (n=110)

* t= 3.90, $p<0.001$

presence of the polymorphic PvuII restriction site (genotypes A1A1 and A1A2), totally eliminated the strong effect of the apoE4 allele on cholesterol level which is observed in population studies (Table 3).

The above observations were confirmed in a new and larger population sample and they are therefore likely to reflect true biological phenomena (Pedersen and Berg, in preparation).

USEFULNESS OF GENETIC INFORMATION

Genetic analyses at the molecular level may contribute significantly to the understanding of mechanisms underlying a disease, an understanding that is necessary for developing rational therapy. Genetic information may, however, be of great practical importance also before one arrives at an understanding of a disease at the molecular level. There is every reason to expect that knowledge of increased personal risk for premature CHD is a powerful message that will strongly motivate people to adhere to preventive measures. Thus, identification relatively early in life of people with a genetically determined, high risk to develop premature CHD should lead to intense preventive efforts in those who need it the most. A system of voluntary predictive genetic testing with respect to CHD risk should become part of the efforts to prevent CHD.

ACKNOWLEDGEMENTS

Work in the author's laboratory is supported by the Norwegian Council on Cardiovascular Disease, the Norwegian Research Council for Science and the Humanities, and Anders Jahres Foundation for the Promotion of Science.

REFERENCES

Berg, K. (1963) 'A new serum type system in man - the Lp system', Acta path. microbiol. scand. 59, 369-382.

Berg, K. (1979) 'Inherited lipoprotein variation and atherosclerotic disease', in A. M. Scanu, R. W. Wissler, and G. S. Getz (eds.), The Biochemistry of Atherosclerosis, Marcel Dekker, New York, pp. 419-490.

Berg, K. (1981) 'Twin research in coronary heart disease', in L. Gedda, P. Parisi, and W. E. Nance (eds.), Twin Research 3: Part C, Epidemiological and Clinical Studies, A. R. Liss, New York, pp. 117-130.

Berg, K. (1983) 'Genetics of coronary heart disease', in A. G. Steinberg, A. G. Bearn, A. G. Motulsky, and B. Childs (eds.), Progress in Medical Genetics, W.B. Saunders Co., Philadelphia, pp. 35-90

Berg, K. (1984) 'Twin studies of coronary heart disease and its risk factors', Acta Genet. Med. Gemellol. 33, 349-361.

Berg, K. (1986) 'DNA polymorphism at the apolipoprotein B locus is associated with lipoprotein level', Clin. Genet. 30, 515-520.

Berg, K. (1987a) 'Genetics of coronary heart disease and its risk factors', in G. Bock and G. M. Collins (eds.), Molecular Approaches to Human Polygenic Disease, Ciba Symposium 130, John Wiley & Sons, Chichester, pp. 14-33.

Berg, K. (1987b) 'Genetics of atherosclerosis', in A.G. Olsson (ed.), Atherosclerosis. Biology and Clinical Science, Churchill-Livingstone, Edinburgh, pp. 323-337.

Berg, K. (1988) 'Variability gene effect on cholesterol at the Kidd blood group locus', Clin. Genet. 33, 102-107.

Berg, K. (1989a) 'Lp(a) lipoprotein - an overview', in A. M. Scanu (ed.), Lipoprotein(a): 25 Years of Progress, Academic Press, New York, in press.

Berg, K. (1989b) 'Genetics of atherogenic Lp(a) lipoprotein', in K. Berg, N. Retterstøl, and S. Refsum (eds.), From Phenotype to Gene in Common Disorders, Munksgaard, Copenhagen, in press.

Berg, K. (1989c) 'Level genes and variability genes in the etiology of hyperlipidemia', in K. Berg, N. Retterstøl, and S. Refsum (eds.), From Phenotype to Gene in Common Disorders, Munksgaard, Copenhagen, in press.

Berg, K. (1989d) 'Molecular genetics and nutrition', in A. Simopoulos (ed.), Proceedings of the International Conference: Genetic Variation and Nutrition, Karger, Basel, in press.

Berg, K., G. Dahlén, and M. H. Frick (1974) 'Lp(a) lipoprotein and pre-ß1-lipoprotein in patients with coronary heart disease', Clin. Genet. 6, 230-235.

Berg, K., C. Hames, G. Dahlén, M. H. Frick, and I. Krishan (1976) 'Genetic variation in serum low-density lipoprotein and lipid levels in man', Proc. Natl. Acad. Sci. USA 73, 937-940.

Berg, K., L. M. Powell, S. C. Wallis, R. Pease, T. J. Knott, and J. Scott (1986) 'Genetic linkage between the antigenic group (Ag) variation and the apolipoprotein B gene: assignment of the Ag locus', Proc. Natl. Acad. Sci. USA 83, 7367-7370.

Berg, K., I. Kondo, D. Drayna, and R. Lawn (1989) '"Variability gene" effect of cholesteryl ester transfer protein (CETP) genes', Clin. Genet. 35, 437-445.

Beynen, A. C. and M. B. Katan (1985) 'Reproducibility of the variations between humans in the response of serum cholesterol to cessation of egg consumption', Atherosclerosis 57, 19-31.

Brown, M. S. and J. L. Goldstein (1987) 'Teaching old dogmas new tricks', Nature 330, 113-114.

Dahlén, G., K. Berg, and M. H. Frick (1976) 'Lp(a) lipoprotein/pre-$ß_1$-lipoprotein, serum lipids and atherosclerotic disease', Clin. Genet. 9, 558-566.

Dahlèn, G., C. Ericson, and K. Berg (1978) '*In vitro* studies of the interaction of isolated Lp(a) lipoprotein and other serum lipoproteins with glycosaminoglycans', Clin. Genet. 14, 36-42.

Drayna, D. T., R. A. Hegele, P. E. Hass, M. Emi, L. L. Wu, D. L. Eaton, R. M. Lawn, R. R. Williams, R. L. White, and J. -M. Lalouel (1988) 'Genetic linkage between lipoprotein(a) phenotype and a DNA polymorphism in the plasminogen gene', Genomics 3, 230-236.

Drayna, D. and R. Lawn (1987) 'Multiple RFLPs at the human cholesteryl ester transfer protein (CETP) locus', Nucl. Acids Res. 15, 4698.

Durrington, P.N., L. Hunt, M. Ishola, S. Arrol, and D. Bhatnagar (1988) 'Apolipoproteins (a), AI, and B and parental history in men with early onset ischaemic heart disease', Lancet i, 1070-1073.

Fielding, C. J. and P. E. Fielding (1982) 'Cholesterol transport between cells and body fluids. Role of plasma lipoproteins and the plasma cholesterol esterification system', Med. Clin. N. Am. 66, 363-373.

Frick, M. H., G. Dahlén, K. Berg, M. Valle, and P. Hekali (1978) 'Serum lipids in angiographically assessed coronary atherosclerosis', Chest 73, 62-65.

Groover, M. E, J. A. Jernigan, and C. D. Martin (1960) 'Variations in serum lipid concentration and clinical coronary disease', Amer. J. Med. Sci. 53, 133-139.

Hajjar, K.A., D. Gavish, J.L. Breslow, and R.L. Nachman (1989) 'Lipoprotein (a) modulation of endothelial cell surface fibrinolysis and its potential role in atherosclerosis', Nature 339, 303-305.

Harpel, P. C., B. R. Gordon, and T. S. Parker (1989) 'Plasmin catalyzes binding of lipoprotein (a) to immobilized fibrinogen and fibrin', Proc. Natl. Acad. Sci. USA 86, 3847-3851.

Katan, M.B. and A. C. Beynen (1987) 'Characteristics of human hypo- and hyperresponders to dietary cholesterol', Amer. J. Epidemiol. 125, 387-399.

Katan, M. B., A. C. Beynen, J. H. M. De Vries, and A. Nobels (1986) 'Existence of consistent hypo- and hyperresponders to dietary cholesterol in man', Amer. J. Epidemiol. 123, 221-234.

Kondo, I. and K. Berg (1989) 'Inherited quantitative DNA variation in the LPA ("apolipoprotein (a)") gene', Clin. Genet., in press.

Law, A., L. M. Powell, H. Brunt, T. J. Knott, D. G. Altman, J. Rajput, S. C. Wallis, R. J. Pease, L. M. Priestley, J. Scott, G. J. Miller, and N. E. Miller (1986) 'Common DNA polymorphism within the coding sequence of the apolipoprotein B gene associated with altered lipid levels', Lancet i, 1301-1303.

Maartmann-Moe, K., P. Magnus, W. Golden, and K. Berg (1981) 'Genetics of the low density lipoprotein receptor: III. Evidence for multiple normal alleles at the low density lipoprotein receptor locus', Clin. Genet. 20, 113-129.

Magnus, P., K. Berg, A.-L. Børresen, and W. E. Nance (1981) 'Apparent influence of marker genotypes on variation in serum cholesterol in monozygotic twins', Clin. Genet. 19, 67-70.

McLean, J. W., J. E. Tomlinson, W.-J. Kuang, D. L. Eaton, E. Y. Chen, G. M. Fless, A. M. Scanu, and R. M. Lawn (1987) 'cDNA sequence of human apolipoprotein (a) is homologous to plasminogen', Nature 330, 132-137.

Miles, L. A., G. M. Fless, E. G. Levin, A. M. Scanu, and E. F. Plow (1989) 'A potential basis for the thrombotic risks associated with lipoprotein (a)', Nature 339, 301-303.

Pedersen, J. C. and K. Berg (1988), 'Normal DNA polymorphism at the low density lipoprotein receptor (LDLR) locus associated with serum cholesterol level', Clin. Genet. 34, 306-312.

Pedersen, J. and K. Berg (1989), 'Interaction between low density lipoprotein receptor (LDLR) and apolipoprotein E (apoE) alleles contributes to normal variation in lipid level', Clin. Genet. 35, 331-337.

Rajput-Williams, J., S. C. Wallis, J. Yarnell, G. I. Bell, T. J. Knott, P. Sweetnam, N. Cox, N. E. Miller, and J. Scott (1988) 'Variation of apolipoprotein-B gene is associated with obesity, high blood cholesterol levels, and increased risk of coronary heart disease', Lancet ii, 1442-1446.

Rhoads, G.G., G. Dahlén, K. Berg, N. E. Morton and A.L. Dannenberg (1986) 'Lp(a) lipoprotein as a risk factor for myocardial infarction', JAMA 256, 2540-2544.

Utermann, G., N. Pruin, and A. Steinmetz (1979) 'Polymorphism of apolipoprotein E. III Effect of a single polymorphic gene locus on plasma lipid levels in man', Clin. Genet. 15, 63-72.

Weitkamp, L. R., S. A. Guttormsen, and J. S. Schultz (1988) 'Linkage between the loci for the Lp(a) lipoprotein (LP) and plasminogen (PLG)', Hum. Genet. 79, 80-82.

10
The type of mutation in apolipoprotein E determines whether type III hyperlipoproteinemia is expressed as a dominant or recessive trait

S.C. RALL, Jr., T.L. INNERARITY, K.H. WEISGRABER, M.R. WARDELL and R.W. MAHLEY

Gladstone Foundation Laboratories for Cardiovascular Disease, Cardiovascular Research Institute, University of California, San Francisco, PO Box 40608, San Francisco, CA 94140-0608, USA

ABSTRACT. We have developed a hypothesis to explain the association of the different binding-defective apolipoprotein E (apo-E) mutants with either the dominant or recessive mode of inheritance of type III hyperlipoproteinemia (type III HLP). The apo-E2(158 Arg → Cys) mutant is the only variant proven to be associated with recessive expression of type III HLP, and the only one for which modulation of receptor binding of the intact protein has been demonstrated. Thus, the ability of this mutant to assume either a receptor-binding-inactive or -active conformation is the key factor that determines recessive expression of type III HLP. In six other, rare apo-E variants the defective binding cannot be modulated, and we believe that this resistance to modulation causes dominant expression of type III HLP. Although recessive expression of type III HLP is much more common than dominant expression in the human population because of the much higher frequency of the apo-E2(158 Arg → Cys) allele, recessive expression may be the exception rather than the rule for the mode of inheritance of type III HLP because of the unique properties of the apo-E2(158 Arg → Cys) variant.

Characteristics of Type III Hyperlipoproteinemia

Type III hyperlipoproteinemia (type III HLP) is an important genetic disorder of lipid metabolism that affects as many as one in every one thousand individuals, primarily adults (1) (see Ref. 1 also for a more complete description of type III HLP). Subjects with type III HLP have both hypercholesterolemia and hypertriglyceridemia and are predisposed to premature development of atherosclerosis, particularly of the peripheral arteries. Xanthomas of the palmar creases are a distinctive clinical feature of this disorder. The primary molecular defect in type III HLP is a mutation(s) in apolipoprotein E (apo-E) that causes the mutant apo-E to bind defectively to lipoprotein receptors. This in turn causes impaired clearance of both intestinally derived chylomicron remnants and hepatically derived very low density lipoprotein (VLDL) remnants. These abnormal lipoproteins, termed collectively as β-VLDL, are cholesteryl ester- and apo-E-enriched and accumulate in the plasma, leading to the characteristic hyperlipidemia.

The vast majority of type III HLP subjects are homozygous for a particular mutant form of apo-E, apo-E2(158 Arg → Cys), which is one of three common genetically determined polymorphic forms of apo-E (2). Apolipoprotein E2(158 Arg → Cys) is defective in binding to lipoprotein receptors, whereas the two other polymorphs, apo-E3 and apo-E4, bind normally (3). Individuals who have only one allele for apo-E2(158 Arg → Cys) almost never develop type III HLP (4), suggesting that apo-E2(158 Arg → Cys) is associated with a recessive mode of inheritance of type III HLP. Furthermore, although about 1% of all individuals are homozygous for apo-E2(158 Arg → Cys), only a fraction of them ever become hyperlipidemic (type III HLP), even though all these homozygous E2/2 subjects demonstrate β-VLDL (primary dysbetalipoproteinemia). Thus, not only is type III HLP fundamentally a recessive trait, it also has a low degree of penetrance. Expression of the disorder requires other factors, environmental and/or genetic, a hypothesis put forth by Utermann a number of years ago to explain the various findings in type III HLP (5).

Rare Apolipoprotein E Variants and Mode of Inheritance of Type III Hyperlipoproteinemia

The discovery over the past several years of rare variants of apo-E that are associated with type III HLP has made it clear that the idea about the recessive mode of expression of type III HLP needs to be modified. More than a dozen naturally occurring rare variants of apo-E are now known (Fig. 1). Seven of these, in addition to apo-E2(158 Arg → Cys), have been found to be associated with type III HLP. These seven apo-E mutants all bind defectively to lipoprotein receptors *in vitro* (6). In fact, defective-binding apo-E variants are invariably associated with type III HLP. In contrast, the apo-E mutants that exhibit normal receptor binding are not associated with type III HLP.

It has been demonstrated that many of the defective-binding apo-E mutants are associated with dominant, rather than recessive, expression of type III HLP; *i.e.*, all individuals who are heterozygous for these functionally defective mutants have type III HLP. One exception is apo-E1(127 Gly → Asp, 158 Arg → Cys). This mutant is functionally identical to apo-E2(158 Arg → Cys) and also is associated with recessive expression of type III HLP, indicating that the mutation at residue 127 is functionally silent. The other six rare apo-E mutants and their association with type III HLP expression are summarized in Table 1. The apo-E2(146 Lys → Gln) mutant has been described in six unrelated probands, all of whom express normal apo-E3 as well as the variant apo-E (7, 8). Family studies have suggested that this mutant has a dominant mode of inheritance and a high degree of penetrance (8). The apo-E1-Harrisburg(146 Lys → Glu) variant has a different substitution at the same site. It has been described in a single family, in which the five affected subjects in three

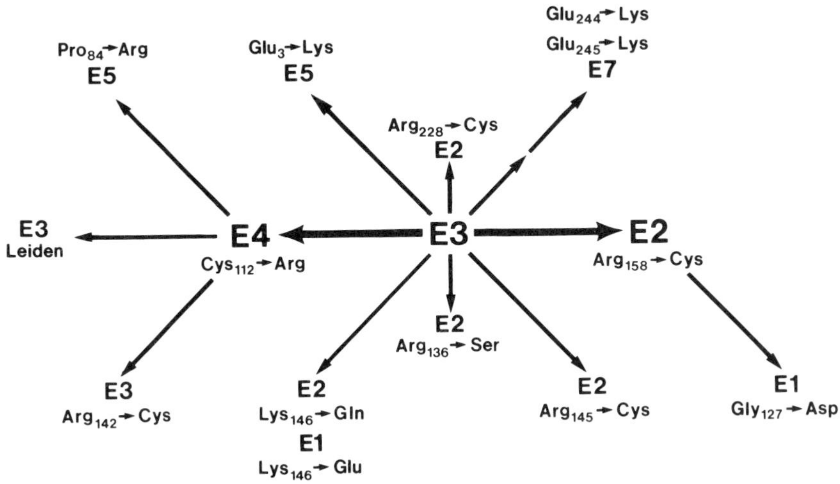

Figure 1. Naturally occurring variants of human apo-E. Each variant is defined relative to the most commonly occurring isoform, apo-E3. For each variant, the isoelectric focusing position and the amino acid substitution(s) are given. Apolipoprotein E3-Leiden has a seven-amino acid insertion that is a direct repeat of the preceding seven residues (121-127).

generations are all heterozygous (having normal apo-E as well as the variant), indicating a dominant mode of transmission (9). Four of the five affected subjects have type III HLP, and the fifth has dysbetalipoproteinemia without the hyperlipidemia. Other members of the kindred have neither the apo-E variant nor type III HLP. Similarly, the apo-E3(112 Cys → Arg, 142 Arg → Cys) variant has been described in a single family in which seven members (four generations) heterozygous for this variant all express type III HLP, including non-adults, while unaffected members do not have the apo-E variant (10). The apo-E3-Leiden variant (11) has an unusual mutation: near the receptor-binding region is an insertion of seven amino acids that are a tandem duplication of residues 121-127 (12, 13). This variant also contains the "E4-like" substitution, 112 Cys → Arg, and, like apo-E4, lacks cysteine. This variant has been shown by Havekes *et al.* (11, 13) to be associated with dominant transmission of type III HLP in at least three families.

In the cases of two other rare mutants associated with type III HLP, an assignment of dominant or recessive inheritance cannot be made on the basis of current knowledge. Four unrelated individuals with apo-E2(145 Arg → Cys) all have type III HLP (14, 15), but two of them are homozygous for this mutant apo-E, while two of them are heterozygous but have apo-E2(158 Arg → Cys) as the other apo-E gene product. Likewise, two subjects with type III HLP that are heterozygous for apo-E2-Christchurch(136 Arg → Ser) both have apo-E2(158 Arg → Cys) as well (15, 16). Because apo-E2(158 Arg → Cys) is itself associated with type III HLP, it is not pos-

TABLE 1. Apolipoprotein E variants and mode of expression of type III hyperlipoproteinemia

IEF[a]	Responsible Abnormality	Instances	Mode of Inheritance
E2	158 Arg→Cys	Many	Recessive
E2	146 Lys→Gln	6	Dominant
E1	146 Lys→Glu	1	Dominant
E3	142 Arg→Cys	1	Dominant
E3	7-amino acid insertion[b]	3	Dominant
E2	145 Arg→Cys	4	Unknown
E2	136 Arg→Ser	2	Unknown

[a] IEF, isoelectric focusing position.
[b] Apo-E3-Leiden, with seven-amino acid insertion that directly repeats the preceding seven residues (121-127).

sible to determine the individual effects of these other two mutants on the expression of the disorder. Also, the absence of family studies in these cases, the mode of inheritance of type III HLP cannot be determined.

Properties of Apolipoprotein E Mutants Responsible for Dominant versus Recessive Mode of Inheritance of Type III Hyperlipoproteinemia

The basic amino acids arginine and lysine have been shown to be crucial for the binding of apo-E to lipoprotein receptors, and it is thought that the basic amino acids in a predicted α-helical segment (residues 131-150) provide direct ionic interaction with acidic residues in the ligand-binding repeats of the low density lipoprotein (LDL) receptor (6). This ionic interaction provides the primary, if not total, force for the ligand–receptor binding. In five of the apo-E variants listed in Table 1, a neutral or acidic amino acid substitutes for a basic one in this putative α-helical segment. In contrast, the substitution in apo-E2(158 Arg → Cys) lies beyond this helical segment and occurs after a predicted β-turn (residues 151-154).

We hypothesize that any substitution of a neutral or acidic amino acid for a basic amino acid within the putative α-helical segment 131-150 affects the binding activity of apo-E by reducing the strength of the ionic interaction with the LDL receptor. Because the helix-forming potential of the 131-150 region is so strong, it is unlikely that single mutations could disrupt the conformation of the apo-E molecule. This reduced ionic bonding potential is unlikely to be influenced by other factors, essentially making the defect in receptor binding "permanent." As a result, the mode of inheritance of type III HLP would be dominant, requiring the expression of only one defective-binding apo-E allele product.

The mutation in apo-E2(158 Arg → Cys) not only lies outside the helical segment, but there is also evidence that its receptor-binding activity can be modulated *in vitro*. It has been shown that after certain chemical manipulations of this variant and its recombination into artificial phospholipid complexes, this mutant can demonstrate normal, or nearly normal, binding (17). For example, treatment of apo-E2(158 Arg → Cys) with cysteamine, a sulfhydryl reagent that converts cysteine residues into positively charged lysine analogues, increases the *in vitro* binding by more than an order of magnitude. The reversal of the cysteamine modification with β-mercaptoethanol, which eliminates the positive charge at residue 158, does not result in an immediate loss of the increased binding activity. This demonstrates that the positive charge at residue 158 is not directly involved in mediating the interaction of apo-E with the LDL receptor, but is instead important in obtaining the proper conformation of the binding region. In contrast, cysteamine treatment has no effect on the binding of the apo-E3(112 Cys → Arg, 142 Arg → Cys) mutant that is associated with dominant expression of type III HLP (10). This indicates that the arginine side chain at residue 142 is essential for normal binding and that positive charge alone is not a sufficient substitute for this residue.

A more dramatic demonstration of the capacity of the receptor binding of apo-E2(158 Arg → Cys) for modulation comes from a study of the lipoproteins from a type III subject homozygous for this variant (18). A comparison was made of the receptor-binding activities of native β-VLDL isolated before and after dietary treatment. Prior to dietary treatment, the subject's plasma cholesterol and triglyceride levels were 725 mg/dl (18.78 mmol/l) and 670 mg/dl (7.64 mmol/l), respectively. After adherence to a dietary regimen, the subject lost a significant amount of weight (15 kg) and his plasma cholesterol and triglyceride levels dropped dramatically, to 92 mg/dl (2.38 mmol/l) and 77 mg/dl (0.88 mmol/l), respectively. The β-VLDL isolated post-diet had significantly different chemical composition from the pre-diet β-VLDL, with a threefold lower cholesterol/triglyceride ratio; *i.e.*, the post-diet β-VLDL were not nearly so cholesterol-enriched. The results of the binding study of the β-VLDL are shown in Figure 2. The pre-diet β-VLDL behaved like the artificial apo-E phospholipid complexes, *i.e.*, they bound with low affinity and could be significantly activated with cysteamine. In contrast, the post-diet β-VLDL bound with 30-fold higher affinity (all the binding was shown to be due to apo-E) and were not significantly activated with cysteamine (Fig. 2). These results suggest that the conformation of apo-E2(158 Arg → Cys) is very sensitive to its environment (such as the lipid composition of the lipoprotein particle), and this conformational sensitivity is reflected in the change in receptor-binding activity. Because this modulation of receptor-binding activity can be demonstrated *in vitro*, we believe that it also occurs

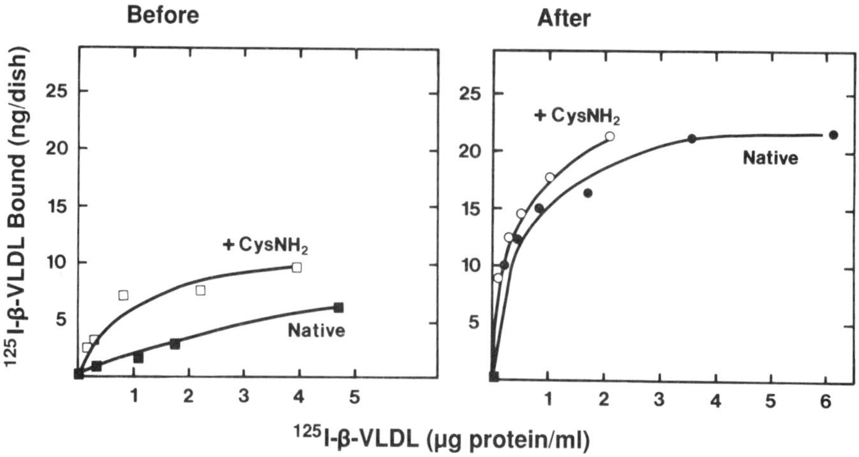

Figure 2. Receptor-binding activity of β-VLDL from a subject homozygous for apo-E2(158 Arg → Cys). Activity was measured in an *in vitro* assay using normal human fibroblasts. In the left panel is the activity of β-VLDL isolated from the subject when he was hyperlipidemic (before diet), without (native) or with (+CysNH$_2$) cysteamine treatment of the β-VLDL. In the right panel is the activity of β-VLDL isolated from the subject when he was hypolipidemic (after diet), without or with cysteamine treatment of the β-VLDL. (Modified, with permission, from Innerarity *et al.* (18)).

in vivo. This property is very likely to be the explanation for the recessive mode of inheritance of type III HLP in subjects homozygous for apo-E2(158 Arg → Cys) and also may explain the requirement for additional environmental and/or genetic factors for expression of the disorder. We hypothesize that in subjects heterozygous for apo-E2(158 Arg → Cys), *e.g.*, E3/2 subjects, and in homozygous subjects (E2/2) who are not hyperlipidemic, the receptor-binding activity of apo-E2(158 Arg → Cys) on β-VLDL is nearly normal and allows for enough catabolism of these particles so that hyperlipidemia is avoided. When exacerbating factors are present, the β-VLDL receptor-binding activity decreases, leading to their accumulation in the plasma and resulting in severe hyperlipidemia.

The apo-E3-Leiden variant, which is associated with dominant expression of type III HLP, has an interesting property that may or may not be paradoxical. The intact apo-E3-Leiden mutant exhibits defective binding *in vitro*, but when the carboxy-terminal structural domain is removed enzymatically, the amino-terminal structural domain (which contains the seven-amino acid insertion near the receptor-binding region) has almost normal receptor-binding activity (12). This increase in binding upon removal of the carboxy-terminal domain also occurs with apo-E2(158 Arg → Cys) and is another piece of evidence that there is a conformational disruption in that mutant (17). However, we believe that the conformational disruption and subsequent defective receptor binding of intact apo-E3-Leiden are probably "permanent" *in vivo* as a result of the seven additional amino acids causing an aberrant interaction with the carboxy-terminal domain, leading to dominant expression of type III HLP.

REFERENCES

1. Mahley, R. W., and Rall, Jr., S. C. 1989. Type III hyperlipoproteinemia (dysbetalipoproteinemia): the role of apolipoprotein E in normal and abnormal lipoprotein metabolism, in C. R. Scriver, A. L. Beaudet, W. S. Sly, and D. Valle (eds.), The Metabolic Basis of Inherited Disease, 6th Edition, McGraw-Hill, New York, pp. 1195-1213.
2. Utermann, G., Hees, M., and Steinmetz, A. 1977. Polymorphism of apolipoprotein E and occurrence of dysbetalipoproteinaemia in man. *Nature* 269:604-607.
3. Weisgraber, K. H., Innerarity, T. L., and Mahley, R. W. 1982. Abnormal lipoprotein receptor-binding activity of the human E apoprotein due to cysteine-arginine interchange at a single site. *J. Biol. Chem.* 257:2518-2521.
4. Utermann, G., Vogelberg, K. H., Steinmetz, A., Schoenborn, W., Pruin, N., Jaeschke, M., Hees, M., and Canzler, H. 1979. Polymorphism of apolipoprotein E. II. Genetics of hyperlipoproteinemia type III. *Clin. Genet.* 15:37-62.
5. Utermann, G. 1985. Genetic polymorphism of apolipoprotein E. Impact on plasma lipoprotein metabolism, G. Crepaldi, A. Tiengo, and G. Baggio (eds.), Diabetes, Obesity and Hyperlipidemias - III, Elsevier Science Publishers, Amsterdam, pp. 1-28.
6. Mahley, R. W. 1988. Apolipoprotein E: cholesterol transport protein with expanding role in cell biology. *Science* 240:622-630.
7. Rall, Jr., S. C., Weisgraber, K. H., Innerarity, T. L., Bersot, T. P., Mahley, R. W., and Blum, C. B. 1983. Identification of a new structural variant of human apolipoprotein E, E2($Lys_{146} \rightarrow Gln$), in a type III hyperlipoproteinemic subject with the E3/2 phenotype. *J. Clin. Invest.* 72:1288-1297.
8. Smit, M., de Knijff, P., van der Kooij-Meijs, E., Groenendijk, C., van den Maagdenberg, A. M. J. M., Gevers Leuven, J. A., Stalenhoef, A. F. H., Stuyt, P. M. J., Frants, R. R., and Havekes, L. M. 1990. Genetic heterogeneity in familial dysbetalipoproteinemia. The E2(lys146→gln) variant results in a dominant mode of inheritance. *J. Lipid Res.* 31:45-53.
9. Mann, W. A., Gregg, R. E., Sprecher, D. L., and Brewer Jr, H. B. 1989. Apolipoprotein E-$1_{Harrisburg}$: a new variant of apolipoprotein E dominantly associated with type III hyperlipoproteinemia. *Biochim. Biophys. Acta*

1005:239-244.

10. Rall, Jr., S. C., Newhouse, Y. M., Clarke, H. R. G., Weisgraber, K. H., McCarthy, B. J., Mahley, R. W., and Bersot, T. P. 1989. Type III hyperlipoproteinemia associated with apolipoprotein E phenotype E3/3: structure and genetics of an apolipoprotein E3 variant. *J. Clin. Invest.* 83:1095-1101.
11. Havekes, L., de Wit, E., Gevers Leuven, J., Klase, E., Utermann, G., Weber, W., and Beisiegel, U. 1986. Apolipoprotein E3-Leiden. A new variant of human apolipoprotein E associated with familial type III hyperlipoproteinemia. *Hum. Genet.* 73:157-163.
12. Wardell, M. R., Weisgraber, K. H., Havekes, L. M., and Rall, Jr., S. C. 1989. Apolipoprotein E3-Leiden contains a seven-amino acid insertion that is a tandem repeat of residues 121 to 127. *J. Biol. Chem.* 264:21205-21210.
13. van den Maagdenberg, A. M. J. M., de Knijff, P., Stalenhoef, A. F. H., Gevers Leuven, J. A., Havekes, L. M., and Frants, R. R. 1989. Apolipoprotein E*3-Leiden allele results from a partial gene duplication in exon 4. *Biochem. Biophys. Res. Commun.* 165:851-857.
14. Rall, Jr., S. C., Weisgraber, K. H., Innerarity, T. L., and Mahley, R. W. 1982. Structural basis for receptor binding heterogeneity of apolipoprotein E from type III hyperlipoproteinemic subjects. *Proc. Natl. Acad. Sci. USA* 79:4696-4700.
15. Emi, M., Wu, L. L., Robertson, M. A., Myers, R. L., Hegele, R. A., Williams, R. R., White, R., and Lalouel, J. M. 1988. Genotyping and sequence analysis of apolipoprotein E isoforms. *Genomics* 3:373-379.
16. Wardell, M. R., Brennan, S. O., Janus, E. D., Fraser, R., and Carrell, R. W. 1987. Apolipoprotein E2-Christchurch (136 Arg → Ser). New variant of human apolipoprotein E in a patient with type III hyperlipoproteinemia. *J. Clin. Invest.* 80:483-490.
17. Innerarity, T. L., Weisgraber, K. H., Arnold, K. S., Rall, Jr., S. C., and Mahley, R. W. 1984. Normalization of receptor binding of apolipoprotein E2. Evidence for modulation of the binding site conformation. *J. Biol. Chem.* 259:7261-7267.
18. Innerarity, T. L., Hui, D. Y., Bersot, T. P., Mahley, R. W. Type III hyperlipoproteinemia: a focus on lipoprotein receptor-apolipoprotein E2 interactions, A. Angel and J. Frolich (eds.), Lipoprotein Deficiency Syndromes, Plenum Publishing Co., New York, pp. 273-288.

THE VEGETATIVE NERVOUS SYSTEM AND CARDIOVASCULAR DISEASE

11
The sympatho-vagal balance and arterial hypertension

A. MALLIANI

Instituto Ricerche Cardiovascolari, Centro Ricerche Cardiovascolari, CNR; Ospedale "L. Sacco", "Centro Fidia", Patologia Medica, Università Milano, via Bonfadini 214, 20138 Milano, Italy

The view of arterial hypertension as an abnormal "quantity" is the well known milestone introduced by Pickering (1) in modern pathophysiological thinking. This provocative hypothesis opened the door to the search for factors capable of explaining the "continuum" between normal and abnormal values. Alterations in neural regulatory activities could be one of these factors (2-4), if not the prevailing one, at least in the early phases of this disorder of regulation. Along this line of reasoning, attention was focused on the sympathetic tone and on the direct or indirect signs of its possible enhanced level (2-4).

The evaluation of the sympathetic tone in the frequency domain.

The possibility recently offered by computer techniques of quantifying the small spontaneous beat by beat oscillations present in cardiovascular variables and in particular in the electrocardiographic R-R interval aroused a growing interest in view of the hypothesis that these rhythmical oscillations could provide some insight into neural regulatory mechanisms operating in the intact organism under various real life conditions.

Indeed, the application of computationally efficient spectral techniques (5) offered the opportunity of assessing specifically the non random components of heart rate variability thus quantifying the possible different rhythms hidden in the signal. Sayers (6), for instance, employing the Fast Fourier Transform technique reported the existence in humans of three major components in R-R variability that he observed in specific bands of predetermined frequencies around 0.25, 0.10, 0.03 Hz respectively: i.e. a component related to respiration (0.25 Hz) and two others at lower frequencies. Following this pioneering work several other investigators applied this technique and, in spite of the fact that the heart rate variability signal is not strictly periodical, as requested by the deterministic nature of the FFT algorithm, it became clear that it could be used as a quantitative probe to assess heart rate fluctuations (7).

METHODS According to the methodology used in our laboratory (8-12) two major components are recognized in either heart rate or arterial pressure beat by beat variabilities: one synchronous with respiration and indicated as high frequency (HF) and one at a low frequency (LF) of about 0.1 Hz. From sections of tachogram of 512 or less successive R-R intervals the computer automatically calculates the model. i.e. the autoregressive coefficients, that provide the best statistical estimate of the spectral distribution (see the Appendix in ref 9). Each spectral component is presented in absolute units as well as in normalized form (in order to facilitate comparisons between spectra with large differences in total power): normalized data (9) are calculated by dividing the power of each spectral component by total variance (i.e. total power) minus the very low frequency DC component, when present.

It should be pointed out that in order to properly apply spectral analysis to cardiovascular variables, the series must be stationary, a fact that can be assessed with appropriate procedures. As a corollary, the very slow oscillations, i.e. those with a frequency of less than 0.02-0.03 Hz, which may contain significant physiological information and that on short time recordings appear as slow trends, cannot be properly assessed with this methodology, but require different algorithms (13).

A recent development of the methodology refers to the possibility of analyzing long periods of analog recordings, by using a recursive version (12,14) of the program of spectral analysis. For instance, Holter tapes can furnish a quantitative assessment of R-R or SAP variability throughout the 24 h period of the recording (14).

RESULTS With this approach we have explored the possibility of obtaining markers of the sympatho-vagal interaction conceived as a simple push-pull or balance. Partly on the basis of the literature and partly as our hypothesis, we propose that a broad appraisal of the state of this balance can be based on the following elements:

a) heart rate variability.

i) Total variance, i.e. total power: it is commonly accepted as an indicator of vagal "tone" (15). In our opinion, it is a rather indirect indicator of vagal tone as it can remain unchanged when the balance is shifted towards sympathetic predominance (16). Thus, it seems rather to reflect both vagal and sympathetic modulations.

ii) HF component: is generally accepted as a marker of vagal activity (7,9,17).

iii) LF component: we proposed it as a marker of sympathetic activity (9,12,14,16,18,19). The LF/HF ratio would obviously further emphasize the concept of balance (9).

b) arterial pressure variability

iv) LF component (Mayer waves, [20]) seems to represent a good marker of the sympathetic activity impinging upon arterial smooth muscle tone (9,12,14,16,18,19).

The methodological soundness of this simple attributitive stage has been checked through a variety of experimental and clinical states. In human studies, LF component of both heart rate and arterial pressure variabilities was increased with tilt (8,9), mental stress, moderate physical exercise (12,21). In experimental studies, LF component was increased by moderate hypotension (9,19), coronary artery occlusion

(19), carotid artery occlusion and physical exercise.

Conversely, the HF component of heart rate variability was increased by controlled respiration (9). The HF component of arterial pressure, being largely influenced by mechanical changes induced by respiration, cannot be considered a marker of vagal activity.

As to the pathophysiological conditions that we have examined, this article will only briefly summarize the results concerning patients with arterial essential hypertension.

R-R Variability in hypertensive patients

Under the hypothesis that an increased sympathetic activity has a pathogenetic role in this abnormal "quantity" (1), we studied (18) the heart rate variability in a population of hypertensive subjects with a diastolic blood pressure consistently above 95 mmHg. When comparing hypertensives with normotensive age matched controls, it was found that LF was greater (LF:68±3 versus 54±3 n.u.) and HF smaller (HF:24±3 versus 33±2 n.u.) in hypertensive patients, hence suggesting an enhanced sympathetic and a reduced vagal activity. Additionally, passive tilt produced in hypertensive patients smaller increases in LF (LF: 6.3±3 versus 26±2) and decreases in HF (HF: -7.5±2 versus -22±2) than in the normotensive controls. Furthermore, the values of LF at rest and the altered effects of tilt on LF and HF were significantly correlated with the degree of the hypertensive state. In short, Pickering's concept of continuum would be supported by the continuum that we found from normotension to hypertension in the markers of sympathetic activity.

After chronic ß-adrenergic receptor blockade (100 mg of atenolol, given orally, once daily for 2 weeks), we observed in hypertensive patients a reduction in heart rate (from 74±3 to 56±2 beat/min) and in diastolic arterial pressure (from 103±3 to 88±2 mmHg). During ß-blockade the R-R interval variance augmented, at rest, on average but with a wide dispersal among the single subjects so that the increase was not significant. Viceversa, marked changes were observed in autospectra of R-R variability at rest: LF was significantly reduced to 50±5 n.u. and HF increased to 39±5 n.u. These values were similar to those observed in the control population. With tilt, LF increased to a value (68±6 n.u.) which was smaller than that observed before treatment (77±4 n.u.) in the same subjects. On the contrary, HF decreased to a value (22±5 n.u.) which was greater than that observed before treatment (13±2 n.u.). In normal subjects as well, after chronic ß-adrenergic receptor blockade, the values of LF were significantly reduced in respect to control conditions both at rest and during tilt (9).

Simultaneous evaluation of heart rate and arterial pressure variabilities

In our protocol for suspected hypertension at times we include a continuous ambulatory direct high fidelity recording of arterial pressure and ECG (22).

A dynamic analysis of the complex instantaneous relationship between heart rate and arterial pressure can be attempted (23). Usually the slope of the linear regression of the heart period, as a function of systolic arterial pressure plotted during the rise produced by the i.v.

injection of a pressor agent like phenylephrine, is taken as a measure of the gain of the baroreflex control of heart rate (24). This model however, does not take into account that changes in heart period can also induce changes in systolic arterial pressure, such as those related to variations in stroke volume and hence in systolic arterial pressure, which accompany beat-to-beat changes in heart period.

For these reasons we used (12) a closed loop model for the analysis of the relationship between the beat-to-beat variability of R-R and SAP. An important consequence of this model is that it provides a way of computing by spectral and cross-spectral analysis of spontaneous variabilities an index (called α) of the overall gain of this neural interaction . This index (α) is usually computed both in correspondence of LF and HF components, provided the coherence function between R-R and SAP variabilities is high (i.e. >0.50) (for more details see 12). We have proven that this approach furnishes, both at rest and during physical exercise, clinical results comparable to those obtained with the phenylephrine method (24).

By applying this approach in a group of mild hypertensive patients we observed an increase in the gain after physical training. In a second group of normotensive (n=9; systolic arterial pressure 133±3 mmHg) and hypertensive (n=9; systolic arterial pressure 177±9 mmHg) subjects undergoing 24 hour diagnostic continuous recording of ECG and high fidelity arterial pressure monitoring, the index α was significantly reduced in the hypertensive group at rest (α_{LF}=4±1 vs 10±2 msec/mmHg).

Furthermore, this methodology allowed us to describe the behavior of the gain of the heart period - arterial pressure relationship throughout the 24h period: such gain undergoes large changes during the 24h recording period, being higher during the night and lower during the day.

CONCLUDING REMARKS This approach in the frequency domain seems to provide a reliable tool to investigate the state of the sympatho-vagal balance both in the so-called resting conditions (9) and through the continuous changes which occur during the whole day (9,14). When this tool is employed in the evaluation of patients with primary arterial hypertension the conclusion seems inescapable of a higher than normal sympathetic tone.

BIBLIOGRAPHY

1) Pickering G: The nature of essential hypertension. London, Churchill-Livingstone. 1961
2) Julius S: Role of the autonomic nervous system in mild human hypertension. Am Heart J 1975;48:243s-252s
3) Folkow B: Physiological aspects of primary hypertension. Physiological Reviews 1982;62:347-504
4) Malliani A, M. Pagani, F. Lombardi: Positive feedback reflexes. In Handbook of Hypertension, vol 8 Pathophysiology of Hypertension. Zanchetti A, Tarazi RC eds. Amsterdam Elsevier 1986 pp69-81
5) Cooley, J.W. and J.W. Tukey: An algorithm for the machine calculation of complex Fourier Series. Math. Comput. 1965,19:297-301
6 Sayers, B. McA: Analysis of heart rate variability. Ergonomics

1973,16:17-32

7) Akselrod, S., D. Gordon, F.A. Ubel, D.C. Shannon, A.C. Barger and R.J. Cohen: Power spectrum analysis of heart rate fluctuation: A quantitative probe of beat-to-beat cardiovascular control. Science 1981,213:220-222.

8) Brovelli M, G. Baselli, S Cerutti, S Guzzetti, D Liberati, F Lombardi, A Malliani, M Pagani, P Pizzinelli: Computerized analysis for an experimental validation of neurophysiological models of heart rate control. Comps in Cardiol IEEE, Computer Society, Aachen 1983 pp205-208.

9) Pagani, M., F. Lombardi, S. Guzzetti, O. Rimoldi, R. Furlan, P. Pizzinelli, G. Sandrone, G. Malfatto, S. Dell'Orto, E. Piccaluga, M. Turiel, G. Baselli, S. Cerutti and A. Malliani: Power spectral analysis of heart rate and arterial pressure variabilities as a marker of sympatho-vagal interaction in man and conscious dog. Circ. Res. 1986,59:178-193

10) Cerutti, S., G. Baselli, S. Civardi, R. Furlan, F. Lombardi, A. Malliani, M. Merri and M. Pagani: Spectral analysis of heart rate and arterial blood pressure variability signals for physiological and clinical purposes. Computers in Cardiology, IEEE Computer Society Press, Washington D.C. 1987 pp 435-438

11) Baselli, G., S. Cerutti, S. Civardi, A. Malliani, M. Pagani: Cardiovascular variability signals: Towards the identification of a closed-loop model of the neural control mechanisms. IEEE Transactions on Biomed Eng. 1988,35:1033-1046.

12) Pagani, M., V. Somers, R. Furlan, S. Dell'Orto, J. Conway, G. Baselli, S. Cerutti, P. Sleight, And A. Malliani: Changes in autonomic regulation induced by physical training in mild hypertension. Hypertension 1988,12:600-610

13) Saul J.P., P. Albrecht, R.D. Berger, R.J. Cohen: Analysis of long term heart rate variability: methods, 1/f scaling and implications. Computers in Cardiology, IEEE Computer Society Press Washington D.C. 1988 pp419-422

14) Furlan R, S. Guzzetti, W Crivellaro, S Dassi, M Tinelli, G Baselli, S Cerutti, F Lombardi, M Pagani, A Malliani: Continuous 24 h assessment of the neural regulation of systemic arterial pressure and R-R variabilities in ambulant subjects. Circulation (in press)

15) Fouad FM, RC Tarazi, CM Ferrario, S Fighaly, C Alicandri: Assessment of parasympathetic control of heart rate by a non-invasive method. Am J Physiol 1984,246:H838-H842

16) Lombardi, F., G. Sandrone, S. Pernpruner, R. Sala, M. Garimoldi, S. Cerutti, G. Baselli, M. Pagani and A. Malliani: Heart rate variability as an index of sympathovagal interaction after acute myocardial infarction. Am. J. Cardiol. 1987,60:1239-1245.

17) Pomeranz, P., R.J.B. Macaulay, M.A. Caudil, I. Kutz, D. Adam, D. Gordon, K.M. Kilborn, A.C. Barger, D.C. Shannon, R.J. Cohen and H. Benson: Assessment of autonomic function in humans by heart rate spectral analysis. Am. J. Physiol. 1985,248:H151-H153.

18) Guzzetti, S., E. Piccaluga, R. Casati, S. Cerutti, F. Lombardi, M. Pagani and A. Malliani: Sympathetic predominance in essential hypertension: a study employing spectral analysis of heart rate

variability. J. Hypert. 1988,6:711-717

19) Rimoldi, O, S Pierini, A Ferrari, S Cerutti, M Pagani, A Malliani: Analysis of the short term oscillations of R-R and arterial pressure in conscious dogs. Am J Physiol (in press)

20) Mayer, S: Studien zur Physiologie des Herzens und der Blutgefässe: 5. Abhandlung: Über spontane Blutdruckschwankungen. Sber. Akad. Wiss. Wien, 3. Abt., 1876,74:281-307.

21) Furlan, R., S. Dell'Orto, W. Crivellaro, P. Pizzinelli, S. Cerutti, F. Lombardi, M. Pagani, A. Malliani: Effects of tilt and treadmill exercise on short-term variability in systolic arterial pressure in hypertensive men. J. Hypert. 1987,5:S423-S425

22) Pagani, M., R. Furlan, S. Dell'Orto, P. Pizzinelli, G. Lanzi, G. Baselli, C. Santoli, S. Cerutti, F. Lombardi and A. Malliani: Continuous recording of direct high fidelity arterial pressure and electrocardiogram in ambulant patients. Cardiovasc. Res. 1986,20:384-388

23) De Boer, R.W., J.M. Karemaker and J. Strackee: Hemodynamic fluctuations and baroreflex sensitivity in humans: a beat-to-beat model. Am. J. Physiol. 1987,253:H680-H689.

24) Smyth, H.S., P. Sleight and G.W. Pickering: Reflex regulation of arterial pressure during sleep in man. Circ. Res. 1969,24:109-121.

12
The autonomic disturbance accompanying myocardial infarction

F. LOMBARDI, G. SANDRONE, R. SALA, S. CERUTTI and A. MALLIANI

Istituto Ricerche Cardiovascolari, CNR; Patologia Medica, Centro "Fidia", Ospedale "L. Sacco", Università di Milano, via Bonfadini 214, 20138 Milano, Italy

ABSTRACT To evalauate the alteration of sympatho-vagal balance after myocardial infarction we compared the spectral components of heart variability of 70 patients at 2 weeks, 6 and 12 months after myocardial infarction with 26 age matched control subjects. Spectral analysis of heart rate variability was characterized in control subjects by two major components at low (LF,~0.10 Hz) and high (HF,~0.25 Hz) frequency. According to several clinical and experimental observations they can be considered appropriate indices of, respectively sympathetic and vagal neural activities directed to the heart and their ratio an indirect measure of sympatho-vagal balance. In patients at 2 weeks after myocardial infarction there was a significant increase in LF (69±2 versus 53±3 nu) and LF/HF ratio (8±1.1 versus 2±0.3) as well as a diminished HF (17±1 versus 35±3 nu) thus indicating an increased sympathetic and a reduced parasympathetic tone. At 6 and 12 months after myocardial infarction we observed a progressive reduction of LF and LF/HF ratio as well as an increase in HF which suggested a normalization of sympatho-vagal interaction.

INTRODUCTION. The clinical management of patients after myocardial infarction has been profoundly influenced by the result of several clinical trials (1-3) that have shown the beneficial and protective effects of beta adrenergic receptor blockade. Even if the understanding of the mechanisms of action of these drugs are still incomplete, then beneficial and protective effects are further proof of the importance of adrenergic mechanisms in determining the prognosis of patients after myocardial infarction. Regarding this it is important to mention that more than 20 years ago the group of Pantridge (4) by analyzing the heart rate and systolic arterial pressure of patients within 60 minutes from the onset of chest pain, was able to detect signs of autonomic inbalance in more than 60% of the patients with an acute myocardial infarction. According to the presence of sinus tachycardia and hypertension signs of sympathetic overactivity were found more frequently in patients with an anterior myocardial infarction, while bradycardia and hypotension i.e. signs of parasympathetic activation were more frequently observed with an inferior myocardial infarction.

These preliminary observations were however, followed by a limited number of investigations with the objective of assessing the autonomic changes in patients after a myocardial infarction as a consequence of both the growing diffusion of early pharmacological or invasive interventions to reduce infarct size and the awareness of the limits of the techniques available for clinical assessment of sympathetic and vagal tone. Moreover, even if the elevated concentration of plasma catecholamines suggested the existence of an elevated adrenergic tone it was quite evident that the absolute values of heart rate and of arterial blood pressure were parameters inadequate to characterize an autonomic tone.

Recently however, attention has been focused not only on the responses of heart rate but on its variability and, in particular, it has been demonstrated that the power spectral analysis of heart rate variability can provide adequate information on sympatho-vagal interaction in different clinical conditions (5-7). Therefore, we applied this non-invasive approach to the study of heart rate variability in patients at 2 weeks 6 weeks and 12 months after the first myocardial infarction (8).

METHODS. We studied 70 patients discharged from the Coronary Care Unit of our hospital with the clinical electrocardiographic and enzymatic diagnosis of myocardial infarction. The group included 63 men and 7 women with a mean age of 54±2 years. The localization of myocardial infarction was anterior in 33 and posterior in 37 of the patients non Q wave infartion was present in 16 of 70 subjects.

All subjects were placed on an electrically driven tilt table connected to a conventional electrocardiographic amplifier and FM tape recorder for 30 minutes during resting conditions. The effects of sympathetic stimulation induced by 90° head up tilt was assessed in 24 patients at 2 weeks and 1 year after myocardial infarction. Off-line analysis was performed on a PDP11/24 minicomputer. Electrocardiographic data were played back from the FM tape, digitized at 300 samples/sec and processed as previously reported (7,8). After selection of stationary sections of data, the computer program computed the interval tachogram, simple statistics (mean and variance), and then the autoregressive coefficients necessary to define the power spectral density estimate. The power and frequency of every spectral component is calculated in absolute as well as in normalized units. The latter are obtained by dividing the power of each component by the total variance less the direct current component.

RESULTS. The variance of the R-R interval of the whole group of patients at two weeks after myocardial infarction was only slightly reduced in comparison to control subjects, however it was significantly diminished (323±68 versus 111+100 $msec^2$) in 9 patients who had signs and symptoms of heart failure at the time of the study and was even more markedly reduced (231±63 $msec^2$) in 3 patients who died during the first 3 months of observation (Fig. 1). Spectral analysis of heart rate variability (Fig 2) revealed a predominant low frequency (LF: 69±2 nu) and a reduced high frequency (HF: 17±1 nu) respiration related component with a marked increase of the LF/HF ratio (8±1.1). All values were significantly different from those observed in the control group (LF 53±3 nu;, HF 35±3 nu; LF/HF 2±0.3). In patients at 2 weeks after myocardial infarction, in addition, tilt did not modify the already predominant low frequency component (Fig 2). At 6 and 12 months after myocardial infarction (Fig 3) there was a progressive reduction of LF (62±2 and 54±3 nu) and an increase of HF component (23±2 and 30±2) with the consequent normalization of LF/HF ratio.

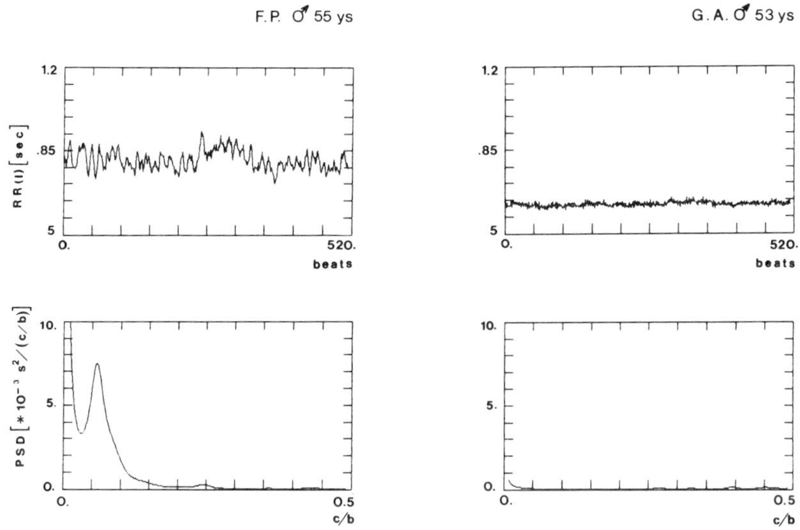

Fig 1. Spectral analysis of R-R variability in a patient with an uncomplicated outcome (left panel) and in a patient who died within 3 months from acute myocardial infarction (right panel). Note in the latter the low variance of R-R intervals and the absence of detectable spectral components (from Ref 8, unpublished).

One year after myocardial infarction there was, in addition, a marked increase of the low frequency component (from 55±3 to 73±3 nu) in response to tilt as observed in control subjects.

DISCUSSION. These data indicate that signs of an increased sympathetic tone and of a diminished parasympathetic activity characterize the acute phase of myocardial infarction and that a normalization of sympatho-vagal balance occur within one year from the acute episode (8).

In the present study we analyzed the beat by beat oscillations of cardiac cycle in patients with a previous myocardial infarction according to the hypothesis that changes in sympathetic and vagal efferent activities directed to the heart might be reflected by cardiac beat to beat oscillations. While peak to peak variation of heart period has been previously used as an index of parasympathetic activity (10-11), we (7,8,12) have recently suggested that spectral analysis of heart rate variability could also provide information on changes in efferent sympathetic activity and therefore on the interaction of the two neural regulatory outflows. The low frequency component has been proven to represent an index of sympathetic activity (7). It not only corresponds to the Mayer waves and to the main frequency of discharge of cardiac preganglionic fibers (13) but can be altered by all the maneuvers that increase functionally or block pharmacologically the sympathetic drive to the heart. The high frequency component instead is synchronous with respiration and is considered an index of vagal activity (5-7).

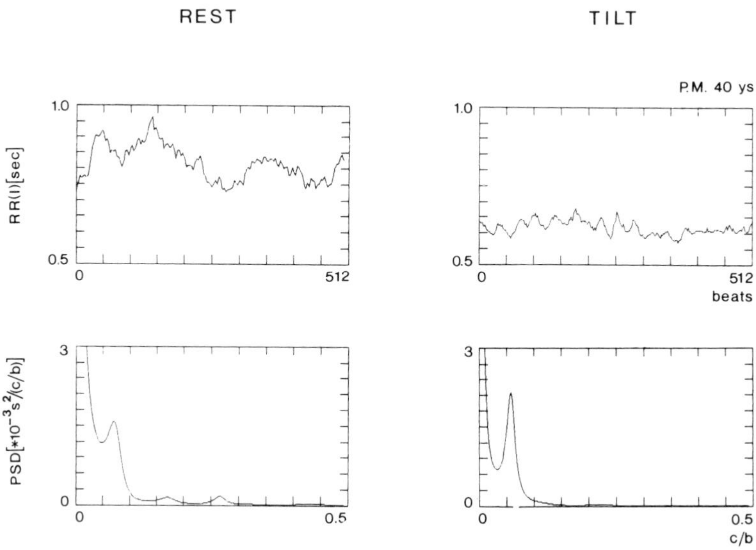

Fig. 2 R-R interval series, i.e. tachogram (top) and autospectra (bottom) at rest and during passive upright 90° tilt in a patient at two weeks after acute myocardial infarction. At rest there is a predominant low frequency component which is not modified by tilt (from Ref 8 unpublished).

Our data indicate that independently of the localization of the infarction signs of sympathetic activation are still detectable in patients at 2 weeks after myocardial infarction, at the time of discharge from the hospital, while the decrease in the high frequency component confirms a concomitant reduction of parasympathetic activity (14). The existence of an alteration of sympatho-vagal balance is further supported by the absence of a normal response to 90° head up tilt, a stimulus adequate to produce signs of sympathetic activation in control subjects and in patients at one year after myocardial infarction. An impaired parasympathetic control of heart rate has been previously reported in patients after myocardial infarction (14); in the present study, in addition, we have been able to detect signs of a concomitant sympathetic predominance, a condition which may well be relevant to explain the protective effects of beta adrenergic receptor blockade after myocardial infarction.

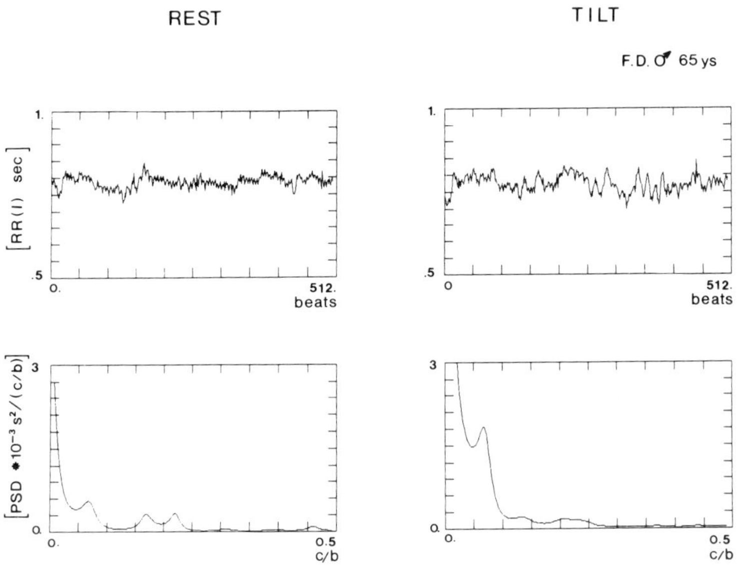

Fig. 3 R-R interval series, i.e. tachogram (top) and autospectra (bottom) at rest and during passive upright 90° tilt in a patient at 1 year after acute myocardial infarction. Two clearly separate low and high frequency components are present at rest. During tilt, the low frequency component becomes predominant (from ref 8, unpublished).

Regarding the clinical possibility of using measurement of heart rate variability, such as variance or standard deviation of R-R interval as markers of alterations of neural regulatory mechanisms, it is important to mention that in a recent report Kleiger et al (15) demonstrated a significant association between decreased heart rate variability and increased mortality after acute myocardial infarction. In the light of our results however, this strong association could not be explained only as a consequence of a diminished parasympathetic tone. Indeed, spectral analysis revealed in patients with a marked reduction of heart rate variability the existence of a greater alteration of neural control of the heart rate as a likely result of a diminished responsiveness of target function to efferent neural regulatory activities.

As to mechanisms responsible for the alteration in sympatho-vagal balance it is important to mention that no direct information can be derived from the analysis of heart rate variability.

Even if the reduction of baroreceptive mechanisms (16,17) or change in central "command" have been frequently advocated, to explain an increased adrenergic tone, it was worth considering the fact that an augmented sympathetic drive to the heart could be the result of prevailing excitatory sympathetic reflexes elicited by the continuous excitation of cardiac sympathetic afferent fibers activated by an abnormal mechanical or chemical stimulus locate in the heart (18).

ACKNOWLEDGEMENTS. We should like to thank Mr. Ugo Boccaccini for his technical assistance and Ms. Yvonne Stewart for her help in typing the manuscript.

REFERENCES

1) Hjalmarson, Å., Herlitz, J., Holmberg, S., et al. (1983) 'The Göteborg metoprolol trial: Effetcs on mortality and morbidity in acute myocardial infarction'. Circulation, 67:126-132
2) Furberg, CD., Hawkins, CM., Lichstein, E., the Beta-Blocker Heart Attack Trial Study Group. (1984) 'Effect of propranolol in post infarction patients with mechanical or electrical complications. Circulation, 69:761-765
3) Olsson, G., Rehnqvist N, Sjögren, A. et al. (1985) 'Long-term treatment with metoprolol after myocardial infarction: Report on three year mortality and morbidity'. J Am Coll Cardiol, 5:1428-1437
4) Webb, SW., Adgey, AAJ., Pantridge, JF. (1972) 'Autonomic disturbance at onset of acute myocardial infarction'. Br Med J, 3:89-92
5) Akselrod, S., Gordon, D., Ubel, FA., Shannon, DC., Barger, AC., Cohen, RJ. (1981) 'Power spectrum analysis of heart rate fluctuation: A quantitative probe of beat to beat cardiovascular control'. Science 213:220-222
6) Pomeranz, M., Macaulay, RJB., Caudill, MA., Kutz, I., Adam, D., Gordon, D., Kilborn, KM., Barger, AC., Shannon, DC., Cohen, RJ., Benson, M. (1985) 'Assessment of autonomic function in humans by heart rate spectral analysis'. Am J Physiol, 248:H151-H153
7) Pagani, M., Lombardi, F., Guzzetti, S., Rimoldi, O., Furlan, R., Pizzinelli, P., Sandrone, G., Malfatto, G., Dell'Orto, S., Piccaluga, E., Turiel, M., Baselli, G., Cerutti, S., Malliani, A. (1986) 'Power spectral analysis of heart rate and arterial pressure variabilities as a marker of sympatho-vagal interaction in man and conscious dog'. Circ Res, 59:178-193
8) Lombardi, F., Sandrone, G., Pernpruner, S., Sala, R., Garimoldi, M., Cerutti, S., Baselli, G., Pagani, M., Malliani, A. (1987) 'Heart rate variability as an index of sympathovagal interaction after acute myocardial infarction'. Am J Cardiol 60:1239-1245
9) Brovelli, M., Baselli, G., Cerutti, S., Guzzetti, S., Liberati, D., Lombardi, F., Malliani, A., Pagani, M., Pizzinelli, P. (1983) 'Computerized analysis for an experimental validation of neurophysiological models of heart rate control'. Comps in Cardiol 205-208

10) Ewing, DJ., Neilson, JMM., Travis, P. (1984) 'New method for assessing cardiac parasympathetic activity using 24-hour electrocardiograms'. Br Heart J, 52:396-402
11) Fouad, FM., Tarazi, RC., Ferrario, CM., Fighaly, S., Alicandri, C. (1984) 'Assessment of parasympathetic control of heart rate by a non-invasive method'. Am J Physiol 246:H838-H842
12) Furlan, R., Guzzetti, S., Crivellaro, W., Dassi, S., Tinelli, M., Baselli, G., Cerutti, S., Lombardi, F., Pagani, M., Malliani, A. (1990) 'Continuous 24H assessment of the neural regulation of systemic arterial pressure and R-R variabilities in ambulant subjects'. Circulation (in press)
13) Lombardi, F., Montano, N., Finocchiaro, ML., Gnecchi Ruscone, T., Baselli, G., Cerutti, S., Malliani, A. (1990) 'Spectral analysis of sympathetic discharge in decerebrate cats'. J Autonom Nerv Syst, (in press)
14) Eckberg, DL., Drabinsky, M., Braunwald, E. (1971) 'Defective cardiac parasympathetic control in patients with heart disease'. N Eng J Med, 285:877-881
15) Kleiger, RE., Miller, JP., Bigger, JT., Moss, AJ., and the multicenter post-infarction research group. (1987) 'Decreased heart rate variability and its association with increased mortality after acute myocardial infarction'. Am J Cardiol 59:256-262
16) La Rovere, MT., Specchia, G., Mortara, A., Schwartz, PJ. (1988) 'Baroreflex sensitivity, clinical corelates and cardiovascular mortality among patients with a first myocardial infarction. A prospective study'. Circulation, 78:816-824
17) Schwartz, PJ., Zaza, A., Pala, M., Locati, E., Beria, G., Zanchetti, A. (1988) 'Baroreflex sensitivity and its evolution during the first year after myocardial infarction'. J Am Coll Cardiol, 12:629-636
18) Malliani A. (1982) 'Cardiovascular sympathetic afferent fibers'. Rev Physiol Biochem Pharmacol, 94:11-74

13
The vegetative nervous system and atrial natriuretic factor

F. FONTANA and P. BERNARDI

Institute of Medical Pathology, Bologna University, Policlinico S. Orsola, via Massarenti 9, 40138 Bologna, Italy

ABSTRACT. The vegetative nervous system (VNS) and atrial natriuretic factor (ANF) are linked in various ways: 1) the VNS affects ANF release; 2) ANF changes some VNS activities and 3) the VNS influences the effects of ANF. These functional relationships have been confirmed by literature reports. Our studies on the effects of Dopamine infusion on ANF and noradrenaline (NA) plasma levels in healthy subjects and in congestive heart failure patients suggested that NA may be involved in ANF release. In diseases characterized by an increase in sympathetic tone we found that hypersympathicotonia does not appear to modify plasma ANF levels if central venous pressure (CVP) is normal as in hypovolemic shock due to melena. On the other hand, in patients with acute myocardial infarction (AMI) during bradycardia and hypotension syndrome characterized by an increase in parasympathetic tone we observed normal ANF and CVP values; this suggests that hypervagotonia curbs peptide secretion because ANF release is usually high during AMI.

The vegetative nervous system (VNS)and atrial natriuretic factor (ANF) are known to be linked in various ways: 1) the VNS affects ANF release; 2) ANF changes some VNS activities and 3) the VNS influences the effects of ANF.

1. VNS and plasma ANF release.

1.1. Adrenergic stimulation of ANF release in vitro, in animals and man under physiological conditions.

That a functional relationship exists between the VNS and ANF release has been established by studies in chronic spinal animals [1] with severely impaired autonomic control. These experiments demonstrated reduced basal ANF release and an absent atrial secretory response following hydrosaline infusion [1].

However, the VNS does not appear to play a major role in ANF release under basal conditions since administration of atropine and ganglioplegic drugs in non-lesioned animals [2], and beta-blockers at subpressor doses in animals [2] and man [3] had no effect. On the other hand, numerous studies have demonstrated that adrenergic stimulation triggers peptide release [4,5,6,7]. Experiments with atrial specimens [4] and perfused isolated rat heart [5] showed enhanced ANF release after administration of sympathomimetic agents, especially α-agonists [6]. The only adrenergic agonist to be studied in vivo in the rabbit is isoproterenol which was shown to stimulate ANF release [7].

Different experimental models have been adopted to assess the influence of the VNS on ANF secretion in man under physiological conditions. During hypersympathicotonia induced by physical exercise [8] or atrial pacing [9], and after administration of noradrenalin and angiotensin [10] ANF plasma levels were raised. However, the ANF increase was accompanied by hemodynamic changes such as heart rate (HR), blood pressure (BP), central venous pressure (CVP) which could have triggered ANF secretion in all these experiments as well as in perfused isolated rat heart [5,6] and in vivo in animal [7] studies. Only the in vitro experiments using atrial specimens [4] demonstrate the direct effect of VNS sympathomimetic agonists on ANF release.

The importance of hemodynamic alterations was confirmed by experiments in man using drugs known to reduce or raise CVP. ANF values normalized in these studies after administration of vasodilators able to prevent a rise in CVP when subjects underwent physical exercise [11], atrial pacing [9] or received noradrenalin (NA) [12]. On the other hand, administration of ß-blockers during physical exercise [8] and atrial pacing [9] reducing myocardial contractility and hence raising pressure and atrial dilatation further stimulates ANF secretion.

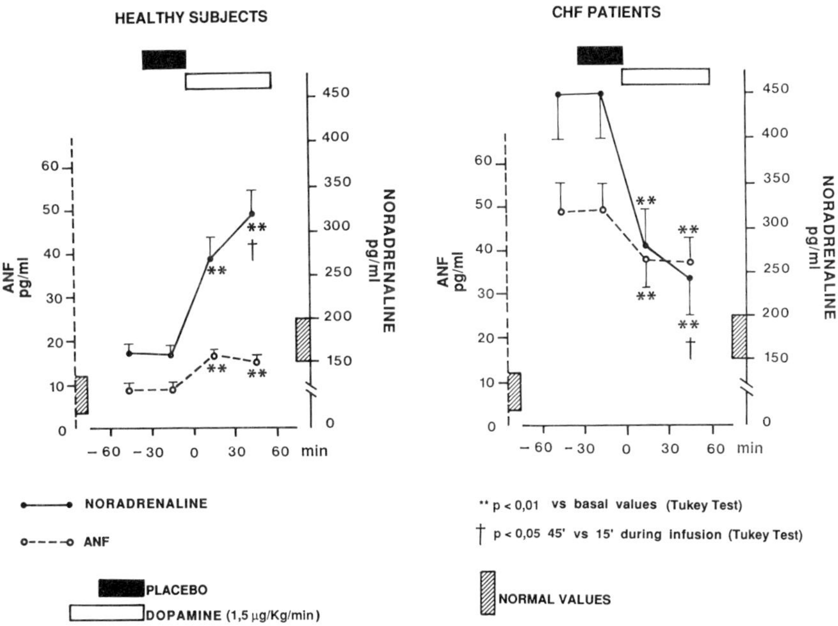

Fig.1 Effects of DA infusion on plasma ANF and NA levels in healthy subjects and in congestive heart failure patients.

Our studies on the effects of dopamine (DA) on ANF release have demonstrated that NA is involved in ANF secretion control irrespective of hemodynamic changes.

We aimed to evaluate the short-term effects of DA infusion on release of ANF and NA using doses which do not affect basal BP. We studied 10 healthy subjects (HS) and 10 patients with congestive heart failure (CHF) (NYHA Classes III,IV) due to chronic ischemic heart disease or idiopathic dilated cardiomyopathy.

The protocol included four thirty-minute clearance periods: first basal, second during placebo infusion, third and fourth during dopamine infusion (1.5 μg/k/min for 60 min). Blood samples for assessment of ANF and NA levels were drawn at the midpoint of each urine collection period after measuring BP, HR and CVP. ANF was determined by radioimmunoassay after chromatographic extraction; NA was measured fluorometrically.

DA infusion modified plasma ANF levels in both groups (Fig.1). In HS, DA determined a significant ANF rise compared with basal values at 15 and 45 minutes after the start of infusion. In CHF patients the high ANF values dropped significantly at the same times. These trends were also evident for plasma NA levels in both groups.

In HS DA led to a significant increase in NA levels at 15 and 45 minutes after the beginning of infusion while in CHF patients the high basal values dropped significantly at the same times.

There was a statistically significant correlation between plasma ANF and NA levels, before and during DA infusion in both HS ($r=0.66, p<0.01$) and CHF patients ($r=0.80, p<0.01$).

No change in systolic or diastolic BP, HR or CVP values were observed during DA infusion in either group. Changes in plasma ANF levels during DA infusion do not appear to be related to a direct DA action on the heart cells secreting ANF since dopaminergic receptors have not been demonstrated in atrial myocardial fibers in man. The significant correlation found between plasma ANF and NA levels in HS and CHF patients suggests that NA may be involved in ANF release. The presence of D2 receptors on the NA containing nerve terminals [13] suggests that the effect of DA on ANF release may be mediated by control of NA release.

1.2. Adrenergic and vagal effects on ANF release in man under pathologic conditions.

The relation between plasma ANF levels and VNS function has been studied in diseases which usually present increased sympathetic tone as in hypertension [14] and cardiogenic and hypovolemic shock, or hypervagotonia as in the bradycardia with hypotension syndrome occurring during acute myocardial infarction (AMI).

Plasma ANF levels are raised in hypertension except when it is borderline [15]. The direct effect of the hypersympathicotonia present in hypertension on ANF secretion seems to be of scant importance since ANF is normal in the only form of hypertension presenting slight hemodynamic changes (borderline). Moreover, among patients with essential hypertension, those with high renin levels characterized by marked resistance and hence sympathetic hypertonia [14], have lower ANF values than patients with low renin levels.

We investigated 10 patients with cardiogenic shock due to AMI of the anterior wall, 10 with hypovolemic shock due to melena from peptic ulcer and 10 with hypotension with bradycardia syndrome due to AMI of the inferior wall which occurred in the coronary care unit at the 12th to 48th hour after onset of myocardial infarction.

In patients with cardiogenic shock hypersympathicotonia was associated with marked hemodynamic changes as well as high HR (119.7 ± 1.2 b/min), low BP (SBP 56 ± 3, DBP 40 ± 2 mmHg) and high CVP (16.2 ± 0.6 cm H_2O). Impaired ventricular performance reflected by acute pulmonary edema and the increase in CVP raised plasma ANF levels (102.4 ± 7.4 pg/ml) to 12-13 times the levels in healthy subjects (8.4 ± 0.3 pg/ml).

In hypovolemic shock hypersympathicotonia was accompanied by high HR (111.0 ± 1.4 b/min), low BP (SBP 74 ± 1, DBP 57 ± 2 mmHg) and normal CVP (6.3 ± 0.5 cm H_2O). In these patients raised HR had a negligible effect on plasma ANF levels (8.8 ± 0.7 pg/ml) which did not differ from the healthy volunteer group.

In the bradycardia with hypotension syndrome, reduced CVP values (4.6 ± 0.4 cm H_2O) were found while plasma ANF levels were normal (8.7 ± 0.6 pg/ml). This is noteworthy since the syndrome was a complication of AMI due to hypervagotonia, as atropine effectively antagonized symptoms. In uncomplicated AMI we recently showed high plasma ANF values persisting for over a week after onset of infarction [16]. The normal plasma ANF values obtained in bradycardia with hypotension syndrome mainly reflect the impaired hemodynamic conditions (i.e. a drop in left ventricular and right atrial filling pressure). A direct effect of the parasympathetic nervous system has yet to be established and current findings report conflicting data. In vitro studies have demonstrated that acetylcholine stimulates ANF release [4] whereas in man several investigations into the nyctohemeral rhythm of ANF suggest that the vagus has an inhibiting effect [17].

In conclusion, these results show that in the above low output heart failure syndromes characterized by severe VNS impairment, hypersympathicotonia does not appear to stimulate ANF release unless endoatrial pressure is raised. Hypervagotonia, on ther other hand, appears to curb ANF secretion by reducing endoatrial pressure.

2. ANF influences some VNS activities.

Experimental evidence suggests that ANF has a substantial effect on VNS function. Experiments on atrial fragments incubated with ANF revealed a drop in NA secretion by inhibition of dopamine ß-hydroxylase [18]. In dogs, the ANF-induced reduction in NA plasma levels seems to confirm that the peptide inhibits adrenergic activity [19]. That the fall in BP is not accompanied by a rise in HR is further indirect evidence of the same effects [20]. However, a more complex interaction between ANF and the VNS emerges from some findings such as the inability of ß-blockers and atropine to curb the drop in BP following ANF infusion and, conversely, the disappearance of ANF effects after vagotomy [21]. Data obtained in animals have been confirmed in man [22]. Some patients present marked vascular sensitivity to ANF which may lead to severe hypotension and bradycardia following synthetic ANF administration [22], as we found in some patients with hypervagotonia receiving digitalis (unpublished data).

Although in vitro studies have demonstrated the peripheral effect of ANF on adrenergic nerve endings [18], its effects are better interpreted at the nerve centers responsible for cardiocirculatory control [20]. ANF stimulation of cardiopulmonary receptors would increase the vagal afferent impulses which at CNS level would trigger a reflex drop in adrenergic activity and an increase in that of the vagus.

The hypotensive effect of ANF is thought to be caused by vasodilation due to reduced adrenergic tone, whereas the bradycardia or the absent rise in HR which accompanies hypotension during ANF infusion is ascribed to vagal hypertonus. This mechanism of action fits in with the finding that vagotomy abolishes ANF-induced hypotension in animal [21]. Beta-blockers and atropine fail to counteract the hypotensive effect of ANF as the vasodilation is not induced by stimulation of ß-adrenergic or cholinergic receptors, but by a fall in basal adrenergic tone.

3. VNS influences ANF effects.

Experimental data on this topic are scanty and difficult to demonstrate. However, some evidence suggests that enhanced ANF effects were found under conditions of hypervagotonia, as observed in patients treated with digitalis. On the other hand, hyperadrenergic tone may curb the effects of ANF as witnessed in patients with hypertension, frequently associated with increased sympathetic tone and high plasma ANF levels, in whom ANF administration has a scant hypotensive effect [23]. These findings suggest that spontaneous or drug-induced changes in vagal or sympathetic tone may affect kidney function and/or BP by interfering with the effects of ANF. If this is the case, increased vagal tone or decreased sympathetic tone may enhance the effects on kidney function and/or BP in diseases presenting high ANF plasma levels (hypertension, CHF, etc.). Among others, two questions arise in this connection: do ß-blockers enhance the hypotensive effect of ANF by reducing adrenergic tone? If so, does the hypotensive effect of ß-blockers depend on ANF plasma levels?

REFERENCES.

1) Pettersson, A., Ricksten, S.E., Towle, A.C., Hedner, J. and Hedner, T. (1985) 'Effect of blood volume expansion and sympathetic denervation on plasma levels of atrial natriuretic factor (ANF) in the rat', Acta Physiol. Scand. 124, 309-311.
2) Haass, M., Zukowska-Grojec, Z., Kopin, I.J. and Zamr, N. (1987) 'Role of autonomic nervous system and vasoactive hormones in the release of atrial natriuretic peptides in conscious rats', J. Cardiovasc. Pharmacol. 10, 424-432.
3) Nguyen, P.V., Smith, D.L. and Leenen, F.H.H. (1988) 'Acute volume loading, atrial natriuretic peptide release and cardiac function in healthy men. Effects of beta-blockade', Life Sci. 43, 821-830.
4) Sonnenberg, H. and Veress, A.T. (1984) 'Cellular mechanism of release of atrial natriuretic factor', Biochem. Biophys. Res. Commun. 124, 443-449.
5) Currie, M.G. and Newman, W.H. (1986) 'Evidence for α-1 adrenergic receptor regulation of atriopeptin release from the isolated rat heart', Biochem. Biophys. Res. Commun. 137, 94-100.
6) Wong, N.L.M., Wong, E.F.C., Au, G.H. and Hu, D.C.K. (1988) 'Effect of α- and ß-adrenergic stimulation on atrial natriuretic peptide release in vitro', Am. J. Physiol. 255, E260-E264.
7) Rankin, A.J., Wilson, N. and Ledsome, J.R. (1987) 'Influence of isoproterenol on plasma immunoreactive atrial natriuretic peptide and plasma vasopressin in the anesthetized rabbit', Pflugers Arch. 408, 124-128.
8) Tsai, R., Yamaji, T., Ishibashi, M., Takaku, F., Hsu, S., Lai, C., Yeh, S., Hung, J., Wu, D. and Lee, Y. (1988) 'Effect of ß-adrenergic blockade on plasma levels of atrial natriuretic peptide during exercise in humans', J. Cardiovasc. Pharmacol. 11, 614-618.
9) Haufe, M.C., Weil, J., Ernst, J., Gerzer, R. and Theisen, K. (1987) 'Secretion of atrial natriuretic factor (ANF) is suppressed by verapamil and unaffected by atenolol in man' (Abstract), Circulation 76 (Suppl.IV), 270.
10) Tunny, T.J., Klemm, S.A. and Gordon, R.D. (1987) 'Effects of angiotensin and noradrenalin on atrial natriuretic peptide levels in man', Clin. Exper. Pharmacol. Physiol. 14, 221-225.
11) Keller, N., Moller, T., Sykulski, R., Storm, T.L. and Thamsborg, G.M. (1987)

'Effect of alpha 1-adrenoceptor blockade on plasma levels of atrial natriuretic peptide during dynamic exercise in normal man', Horm. Metabol. Res. 19, 344-349.
12) Vehlinger, D.E., Zaman, T., Weidmann, P., Shaw, S. and Gnädinger, M. (1987) 'Pressure dependence of atrial natriuretic peptide during norepinephrine infusion in humans', Hypertension 10, 249-253.
13) Goldberg, L.I. and Rajfer, S.I. (1985) 'Dopamine receptors: applictions in clinical cardiology', Circulation 72, 245-248.
14) Larochelle, P., Cusson, J.R., Gutkowska, J., Schiffrin, E.L., Hamet, P., Kuchel, O., Genes, J. and Cantin, M. (1987) 'Plasma atrial natriuretic factor concentrations in essential and renovascular hypertension', Br. Med. J. 294, 1249-1252.
15) Kohno, M., Yasunari, K., Matsuura, T., Murakawa, K. and Takeda, T. (1987) 'Circulating atrial natriuretic polypeptide in essential hypertension', Am. Heart J. 113, 1160-1163.
16) Fontana, F., Spagnolo, N., Guardigli, G., Ventura, C., Cavazza, M., Bastagli, L., Capelli, M., Martelli, E., Bernardi, P and Lenzi, S. (1987) 'Analysis of the plasmatic levels of atrial natriuretic factor in patients with acute myocardial infarction (AMI)', in: S. Lenzi and G.C. Descovich (eds.), Atherosclerosis and Cardiovascular Disease, Editrice Compositori, Bologna, pp. 961-963.
17) Orlandini G., Bruschi, G., Cavatorta, A., Ceresini, M.B., Manca, C., Pucci, F. and Borghetti, A. (1987) 'Physiological stimuli to atrial natriuretic peptide secretion in normal humans', J. Hypertension 5(5), S67-S70.
18) Racz, K., Kuchel, O., Buu, N.T., Debinski, W:, Cantin, M. and Genest, I. (1986) 'Atrial natriuretic factor, catecholamines and natriuresis', N. Engl. J. Med. 314, 321-322.
19) Holtz, J., Sommer, O. and Bassenge, E. (1987) 'Inhibition of sympathoadrenal activity by atrial natriuretic factor in dogs', Hypertension 9, 350-354.
20) Volpe, H., Cuocolo, A., Vecchione, F., Melea, F., Condorelli, M. and Trimarco, B. (1987) 'Vagal mediation of the effects of atrial natriuretic factor on blood pressure and arterial baroreflexes in the rabbit', Circ. Res. 60, 747-755.
21) Schultz, H.D., Gardner, D.G., Deschepper, C.F., Coleridge, H.M. and Coleridge C.G. (1988) ' Vagal C-fiber blockade abolishes sympathetic inhibition by atrial natriuretic factor', Am. J. Physiol. 255, R6-R13.
22) Weder, A.B., Sekkarie, H.A., Takiyyuddin, H., Schork, N.J. and Julius S. (1987) 'Antihypertensive and hypotensive effects of atrial natriuretic factor in man', Hypertension 10, 582-589.
23) Lang, R.E., Unger, T. and Ganten, D. (1987) 'Atrial natriuretic peptide: a new factor in blood pressure control', J. Hypertension 5, 255-271.

NOSOLOGY OF HYPERLIPOPROTEINAEMIAS

14
Apolipoproteins and metabolism in atherosclerosis

A.M. GOTTO, Jr.

Department of Medicine, Chief, Internal Medicine Service, The Methodist Hospital, 6565 Fannin, M.S. A-601, Houston, TX 77030, USA

The term "apolipoproteins" was initially coined by John Oncley in the 1940s to refer to the protein constituents of the plasma lipoproteins. Since then, we have learned a great deal about the structures, functions, and in some cases, the mechanisms of apolipoproteins.

One of the more important functions of apolipoproteins is to help bind and emulsify the water-insoluble lipids in lipoprotein packages. However, the apolipoproteins are not limited to structural functions. They also contribute to the regulation of lipoprotein metabolism.

With the exception of apolipoprotein B or apo B, the apolipoproteins are located on the surface of the lipoproteins. The apolipoproteins contain unique structures called amphipathic helices. These helices were first described by Segrest, et.al in 1974.[R1] Amphipathic helices allow the apolipoproteins to reside on the surface of the lipoprotein particle. Table 1 summarizes the apolipoproteins and some of their important properties.

Apo A's

Apo A is secreted by the liver and intestine. It is found in HDL and is also present in chylomicrons. Apo A-I is an activator of LCAT and is believed to play an important role in reverse cholesterol transport. Like Apo A-I, Apo A-II is secreted by the liver, but its intestinal origin is unclear. In addition to binding lipid, it has been suggested that apo A-II serves as an activator of the enzyme hepatic triglyceride lipase. Apo A-IV is secreted by the intestine and is present in chylomicrons and HDL. Some investigators have suggested that apo's A-I, A-IV and possibly A-II are involved in reverse cholesterol transport since these apolipoproteins are able to bind to 'HDL receptors' on the surface of cells and subsequently to promote cholesterol removal.

Apo B's

Apo B is the major protein constituent of LDL, but it is also found in chylomicrons and VLDL. Human apo B is a glycoprotein which occurs in two forms, apo B and apo B-100. In man, Apo B-48 is synthesized by the intestine, while apo B-100 is synthesized by the liver. The human gene for apo B contains 43 kilobases with 9.8 introns and is located on chromosome 2. Apo B-48 occurs because of the insertion of a stop codon in the editing of DNA.[R2] Most of the MRNA of the intestine is about 15 kilobases in size. This is the same as that for the MRNA for apo B-100. However, the stop codon is triggered by a CAA substitution for an UAA sequence. This substitution results in an aborted synthesis of the apolipoprotein and in the absence of the LDL receptor binding region.

Apo C's

Apo C-I, C-II and C-III are secreted by the liver. They are found in HDL and may also be transferred to VLDL and chylomicrons. Apo C-I can serve as an activator of LCAT; its other functions are unknown. Apo C-II is required to activate lipoprotein lipase. In certain kindreds, apo C-II is defective or deficient and is associated with a severe form of fasting chylomicronemia called Type I hyperlipoproteinemia. The clinical and lipoprotein abnormalities are very similar to those seen in familial lipoprotein lipase deficiency. Although the function of apo C-III is unknown, some investigators have suggested that apo C-III prevents a premature uptake of remnant particles by the liver.

Apo D's

Apo D is a minor protein which appears to be able to form complexes with HDL and the cholesteryl ester transfer protein (CETP), also called the lipid transfer protein (LTP). CETP catalyzes the exchange of cholesteryl ester and triglyceride between HDL and the lower-density lipoproteins.

ApoE's

Apo E is mainly synthesized in the liver, although a number of other tissues, including the brain, kidney and adrenal gland, are capable of making it. Synthesis and secretion of apo E has been shown in macrophages. Apo E serves as a ligand for the LDL or apo B/E receptor present on hepatic and extrahepatic tissues. Apo E also serves as a ligand recognized by liver receptors for chylomicron remnants.

Apo E exists in three primary isoproteins which differ in size and/or charge. Apo E-2 has two cysteines replacing two arginines from apo E-4 and one arginine from apo E-3. Apo E has the lowest affinity for the hepatic receptors. The closely-related apo E-3 and apo E-4 proteins have increasingly greater affinity with hepatic receptors.

Evolutionary Family of Apolipoproteins

Chan, et al suggested that the apolipoproteins represent a gene family, with Apo A-I the primordial apolipoprotein.[R3] According to this concept, the apolipoprotein represents inter-related families that have evolved through a series of complete or incomplete gene duplications, primarily involving the amphipathic helical regions of the protein. In 1977, Barker and Dayhoff predicted that the amphipathic helical regions were repeated throughout the various apolipoproteins.[R4] Their prediction was based on the structual knowledge of apos A-I, A-II and C-III.

Apo A-I is the prototypic protein with amphipathic regions which are represented in the MRNA or CDNA by 66 bp tandem DNA repeats.[R5] This translates into amphipathic helical regions of 22 amino acid residues, which may be subdivided into regions of 11 amino acids. The separate amphipathic helical regions tend to begin or end with a protein which serves as an alpha-helix breaker.

Apos A-I and C-III, on chromosome 11, are on opposite strands of DNA. Apo A-IV is downstream from apo A-I. The gene for Apo A-II is on chromosome 1. Genes for apo E and apo C-I are found on chromosome 19. Furthermore, there is extensive homology between the amphipathic helical regions of apos A-I, A-IV and E. Homology has also been shown between by the 5' region of apo A-I and a segment of apo C-II. If one lines up the mRNAs of these various apolipoproteins so that there is an approximate alignment between the regions coding for the protein, the introns have a remarkable degree of similarity in their location.

Apo B is quite different in its structure and whether it is part of the same apolipoprotein gene family is not yet determined.

HDL Function: Reverse Cholesterol Transport

The postulated role of apo A-I in reverse cholesterol transport as follows: apo A-I and its HDL particle are taken up by receptors on the cell's surface, but they do not participate in intracellular degradation. Instead, cholesterol is removed from the cell and transferred to particles. Since apo A-I is an activator of LCAT, it can also promote the conversion of cholesterol to cholesteryl ester, a necessary step in the transformation of nascent to mature HDL.

Some HDL particles contain only apo A-I. Fielding[R6] has recently described a particle with only apo A-I pre-beta electrophoretic mobility which he believes may be involved in reverse cholesterol transport. Some HDL particles contain apo A-I and apo A-II, while others also contain apo E. HDLs with apo E may transfer cholesteryl ester directly to the liver. The cholesteryl ester in the HDL particles without apo E is transferred to VLDL, IDL or LDL by the CETP.

As mentioned earlier, Apo A-I is synthesized by the intestine and liver, while Apo A-IV is synthesized by the intestine, and apos A-II and E by the liver. These apolipoproteins are secreted with phospholipid, and form the nascent HDL particle. The nascent HDL particle is then converted to a mature particle as cholesterol is removed from tissues and by converted cholesteryl ester.

In one study, measurements of apo A-I were reported to be superior to those of lipoprotein cholesterol is predicting coronary disease, but this generally has not been the case.

HDL deficiency, Apo A-I mutants and polymorphism

A fascinating disorder, in which a portion of the chromosome 11 coding region for Apo C-III was displaced into the coding region for apo A-I, was reported in two sisters. This mutation severely disrupted the synthesis of both apos A-I and C-III. As a result, the two sisters had essentially no HDL and overwhelming atherosclerosis.

There are other diseases associated with deficiencies of HDL, not all of which produce severe overwhelming atheroslcerosis. The classical disease in which HDL deficiency occurs is Tangiers' Disease.[R7] It has recently been suggested that the defect in Tangiers' Disease is due to a defect in HDL. Coronary disease certainly occurs in patients with Tangiers' Disease but generally not until middle age. The deposition of cholesteryl esters occur mainly in the reticular endothelial cells of Tangier's patients resulting in orange tonsils, hepatosplenomegaly, and the deposition in the Schwann cells. The latter may contribute to the neuropathy of this disease. While levels of apo A-I and HDL are extremely low in Tangiers' Disease, it's possible that the HDL that is present can function in reverse cholesterol tranport.

The HDL deficiency called apo A-I Milano is linked to a substitution of cysteine at residue 173. This HDL deficiency is associated with low levels of HDL, but not with accelerated coronary disease. In fact, in one Italian town where the apo A-I Milano mutant is common, many affected individuals have been reported to live into their 80's and 90's. It may be that with apo A-I Milano, HDL's are more rapidly catabolized. Thus, a low concentration of HDL in the blood does not necessarily mean a deficiency in reverse cholesterol transport.

HDL deficiency has been linked to corneal opacities as in Fish Eye Disease. Also, a primary deficiency of HDL has been described in other kindreds.

The variety of HDL mutants has been extensively reviewed by the Munster Laboratory in West Germany. Most of the HDL mutants are the result of amino acid substitutions which increase the negative charge and acidity or the positive charge and basicity of the protein.

The most frequent mutant is associated with a proline substitution causing depressed levels of HDL concentrations. Another mutation associated with a proline substitution involving residue 4 increases levels of pro apo A-I. In general, most of the mutations do not result in serious pathological conditions or in disruptions of HDL or apo A-I function.

Three prominent forms of apo A-I polymorphism have been described. In one form, the polymorphism occurs approximately 2.7 kilobases downstream from the A-I gene. In a second, the polymorphism is about 0.7 kilobases downstream. In a third, the polymorphism is approximately 8 kilobases upstream. Using the SST1 restriction enzyme, a group of investigators reported that the P2 allele was associated with a higher incidence of CHD and with HDL levels in the lowest 10th percentile of the population.

These findings have not been repeated in other populations. The inability to reproduce these results from one population to another raises the question of whether the mutations are really associated with CHD or dyslipidemia, or whether they indicate a genetic disequilibrium between genes. The development of a series of genetic markers to identify individuals who are susceptible to early atherosclerosis, and particularly to dietary-induced lipidemia, would be extremely valuable in targeting therapy and in identifying high-risk individuals early in life for intervention.

Apo B and CHD

The lipoprotein and apolipoprotein which have most clearly been associated with atherosclerosis are LDL and apo B-100. It is thought that VLDL is secreted with one apo B-100 molecule and that this apo B-100 molecule is passed on down to LDL. Apo B-100 differs from the other apolipoproteins because it contains a greater quantity of beta or pleated sheet structure. The amphipathic helical structure is also present, but its relatively smaller content sets it apart from other apolipoproteins. The high beta sheet content of apo B-100 contributes to the relative insolubility of the protein once its lipid constituents are stripped away. In this regard, the protein resembles amyloid which also has a high content of beta structure. Apo B also has a higher hydrophobicity of apo B and its beta-structure permit more of this apolipoprotein to be submerged below the surface of the LDL particle.

Yang, et al, had proposed a model for apo B-100 on the surface of LDL which differs from the classical one (Figure 1).[R8] In their model, apo B exists as an extended structure so that portions of the apo B are on the surface while other portions are buried. Yang's structure is consistent with the relative distribution of peptides released when LDL is treated with trypsin. This finding would also explain the antigenecity of apo B with the carbohydrates on the surface of the apolipoprotein.

A major function of apo B-100 is to bind the LDL to the LDL receptors on the cell surfaces. Apo B-100 contains a region between approximately residues 3300 and 3800 that is very positively charged. This region of positive charge is thought to interact with a region of negative charge on the surface of the LDL receptor.

The structure of apo B-100 was solved simultaneously in three laboratories. Chen, et al, reported the structure of over one-half of the amino acids residues by direct sequencing which agreed with the C-DNA structure.[R9] These investigators also produced synthetic peptides of a putative lipid-binding region, which was able to bind to the B/E receptor.[R10] Synthetic peptides from other regions of apo B did not bind to the receptor. Scott, et al, had earlier pointed out that a homology between the putative binding regions between residues 140 and 150 of apo B-100 and apo E.[R11] Soria, et al, have identified a mutant at amino acid 3500 in the binding region, which reduces binding to the LDL receptor, and results in moderate elevations of plasma LDL.[R12]

This finding of a defective apo B-100 illustrates that a patient may have an elevation of LDL either due to a defective or abnormal LDL receptor, as in familial hypercholetserolemia, or due to a defect in the binding region of the apolipoprotein.

However, apo B-48 appears to play a role in lipid transport in normotriglyceridemic patients. In one varient of abetalipoproteinemia, apo B-48 is present while apo B-100 is absent. Individuals with this disorder do not have the degree of malabsorption of dietary fat that is typically seen in patients with a classical form of abetalipoproteinemia.

Apo B-100 is required for the secretion of VLDL. In the absence of apo B-100, the liver fails to produce VLDL, and VLDL, IDL, and LDL are all missing from the blood. Individuals with classical abetalipoproteinemia or with homozygous hypobetalipoproteinemia have a total deficiency of apo B-100 or apo B-48, and subsequently of chylomicrons as well as VLDL, IDL and LDL.

In abetalipoprotein the gene for apo B appears to be normal and in some cases apo B-48 may be shown in intestinal cells. The defect appears to be in assembling the intact chylomicron particle or VLDL particle in the liver.

Apo B-100 is also bound in a disulfide linkage to Lp(a). The structure of Lp(a) has a high degree of homology with plasminogen. Lp(a) may be a promoter of atherogenesis for coronary disease since it has an anti-fibronolitic action due to its homology to plasminogen. Concentrations of Lp(a) greater than 30 mg/dl have been associated with a much higher incidence of coronary disease. Lp(a) may interact with the receptors on the surface of the endothelial cells and prevent their binding to plasmin. Lp(a) appears to contain two apo B proteins which are linked together in a disulfide linkage.

Thus, combined with vitamins, Lp(a) has the potential for inhibiting thrombolysis and for carrying cholesterol. Interesting possibilities are raised for linking thrombosis and apolipoprotein metabolism in the pathogenesis of coronary heart disease.

Sniderman, et al, have described a condition common in CHD patients which they called hyperapo B.[R13] This trait appears to run in families and is characterized by an increased proportion of apo B-100 in VLDL, IDL and LDL. Hyperapo B is particularly common in patients who have normal or only slightly elevated levels of LDL and total cholesterol, but who suffer from premature coronary disease. Figure 2 shows that the levels of apo B are just as high in hyperapo B as in familial hypercholesterolemia. However, the concentration of LDL is much higher in patients with familial hypercholesterolemia.

There are several conditions which may be related to hyperapo B. One is a genetically-determined hyperlipidemia first described by Goldstein, et al, called familial combined hyperlipidemia or familial multiple lipoprotein-type hyperlipidemia.[R14] This appears to be a dominantly-inherited trait that may be caused by an overproduction of apo B and subsequently of VLDL. Early coronary disease and atherosclerosis are characteristics of familial combined hyperlipidemia. The lipoprotein pattern in this condition may be one in which LDL or VLDL is increased. Any one pattern may predominate in a given individual. Related conditions include dyslipidemic hyperlipidemia, recently described in Utah kindreds by Williams, et al.[R15] They may also include syndrome x, in which hyperinsulinemia, insulin resistance and small, dense LDL particles are present.

Krause recently described the LDL particles in hypertriglyceridemic subjects as small, dense proteins enriched with apo B.[R16] It is speculated that these particles may be more atherogenic. The presumed mechanism for the formation of these dense LDL particles is analogous to that by which the HDL particle size and concentration is reduce in hypertriglyceridemia. When the concentration of lipoprotein lipase is diminished, CETP or LTP causes an increased transfer of triglyceride from the remnant particles into LDL and HDL in exchange for cholesteryl ester. In this exchange, the remnant particles become enriched in cholesteryl ester while the HDL or LDL particles become enriched in triglyceride. The triglyceride-enriched HDL or LDL particles are thought to be enhanced substrates for hepatic lipase. The triglyceride is hydrolyzed, producing small, dense LDL and HDL particles and decreased concentration of HDL. Prolonged postprandial lipemia would favor this process. In fact, it is well known that the concentration of HDL is inversely related to those of triglycerides and postprandial lipemia.

In theory, hyperapo B could result from an increased porportion of apo B in VLDL, as in familial combined hyperlipidemia, or from and exchange of triglyceride into LDL which ultimately results in smaller apo B-enriched LDL particles. The latter scenario is presumed to be the case in hypertriglyceridemia. Data are not available for determining whether the small, dense LDL particles have an impaired interaction with the LDL receptor or an increased interaction with the macrophage receptors which recognize oxidized LDL. Frushar showed that in dysbetalipoproteinemia, some LDL particles contain apo C-III or apo E in addition to apo B, and that the apo C-III particles have diminished binding to the LDL receptor.[R17]

While LDL binds readily to the LDL receptor through the

interaction of apo B, it binds poorly to the scavenger or macrophage receptor.(Figure 3) However, LDL that has been modified in various ways readily binds to scavenger receptors. Such is the case when LDL is oxidated on reaction with molondialdehyde. This uptake may stimulate the conversion of macrophages to foam cells. The scavenger receptor may play a role in the development of the atherosclerotic plaque by promoting cholesterol uptake in a unregulated way. Its structure has been recently described by Kodama, et al, and contains helical and collagen-like coiled coils and exists as a trimeric membrane glycoprotein.[R18] Interestingly, probucol appears to block this uptake. In the wanatabe rabbit, probucol retards the progression of atherosclerosis apart from any LDL-lowering factor. This may be due to an anti-oxidant effect of the drug, although the mechanism for this effect is not clear. What does seem to be clear is that the oxidation of LDL is caused by oxygen radicals. Steinberg suggested that the initial oxidation of LDL may be the effect of double-bonds in the polyunsaturated fatty acids, but that there may also be a breakdown of apo B and of phospholipid.[R19] Oxysterols are very potent inhibitors of cholesterol synthesis, and may also be toxic to endothelial cells and smooth muscle cells.

In summary, apo B may be related to atherosclerosis in a number of ways, most of which are only poorly understood. As a carrier of cholesterol, the apolipoprotein directly contributes to atherogenesis. Alterations in the structure of apo B which affect its binding to the LDL receptor may also cause atherogenesis by increasing the concentration of LDL. A change in the concentration of apo B, itself, or its content within IDL and LDL as in hyperapo B, may increase its atherogenecity as well. In addition, the binding of apo B-100 to apo Lp(a) in Lp(a) may link together cholesterol transport thrombosis or an anti-thrombolytic effect. Finally, changes in the LDL structure through oxidation or other modification may result in an enhanced uptake of LDL by scavenger receptors and macrophages present in the arterial wall.

In conclusion, over the past 20 years we have learned a great deal about the structure and the function of the apolipoproteins. This knowledge has permitted us to test new hypotheses concerning the relationship to atherosclerosis. We believe that this knowledge will be of benefit in devising more rational approaches for the treatment and prevention of coronary heart disease, and its complications.

References:

1. Segrest JP, Jackson RL, Morrisett JD, Gotto AM, Jr. A molecular theory of lipid-protein interactions in the plasma

lipoproteins. FEBS Lett 1974;38(3):247-258.

2. Chen SH, Habib G, Yang CY, Gu ZW, Lee BR, Weng SA, Silberman SR, et al. Apolipoprotein B-48 is the product of a messenger RNA with an organ-specific inframe stop codon. Science 1987;238(4825):363-366.

3. Chan L, VanTuinen P, Ledbetter DH, Daiger SP, Gotto AM, Jr., Chen SH. The human apolipoprotein B-100 gene: A highly polymorphic gene that maps to the short arm of chromosome 2. Biochem Biophy Res Commun 1985;133(1):248-255.

4. Baker WC, Dayhoff MO. Evolution of lipoproteins deduced from protein sequence data. Comp Biochem Physiol 1977;57(4):309-315.

5. Karathanasis SK, Zannis VI, Breslow JL. Isolation and characterization of the human apolipoprotein A-I gene. Proc Natl Acad Sci USA 1983;80(20):6147-6151.

6. Fielding CJ. Monoglyceride hydrolase activities of rat plasma and platelets. Their properties and roles in the activity of lipoprotein lipase. J Biol Chem 1981;256(2):876-881.

7. Schmitz G, Assmann G, Robenek H, Brennhausen B. Tangier disease: A disorder of intracellular membrane traffic. Proc Natl Acad Sci USA 1985;82(18):6305-6309.

8. Yang CY, Lee FS, Chan L, Sparrow DA, Sparrow JT, Gotto AM, Jr. Determination of the molecular mass of apolipoprotein B-100. A chemical approach. Biochem J 1986;239(3):777-780.

9. Chen SH, Yang CY, Chen PF, et al. The complete cDNA and amino acid sequence of human apolipoprotein B-100. J Biol Chem 1986;261(28)12918-12921.

10. Sparrow JT, Sparrow DA, Culwell AR, Gotto AM, Jr. Apolipoprotein E: Phospholipid binding studies with synthetic peptides containing the putative receptor binding region. Biochemistry 1985;24(24):6984-6988.

11. Forgez P, Gregory H, Young JA, Knott T, Scott J, Chapman MJ. Identification of surface-exposed segments of apolipoprotein B-100 in the LDL particle. Biochem Biophys Res Commun 1986;140(1):250-257.

12. Soria LF, Ludwig EH, Clarke HR, Vega GL, Grundy SM, McCarthy BJ. Association between a specific apolipoprotein B mutation and familial defective apolipoprotein B-100. Proc Natl Acad Sci USA 1989;86(2):587-591.

13. Teng B, Sniderman AD, Soutar AK, Thompson GR. Metabolic basis of hyperapobetalipoproteinemia. Turnover of apolipoprotein B in low density lipoprotein and its precursors and subfractions compared with normal and familial hypercholesterolemia. J Clin Invest 1986;77(3):663-672.

14. Kita T, Brown MS, Bilheimer DW, Goldstein JL. Delayed clearance of very low density and intermediate density of lipoproteins with enhanced conversion to low density lipoprotein in WHHL rabbits. Proc Natl Acad Sci USA 1982;79(18):5693-5697.

15. Williams RR, Hunt SC, Hopkins PN, Stults BM, Wu LL, et al. Familial dyslipidemic hypertension. Evidence from 58 Utah families for a syndrome present in approximately 12% of patients with essential hypertension. JAMA 1988;259(24):3579-3586.

16. Krause BR, Newton RS. Apolipoprotein changes associated with the plasma lipid-regulating activity of gemfibrozil in cholesterol-fed rabbits. J Lipid Res 1985;26(8):940-949.

17. Lussier Cacan S, Bard JM, Boulet L, Nestruck AC, Grothe AM, Fruchart JC, et al. Lipoprotein composition changes induced by fenofibrate in dysbetalipoproteinemia type III. Atherosclerosis 1989;78(2-3):167-182.

18. Kodama T, Freeman M, Rohrer L, et al. Type I macrophage scavenger receptor contains a-helical and collagen-like coiled coils. Nature 1990;343:531-535.

19. Steinbrecher UP, Witztum JL, Parthasarathy S, Steinberg D. Decrease in reactive amino groups during oxidation or endothelial cell modification of LDL. Correlation with changes in receptor-mediate catabolism. Arteriosclerosis 1987;7(2)135-143.

Figure 1

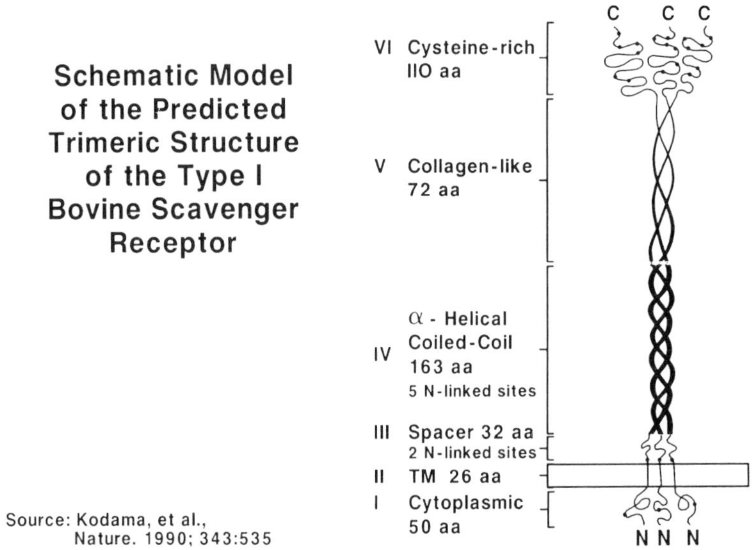

Figure 2

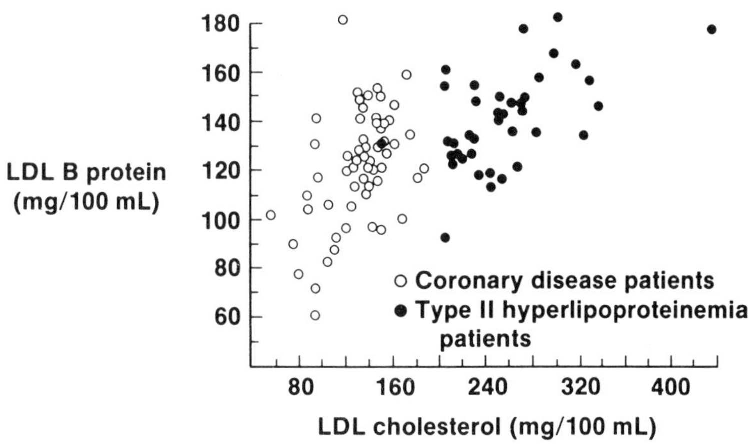

Data for plasma LDL cholesterol and B protein compared between patients with coronary disease (O, group II) and with type II hyperlipidemia (10) (●, group D). Many of the patients with coronary disease have LDL B protein levels similar to those in patients with type II hyperlipidemia.
Source: Sniderman A, et al. Proc Natl Acad Sci USA 1980;77:606.

Figure 3

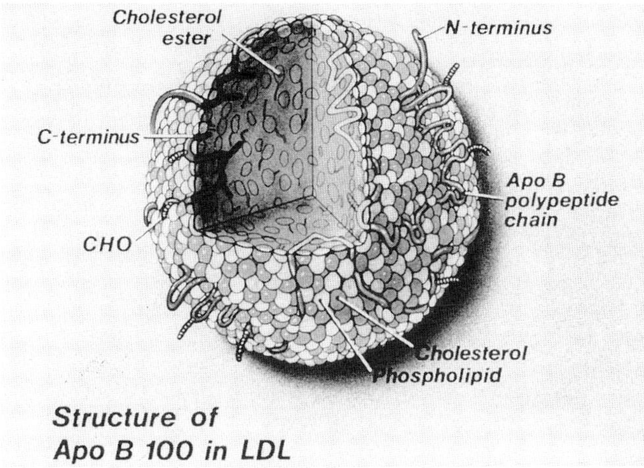

Schematic Structure of Apo B-100 in LDL.

TABLE 1

Apolipoproteins and their association with human diseases

Apo-protein	Plasma concentration (mg/ml)	Isoelectric point (pI)	M.W.	Function	Association with clinical disorders
A-I	1.0 – 1.2	5.85 – 5.40[a]	28K	Activates LCAT	Tangier disease; apoA-I – apoCIII deficiency; athero-sclerosis
A-II	0.3 – 0.5	5.0	8.5K	–	–
A-IV	0.16	5.5	46K	–	–
B-100	0.7 – 1.0	–	550K	Receptor-mediated catabolism of LDL	Abetalipopro-teinemia; normo-triglyceridemic abetalipoproteine-mia (B-100 defi-ciency); athero-sclerosis
B-48		–	275K	Chylomicron produc-tion	–
CI	0.04 – 0.06	7.5	6.5K	Activates (moder-ately) LCAT	–
CII	0.03 – 0.05	4.9	9K	Activates lipoprotein lipase	Familial Type I hyperlipopro-teinemia
CIII	0.12 – 0.14	4.7 – 5.0[b]	9K	Inhibits catabolism of triglyceride-rich lipoproteins	ApoA-I – apoCIII deficiency
E	0.025 – 0.050	6.0 – 5.7[c]	34.2K	Receptor-mediated catabolism of apoE-containing lipoproteins	Familial Type III hyperlipopro-teinemia

[a] The isoelectric points of apoA-I isoproteins are: apoA-I_2 = 5.85; apoA-I_3 = 5.74; apoA-I_4 = 5.65; apoA-I_5 = 5.52; apoA-I_6 = 5.40. The major plasma isoprotein is apoA-I_4.

[b] The isoelectric points of individual apo CIII isoproteins are: apoCIII-0 = 5.0; apoCIII-1 = 4.85; apoCIII-2 = 4.65.

[c] The isoelectric points of individual apoE3 isoproteins are: apoE3 = 6.02; apo $E3_{s-1}$ = 5.89; apo$E3_{s-2}$ = 5.78; apo$E3_{s-3}$ = 5.68. The isoelectric points of the common apoE variants are apoE2 = 5.89; apoE4 = 6.18.

Source: Breslow JL: Lipoprotein genetics and molecular biology. A.M. Gotto, Jr., Ed. Plasma Lipoproteins. Elsevier. Science Publishers B.V. Amsterdam, 1987:360 (Reprinted with permission)

15

Lipoprotein(a) and the LDL receptor (LDL-R): examination of the problem in a pedigree of rhesus monkeys with a familial hypercholesterolemia secondary to LDL-R deficiency

A.M. SCANU

Departments of Medicine, Biochemistry and Molecular Biology, University of Chicago Pritzker School of Medicine, 5841 South Maryland Avenue, Box 231, Chicago, IL 60637, USA

ABSTRACT

A rhesus monkey model for familial hypercholesterolemia was established. The affected animals were heterozygous for a nonsense mutation of the LDL-receptor gene in a position 284 of exon 6 and presented with high plasma levels of total cholesterol, LDL cholesterol and apo B. Plasma concentration of Lp(a) did not correlate with LDL-R deficiency but rather with apo(a) phenotype. The results support the concept that the metabolism of Lp(a) is independent of that of LDL.

INTRODUCTION

Until now the Watanabe rabbit (1) has been the only well characterized model for LDL-R-dependent familial hypercholesterolemia (FH). This model represents a class 2 mutation that removes four residues (Asp-Gly-Ser-Asp) from the third repeat in the binding domain and causes a transport defect of the LDL-R between the endoplasmic reticulum and the Golgi apparatus (2). However, the rabbit is philogenetically distant from man and its lipoprotein metabolism is substantially different from that of human subjects. Thus, the Watanabe-heritable hyperlipidemic rabbit, although it has proven of a great biological importance, may not represent a true model of human FH.

MATERIALS AND METHODS

Recently, we described a pedigree of rhesus monkeys in which some of its members have a hypercholesterolemia while fed a cholesterol-free Purina Chow diet (3). We also found that this hypercholesterolemia is related to a deficiency of the LDL-R based on the results of binding, ligand and immunoblot analyses carried out in cultured skin fibroblasts (3). In subsequent breeding experiments involving one of the affected males and several unrelated females, this defective phenotype was transmitted successfully to second generation animals (4). More recent studies by this laboratory (5) have established that the LDL-R defect is caused by a point mutation involving the replacement of codon TGG (tryptophan) in position 284 of exon 6 by a stop codon (TAG) resulting in a class

1 defect (null allele) according to the classification proposed by Goldstein and Brown for the human LDL-R mutations (2). In our monkey pedigree the abnormal genotype segregated with the abnormal phenotype indicating a relationship between LDL-R deficiency and spontaneous hypercholesterolemia. Thus, this pedigree represents a good model for human FH also based on the close phylogenetic relationship between non-human primates and man. Stimulated by these observations we have embarked on a study of Lp(a) based on the early finding (3) that these animals have high plasma levels of this lipoprotein differing from animal to animal. We first established that the overall structural organization of rhesus Lp(a) is similar to that of man, namely an LDL-like particle having as a protein moiety an apo B-apo(a) complex. Second, we established that rhesus apo(a) is made of several size polymorphs identifiable by SDS-polyacrylamide density gradient electrophoresis with molecular weight higher, equal to or lower than that of apo B_{100} (4). Third, we looked into the issue as to whether the LDL-R participates in the uptake and degradation of Lp(a) an unsettled question based on the published results from cell culture studies (6).

RESULTS

The first thing that became apparent is that the levels of plasma Lp(a) correlated with neither total plasma cholesterol, LDL cholesterol or apo B. Moreover, there were animals where high plasma Lp(a) correlated positively with LDL-R deficiency, but others where such a correlation was absent. Namely we saw animals with normal plasma Lp(a) associated with LDL-R deficiency and animals with high plasma Lp(a) and no LDL-R deficiency. Because earlier studies by Utermann et al. (7) had indicated that a correlation exists between size polymorphism of apo(a) and plasma Lp(a) levels we looked into the possible occurrence of such a correlation in our monkeys. We observed that a fair correlation existed between homozygosity for one of the electrophoretically fast apo(a) isoforms (single band) and high levels of Lp(a). Vice versa, homozygosity for the electrophoretically slow apo(a) isoforms was associated with low plasma levels of Lp(a). However, we also observed that a given apo(a) phenotype was not a good quantitative predictor of plasma Lp(a) levels suggesting that factors other than apo(a) genotype play a role in regulating Lp(a) concentration in the plasma (4). This conclusion was particularly true for animals heterozygous for apo(a) exhibiting a double band by SDS-polyacrylamide gradient gel electrophoresis and also a marked variability between apo(a) phenotype and plasma Lp(a) levels.

DISCUSSION

The above results invite several considerations. In the first place, our rhesus monkey pedigree represents a good model of human FH in terms of class 1 mutation resulting in a null allele. The heterozygous state of FH has not been as extensively studied as the homozygous one. Since our animals have a 50% decrease of LDL-R function due to the presence of only the normal allele it should be possible to assess the metabolic responsiveness of this allele to a number of environmental factors inclusive of drugs. For instance, we have recently established that the animals heterozygous for the LDL-R defect are hyperresponsive to a high fat dietary challenge as reflected by the doubling of their total plasma cholesterol, LDL cholesterol and apo B. Yet we saw no significant changes in the plasma Lp(a) levels indicative of a relative independence between LDL and Lp(a) metabolism. This conclusion is supported by the observation that some LDL-R deficient animals had normal levels of plasma Lp(a) and, conversely, that normocholesterolemic animals had a marked elevation of plasma Lp(a). It may be noted that those animals who had elevated plasma levels of Lp(a) were homozygous for one of the fast originating apo(a) isoforms which, according to current notions, could have been responsible for the Lp(a) elevation. Overall, our animals do not support a major participation of the LDL-R in uptake and degradation of Lp(a), a conclusion in keeping with the results of skin fibroblast culture studies indicating that the Lp(a) has a limited capacity to bind to these cells as compared to Lp(a)-free LDL. This conclusion is also in keeping with the reports showing that HMGCoA reductase inhibitors that act through the LDL-R, do not significantly modify the levels of Lp(a) even in the presence of a marked drop of the plasma LDL levels (8). It follows that apo B_{100}-containing particles as a consequence of their covalent attachment to apo(a), acquire metabolic properties different than those exhibited by LDL. As a consequence synthesis more than degradation may play a role in determining the levels of Lp(a) in the plasma.

ACKNOWLEDGEMENTS:

The original work mentioned in this account was supported by USPHS Program Project HL 18577. The Author is grateful to Ms. Sue Hutchison for help in preparing the manuscript.

REFERENCES:

1. Watanabe, Y. 1980. Serial inbreeding of rabbits with hereditary hyperlipidemia (WHHL rabbit) - Incidence and development of atherosclerosis and xanthoma. *Atherosclerosis* 36:261-268.

2. Russell, D. W. Lehrman, M.A., Sudhof, T.C., Yanamt, T., Davis, C.G., Hobbs H.H., Brown, M.S. and Goldstein, J.L. 1986. The LDL receptor in familial hypercholesterolemia: use of human mutations to dissect a membrane protein. *Cold Spring Harbor Symp. Quantit. Biology,* 51:811-819.

3. Scanu, A.M., Khalil, A., Neven, L.G., Tidore, M., Dawson, G., Pfaffinger, D., Jackson, E., Carey, K.D., McGill, H.C., and Fless, G.M. 1988. Genetically determined hypercholesterolemia in a rhesus monkey family due to a deficiency of the LDL receptor. *J. Lipid Res.* 29:1671-1681.

4. Neven, L.G., Khalil, Al, Pfaffinger, D., Jackson, E., and Scanu, A.M. 1990. Rhesus monkey model of familial hypercholesterolemia: relation between plasma Lp(a) levels, apo(a) isoforms and LDL receptor function. *J. Lipid Res.* In Press.

5. Hummel, M., Zhigao Li, Neven, L.G., and Scanu, A.M. 1988. Definition of the molecular basis of the LDL receptor deficiency in a rhesus monkey pedigree with familial hypercholesterolemia. *Proc. Natl. Aca. Sci., USA.* In Preparation.

6. Scanu, A. 1988. Lipoprotein(a): A genetically determined lipoprotein containing a glycoprotein of the plasminogen family. *Sem. in Thromb. and Hemost.* 14: 266-270.

7. Utermann, G., Menzel, H.J., Kraft, H.G., Duba, C., Kemmler, H.G. and Seitz, C. 1987. Lipoprotein(a) glycoprotein phenotype inheritance and relation to Lp(a) concentration in plasma. *J. Clin. Invest.* 80: 458-465.

8. Brewer H.B., 1990. Effectiveness of Diet and Drugs in the treatment of patients with elevated Lp(a) levels. *In* Lipoprotein(a): 25 years of progress. Scanu, A.M. Editor. *Acad. Press, N.Y.* In press.

16
Clinical significance of apolipoprotein B containing lipoprotein particles

J.C. FRUCHART, J.M. BARD, H.J. PARRA, I. JUHAN-VAGUE and V. CLAVEY

Institut Pasteur, SERLIA et U. Inserm 325, 1 rue Calmette, 59019 Lille Cédex, France

ABSTRACT. Apolipoprotein B (Apo B) exists in different types of particles in human plasma : Lp B containing only Apo B, Lp B:E containing Apo B and Apo E, Lp B:C-III containing Apo B and Apo C-III, Lp B:(a) containing Apo B and Apo (a) and soon. The physicochemically defined lipoproteins were found to be heterogeneous with respect to this concept. A particle such as Lp B, for example, may occur in any segment of the density spectrum depending on the composition and content of its lipid complement. These particles are metabolically distinct and their quantification is essential for better understanding of lipid transport disorders. Using new immunological procedures, we have identified some subpopulations of Apo B containing lipoproteins which are more abondant in atherosclerotic patients and which characterize some dyslipoproteinemic states. Drugs decreasing Apo B act differently on these different types of particles. The results presented substantiate the usefulness of the study of lipoprotein particles defined by their apolipoprotein composition for future clinical, pharmacological and epidemiological studies.

INTRODUCTION

Epidemiological studies have shown a strong positive relationship between plasma apolipoprotein (apo) B levels and the incidence of coronary artery disease. Apo B containing lipoproteins, are often classified according to their physicochemical properties such as electrical charge, hydrated density, size or interaction with polyanions. However, the recent discovery of molecular properties of the apolipoproteins (enzyme co-factors, ligands for receptors) led to their use as specific markers for the classification of lipoprotein species. As suggested by P. Alaupovic, apo B exists in different types of particles : LpB containing only apo B, LpB:E containing apo B and apo E, Lp B:C-III containing apo B and apo C-III, LpB:(a) containing apo B and apo (a), LpB:A-II containing apo B and apo A-II and so on [Alaupovic (1982)]. The physicochemically defined lipoproteins such as VLDL, IDL or LDL were found to be heterogeneous with respect to this concept. A particle such as LpB, for example, may occur in any segment of the density spectrum depending on the composition and content of its lipid complement.

PURIFICATION, PROPERTIES AND QUANTITATION OF APO B CONTAINING LIPOPROTEINS

The main apo B containing particles have been purified by sequential immunoaffinity chromatography and their binding properties have been studied using Hela Cells (Table I) [Bard et al. (1989)].

Figure 1. Changes in apo B containing particles on various therapies

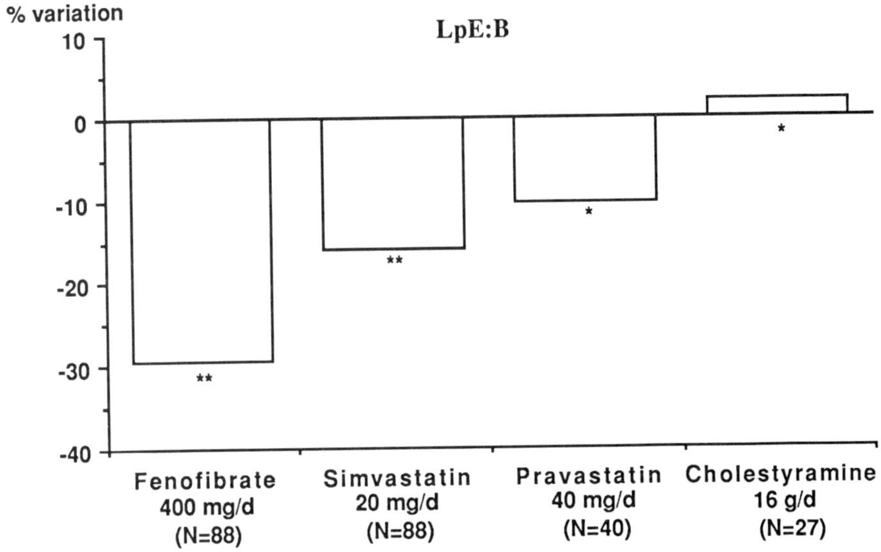

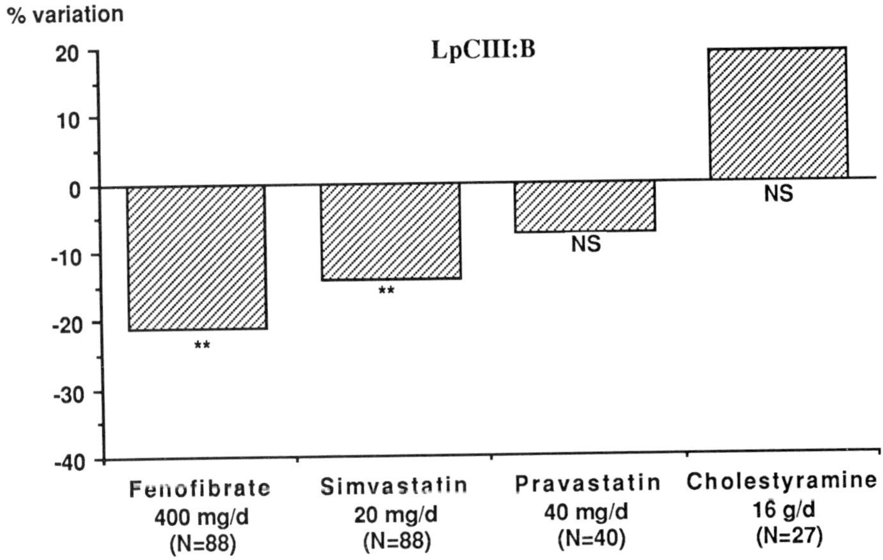

Table I : Binding properties of different apo B containing particles on HeLa cells

	E/B	Site number per cell	KD pmoles/ml
LDL	0,25	40 000	10,5
LpB:CIII	0	-	●
LpB	0	70 000	18,9
LpB:E E3/E3	1,5	18 000	2,9
LpB:CIII:E 1:6:3	3	18 500	2,7
LpB:CIII:E 1:13:10	10	12 500	0,75
LpB:E E4/E4	1,1	68 300	9,1
LpB:E E2/E2	nd	-	●

Lipoprotein affinity increases when the E:B ratio increases. On the other hand, the apparent number of binding sites on cells decreases when the E:B ratio increases. How to explain that in addition the apo E phenotypes may still modulate the affinity. LpB:E from the E2/E2 phenotype do not bind the receptor, while E3 phenotype has a maximum effect on the affinity. E4 phenotype has an intermediate effect on the binding properties of the particles. The presence of apo (a) modifies the organization and function of apo B in Lp(a) particles. The binding of the (a) antigen to apo B via disulfide bridges causes profound conformational changes of the apo B region exposed to the surface and leads to a decrease binding to the LDL receptor (figure 1). The B:C-III particles, free of apo E and the LpB:(a) have a very weak affinity for the B:E receptor and the number of their potential binding sites on cells is very low.
So apo B containing particles apparently represents metabolically distinct subpopulations and this difference could be clinically important. As then quantification in human plasma was essential for further clarification of the diagnostic value of measuring apo B, we have recently developed and immunoenzymometric assay for the measurement of LpB:C-III, LpB:E [Fruchart et al. (1985)], LpB:(a) [Vu Dac et al. (1989)].

CLINICAL SIGNIFICANCE OF APO B CONTAINING LIPOPROTEINS

- the examination of lipoprotein particle profiles of subjects with coronary artery disease as assessed by coronarography and controls, suggests that not only LpB but also some particular subpopulations of apo B containing particles such LpB:(a), LpB:E and LpB:C-III are important risk factors for atherosclerosis.
- some dyslipoproteinemias have specific lipoprotein particle profiles. For example, type III dyslipoproteinemia, a disorder with accelerated atherosclerosis, is characterized by a drastically increased concentration of LpB:E and to a lesser extent of LpB:C-III while the concentrations of LpB are negligeible. In a group of type IIA hypercholesterolemic patients, we have found that besides the increase in LpB, both LpB:E and LpB:C-III are significantly increased. Another example is given by the study of patients with chronic renal disease leading to hemodialysis. We have found a very significant increase in LpB:C-III and in LpB:(a) in patients on hemodialysis when compared to matched controls.

- we have recently studied LpB:(a) in angina pectoris. Patients had significantly higher concentrations as compared to controls but no link was found between elevated LpB:(a) and previous myocardial infarction or severe coronarography score. As a structural homology has been shown between plasminogen and apo (a), the possibility of a relationship between this lipoprotein and the plasma fibrinolytic system was investigated in 66 patients with angina pectoris. No relationship was found between LpB:(a) and fibrinolytic factors (t-PA activity, t-PAAg, PAI activity and antigen, functional plasminogen concentration, global fibrinolytic activity). So the pathogenic role of LpB:(a) does not seem to be mediated by its effect on the plasma fibrinolytic system. In fact, recent data suggest that LpB:(a) promots thrombosis because of its competition with plasminogen for cellular receptors.
- the determination of lipoprotein particles may offer not only a new diagnostic tool but also a means for highly selective therapeutic intervention in patients with dyslipoproteinemia. Hypolipidemic drugs seem to affect discrete apo B containing lipoprotein particles in a specific manner [Lussier-Cacan et al. (1989)] [Bard (1989)] [Bard et al. (1989)]. Fenofibrate, administered to hypercholesterolemic subjects, or to patients with type III dyslipoproteinemia produced a very significant reduction in LpB:E and LpB:C-III particles but less change in the levels of LpB particles. HMG CoA reductase inhibitors (simvastatin, pravastatin) in primary hypercholesterolemia, induced highly significant decrease of LpB particles and have a less pronounced effect on LpB:E and LpB:C-III. On the other hand, the administration of cholestyramine to hypercholesterolemic subjects caused significant decrease of LpB particles accompanied by a significant decrease of LpB particles accompanied by a simultaneous increase in LpB:E and LpB:C-III. None of the drugs had a significant effect on LpB:(a) particles (figure 2).

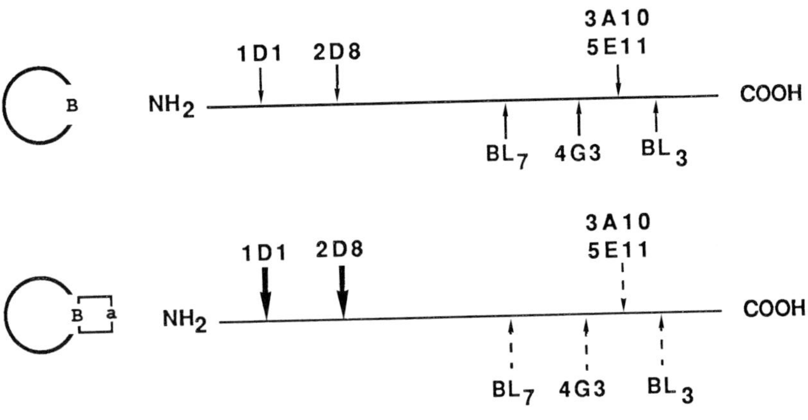

(1) Zawadzki, F. Tercé, L. Seman, R. Theolis, C. Brechendridge, R. Milne, Y. Marcel Biochemistry, 1988 ; 27.8474-0481
(2) A. Gries, C. Fievet, S. Marcovina, J. Nimpf, H. Mezdour, J.C. Fruchart, G.M. Kostner Journal of Lipid Research 1988, 29:1-7

CONCLUSION

The introduction of new immunological methods for differentiating apolipoprotein B containing lipoprotein particles reveals the existence of subpopulations with different lipid and apolipoprotein composition and different metabolic function.

The quantification of discrete lipoprotein particles will allow more accurate prediction of risk of developing premature atherosclerotic vascular disease. This approach may also provide a new basis for classifying dyslipoproteinenias and following the effect of hypolipidemic drugs.

REFERENCES

Alaupovic, P. (1982) 'The role of apolipoproteins in lipid transport processes', Ric. Clin. Lab. 12, 3-21.

Bard, J.M., Agnani, G., Candelier, L., Clavey, V., Fruchart, J.C. (1989)'Influence of apolipoprotein composition on the lipoprotein binding properties for the B:E receptor of Hela Cells' International Atherosclerosis Congress, Vienna, april 20-22.

Bard, J.M. (1989) 'Effect of bile acid sequestrants, fibrates, and HMG CoA reductase inhibitors on lipoprotein particles' 36th Colloquium on Protides of the Biological Fluids, London April 3-5 1989, in press.

Bard, J.M., Parra, H.J., Douste-Blazy, P., Fruchart, J.C. (1989) 'Effect of pravastatin, on HMG CoA reductase inhibitor, and cholestyramine, a bile acid sequestrant on lipoprotein particles defined by their apolipoprotein composition' Metabolism, in press.

Lussier-Cacan, S., Bard, J.M., Boulet, L., Nestruck, A.L., Grothe, A.M., Fruchart, J.C., Davignon, J. (1989) 'Lipoprotein composition changes induced by fenofibrate in dysbetalipoproteinemia type III' Atherosclerosis 78, 167-182.

Fruchart, J.C., Kandoussi, A., Parsy, D., Koren, E., Puchois, P. (1985) 'Measurement of lipoprotein particles defined by their apolipoprotein composition using immunosorbent asssay' annual Meeting on Clinical Chemistry, Mannheim September 25-28 1985 (abstr) J. Clin. Chem. Clin. Biochem. 23, 619.

Vu Dac, N., Mezdour, H., Parra, H.J., Luyeye, I., Fruchart, J.C. (1989) 'A selective bi-site immunoenzymatic procedure for human Lp(a) lipoprotein quantification using monoclonal antibodies against apo(a) and apo B' J. Lipid Res. 30.

17
Hyperlipoproteinemia of lipoprotein Lp(a)

G.M. KOSTNER
Institute of Medical Biochemistry, University of Graz, Harrachgasse 21/III, A-8010 Graz, Austria

ABSTRACT

Lp(a) is a lipoprotein with unknown physiological role. All we know for sure is that individuals with high Lp(a) levels are at an increased atherosclerosis risk. The Lp(a) plasma concentration correlates inversly with the molecular weight of the apo-a isoform; this is valid , however, only in healthy persons belonging to one ethnic group. Diseases, e.g. liver or kidney damage, pregnancy and menopause profundly alter plasma Lp(a) levels, and it also appears that fertile women have higher levels as compared to man.
Many studies of various laboratories demonstrate that plasma Lp(a) concentrations correlate with the incidence of atherosclerosis and myocardial infarction. In the healthy white western population, a treshold level of approx. 25 mg/dl seems to exist below which no increased atherosclerosis risk may be evident. This value certainely has to be adapted for different ethnic groups, as well as for individuals suffering from diseases known to influence Lp(a). Unfortunately we know today only little about the possible therapeutic manipulation of plasma Lp(a) concentrations.

INTRODUCTION

Lipoprotein-a (Lp-a) has been detected in 1963 by Berg [1] Its close relation to LDL has been recognized already at this time, as it was described as a genetic variant of Lp B. Numerous publications of Lp(a) research appeared until today (for reviews see Ref. 2 - 4). After cloning of apo-a and the elucidation of its similarity of the apo-a gene with that of plasminogen [5], a new era of Lp(a) research begun. The interest in Lp(a) is well justified by the fact, that it represents one of the most atherogenic lipoprotein known today. Nevertheless, all the efforts in various laboratories failed to uncover a possible physiological function for this lipoprotein. All what is known today is that individuals with Lp(a) plasma concentrations exceeding 20 - 30 mg/dl are at an 2 - 3 fold risk for atherosclerosis and myocardial infartion (M.I.). An exact figure for a possible treshold value for Lp(a), above which this lipoprotein might be atherogenic cannot be given at present time, because of the difficulties arising in the standardization of Lp(a) measurements.

Quantification of Lp(a)

The quantification of Lp(a) is not a straight forward procedure because of its polymorphic nature: i) Lp(a) consists in its protein moiety of apo B plus the specific antigen (apo-a), the latter being a glycoprotein with variable carbohydrate content; ii) There exist 6 - 10 genetic isoforms of apo-a which exhibit a great variation in the molecular weight ranging from 270 - 1000 kD [6]. iii) Apo-a is composed of a variable number of protein segments which are repeated more than 30 times; these repeats cross react immunochemically with plasminogen, (kringle 4). In spite of all these difficulties it is remarkeable that most of the Lp(a) values published from numerous laboratories using different methodology match each other quite well.
The standardization of Lp(a) measurements in clinical chemistry is currently worked out by many groups. Until firm recommendations may be given it is safe enough to use a commercial standard (e.g. from Immuno AG, Vienna) and express Lp(a) values in mg/ml of Lp(a) lipoprotein mass. There seems to be little difference in the results by either using ELISA, rocket electrophoresis or nephelometry; only radial immuno-diffusion may cause problems because of the large size of the antigen.

Lp(a) as a Risk Indicator for Vascular Diseases

Early reports on the link of increased Lp(a) levels with premature atherosclerosis and MI were published by the group of Dahlen [7]. In their assays based on simple agarose gel electrophoresis, distinctions were only made by the presence or absence of an "extra pre-ß-1 band". Those individuals exhibiting this band were called Lp(a)+, and those without the band Lp(a)-. We have re-evaluated this method and compared with our quantitative assays and found out that it had a sensitivity of approx. 25 - 30 mg/dl, i.e. individuals with < 30 mg/dl of Lp(a) were "Lp(a)-"
The first quantitative report on the distribution of Lp(a) plasma concentrations among post-M.I. individuals and controls was published by our laboratory in collaboration with the group of Avogaro in Venice [8]. In this study, Lp(a) plasma levels of 76 male post-M.I. patients were measured and compared with that of a control group matched for age and sex. Patients and controls were subdivided into "normolipemics" and hyperlipemics of Fredrickson Types II-IV. The results obtained in that study are shown in Table I.
From this early study we may deduce several rather striking facts:

1) The distribution of Lp(a) plasma concentration is far from normal with median values around 8 - 9 mg/dl.

2) Lp(a) is higher in post-M.I. individuals as compared to a control group. Because of the skew frequency distribution, simple statistics may not be applied to calculate cut-off values. Although it appears that the atherosclerosis risk increases with increasing Lp(a) concentrations, a simple formula considering this observation cannot be calculated. But from this and some consecutive studies we may deduce that Lp(a) levels < 20 - 25 mg/dl may be harmless.

TABLE-I : Lp(a) Values of Post-M.I. Patients and Controls Matched for Age, Sex and HLP-Subtype.

		Lp(a)<25 mg%	Lp(a) 25-50 mg%	Lp(a)>50 mg%
HLP-TYPE	n	% DISTRIBUTION of INDIVIDUALS in the 3 GROUPS		
<u>NL:</u>				
CONTROLS	55	69 %	20 %	11 %
M.I.	36	53 %	22 %	25 %
<u>TYPE-IIA:</u>				
CONTROLS	15	53 %	47 %	0 %
M.I.	1644 %	37 %	19 %	
<u>TYPE-IIB:</u>				
CONTROLS	12	67 %	25 %	8 %
M.I.	11	54 %	27 %	18 %
<u>TYPE-IV</u>				
CONTROLS	25	56 %	28 %	16 %
M.I.	13	61 %	31 %	8 %
<u>ALL SUBJECTS</u>				
CONTROLS	107	64 %	26 %	10 %
M.I.	76	52 %	27 %	21 %

3) Most importantly, however seemed to me the finding that the relative risk at given Lp(a) concentrations depends very much upon the prevalence of other lipoprotein abnormalities: In "normolipemics" and HLP Type-II B, a 2 - 2.5 fold relative risk for Lp(a)+ individuals may be calculated. In the Type-II A group, all of the investigated individual with Lp(a) > 50 mg/dl suffered from M.I. Most surprisingly was the observation that in the group of HLP Type-IV Lp(a)+ individuals were at al <u>lower</u> risk for M.I as compared to controls. We have no explanations for this finding which was consistently observed also in subsequent trials.

From these facts we must conclude that for the evaluation of the individual risk of a given person it is necessary, to analyze in addition to Lp(a) also the whole lipoprotein spectrum.

In addition to this early report we performed several other studies, two of them seem worth noting. 190 individuals, who undervent coronary angiography were assayed for Lp(a). The Results are shown in Tab. II.

It was surprising how similar the results of this study were in comparison to the post-M.I. study. Patients with 1-2- or 3 vessel diseases had much higher Lp(a) values as compared to controls.

TABLE II: Distribution of Lp(a) Values in a Coronary Angiography Study

STENOSIS	n	% Distribution of individuals in the 3 groups Lp(a)<5mg/dl	Lp(a) 5-30 mg/dl	Lp(a)>30 mg/dl
1-2-3 V.D.	126	49 %	19 %	32 % ***
NEGATIVE	64	61 %	22 %	17 %

Finally we asked the question whether or not high Lp(a) values are in fact a genetic marker for M.I. [9]. 1500 young male individuals who undervent routine physical examinations for the Austrian military service were assayed for Lp(a) by a semiquantitative method, counter immunoelectrophoresis . The probands were divided into 2 groups: Group 1 , whose father or mother suffered from M.I., and group 2, whose parents were free of M.I.

TABLE III: Lp(a) Distribution in Young Solders in Relation of the Incidence of M.I. of Their Parents.

Probands with Parents	n	$Lp(a)^-$ (< 30 mg/dl)	$Lp(a)^+$ (> 30 mg/dl)
M.I.+	52	77 %	33 %
M.I.-	1434	87 %	13 %
M.I.-(age matched)	244	85 %	15 %

This study to our mind demonstrate in a most impressive way, not only that Lp(a) is inherited in a dominant way, but also that there is a familial aggregation of high Lp(a) with premature M.I.

Distribution of Lp(a) Values in the Male and Female Population of Styria

In a recent study we have quantified Lp(a) in > 300 male and > 200 female individuals of our county in the age group of 18 - 55 years, using an ELISA technique (paper in preparation). The results are shown in Tab. II and Figs 1 A and 1 B.

TABLE IV: Lp(a) Levels in > 500 Men and Women assayed by ELISA

SEX	Lp(a) Levels, mg/dl MEAN	MEDIAN
MEN (n=317)	14.2 **)	5.5
WOMEN (n=203)	18.0	6.0

***) $p < 0.01$

Men exhibited significantly lower mean Lp(a) levels as compared to women of a similar age group.

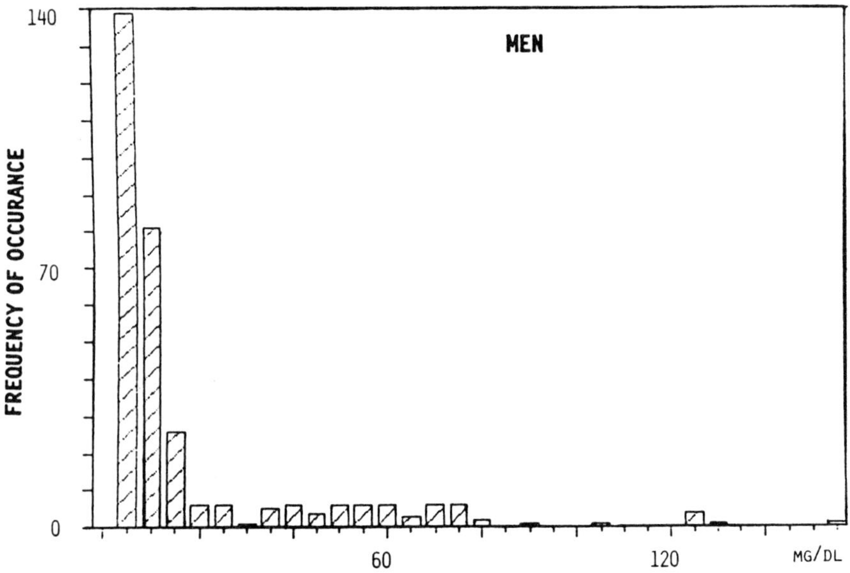

Fig.1 A: Distribution of Plasma Lp(a) Concentration in a Male Styrian Population as Measured by an ELSIA Assay.

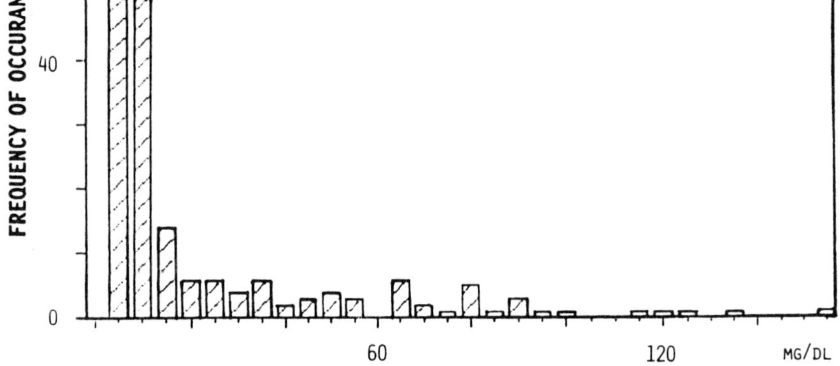

Fig.1 B: Distribution of Plasma Lp(a) Concentration in a Female Styrian Polulation as Measured by an ELISA Assay.

SECONDARY FACTORS INFLUENCING Lp(a) LEVELS

It is known for a long time that Lp(a) plasma levels remain relatively constant over long periods of time. Lp(a) is very low at birth ans raises only slowly in the first months after birth in comparison to Lp B [10]. There is a trend, that Lp(a) is lower in young individuals as compared to an older generation [11]. Lp(a) plasma levels are hardly influenced by diet, although vegetarians appear to have significantly low Lp(a) levels. It is also a known fact that common lipid lowering drugs reducing significantly plasma LDL have little effect on Lp(a) [4]. There are, however, factors known which profundly influence the plasma levels of Lp(a).

Lp(a) in Pregnancy:

We have shown that plasma Lp(a) raise 2 - 3 fold during pregnancy, reaching a maximum at the 20th week of gestation, and coming down again thereafter [12]. There is neither correlation of the extent of Lp(a) increase with the starting plasma level, nor is there any correlation with the fluctuation of hormons e.f. E-2, progesteron, insulin and others. We are also currently studying Lp(a) in post menopausal women and current results suggest that Lp(a) increases significantly in menopause. It thus appears that sex hormons or secundary factors triggered by sex hormons regulate to a certain extent the concentration of Lp(a).

Lp(a) in Alcoholics and Liver Diseases

Studying the frequency distribution of plasma Lp(a) values in heavy chronic alcohol drinkers we noticed a significant shift towards lower values [13]. This was found in persons drinking > 200 g of ethanol per day even before any sign of liver damage was evident. Individuals with signs of liver cirrhosis, Lp(a) was reduced even more strikingly.

Independent from drinking alcohol we als found a profound reduction of plasma Lp(a) in other forms of liver disease, notably in cholestatic patients with high LP-X concentrations. During the course of regenertion of the liver, Lp(a) increased steadily .

Other Factors Influencing Lp(a) Levels

There are several studies currently underway asaying Lp(a) in patients suffering from different forms of renal diseases. In chronic renal failure Lp(a) are more than doubled in comparison to healthy controls. This may reflect the genaral increase of protein synthesis in the liver und this condition, or may have even specific effects. Lp(a) was also postulated to be an acute phase protein and to increase shortly after an myocardial infarction. Also in diabetics Lp(a) tends to rise. Lp(a) Levels in Different Ethnic Groups.
According to findings of Utermann et al [6] there is a striking negative corrlation of Lp(a) plasma concentrations with the molecular weight of the apo-a isoform. This however is valid only among individuals of single ethnic groups. In the black generation

for example, Lp(a) plasma concentrations of individuals with a given isoform are higher as compared to whites . A similar finding might be also true in chineses. It has also been reported that there is a shift of Lp(a)-subtypes towards higher values in familiar hypercholesterolemia.

In conclusion we may say that although Lp(a) levels stay relatively constant, over time, there are many situations known today which have a profound influence on their plasma concentration. The actual mechanism regulating the metabolism of Lp(a), as well as the possible physiological function of this lipoprotein remains a mystery until now.

ACKNOWLEDGEMENTS

These studies were supported by grants from the Österreichischen Forschungsfonds, project programme, S-46 (principal investigator GMK), project number S-4601 and S.4602.

REFERENCES

1. Berg, K. (1963) 'A new serum type system in man - the Lp system', Acta Pathol. Microbiol. Scand. 59, 369 - 382.

2. Kostner, G. M. (1976) 'Lp(a) lipoproteins and the genetic polymorphisms in of lipoprotein B', C.E. Day and R. S. Levy eds, Low Density Lipoproteins, Plenum Press ,229 - 269.

3. Kostner, G. M., Krempler, F. and Sandhofer, F. (1981) 'The lipoprotein Lp(a): Structure, metabolism and significance for vascular diseases', Adv. Physol. Sci (Pergamon), 12, 527 - 534.

4. Kostner, G. M. (1988) 'The affection of lipoprotein-a by lipid lowering drugs', Recents Aspects of Diagnosis and Treatment of Lipoprotein Disorders, Alan R. Liss Inc., 255 - 263.

5. McLean J. W.,Tomlinson, J. E., Scanu, A. M. and Lawn, R. M. (1987) 'DNA sequences of humen apolipoprotein-a is homologous to plasminogen', Naturte 300, 132 - 137.

6. Utermann, G., Menzel, H. J., Kraft H. G.,.uba, H. C., Kremmler, H. G., and Seitz, (1987) 'Lp(a) glycoprotein phenotypes', J. Clin. Invest. 80, 458 - 465.

7. Dahlen, G., Erikson, C., Furberg, C. and Lundquist K. (1972) 'Studies on an extra pre-ß lipoprotein fraction',Acta Med. Scand. Suppl.,531, 1 - 35.

8. Kostner, G. M., Avogaro, P., Cazzolato, G., Marth, E., and Bittolo Bob, G., (1981) 'Lipoprotein lp(a) and the risk for myocardial infarction', Atherosclerosis, 38, 51 - 61.

9. Höfler, G., Harnoncourt, F., Paschke, E., Mirt, W., Pfeiffer, K. P., and Kostner, G. M., (1988) 'Lipoprotein Lp(a). A risk factor for myocardial infarctio', Arteriosclerosis, 8, 398 - 401.

10. Strobl, W., Widhalm, K., Kostner, G. M. and Pollak, A. (1983) 'Serum apolipoproteins and Lp(a) in the first week of life', Acta Paediatr. Scand., 72, 505 - 509.

11. Pagnan, A., Kostner, G. M., Braggion, M, and Ziron, L., (1982) 'Relationship between sinking pre-ß-lipoprotein (Lp(a)) and age in a family kindred', Gerontology, 28, 381 - 385.

12. Zechner, R., Desoye, G., Schweditsch, M., Pfeiffer, K. H. and Kostner G. M., (1986) 'Fluctuation of plasma lipoprotein lp(a) levels during pregnancy and post partum', Metabolism, 35, 333 - 336.

13. Marth, E., Cazzolato, G., Bittolo Bon, G., Avogaro, P. and Kostner G. M., (1982) 'Serum concentrations of Lp(a) and other lipoprotein parameters in heavy alcohol consumers', Ann. Nutrit.Metabol., 26, 56 - 62.

18
LDL and atherosclerosis: from quantity to quality

P. AVOGARO, G. BITTOLO BON and G. CAZZOLATO
Regional General Hospital, 30122 Venice, Italy

Dyslipidemia means "a condition of normolipidemia being present subtle variations of composition a/or structure of lipoproteins". A state of dyslipidemia may concern all the major lipoprotein classes. In this paper will be referred only some variations concerning low density lipoproteins (LDL); the observed variations may explain an atherogenetic power of LDL even when there are normal levels of LDL (normo-LDL-lipidemia).

A first information that the content of LDL-apoB can be abnormally high in atherosclerotic patients came by a study of our group (1). We could record increased levels of apoB in patients survivors of myocardial infarction or complaining angina pectoris whether they are hypercholesterolemic (type IIA) or normocholesterolemic. In some of them therefore the increase of apoB was the only biochemical stigmata. This situation was later more clearly defined and named "Hyperapobeta-lipoproteinaemia" (2). HyperapoB is characterized by an elevated plasma level of the major apoprotein of LDL in the presence of a normal, or near normal level of LDL-cholesterol (LDL-C), producing a low ratio of LDL-C to LDL B protein (LDL C/B) (2). In hyperapoB there is an increased number of LDL particles that are denser, smaller and contain a decreased amount of cholesteryl esters but a relatively increased amount of apoB (3).

Familial defective apoB-100. Elevated LDL levels may result from the presence of abnormal apoB on the surface of LDL particles. Vega and Grundy (4) have identified a group of patients with moderate elevation of LDL-C plasma levels, but apparently normal LDL receptors. A possible explanation for the hypercholesterolemia in these patients is that they have functionally abnormal apoB, that is one that interacts poorly with the B-E receptors. Actually most patients had identical turnover rates for both types of LDL but in some autologous LDL was cleared more slowly than homologous LDL.

Such LDL would be expected to be cleared slowly and accumulate in the plasma. Because LDL binding to B-E receptor is mediated by apoB-100, the defective receptor binding is probably due to structural variation in apoB-100 (5); actually the defective receptor binding remained after the mutant LDL was partially delipidated. The defect is likely the result of a mutation in one of the two copies of the apoB-100 gene. The affected members are heterozygotes who possess a normal and a mutant apoB-100 allele; they have therefore subpopulations of both normal and receptor defective LDL. There is some evidence that some aminoacids substitution, deletion or addition within apoB-100 occurs in a region near residue 3249 (5).

Plasma lipoprotein overproduction, the term proposed by Grundy and Vega (6), represent an excess production of apoB. This primary overproduction is at the root of the increased secretion in the number of lipoprotein particles (VLDL, IDL or LDL). Whether the fraction catabolic rate (FCR) is normal, overproduction of lipoproteins alone does not necessary cause hyperlipidemia. A normolipidemic variant of combined hyperlipidemia belongs to this particular group characterized by overproduction of lipoproteins without hyperlipidemia (7). These patients show premature IHD having normal cholesterol, normal LDL-C, normal LDL-apoB, higher than normal apoB:LDL-C, normal LDL FCR but significantly higher apoB synthetic rate.

The possibility of a genetic defect of apoB in premature IHD has been recently claimed. In patients affected by myocardial infarction and controls the Southern blot analysis with apoB gene probes was performed (8). DNA was digested with endonucleases XbaI and EcoRi. Alleles designed as X1, X2, X3 and R1 and R2 were obtained. The frequencies of X1, R1 and ID1 were all significntly higher than in the controls. None of the alleles in this study was significantly associated with plasma levels of LDL or apoB. Recently however in a random sample of subjects people having omozygosity for the X2 allele of the XbaI restriction fragment length polymorphism a higher mean total and LDL cholesterol and a lower FCR were found (9).

Other studies have shown that the individuals LDL are immunochemically different (10); the different apoB immunoreactivities may be explained by the chemical and structural heterogeneity of apoB components in isolated LDL. Insofar some studies have tried to determine whether the employment of monoclonal antibodies may be more hepful than the determination of apoB with the usual assays in discriminating between patients and controls. The employment of the monoclonal antibody LP+22 (10) succeeded in discriminating patients with IHD from people without IHD. The result appears relevant as some of the IHD patients had apoB values well within the normal range.

Another group of people affected by IHD may be characterized by high values of Lp(a) or of apo(a) being normal the plasma values of "historical" parameters (total cholesterol, triglycerides, LDL-C). Lp(a) lipoprotein is a LDL-like particle with the same lipid composition; its protein moiety contains apoB-100 linked to the Lp(a) specific glycoprotein by disulfide bonds. Apo(a) may be higher than normal in normolipidemics (11) being correlated only with a parental history of myocardial infarction. Recently it was raised the interesting possibility that the association of Lp(a) levels with atherosclerosis may due to differences in Lp(a) concentration species rather than to differences in the concentration of lipoprotein (12). A new method has allowed to establish that Lp(a) may present several phenotypes; they are controlled by five allels that code for from B, S1, S2, S3, S4 or Lp(a) glycoprotein and by a "O" allel. The interest of the finding is that Lp(a) type, rather than concentration, is a risk factor for premature IHD.

Recently we succeeded in isolating a modified LDL in humans (13). This abnormal LDL may consistently contribute to the entire mass of LDL. This modified LDL shares many of the features peculiar of LDL modified by endothelial cells studied by Stinberg et al. (14). This LDL binds poorly to the LDL-receptor of fibroblasts and shows a different behaviour when tested with different monoclonal antibodies to apoB; the response is poor with the monoclonal antibodies testing the binding region domain of apoB. This modified LDL may occur in both hyperlipidemic and normolipidemic patients and seems to be more consistently formed in atherosclerotic patients. It is likely that LDL modified "in vivo" by peroxidative processes contribute to the formation of atheroma even when the plasma lipids a/or lipoproteins are normal.

REFERENCES

1. Avogaro, P., Cazzolato, G., Bittolo Bon, G., Quinci, G.B. and Belussi, F. (1978) 'Plasma levels of apolipoprotein A-I and apolipoprotein B in human atherosclerosis', Artery 4, 385-394.
2. Sniderman, A., Shapiro, S., Maropole, D., Skinner, B., Teng, B. and Kwiterovich, P.O., Jr. (1980) 'Association of coronary atherosclerosis with hyperapobetalipoproteinemia (increased protein but normal cholesterol levels in human plasma low density ( ) lipoproteins)', Proc. Nat. Acad. Sc. 77, 604-608
3. Teng, B., Thompson, G.R., Sniderman, A.D., Forte, T.M., Krauss, R.M. and Kwiterovich, P.O., Jr. (1983) 'Composition and distribution of low density lipoprotein fractions in hyperapobetalipoproteinemia, normolipidemia and familial

hypercholesterolemia', Proc. Natl. Acad. Sci. 80, 662-666.
4. Vega, G.L. and Grundy, S.M. (1986) 'In vivo evidence for reduced binding of low density lipoproteins to rceptors as a cause of primary moderate hypercholesterolemia'. J. Clin. Invest. 78, 1410-1414.
5. Innerarity, T.S., Weisgraber, K.H., Arnold, K.S., Mahley, R.W., Krauss, R.M., Vega, G.L. and Grundy, S.M. (1987) 'Familial defective apolipoprotein B-100: low density lipoproteins with abnormal receptor binding'. Proc. Natl. Acad. Sci. USA 84, 6919-6923.
6. Grundy, G.M. and Vega, G.L. (1984) 'Apolipoprotein B and disorders of lipoprotein in man', in De Gennes, J.L. et al. (eds), Latent Dyslipoproteinemias and atherosclerosis, Raven Press, New York 225-246
7. Kesaniemy, Y.A. and Grundy, S.M. (1983) 'Overproduction of low density lipoproteins associated with coronary heart disease', Arteriosclerosis 3, 40-46.
8. Hegele, R.A., Huang, L-S, Herbert, P.N., Baum, C.B., Buring, J.E., Hennekens, C.H. and Breslow, J.L. (1986), 'ApolipoproteinB-gene DNA polymorphism associated with myocardial infarction', N. Engl. J. Med. 315, 1509-1514
9. Houlston, R.S., Turner, P.R., Revill, J., Lewis, B. and Humphries, S.E. (1988) 'The fractional catabolic rate of low density lipoprotein in normal individuals is influenced by variation in the apolipoprotein B-gene: a preliminary study', Atherosclerosis 71, 81-85.
10. Patton, J.G., Badimon, J. and Mao, S.J.T. (1983) 'Monoclonal antibodies to human plasma low density lipoproteins. II. Evaluation for use in radioimmunoassay for apolipoprotein B in patients with coronary artery disease', Clin. Chem. 29, 1898-1903.
11. Darrington, P.N., Ishola, M., Hunt, L., Arrol, S. and Bhatnagar, D. (1988) 'Apolipoproteins(a), A-I and B and parental history in men with early onsed ischaemic heart disease', Lancet i, 1070-1073.
12. Kraft, H.G., Dieplinger, H., Hoye, E. and Uterman, G. (1988) 'Lp(a) phenotyping by immunoblotting with polyclonal and monoclonal antibodies', Arteriosclerosis 8, 212-216.
13. Avogaro, P., Bittolo Bon, G. and Cazzolato, G. (1988) 'Presence of a modified low density lipoprotein in humans'. Arteriosclerosis 8, 79-87.
14. Steinberg, D. (1983) 'Lipoproteins and atherosclerosis. A look back and a look ahead', Arteriosclerosis 3, 283-301.

19
Lipid distribution in human coronary lesions: analysis by digital imaging microscopy

L.C. SMITH and Ž. JERIČEVIĆ

Baylor College of Medicine and The Methodist Hospital, Departments of Medicine and Cell Biology, 6565 Fannin Street, MS A-601 Houston, TX 77030, USA

ABSTRACT. The pathophysiology of atherosclerosis occurs at the cellular level. Using a digital imaging fluorescence microscopy system and computer based methods, the 3-dimensional coordinates for lipid droplets, smooth muscle cells and macrophages in an arterial wall specimen can be obtained by a single experimental protocol. The experimental approach is to acquire at 2 μm intervals, bright field images and fluorescence images using a combination of lipid stains and monoclonal antibodies. After appropriate image processing, the data sets are combined to establish, with 3-dimensional coordinates, the spatial relationships of these components in the arterial wall. Quantitation of fluorescence requires information in three dimensions. It is obvious that the more easily observed two dimensional heterogeneity must also extend to three dimensions. The series of optical sections is usually achieved by moving the specimen along the z axis by computer controlled stage movement. When other fluorescent sources are nearby, but not in the focal plane, their fluorescence extend to overlap the fluorescent emission of the object of interest in the focal plane. The experimental problem of out-of-plane fluorescence is avoided by using a laser scanning confocal fluorescence microscope, which has an aperature in front of the detector to exclude fluorescence originating from locations other than the diffraction-limited excitation point source. We find predominately small intracellular nile red staining lipid droplets dispersed throughout the vessel wall. The larger extracellular droplets are confined largely to the lesion area, presumably in macrophages.

INTRODUCTION

Lipid accumulation is a central feature of atherosclerosis. Transverse sections of human left anterior descending coronary arteries contain grossly normal areas, a visible lesion and transition areas. Our premise is that the changes in the spatial relation-ships of the lipid deposits, the smooth muscle cells and the macrophages in the transition from normal to diseased regions of the vessel can provide insight into the mechanisms by which the lesions become more complex with time. As a working hypothesis, we suggest that the arterial wall has a limited capacity to utilize or store cholesterol associated with lipoprotein flux. As a result of endothelial injury and/or elevated levels of plasma lipo-proteins, this metabolic capacity can be exceeded. Intracellular lipid deposits in both macrophages and smooth muscle cells ensure. With the high lipoprotein flux, extracellular lipid accumulates, principally as cholesteryl ester droplets and crystalline cholesterol deposits in macrophages. We envision that the progression of the lesion to involve initially small cytoplasmic lipid droplets on smooth muscle cells. The appearance of macrophages coincides with the occurrence of large intracellular lipid deposits in smooth muscle cells. As the macrophage population increases, extracellular lipid deposits appear. To obtain experimental data to address the working hypothesis, bright field images and fluorescence images are acquired at 2 μm intervals in arterial wall specimens treated with a combination of lipid stains and monoclonal antibodies. After appropriate image processing, the data sets are combined to establish, with 3-dimensional coordinates, the spatial relationships of these components the fatty streak lesion of the left anterior descending coronary artery.

The inherent difficulty in making quantitative fluorescence measurements arises from the fact that there is no simple relation between the intensity of the excitation light, the intensity of the emitted fluorescent light and the fluorophore concentration.

$$I_{obs} = I_{exc}\,\Phi\,(1-e^{-\varepsilon cl})$$

where I_{obs} is the observed intensity of the fluorescence emission, I_{exc} is the intensity of the excitation light, Φ is the quantum yield of the fluorophore, ε is molar absorptivity of the fluorophore at the excitation wavelength, c is the concentration of the fluorophore and l is the pathlength for light absorption. The quantum yield Φ is defined by the relationship $k_F/(k_F + \Sigma k_{NR})$, where k_F is the rate constant for fluorescence and the Σk_{NR} denotes the collective rate constants for non-radiative processes.

Following excitation, fluorescence light is emitted from the fluorophore in all directions in a spherical envelope. The microscope samples a thin slice as an optical section through this sphere. Quantitation of fluorescence requires this type of information in three dimensions. It is obvious that the more easily observed two dimensional heterogeneity must necessarily extend to three dimensions. The series of optical sections is usually achieved by moving the specimen along the z axis by computer controlled stage movement. The arterial wall specimens are 50 μm thick. With a conventional light microscope, the interference from light scattering increases as the optical section is positioned deeper into the tissue. When other fluorescent sources are nearby, but not in the focal plane, their fluorescence will overlap the fluorescence of the object of interest in the focal plane. Thus, the measured intensity of the object is the sum of fluorescence from all sources, those in focus as well as those located both above and below the plane of focus. The magnitude of the out-of-plane contribution to the observed fluorescence is not known, but has been estimated to be as much as 90% of the total signal, depending on the numerical aperture of the objective and the depth of focus compared to the thickness of the specimen. It is not possible to know that differences in the intensity of signal in the focal plane are only the result of different concentrations of fluorophore and not due to the camera response and/or differences in the illumination, thus precluding quantitative studies.

The raster scanning laser systems with computer-controlled image acquisition (White et al. 1987) have been the key development to allow entry of image processing and quantitative image analysis. The laser scanning confocal optical microscope uses a diffraction limited focal spot as the imaging light source. The principles of confocal imaging have been described by Wilson and Sheppard (1984) and Sheppard (1987). Confocal imaging has applications in reflected light as well as fluorescence imaging. A survey of applications has been provided by Dixon and Benham (1987). The key element of confocal optics is a small aperture positioned at the secondary focus of the objective lens in the reflected light path (Figure 1). The size of this aperture is such that

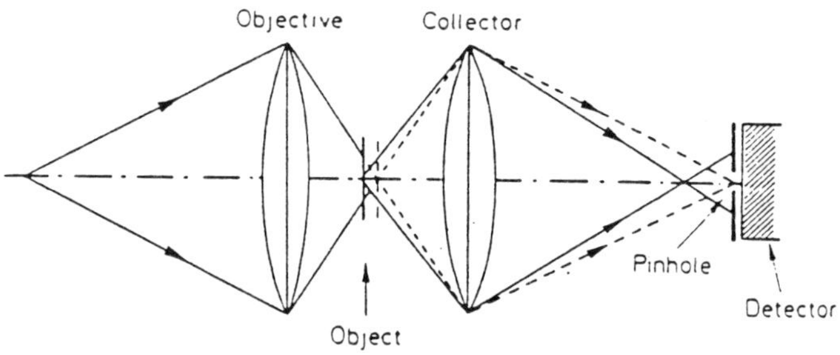

Figure 1. The basic concept of confocal imaging. A spatial filter (pinhole) in front of the detector blocks the out-of-focus light whereas the light from the object in the exact focal plane of the laser excitation (dashed lines), will pass through the pinhole without attenuation.

its virtual image at the sample is approximately the same size as the focal spot. The sharpness of the intensity drop for out-of-focus planes determines the depth contrast. Depending on the numerical aperture of the objective, the "thickness" of the in-focus plane can range between 0.5 - 1.5 μm. The result is an image of high lateral contrast without diffuse background intensity contribution (Wilson and Sheppard, 1984). The exceptionally shallow depth of field of the confocal microscope provides direct optical sectioning. This, together with a spatial resolution of 0.3 μm and existing algorithms, will make confocal scanning laser microscopy the most effective and useful means to obtain the three dimensional information.

MATERIALS AND METHODS

The human LAD specimens were obtained by a common protocol established for the multicenter cooperative study of the pathobiological determinants of atherosclerosis in youth, directed by Dr. Robert W. Wissler, University of Chicago, Chicago, Illinois, USA. The imaging system and analytic procedures for data acquisition and analysis have been described (Plant et al. 1985; Benson et al. 1985; Smith et al. 1987, 1988; Jerecevic et al. 1988, 1989).

RESULTS

Images that are useless in conventional microscopy, because of the scatter associated with ordinary illumination, can be captured clearly by confocal techniques. Coronary artery 37 has been imaged using epi-illumination (Figure 2) and with confocal laser scanning (Figure 3).

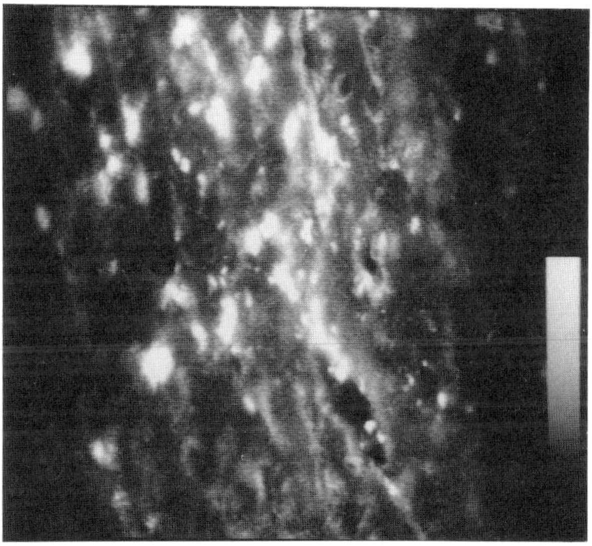

FIGURE 2. LAD 37 was stained with rabbit anti-ATPase that was visualized with FITC-goat anti-rabbit IgG. In addition the specimen was incubated with a nile red/albumin complex to visualize lipid droplets. The intensity levels in the image range from 0 as black to 255 as white on the gray level bar at the right side of the figure.

With an excitation intensity that gave a reasonable definition of the boundaries, the out-of-plane fluorescence saturated the camera. The boundaries are blurred and poorly defined in this image obtained with

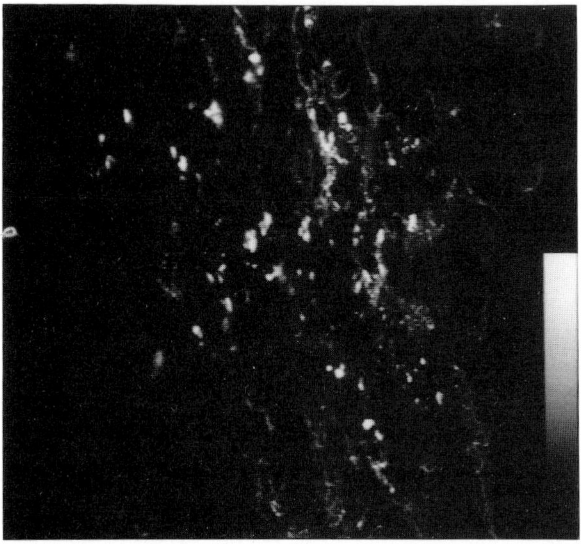

Figure 3. Confocal imaging of FITC goat anti-rabbit anti-ATPase. The configuration of the conventional microscope was changed to the confocal mode to image the same optical section imaged in Figure 2.

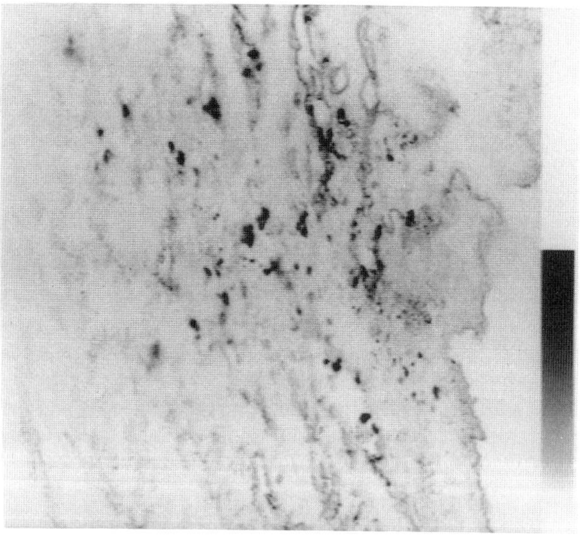

Figure 4. Data from Figure 3 displayed with an inverted gray scale.

conventional microscope optics. Confocal imaging minimizes the out-of-plane contribution and the image is suitable for boundary identification by thresholding without further processing. One advantage of digital imaging is the ease with which the data display can be changed. Figure 4 is the same data that is shown as Figure 3. The display has been changed so that low intensity values are shown as white and high intensity values are black. The spatial relationship of the lipid droplets to other cellular features is much more apparent in Figure 4.

Another LAD specimen was stained simultaneously with propidium iodide to identify the nuclei and nile red to visualize the lipid dropletes. The small bright lipid droplets, as visualized with nile red occur frequently and have an intracellular location (Figure 5).

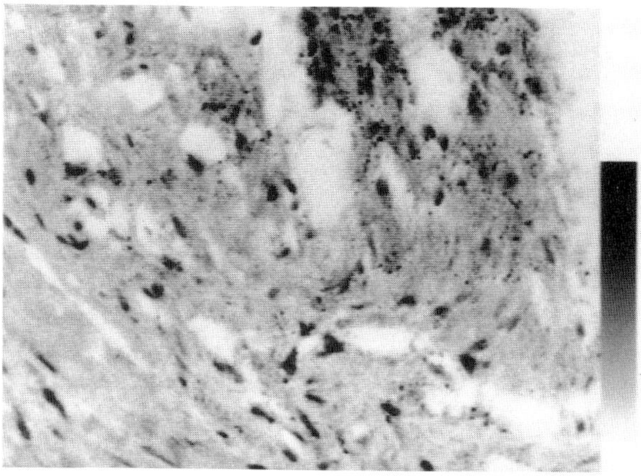

Figure 5. LAD stained for nuclei and for lipid droplets.

The perinuclear clustering in the upper left region of the image is striking and appears associated with polyploid cells, presumably macrophages.

Photobleaching is a pervasive experimental problem with conventional microscopy and constrains confocal laser scanning microscopy even more severely. An illustration of the inability to obtain quantatitive information because of photobleaching is shown in Figure 6. The loss in information is demonstrated by thresholding the fluorescence intensity values in an image of an arterial specimen, a portion of which had been scanned repeatedly. Thresholding of the image identifies the regions with high fluorescence. The area inside the boundaries had intensity values of 150 or greater. The upper half of the arterial specimen was scanned for 20 images. The lower half of the image was scanned once to record the image. As expected, the loss of fluorescence was not uniform. The severity of photobleaching is an experimental variable that must be evaluated emperically with each specimen. Subtraction of digital images serves as a rough guide for experimentation.

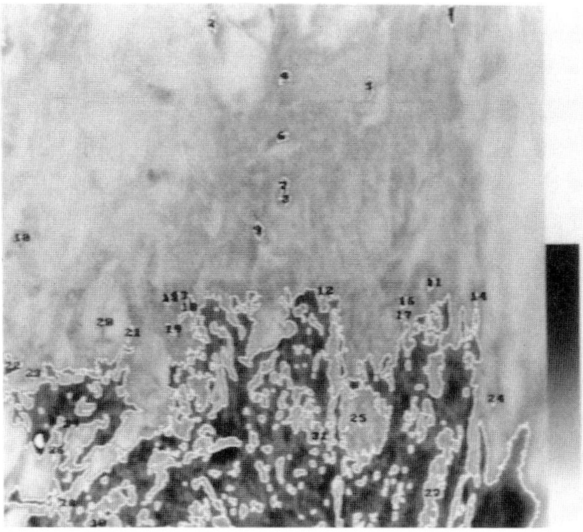

Figure 6. Effect of photobleaching of fluorescence measurements.

DISCUSSION

Computer based methods developed by Cornhill and associates have allowed the creation of and utilization of probability maps of arterial lesions at the macroscopic level. The numerical procedures have overcome the confounding effects of specimen to specimen variability and provided an underlying statistical basis for data analysis. This method will be applicable to our studies at the cellular level and provide the insight obtained from objective statistical methods. Automated computer based methods are necessary, first to obtain the large amounts of data on a cell by cell basis size, and second, to analyze this data in a systematic fashion. The analytical endpoints are: (a) the identity of cells containing lipid droplets, (b) the proportion of smooth muscle cells and macro-phages in each raised lesion, (c) the number of lipid droplets in each lesion, and (d) the 3 dimensional distribution of these cells and droplets in each lesion with respect to the direction of blood flow. The epidemiologic variables are (a) the age and (b) cholesterol values of the donors. Elements of the data base can then be compared with respect to age, race, sex, risk factors, arterial topography and likelihood of lesion progression.

ACKNOWLEDGEMENTS

This work was supported in part by the National Institutes of Health, the Robert A. Welch Foundation (Q-343) and The Methodist Hospital. We are pleased to acknowledge the excellent technical assistance of Brent A. Wise and Faith Strickland.

REFERENCES

Benson, D.M., Plant, A.L., Bryan, J., Gotto, Jr., A.M., and Smith, L.C. (1985) J. Cell Biol. 100:1309-1323.

Dixon, A.J., and Benham, G.S. (1987) Am. Lab. **19**:20-25.

Jericevic, Z., B. Wiese, J. Bryan and L.C. Smith. (1988) Meth. Cell Biol. **30**:47-83.

Jericevic, Z., Wiese, B., Homan, R., Bryan, J., and Smith, L.C. (1989) Adv. Cell Biol. (K.R. Miller, Ed.), in press.

Plant, A.L., Benson, D.M., and Smith, L.C. (1985) J. Cell Biol. 100:1295-1308.

Sheppard, C.J.R. (1987) Adv. Optical and Electron Microscopy, **10**:1-99.

Smith, L.C., Benson, D.M., Gotto, A.M., and Bryan, J. (1986) Methods in Enzymology (J.J. Albers and J. E. Segrest, eds.) Academic Press, New York, NY. **129**: 857-873.

Smith, L.C., Benson, D.M., Plant, A.L., and Gotto, Jr., A.M. (1988) Arztl. Lab. **34**:53-59.

White, J., Amos, W.B. and Fordham, M. (1987) J. Cell Biol. **105**:41-48.

Wilson, T., and Sheppard, C. (1984) Theory and Practice of Scanning Optical Microscopy, Academic Press, London.

NUTRITION: POPULATION STUDIES

20
Time trends of risk factors for coronary heart disease in southern Italy

E. FARINARO, S. PANICO, R. GALASSO, G. FUSCO, F. JOSSA, D. GIUMETTI, E. CELENTANO and M. MANCINI

Institute of Internal Medicine and Metabolic Disease, 2nd Medical School, via Sergio Pansini 5, 80131 Naples, Italy

ABSTRACT. In the last years an unfavourable trend in dietary habits has been observed in Italy, which is recognized to have a low occurrence rate of coronary heart disease. Time trends for some coronary heart disease risk factors related to environmental exposure, have been evaluated using data from the Olivetti longitudinal study. Data of ten year follow-up on one thousand people have been used for this purpose. An unfavourable trend for the average levels of some risk factors was detected in all age groups. Systolic blood pressure (SBP) showed an average increase of 6 mmHg in the population as whole, the greatest increase being experienced in the 20-29 age group. Diastolic blood pressure (DBP) increased from 82 to 89 mmHg. Serum cholesterol (CHOL) at ten years follow-up was 27 mg/dl higher with greatest increase at younger ages. Body mass index (BMI) was almost unchanged over years as well as triglyceride. The unfavourable trend observed in some major risk factors for cardiovascular disease reflects unfavourable changes in lifestyle related to them, including eating habits, have characterized the last thirty years in Italy.

Introduction

In the last decades some differences in coronary heart disease (CHD) mortality trends have been observed when comparing North America, Australia, and Europe [1, 2]. While in North America and Australia a decline in CHD mortality has been consistently found, among European countries some differences have been observed. Interestingly one major finding is related to the Mediterranean side of Europe. In terms of CHD mortality this part of world is experiencing mostly an increasing trend (in some cases a stable one). Italy is a valuable observatory since in the central and in the northern part of the country the trend in CHD mortality seems to be in general stable, whereas in the southern part - the more Mediterranean from the geographical and cultural view point - there is still an increasing trend [3, 4].

In the part of the world where a decline of CHD death rates have been observed, changes in life style and the consequent changes in risk factors related to them, together with the development of a concerned public policy have been claimed as possible reasons to explain this phenomenon. In the United States, in Finland, in Australia - countries where the decline has been consistent over time and dramatic - there have been changes in eating patterns, with a reduction of dietary fat, cholesterol, sugar, salt intake, all added to some efforts to reduce weight. Cigarette smoking has recorded a progressive decrease and leisure time dedicated to physical exercise has been increased by great number of people. In addition, detection, treatment, and control of high blood pressure have reached a very high standard [5].

By contrast, where there is an increase of CHD mortality rates, no such improvements in life style have been observed with negative consequences on risk profile [6]. Few analytical data are available on populations in which a cultural advantage has been registered in the past such as mediterranean ones. This paper present data coming from observations on a southern Italian population followed along the last decade to analyze the trend in risk profile for CHD.

Material and Methods

POPULATION. Employees of the Olivetti factory in the city-area of Naples were first recruited in 1976. Baseline examination was performed on 1,175 men, in the age-range 20-59 years [7, 8]). Two subsequent visits were performed after five and eleven years in 578 individuals on which the analysis of this paper is based.

MEASUREMENTS. The participants were instructed to fast for at least 12 hours the night before the examination. On the next morning the workers were weighted on a standard beam balance scale, with usual indoor clothing and without shoes; height was determined using a fixed ruler attached to the scale, body mass index (BMI) was subsequently calculated - weight (kg) / [height (m)]^2 -.

They were asked to rest at least 10 minutes; the blood pressure was recorded twice - in supine position - with readings made two minutes apart, using a mercury sphygmomanometer, with the mean values of the two readings recorded for SBP, and 5th phase DBP.

Blood was drawn without venostasis and stored; serum lipids - CHOL, and TG - were determined. At first examination the extractive method by Levine and Zak [9] was used for determination of CHOL and Kessler and Lederer method [10] for TG. Both methods were adapted to the automathed analyzer - CLA 1510; Carlo Erba Strumentazione [11] -. In the second and in the third examination serum lipids were determined by enzymatic automated methods adapted to an Hitachi 737-Boheringer Mannheim analyzer [12, 13]. Correction has been made to allow data comparability in trend analysis.

This sample has been divided in 3 age groups, each of them ranging ten years, according to baseline age.

DATA ANALYSIS. Mean values adjusted by age and BMI have been calculated and analysis of variance for multiple measurements were performed using SPSSPC statistical package for personal computer [14].

Results

In tables 1, 2, 3, 4, and 5, mean values of BMI, SBP, DBP, CHOL, and TG, adjusted for age and BMI, observed in the three visits, are shown by baseline decade of age.

Body mass index, SBP, DBP, and CHOL increase with age, either observing the same individuals in the three examinations, and analyzing data of different individuals at the same visit. Body mass index, DBP, and CHOL mean values increase is statistically significant in the same individuals at the three different visits; BMI, SBP at baseline and in the third examination, DBP at baseline mean values show a significant statistical increase from the cross-sectional view. It is also remarkable that groups of people of the same age in different time have higher mean values in 1987 then in 1976. Statistical significance is found when BMI, DBP, and CHOL mean values of individuals aged 30-39 in 1987 are compared with ones of individuals aged 30-39 in 1976.

Triglycerides mean values show slight differences with age and time in the three examinations.

TABLE 1. BMI (kg/m^2) mean values in a free living working population sample of Southern Italy - The Olivetti Survey.

AGE in 1976 (years)		BASELINE 1976 (mean)	FOLLOW-UP 1981 (mean)	1987 (mean)	p
20-29	128	24.4	25.4	25.9°	.000
30-39	320	24.8^	25.9	26.4°°	.000
40-49	130	25.4^^	26.7	27.0	.000
p		.022	.003	.014	
20-49	578	24.8	25.9	26.4	.000

° vs ^ : p = 0.045; °° vs ^^ : p = 0.299

TABLE 2. SBP (mmHg) mean values adjusted by age and BMI, in a free living working population sample of Southern Italy

The Olivetti Survey.

AGE in 1976		BASELINE 1976	FOLLOW-UP 1981	1987	p
20-29	125	121.8	130.2	128.9	ns
30-39	316	125.1	129.6	126.5	ns
40-49	130	126.1	130.7	131.6	ns
p		.003	.738	.051	
20-49	571	125.3	130.0	128.0	ns

TABLE 3. DBP (mmHg) mean values adjusted by age and BMI, in a free living working population sample of Southern Italy

- The Olivetti Survey.

AGE in 1976		BASELINE 1976	FOLLOW-UP 1981	1987	p
20-29	125	79.0	83.5	87.4°	.000
30-39	316	82.3^	83.9	87.3°°	.000
40-49	130	85.8^^	84.7	89.3	.000
p		.033	.689	.331	
0-49	571	82.4	84.0	87.7	.000

° vs ^ : p = 0.012; °° vs ^^ : p = 0.009

TABLE 4. CHOL (mg/dl) mean values adjusted by age and BMI, in a free living working population sample of Southern Italy

- The Olivetti Survey.

AGE in 1976		BASELINE 1976	FOLLOW-UP 1981	1987	p
20-29	122	177.7	190.6	208.3°	.000
30-39	295	189.9^	195.8	211.8°°	.000
40-49	117	200.7^^	200.0	215.2	.000
p		.201	.393	.358	
20-49	534	189.7	195.2	212.1	.000

° vs ^ : p = 0.012; °° vs ^^ : p = 0.009

TABLE 5. TG (mg/dl) mean values adjusted by age and BMI, in a free living working population sample of Southern Italy

- The Olivetti Survey.

AGE in 1976		BASELINE 1976	FOLLOW-UP 1981	1987	p
20-29	119	118.5	107.5	154.6	ns
30-39	291	135.2	127.6	145.7	ns
40-49	116	140.9	153.8	137.9	ns
p		ns	ns	ns	
20-49	534	130.7	129.7	149.8	ns

Discussion

In United States, after a sharp increase in CHD mortality that lasted more than fourty years, mortality rates for this disease have greatly decreased since the 1960s. At the present time male and female CHD mortality is still declining. The magnitude of this decrease is 3% per year. Smaller declines have also occured in some other industrialized countries, particularly in Australia, New Zealand, and Canada [1].

In Europe the figures related to CHD mortality and the geographical distribution of the related risk factors differ from country to country. In general, some European countries in the last few years have registered a decline of the total mortality from 38% to 32% for men aged 25-64 years.

Many European countries, such as the Netherlands, Belgium, Norway, Israel, have shown a decline in CHD mortality and in Finland, were this trend is the strongest, the rates show a 20% decrease in 10 years. On the contrary, an unfavourable trend has been observed in a number of Eastern European countries, Sweden, Spain, and to some extent, in Italy, - were there are local variations between Southern and Northern regions.

Indeed in the Eastern countries since 1970 CHD mortality accounts for more than 50% of the total mortality in 10 years. All these changes were generally confined to the younger age groups.

It has been continuously observed that Southern Italy is a traditionally low risk region for coronary heart disease; this advantage, compared to other industrialized countries depends mostly upon the lifestyle and upon the typical Mediterranean diet [15, 16]. Traditional dietary habits in this region reflect almost entirely the dietary recommendations of various Heart and Nutrition Foundations focusing on Prevention of Coronary Heart Diseases. Nevertheless, an increase in CHD mortality and in the levels of some variables considered risk factors for CHD in the last two decades, in Southern Italy has been registered. This unfavourable change seems to be strictly related to changes in lifestyle. The increased industrialization, the concomitant use of automatic facilities with a consequent reduction of physical exercise, and the overall changes in dietary habits have induced some important modifications in Mediterranean populations.

In the last decade there has been an increase in total calories intake, total fats, saturated fat, dietary cholesterol, which have led to a consequent reduction of complex carbohydrates, vegetables, and fibers. In the meantime the average levels of CHOL have gone up (2 mg/dl per year), average body weight has increased and blood pressure has also shown an upward trend. This issue was raised at the European Consensus Conference organized a few years ago in Naples by the European Atherosclerosis Society [17]. The data from the Olivetti Survey confirm the changes described demostrating that the situation has been deteriorating year by year, indicating that also in a traditional Mediterranean country risk factors need to be approached in a vigorous and widespread way in order to prevent the modern epidemics of coronary heart disease.

References

1- Uemura, K. and Pisa, Z. (1988) 'Trends in cardiovascular disease in industrialized countries', World Health Statistics Quarterly 41, 155-178.
2- Thom, T.J., Epstein, F.H., Feldman, J.J., Leaverton, P.E. (1985) 'Trends in total mortality from heart diseases in 26 countries from 1950 to 1978', International Journal of Epidemiology 14, 510-520.
3- Nicolosi, A., Casati, S., Taioli, E., Polli, E. (1988) 'Death from cardiovascular disease in Italy, 1972-1981: Decline in mortality rates and possible causes', International Journal of Epidemiology 17, 766-772.
4- Arcà, M., Di Orio, F., Forastiere, F., Tasco, C., Perucci, C.A. (1988) 'Years of potential life lost (YPLL) before age 65 in Italy', Am. J. Public Health 78, 1202-1205.
5- Dwyer, T., Hetzel, B.S. (1980) ' A comparison of trends of coronary heart disease mortality in Australia, USA and England and Wales with reference to three major risk factors - hypertension, cigarette smoking and diet', International Journal of Epidemiology 9, 65-71.
6- Research Group ATS-RF2-Ob43 of the Italian National Research Council (1987) 'Time trends of some cardiovascular risk factors in Italy. Results from the Nine Italian Communities Study', American Journal of Epidemiology 126, 95-103.
7- Farinaro, E., Panico, S., Oriente, P., Paggi, E., and Mancini, M. (1978) ' Prevalence of risk factors in an urban working population of Southern Italy', in L.A. Carlson, R. Paoletti, C. R. Sirtori, G. Weber (eds.) International Conference on Atherosclerosis - Milan, 1977, Raven Press, New York, pp. 375-378.
8- Farinaro, E., Panico, S., Oriente, P., Mancini, M. (1979) 'The Olivetti Survey: asymptomatic hyperglicemia and ECG abnormalities at baseline', Journal of Chronic Disease 32, 773-777.
9- Abell, L.L., Levy, B.B., Brodie, B.B., Kendall, F.E. (1952) 'A simplified method for estimation of total cholesterol in serum and demostration of its specificity', J. Biol. Chem. 195, 357-366.
10- Pantulu, G.V.A., Anderson, J.T., Keys, A. (1964) ' A rapid and specific method fro serum triglycerides determination', Fed. Proc. 24, 438-441.
11- Oriente, P., Di Marino, L., Mastranzo, P., Iovine, C., Patti, L. (1979) 'Simultaneous determination of cholesterol and triglycerides in serum and lipoprotein fractions with enzymatic automated methods', in A. Burlina and L. Galzigna (eds.) Clinical enzymology Symposia - vol. II - Piccin Medical Books, Padova, pp. 387-402.

12- Siedel, J., et al. (1981) J. Clin. Chem. Clin. Biochem. 19, 838.
13- Nagele U., et al. (1984) J. Clin. Chem. Clin. Biochem. 22, 165-174.
14- Norusis, M.J. (1986) 'Statistical Package for Social Science - SPSSPC+', SPSS inc., Chicago.
15- Mariani Costantini A. (1983) 'Evoluzione del comportamento alimentare in Italia' Agg. Med. 3, 692-706.
16- Gruppo di Ricerca ATS-RF2 (1980) 'I fattori di rischio dell'arteriosclerosi in Italia', Giornale Italiano di Cardiologia 10 (Supp. 3), 1-184.
17- Study Group, European Atherosclerosis Society (1987) 'Strategies for the prevention of coronary heart disease: A policy statement of the European Atherosclerosis Society', European Heart Journal 8, 77-88.

21
Nutritional aspects in the C.N.R. 'DI.S.CO.' Project

G. RICCI, F. ANGELICO, M. DEL BEN and G.C. URBINATI

Institute of Systematic Medical Therapeutics, University of Rome "La Sapienza", Policlinico Umberto I - Viale del Policlinico, 00161 Roma, Italy

ABSTRACT. This article is concerned with the nutritional intervention in the 'DI.S.CO' Project (Sezze District Community Control of Chronic Dis= eases) of the Italian National Research Council. This project was aimed at reducing morbidity and mortality from certain chronic diseases through an intervention of community medicine intended to modify the lifestyle of an intervention population. The article focuses on description of dietary habits at the baseline survey and on the nutrition intervention activities. Some preliminary data on risk factors changes are also reported.

Dietary interventions play a major role in community medicine for the negative implications that a wrong nutritional approach - either quantitative or qualitative - has on some of the main risk factors for atherosclerosis and its complications, such as plasma lipid levels (total and LDL-cholesterol, triglycerides), arterial blood pressure, body weight, etc.

This is all the more true considering the results of the most recent primary prevention trials of coronary heart disease through drug therapy (cholestyramine, gemfibrozil) (1, 2) which confirmed that each 1% reduction in total or LDL-cholesterol yields approximately a 2% reduction in CHD morbidity and mortality rates.

This unequivocal body of evidence, which allowed blood cholesterol to be considered a 'causal' factor in the pathogenesis of ischemic heart disease and of other complications of atherosclerosis, prompted the Consensus Conferences held in several parts of the world to stress the time has come to take action through population-based strategies, as well as through the patient-based approach, i.e. aimed at high risk subjects. Education campaigns to lower blood cholesterol levels in the population have been launched in the United States and Italy (3, 4, 5). The 'prudent' diet recommended to prevent degenerative cardiovascular diseases is also fit for the prevention of a number of cancers, as shown in several epidemiological studies (6, 7, 8).

The role of non-pharmacological measures in reducing blood pressure values, among which diet ranks first, either alone or combined with drug therapy, cannot be underestimated. As a matter of fact, epidemiological studies have indicated, although less conclusively, that dietary sodium intake is related to arterial blood pressure (9) and that reducing borderline hypertension (SBP 140-159 and/or DBP 90-94 mmHg) will result in a reduced number of total endpoints (10, 11).

The present article is concerned with the nutritional intervention carried out within the 'DI.S.CO.' Project (Sezze District Community Control of Chronic and Degenerative Diseases)in the framework of the Targeted Project 'Preventive Medicine and Rehabilitation' of C.N.R. (National Research Council of Italy) (12). This Project was aimed at starting a pilot study with the object of reducing morbidity and mortality from certain chronic diseases in a population referring to a Health District (Unità Sanitaria Locale = USL), through direct intervention of community medicine intended to modify the lifestyle of three intervention areas (municipalities of Sezze, Bassiano and Roccagorga), as compared to a control area (municipality of Priverno). Since the District had already been included in the surveillance system MONICA (WHO collaborative program for monitoring cardiovascular diseases), the evaluation of morbidity and mortality trends for cardiovascular events, as well as of the efficacy of preventive measures, is likely to be easier. The overall situation, as far as the mean initial levels of the main risk factors influenced by dietary habits are concerned, was found to be worse than might have been expected on the basis of the results of the ATS-RF2 Study of the first Targeted Project 'Preventive Medicine' of C.N.R., carried out in 1978-1979, with the aim of obtaining a map of risk factors for atherosclerosis in Italy (13).

Mean body mass index both in men and women was higher as compared to that observed in nine Italian areas in the framework of the ATS-RF2 Study, as well as to that observed within a further C.N.R. study (Ob. 43 of the Targeted Project 'Preventive Medicine and Rehabilitation') (table 1) (14).

Also serum triglycerides were significantly higher, especially in women (table 2). No significant differences were found in mean serum total cholesterol levels.

Most interesting are the comparisons with the results of the second C.N.R. study (1983-1984), since 'generational' differences may be present in a given area.

A dietary survey was performed by using questionnaires on the frequency of food consumption in subjects who participated in the baseline examination.

A balance sheet survey was also performed in a cluster of 50 families of the municipality of Sezze (for a total of 198 individuals) (15). In this study, the average daily calorie intake was 2,700 kcal, which represents an excess intake of 240 kcal, as compared to dietary allowances for the Italian population (LARN) (tables 3 and 4). Such an excess was mainly due to dietary fat consumption, which was almost twice as high as the recommended levels (108 vs 59 g). In the same dietary survey particalarly high intakes of red and white meat (166 g/day), cheese (60 g/day), bread and pasta (581 g/day), and seasoning and cooking fats (56 g/day, mostly represented by olive oil) were observed. Conversely, fish and legume intakes were rather low. Most interesting is the very high salt intake (>18 g/day), which was also confirmed by the results of a study of the 24-h urinary electrolyte excretion, performed in 8-9 year-old boys of 19 different European countries in the framework of the EURO-NUT-SALT2 Collaborative Study (16). This study did not show favorable results. In fact, as reported in table 5, children in Sezze ranked almost first for Na/K urinary excretion and for mean blood pressure values, as compared to children belonging to other 18 European communities.

On the basis of the food frequency survey performed during the baseline screening of 846 women, 44% reported an habitual butter consumption, although olive oil was the most used seasoning and cooking fat (70.4%). This result appears all the more important since the Sezze District is a mountain rural area with no major local dairy production.
In another survey carried out in the primary schools of Sezze, bread with salami and chips were reported to be the most consumed food snacks at school.

The rather unfavorable situation emerging from the results of field activities urged the responsible investigators of the 'DI.S.CO.' Project to review the already planned activities of nutrition intervention. The most relevant nutrition education activities performed sofar are reported in table 6. The main target groups of these activities were health professionals, schools and the community at large.
A comparative analysis of the results of the baseline and the 1986-1987 screenings as far as dietary changes are concerned, performed on independent population samples, is still under way. Table 7 reports some very preliminary results. In agreement with the results of other community-based intervention studies, such as the North Karelia Project and the Stanford Five City Project, favorable results, particularly for body mass index and dietary habits, have been observed. However, in the evaluation of these preliminary results, it is important to consider that preventive activities lasted only two years. As a matter of fact, a longer follow-up period is necessary for major health status changes to be expected as a consequences of modification in lifestyles. Therefore, nutrition intervention should be continued without interruption and new and original approaches intended to modify lifestyles should be continuously developed.

Some preliminary results on the short-term effectiveness of dietary interventions in achieving desirables cholesterol levels in children are reported in table 8. In this study, simple dietary recommendations, consisting in lists of foods to be avoided and foods to be consumed, given to parents on the occasion of blood drawing, were able to reduce the proportion of children with serum cholesterol levels above the desirable level of 180 mg/dl from 44% to 11%.

REFERENCES

(1) Lipid Research Clinics Program: The Lipid Research Clinics Coronary Prevention Trial results: I. Reduction in incidence of coronary heart disease. II. The relationship of reduction in incidence of coronary heart disease to cholesterol lowering. J. Am. Med. Assoc. 251: 351-374, 1984.

(2) Frick H.M., Elo O., Haapa K., Heinonen O.P., Heinsalmi P., Helo P., Ussi J., Huttunen K., Kaitaniemi P., Koskinen P., Manninen V., Mäenpää H., Mälkönen M., Mänttäri M., Norola S., Pasternack A., Pikkarainen J., Romo M., Sjöblom T., Nikkilä E.A.: Helsinki Heart Study: Primary-prevention trial with gemfibrozil in middle-aged men with dyslipidemia. Safety of treatment, changes in risk factors, and incidence of coronary heart disease. N. Engl. J. Med. 317: 1237-1245, 1987.

(3) Consensus Conference on Lowering Blood Cholesterol to Prevent Heart Disease. J. Am. Med. Assoc. 253: 2080-2086, 1986.

(4) Consensus Conference Italiana "Abbassare la colesterolemia per ridurre la cardiopatia coronarica", Roma, 11-12 giugno 1986.

(5) Study Group, European Atherosclerosis Society: Strategies for the prevention of coronary heart disease: A policy statement of the European Atherosclerosis Society. Eur. Heart J. 8: 77-88, 1987.

(6) Lubin F., Wax Y., Modan B.: Role of fat, animal protein, and dietary fiber in breast cancer etiology: A case-control study. J Natl Cancer Inst. 77: 605-612, 1986.

(7) Kritchevsky D., Weber M.M., Buck C.L., Klurfeld D.M.: Calories, fat and cancer. Lipids 21: 272-274, 1986.

(8) Willett W.C., MacMahon B.: Diet and cancer — an overview (part I). N. Engl. J. Med. 310: 633-638, 1984.

(9) Intersalt Cooperative Research Group: Intersalt: An international study of electrolyte excretion and blood pressure. Results for 24 hours urinary sodium and potassium excretion. Br. Med. J. 297: 319-328, 1988.

(10) Hypertension Detection and Follow-up Program Cooperative Group: Five-year findings of the Hypertension Detection and Follow-up Program. I. Reduction in mortality of persons with high blood pressure, including mild hypertension. J. Am. Med. Assoc. 242: 2562-2571, 1979.

(11) Report by the Management Committee: The Australian Therapeutic Trial in Mild Hypertension. Lancet 1: 1261-1267, 1980.

(12) Urbinati G., Ricci G.: The Di.S.Co. Project. In: Muntoni S., Epstein F.H., Lamm G. (Eds): Epidemiology of Atherosclerosis. CIC Edizioni Internazionali, Roma, 1988; pp. 43-53.

(13) Gruppo di Ricerca ATS-RF2: I fattori di rischio dell'arteriosclerosi in Italia. La fase A del Progetto Finalizzato del CNR "Medicina Preventiva-Aterosclerosi-RF2". G. Ital. Cardiol. 10 (Suppl.3): 1-184, 1980.

(14) Gruppo di Ricerca ATS-OB43: I fattori di rischio cardiovascolare in Italia. Aggiornamento agli anni '80 dello studio delle nove comunità. Cardiol. Prev. Riabil. 5: 77-137, 1987.

(15) Urbinati G.C., Menotti A., Giampaoli S., Arca M., Pasquali M. e Gruppo di Ricerca del Progetto Di.S.Co.: Il progetto Distretto Sezze Controllo Comunitario delle malattie cronico-degenerative (Di.S.Co.): dati relativi all'esame iniziale. Rapporto ISTISAN 88/6. Istituto Superiore di Sanità, Roma, 1988; pp. 1-186.

(16) EURONUT Research Group: Blood pressure and excretion of sodium, potassium, calcium and magnesium in 8 and 9 year-old boys from 19 European countries. Eur. J. Clin. Nutr. 18: 5-9, 1988.

	ATS-RF2 (1978-1979)	OB 43 (1983-1984)	DISCO (1983-1984)
MALES	25.29 -----	25.42 -----	26.29 +4% +3.5%
FEMALES	25.34	24.62	28.20 +11.5% +14.5%

Table 1 - BMI mean values.

	ATS-RF2 (1978-1979)	OB 43 (1983-1984)	DISCO (1983-1984)
MALES	132.92 ------	140.68 ------	150.05 +13% +6%
FEMALES	99.03 -----	102.62 ------	115.82 +17% +11%

Table 2 - Serum triglyceride mean levels.

NUTRIENTS		daily dietary intake
Total proteins	g	110.8
Animal proteins	g	54.9
Vegetable proteins	g	55.9
Total fat	g	108.5
Saturated fat	g	25.2
Oleic acid	g	44.2
Linoleic acid	g	13.0
Linolenic acid	g	1.3
Arachidonic acid	g	0.4
Cholesterol	mg	263.5
Total carbohydrates	g	355.5
Fiber	g	7.7
Iron	mg	20.3
Calcium	mg	910.1
Phosphorus	mg	1,538.5
Thiamine	mg	2.7
Riboflavin	mg	2.3
Niacin	mg	19.2
Vitamin A	mg	1,245.3
Vitamin C	mg	216.3
Sodium chloride	g	18.2
	kcal	2,688.5

Table 3 - Mean daily nutrient intake. Results of the family balance sheet survey of 50 families (198 subjects).

FOODS		daily dietary intake
Bread, pasta, rice	g	581.1
Legumes	g	27.4
Vegetables	g	473.1
Fruit	g	219.2
Meat and salami	g	166.1
Fresh and frozen fish	g	27.5
Milk	g	147.1
Cheese	g	59.9
Eggs	g	21.4
Cooking and seasoning fat	g	55.9
Cakes and puddings	g	35.3
Various foods	g	19.9
Alcohol (drinkeers only, n = 140)	g	84.8

Table 4 - Mean daily intake of some foods. Results of the family balance sheet survey of 50 families (198 subjects).

Rank		Na/K	Rank		SBP	Rank		DBP
1	BUD2	3.36	1	SEZZE	105	1	WAG	66
2	SEZZE	3.35	2	LUN	103	2	GHE	66
3	CAT	3.35	3	WAG	102	3	MAD	65
4	BUD1	3.31	4	WAR	101	3	FRE	65
5	WAR	3.25	4	SAN	101	5	SEZZE	63
6	SOF	3.20	4	MAD	101	5	LUN	63
7	HEI	3.02	7	GHE	100	5	SAN	63
8	MIL	2.94	7	BUD1	100	5	SOF	63
9	LIS	2.84	9	BER	99	9	VIE	61
10	ATH	2.80	9	SOF	99	9	MIL	61
11	VIE	2.65	11	HEI	98	11	WAR	60
12	MAD	2.54	11	VIE	98	12	HEI	59
13	FRE	2.39	13	FRE	97	13	ATH	58
14	BER	2.23	13	ATH	97	14	TUR	58
15	SAN	2.22	13	MIL	97	15	LIS	55
16	GHE	2.04	16	TUR	96	16	CAT	54
17	LUN	1.97	16	BUD2	96	17	BUD1	53
18	WAG	1.85	18	CAT	95	17	BUD2	53
19	TUR	1.56	19	LIS	91	19	BER	51

ATH = Athens; BER = Berlin; BUD1 = Budapest 1; BUD2 = Budapest 2; CAT = Catania; FRE = Freiburg; GHE = Ghent; HEI = Heidelberg; LIS = Lisbona; LUN = Lund; MAD = Madrid; MIL = Milano; SAN = Santiago; SEZZE = Sezze; SOF = Sofia; TUR = Turku; VIE = Vienna; WAG = Wageningen; WAR = Warsaw.

Table 5 - EURO-NUT-SALT2: Mean 24-h Na/K urinary excretion ans mean systolic and diastolic blood pressure in groups of boys aged 8-9 years belonging to 19 different European centers.

HEALTH WORKERS

* Course on nutrition for healthy workers

GENERAL POPULATION

* Booklet "Health Series":
    - Health of Heart and Arteries
    - Blood Pressure: Let Us Know It
    - Some Useful Pieces of Advice for Hypertensives
    - A Safe Nutrition for Your Children
* Booklets "Another Taste for a Better Nutrition"
    - Health of Heart and Arteries: Nutrition and Health. Some Useful Piece of Advice
    - A Guide for Buying Foods: Contents in Saturated Fat and Cholesterol
* Articles in newspapers and magazines
* Itinerant exhibition
* Preparation of a book of traditional local recipes with calculation of nutrients
* Setting-up of consulting-rooms in the three municipalities
* Preparation of computerized diets
* Sensitization of foodstuff retailers
* Competitions between restaurants
* "INTERSALT" Study in the municipality of Bassiano (indirect action to draw attention on the problem of blood pressure and hypertension)
* Assessment of nutritional status of elderly subjects

SCHOOLS

* Course of nutrition education for teachers
* Nutrition education in schools
* Lecture-debates in secondary schools with teachers and parents of the pupils
* Preparation of meals for nursery schools
* Preparation of a meal by schoolchildren
* Itinerant exhibition
* Survey on snacks at school
* 3-day food record
* Tale on the fatness written and played by the children
* Competition for the best poster on subjects of prevention (for schoolchildren or classes)
* Production of a picture book on the subject of health (including nutritional aspects), worked out by the children themselves and intended for the youngests
* Production of an obstacle game, worked out by the children themselves, concerned with correct nutrition
* Assessment of plasma lipid levels in schoolchildren
* Detection of apolipoprotein RFLPs in schoolchildren
* EURO-NUT-SALT2 Study in children aged 8-9 years in the three municipalities

Table 6 - Summary of the intervention activities.

	MALES %	FEMALES %
Total cholesterol	+1.5	-0.6
Systolic blood pressure	+0.9	-2.1**
Diastolic blood pressure	+1.5	-0.2
Body mass index	-1.3***	-3.2****
No. of cigarettes/day (smokers and non-smokers)	-5.1	-34.4*
Risk	+1.0	-6.5****

*p<0.05; ** p<0.02; *** p<0.01; **** p<0.001

Table 7 - Net changes in treated versus controls. Paired samples adjusted by initial levels.

	before diet	after diet	
Total cholesterol	173.8 (32.3)	151.2* (23.0)	-13.0%
LDL-cholesterol	103.1 (29.8)	86.0* (19.8)	-16.5
HDL-cholesterol	55.3 (12.4)	50.0* (10.8)	-9.6%
Total/HDL-cholesterol ratio	3.14	3.02*	-3.8%

Table 8 - Mean serum lipoprotein cholesterol (mg/dl) in 45 schoolchildren before and after six weeks on a moderate-fat, moderate-cholesterol diet. * p<0.001. SD in parenthesis.

22
Nutrition habits in free living community: the Brisighella Study

G.L. MAGRI, A. DORMI, G. DE SIMONE, G.B. SISCA, M.A. CAVINA, S. D'ADDATO, A. ROMAGNOLI, Z. SANGIORGI, M.L. BORLOTTI, E. FAGGIOLI, G. NEGRO, G.C. DESCOVICH

Chair of Geriatrics, Atherosclerosis Center, University of Bologna, via Massarenti 9, 40138 Bologna, Italy

ABSTRACT. The aim of this paper is to evaluate the importance of the combination of the major components of lipid intake and the possible interrelationship between vitamin intake and cardiovascular deaths in an observational longitudinal survey: the Brisighella Study. A population sample with diet P/S ratio (polyunsaturated/saturated fatty acids) over the third quintile and saturated fatty acids/1000 calories (C), lipids/1000 C, diet cholesterol under the third quintile was isolated to define an arbitrarily "correct diet" opposite to the "rich diet". The arbitrarily correct diet and the rich diet samples showed clearly different coronary mortality and morbidity rates (no pathology in the correct diet group). These characteristics emphasize the "per se" independent role of diet in the development of coronary heart disease.

Vitamin intakes were divided in quintiles at the 1980 examination and death causes included the period 1980-1987 (in this way the period 1972-1980 was verified and only the apparently healthy subjects at 1980 were considered). The percentage of fatal new events was elaborated for coronary heart disease (CHD) and for all cardiovascular diseases (CVD).

Our observations suggest a possible protective role of vitamins A, C and E dietary intakes against CHD and CVD.

INTRODUCTION

In the development of ischemic disease the "rich diet" risk factor may be defined as a lipid overfeeding but it is difficult to analyze this role in a population where high lipid intake is common.

Epidemiological and clinical studies (1) emphasize the role of nutritional habits in the development of cardiovascular diseases and recently many scientists have emphasized a possible importance of micronutrients over the so-called "rich diet". In pathology the direct damage of free radicals would be promoted by a toxic attack of oxidant molecules (2) and the physiological protective action would be effected by two pathways. Besides the enzymatic route (catalases etc.) the role of "breaking chain" molecules (3) such as tocoferols, ascorbic acid and vitamin A must be stressed in a possible protective action against ischemic pathology (4).

Many clinical studies try to evaluate this connection but there is a lack of data from epidemiological surveys. Some data showing a negative correlation between vitamin C-containing fresh fruit intake and vascular death rates in Great Britain (5) are impressive. Gey (2) in a study on men aged 40-49 in Finland, Scotland, Switzerland and Italy demonstrated the importance of some antioxidant plasma levels in the development of coronary heart disease: in particular he stressed the positive role of the "antioxidant potential" and showed a strong correlation between CHD mortality and the median of the ratio

$$\frac{\text{plasma cholesterol}}{\text{(vitamin C x cholesterol standardized vitamin E x selenium x beta-carotene)}}$$

The aim of this paper is to evaluate the importance of the combination of the major components of lipid intake and the possible interrelationship between vitamin intake and cardiovascular deaths in an observational longitudinal survey: the Brisighella Study.

The Brisighella Study started in 1972 with the aim of obtaining data on a population sample of 2939 subjects (1491 males and 1448 females aged over 14) to evaluate the possible interrelationship between the main cardiovascular risk factors and the incidence of new events.

The spontaneous trend (1972-1984) of the variations of main risk factors levels and daily food intake in Brisighella population are described elsewhere (6). The observation that daily food intake levels are clearly higher than Italian dietary recommandations (LARN) (7) suggested testing the promoting action of the contemporary slight increase or decrease of some diet lipid components.

MATERIALS AND METHODS

Over 70 parameters were recorded for each subject.

Dietary intakes were evaluated by a "Seven day questionnaire" given to each subject and data were elaborated by a computer system applying the contents tables of the Italian National Institute of Nutrition; death causes were recorded according to the classification of the eighth revision of the WHO.

The population sample was aged 35-69 because 35 years was the age of the youngest CHD patient and our studies with Multiple Logistic Function indicate that no significances are available over 69 (except for age).

A study

A population sample with diet P/S ratio (polyunsaturated/saturated fatty acids) over the third quintile and saturated fatty acids (SFA) /1000 C, lipids/1000 C, diet cholesterol under the third quintile was isolated to define an arbitrarily "correct diet" opposite to the "rich diet". This sample was defined in the 1980 follow up to enrol only the apparently health subjects and to consider the pathology incidence at 1984.

B study

Vitamin intakes were divided in quintiles at 1980 and death causes included the period 1980-1987 (in this way the period 1972-1980 was verified and only the apparently healthy subjects at 1980 were considered). The percentage of fatal new events was elaborated for coronary heart disease (CHD) and for all cardiovascular diseases (CVD).

RESULTS

A study

Cut-off points obtained at the third quintile were:

	MALES	FEMALES
Lipid day C/1000 C	304	329
SFA day C/1000 C	116	122
Diet Chol. mg/day	323	266
P/S x 100	31	31

Males of the arbitrarily "correct diet" had contemporary Lipid day C/1000 C <304, SFA day C/1000 C <116, Diet Chol. mg/day <323 and P/S * 100 >31.
Females of the arbitrarily "correct diet" had contemporary Lipid day C/1000 C <329, SFA day C/1000 C <122, Diet Chol. mg/day <266 and P/S * 100 >31. These data are partially explained by the high consumption of olive oil; olive oil production is in fact the "main business" of Brisighella farmers.
It must be considered that these values are far from desirable amounts.

The two samples presented similar main risk factor mean levels and the same mean age (almost 45).
The arbitrarily "correct diet" group was almost 6% of the entire "health" population.

Fatal new events

In the "correct diet" group, at the four year follow up (1980-1984), a mortality rate of 44/10000/year was observed in males; no deaths were observed in females. No coronary deaths were observed in this group.
In the opposite arbitrarily "rich diet" sample mortality rates excepting CHD were 124/10000/year in males and 51/10000/year in females. Coronary deaths incidence (myocardial infarction were registered only in the rich diet group) was 31/10000/year in males and 3/10000/year in females.

Non-fatal new events

No coronary pathology was observed in the correct diet sample. In the rich diet group angina new events showed incidence data of 10/10000/year in males and of 16/10000/year in females; non-fatal myocardial infarctions showed incidence data of 7/10000/year in males and of 3/10000/year in females.

B study

Dietary recommended allowances for vitamins A, C and E in our population [Age adjusted (vitamin A: 2300 IU for males and 2000 IU for females; vitamin C: 45 mg/day; vitamin E: 10 mg/day for males and 8 mg/day in females)] were satisfied because in the entire population only people aged over 69 showed marked low levels.
The mean dietary intake of vitamin A was 1826 IU in males and 1940 IU in females.
The mean dietary intake of vitamin C was 54.3 mg/day in males and 55.9 mg/day in females.
The mean dietary intake of vitamin E was 10 mg/day in males and 8.2 mg/day in females.

Vitamin A

Males (fig.1)
The highest percentage of deaths (respectively 6.8% for CHD and 9.1% for CVD) was observed in the first dietary intake quintile (mean value of 680 IU) while in the fifth quintile (mean value of 4497 IU) the lowest percentage of deaths was observed (1.4% of CHD and 2.1% of CVD .

Females (fig.2)
The most CHD deaths were observed in the first, second and third quintile (2.1% in each one) and CVD deaths showed the highest percentage in the second quintile (2.8%). In the fifth quintile no coronary deaths were observed but CVD deaths showed a percentage of 2.1% and the highest plasma cholesterol mean level.

Vitamin C

Males (fig.3)
The highest percentage of deaths (respectively 6.7% for CHD and 10.1% for CVD) was observed in the first dietary intake quintile (mean value of 15.2 mg/day) while in the fifth quintile (mean value of 114.2 mg/day) 3.3% of CHD deaths and 4.6% of CVD deaths were verified.

Females (fig.4)
The most deaths (3.3% for CHD and 3.9% for CVD) were observed in the first quintile but CVD deaths showed a high percentage in the fifth quintile too (3.2%); CVD deaths of the last quintile presented the highest total plasma cholesterol mean value (304 mg/dl) and no significative differences in blood pressure values.

Vitamin E

Males (fig.5)
The most fatal events were observed in the first (intake mean value of 5.9 mg/day) and second quintiles (respectively 8.2% and 7.3% for CHD and 16.4% and 8.5% for CVD); therefore no CHD deaths were recorded in the fifth quintile (intake mean value of 15.1 mg/day).

Females (fig.6)
The most fatal events were verified in the fourth quintile (2.5% for CHD and 4.9% for CVD) and then in the first quintile (2.2% for CHD and for CVD, namely only coronary deaths were observed).
In the face of these results it was ascertained that coronary deaths of the fourth quintile presented the highest total plasma cholesterol mean value (301 mg/dl) in 1980.

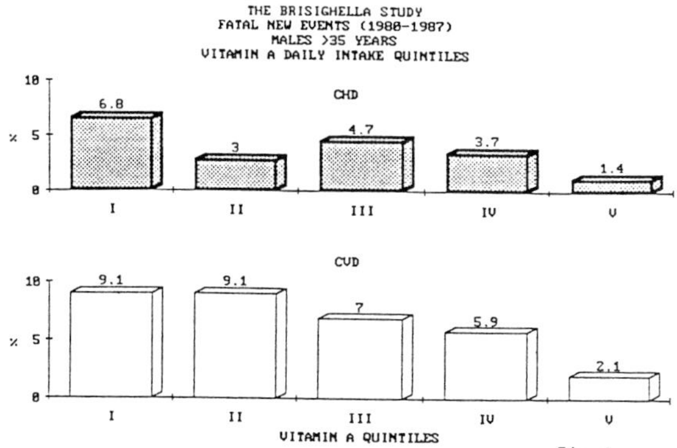
THE BRISIGHELLA STUDY
FATAL NEW EVENTS (1980-1987)
MALES >35 YEARS
VITAMIN A DAILY INTAKE QUINTILES
CHD
CVD
%
6.8
3
4.7
3.7
1.4
9.1
9.1
7
5.9
2.1
I
II
III
IV
V
VITAMIN A QUINTILES

Fig.1

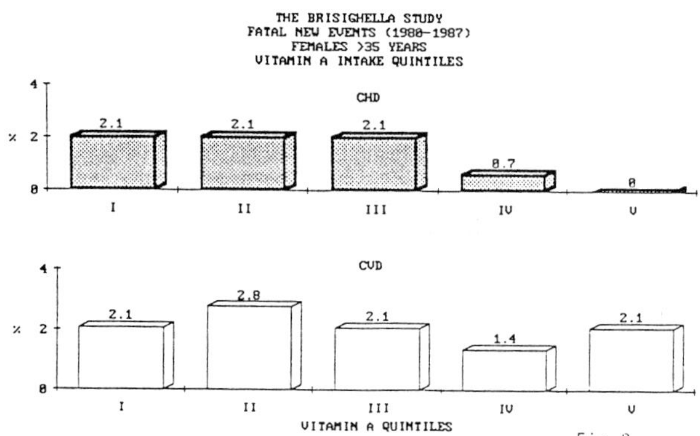
THE BRISIGHELLA STUDY
FATAL NEW EVENTS (1980-1987)
FEMALES >35 YEARS
VITAMIN A INTAKE QUINTILES
CHD
CVD
%
2.1
2.1
2.1
0.7
0
2.1
2.8
2.1
1.4
2.1
I
II
III
IV
V
VITAMIN A QUINTILES

Fig.2

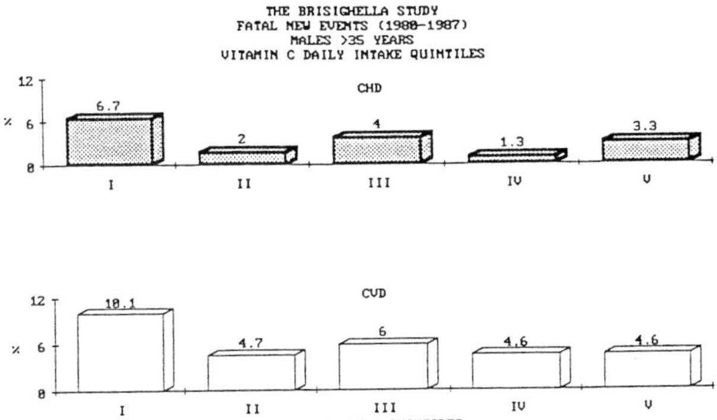
THE BRISIGHELLA STUDY
FATAL NEW EVENTS (1980-1987)
MALES >35 YEARS
VITAMIN C DAILY INTAKE QUINTILES
CHD
12
%
6
0
6.7
2
4
1.3
3.3
I
II
III
IV
V
CVD
10.1
4.7
6
4.6
4.6
VITAMIN C QUINTILES

Fig.3

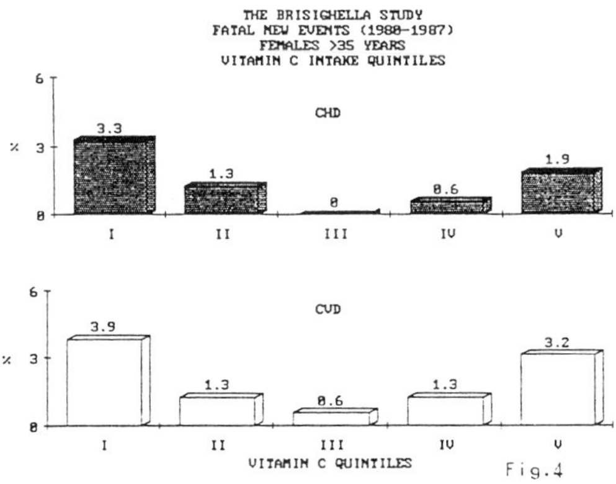
THE BRISIGHELLA STUDY
FATAL NEW EVENTS (1980-1987)
FEMALES >35 YEARS
VITAMIN C INTAKE QUINTILES
CHD
6
%
3
0
3.3
1.3
0
0.6
1.9
I
II
III
IV
V
CVD
3.9
1.3
0.6
1.3
3.2
VITAMIN C QUINTILES

Fig.4

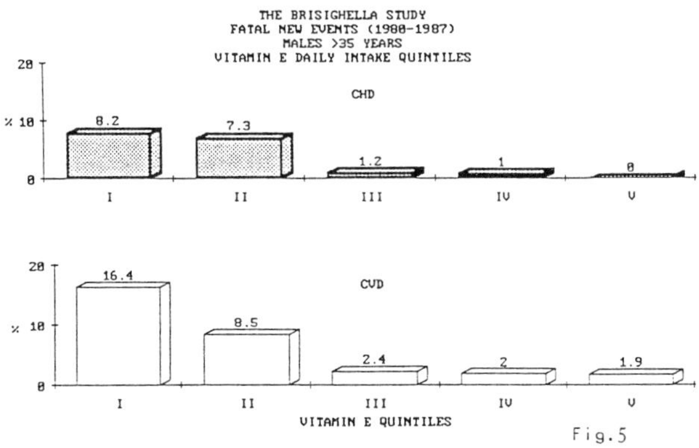
THE BRISIGHELLA STUDY
FATAL NEW EVENTS (1980-1987)
MALES >35 YEARS
VITAMIN E DAILY INTAKE QUINTILES
CHD
% 10
20
0
8.2
7.3
1.2
1
0
I
II
III
IV
V
CVD
16.4
8.5
2.4
2
1.9
VITAMIN E QUINTILES

Fig.5

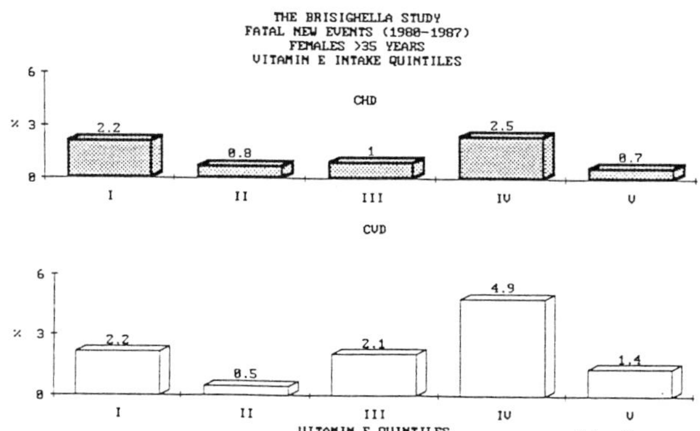
THE BRISIGHELLA STUDY
FATAL NEW EVENTS (1980-1987)
FEMALES >35 YEARS
VITAMIN E INTAKE QUINTILES
CHD
% 3
6
0
2.2
0.8
1
2.5
0.7
I
II
III
IV
V
CVD
2.2
0.5
2.1
4.9
1.4
VITAMIN E QUINTILES

Fig.6

DISCUSSION

A study
Two observations are very impressive:
1) The cut off points to define the correct diet are far from desirable values and so a "mix" effect may be underlined.
2) The arbitrarily correct diet and the rich diet samples showed similar mean values of age, total plasma cholesterol, triglycerides, blood pressure; the smoking habit percentage was almost the same. These characteristics emphasize the "per se" independent role of diet in the development of coronary heart disease.

B study
Our observations suggest a possible protective role of vitamins A, C and E dietary intakes against CHD and CVD. However these results need thorough examination and above all the possible connections with the so-called "major risk factors" and with lipid metabolism must be examined.

REFERENCES

1) Council on Scientific Affairs: Vitamin preparation as dietary supplements and as therapeutic agents. JAMA 1987; 257: 1929-1936.
2) Gey K.F.: On the antioxidant hypothesis with regard to arteriosclerosis. Biblthca Nutr. Dieta 1986, No.37, pp.53-91.
3) Niki E., Saito T., Kawakami A., Kamiya Y.: Inhibition of oxidation of methyl linoleate in solution by vitamin E and vitamin C. J. Biol. Chem. 1984, 259: 4177-4182.
4) Labadarios D., Brink P.A., Weich H.F.H., et al.: Plasma vitamin A, E, C and B6 levels in myocardial infarction. SAMJ 1987, Vol. 71: 561-564.
5) Acheson R.M., Williams D.R.R.: Does consumption of fruit and vegetables protect against stroke? Lancet 1983, i: 1191-1193.
6) Descovich G.C., Dormi A., Gaddi A., Magri G.L., et al.: From observational to intervention programmes. The Brisighella study in Lenzi S. and Descovich G.C. "Atherosclerosis and Cardiovascular diseases". MTP Press Limited 1987, 215-222.
7) Società Italiana di Nutrizione Umana (S.I.N.U.): Livelli di assunzione giornalieri di energia e nutrienti per la popolazione italiana (LARN)-Revisione 1986-87. 1989 Nutrizione Umana.

NUTRITION: SPECIAL DIETS AND METABOLIC EFFECTS OF FATS AND PROTEINS

23
Experimental atherosclerosis: anomalous fats

D. KRITCHEVSKY

The Wistar Institute of Anatomy and Biology, 3601 Spruce Street, Philadelphia, PA 19104, USA

ABSTRACT. Some fats in common use do not fit the generalization concerning effects of unsaturation on cholesterolemia and atherosclerosis. Cocoa butter is not as hypercholesterolemic or atherogenic as would be expected from its iodine value of 35. The reason for this anomaly is the high level (>35%) of stearic acid present in this fat. Rats fed oil from a soybean cultivar (A6) which contains 28% stearic acid (rather than the 4% found in soybean oil) exhibit lower levels of serum cholesterol and liver cholesteryl ester. Peanut oil (iodine value, 102) is unexpectedly atherogenic. Randomization of peanut oil reduces significantly its atherogenicity. Comparison of peanut oil from three sources showed that the oil with the highest amount of linoleic acid in the 2 position was the most atherogenic. Oil from a corn cultivar (Coker 776) whose 18:1/18:2 ratio is 1.05 is less atherogenic than corn oil whose 18:1/18:2 ratio is 0.43. More must be learned about the influence of triglyceride structure on lipid metabolism and atherosclerosis.

The equation formulated by Keys and his colleagues [1-4] to predict effects of fats of different fatty acid composition on serum or plasma cholesterol levels has served generally to explain the lipidemic effects of saturated and polyunsaturated fats. However, some fats have not conformed to the generalization and a few of these are the subject of the ensuing discussion.

Keys et al. [4] found that cocoa butter, a stearic acid-rich fat, did not elevate human cholesterol levels to the extent predicted by their equation. Comparison of the atherogenic effects of corn oil (iodine value 130), palm oil (iodine value 53), cocoa butter (iodine value 35) and coconut oil (iodine value 9) in cholesterol-fed rabbits showed that cocoa butter was less atherogenic than palm oil or coconut oil (by 16 and 18%, respectively) but 24% more atherogenic than corn oil [5]. When these fats were compared using a cholesterol-free, semipurified diet [6], cocoa butter was less cholesterolemic and atherogenic than either palm oil or coconut oil [7]. These results would not be anticipated from the iodine numbers of the fats used and may be attributable to the fact that cocoa butter contains about 35% stearic acid (Table 1).

Serum cholesterol levels of rats fed cocoa butter are not different than those of rats fed corn oil, but liver cholesterol levels are considerably lower. This finding is true in rats fed cholesterol-free diets [8] as well as in those fed 0.4% cholesterol [9].

Soybean oil (4.4% stearic acid, 42.8% oleic acid, 36.7% linoleic acid; P/S, 2.66) was compared with oil from a special cultivar of soybean (A6) which contained 28.1% stearic acid, 19.8% oleic acid and 35.5% linoleic acid (P/S, 0.93). Cholesterol levels in rats fed soybean oil were 83 ± 6 mg/dl whereas those in rats fed A6 were 54 ± 3 mg/dl ($p < 0.05$). Liver total cholesterol was the same in the two groups but liver cholesteryl ester levels were $12.4 \pm 1.3\%$ in rats fed A6 and 23.4 ± 1.4 in rats fed soybean oil ($p < 0.01$) [10].

Peanut oil has long been known to be unexpectedly atherogenic for monkeys [11], rabbits [12] and rats [13]. The effect in rabbits and monkeys is evident even in the absence of dietary cholesterol [14,15]. Randomization of peanut oil reduces significantly its atherogenic potential [16]. We have compared peanut oils from three different sources for their effects on atherogenicity in cholesterol-fed rabbits [17]. The oils came from North America (N), Africa (A) or South America (S). Average atherosclerosis (thoracic + arch/2) in the three groups was: N, 1.59; A, 1.75; and S, 1.88. Serum cholesterol levels (mg/dl) were: N, 2404; A, 2473; and S, 2567. Fatty acid analysis of the three fats showed the ratio of oleic to linoleic acid to be: N, 1.65; A, 2.70; and S, 0.89. This raised the possibility that the ratio of oleic to linoleic acid or the position of these fatty

TABLE 1. Serum lipids and atherosclerosis in rabbits fed different fats*

	Fat			
	Corn oil [12][a]	Palm kernel oil [8]	Cocoa butter [8]	Coconut Oil [5]
Serum lipids (mg/dl)				
Cholesterol	64 ± 6	436 ± 57	220 ± 32	474 ± 104
% HDL-C	38 ± 2	9 ± 1	25 ± 4	7 ± 2
Triglycerides	31 ± 4	174 ± 60	107 ± 21	136 ± 37
Phospholipids	75 ± 9	164 ± 15	148 ± 15	146 ± 12
Liver lipids (g/100 g)				
Cholesterol	0.79 ± 0.06	1.47 ± 0.13	1.62 ± 0.19	1.07 ± 0.16
Triglycerides	0.97 ± 0.12	1.52 ± 0.19	0.61 ± 0.06	0.48 ± 0.11
Atherosclerosis[b]				
Arch	0.21 ± 0.07	1.69 ± 0.30	0.81 ± 0.21	2.10 ± 0.51
Thoracic	0.08 ± 0.06	0.88 ± 0.21	0.25 ± 0.09	1.10 ± 0.24

* Fed cholesterol-free, semipurified diet containing 14% fat for 9 months.
[a] Number.
[b] Graded on a 0-4 scale.

TABLE 2. Differences in positional isomers in peanut oils
North American = 1.00

	South American	African
Position 1		
18:1	0.86	1.32
18:2	0.89	0.51
Position 2		
18:1	0.55	1.16
18:2	1.66	0.74
Position 3		
16:0	1.19	0.77
18:1	0.84	1.13
18:2	1.52	0.89

acids in the triglyceride molecule might affect atherogenicity. The acylglycerol structures of the three fats were determined [18].

Table 2 shows the differences of positional isomerism in the three fats. Relative to North American peanut oil, the African peanut oil has more oleic and less linoleic acid in positions 1 and 2. The South American peanut oil, on the other hand, has less of both oleic and linoleic in position 1 and, much less oleic and much more linoleic acid in position 2. The possibility arises that there may be a threshold level of linoleic acid in the 2 position beyond which a fat becomes increasingly atherogenic. The ratio of oleic to linoleic acid in the 2 position of glycerol may also influence atherogenicity. It will be necessary to test model triglycerides to realize the various possibilities.

Another study was carried out in rabbits fed 1% cholesterol and 4% of either corn oil or oil from a corn cultivar (Coker 77B) [19]. The levels of oleic and linoleic acids present in corn oil are 25.4 and 59.6% respectively (ratio 0.43) whereas Coker 77B contains 42.6% oleic acid and 40.5% linoleic acid (ratio 1.05). Rabbits fed the two fats showed similar weight gain, liver weight and serum and liver lipids.

However, rabbits fed Coker 77B exhibited 24.7% less aortic sudanophilia than did those fed commercial corn oil. The exact levels of sudanophilia were: Coker 77B, 37.2 ± 6.4% and corn oil, 49.4 ± 8.9%.

Fats containing trans-unsaturated fatty acids (trans fats) are present in some plants and in animal tissue but most of the trans fats available in the diet are present in margarines which are made by hydrogenation of soybean oil or other oils. Trans fats are in general transported and metabolized like other naturally occurring fats at high levels in the diet they may be hypercholesterolemic compared to cis-fats but are not more atherogenic. It has been suggested that trans-fats be regarded as saturated fats. Tissues of humans who died of cardiovascular disease contain no more trans fats than those of subjects who succumbed from other causes. The subject has been reviewed recently [20].

While the basic premise of effects of saturated and unsaturated fats on cholesterolemia are well established, it must be recognized that we still have much to learn about the effects of positional isomerism. With emerging capabilities to engineer genetically fat contents of plants and possibly the ability to direct positional isomerism it is mandatory that we begin to learn more about the effects of triglyceride structure on lipid metabolism and atherosclerosis.

Acknowledgements

Supported, in part, by a grant (HL03299) and a Research Career Award (HL00734) from the National Institutes of Health, and by funds from the Commonwealth of Pennsylvania.

References

1. Keys, A., Anderson, J.T., and Grande, F. (1965) 'Serum cholesterol response to changes in the diet. I. Iodine value of dietary fat versus 2S-P', Metabolism 14, 747-758.
2. Keys, A., Anderson, J.T., and Grande, F. (1965) 'Serum cholesterol response to changes in the diet. II. The effect of cholesterol in the diet', Metabolism 14, 759-765.
3. Keys, A., Anderson, J.T., and Grande, F. (1965) 'Serum cholesterol response to changes in the diet. III. Differences among individuals', Metabolism 14, 766-775.
4. Keys, A., Anderson, J.T., and Grande, F. (1965) 'Serum cholesterol response to changes in the diet. IV. Particular saturated fatty acids in the diet', Metabolism 14, 776-787.
5. Kritchevsky, D. and Tepper, S.A. (1965) 'Cholesterol vehicle in experimental atherosclerosis. VII. Influence of naturally occurring saturated fats', Med. Pharmacol. Exp. 12, 315-320.
6. Kritchevsky, D. and Tepper, S.A. (1965) 'Factors affecting atherosclerosis in rabbits fed cholesterol-free diets', Life Sci. 4, 1467-1471.
7. Kritchevsky, D., Tepper, S.A., Bises, G., and Klurfeld, D.M. (1982) 'Experimental atherosclerosis in rabbits fed cholesterol-free diets. 10. Cocoa butter and palm oil', Atherosclerosis 41, 279-284.

8. Kritchevsky, D., Tepper, S.A., Bises, G., and Klurfeld, D.M. (1983) 'Influence of cocoa butter on cholesterol metabolism in rats: Comparison with corn oil, coconut oil and palm kernel oil', Nutr. Res. 3, 229-236.
9. Kritchevsky, D., Tepper, S.A., Lloyd, L.M., Davidson, L.M., and Klurfeld, D.M. (1988) 'Serum and liver lipids of rats fed cocoa butter, corn oil, palm kernel oil, coconut oil and cholesterol', Nutr. Res. 8, 287-294.
10. Kritchevsky, D., Tepper, S.A., Klurfeld, D.M., Fehr, W.R., and Hammond, E.G. (1987) 'Influence of A6 soybean oil on cholesterol metabolism in rats', Nutr. Rep. Int. 35, 265-268.
11. Vesselinovitch, D., Getz, G.S., Hughes, R.H., and Wissler, R.W. (1974) 'Atherosclerosis in the Rhesus monkey fed three food fats', Atherosclerosis 20, 303-321.
12. Kritchevsky, D., Tepper, S.A., Vesselinovitch, D., and Wissler, R.W. (1971) 'Cholesterol vehicle in experimental atherosclerosis. XI. Peanut oil', Atherosclerosis 14, 53-64.
13. Gresham, G.A., and Howard, A.N. (1960) The independent production of atherosclerosis and thrombosis in the rat', Br. J. Exp. Pathol. 41, 395-402.
14. Kritchevsky, D., Tepper, S.A., Kim, H.K., Story, J.A., Vesselinovitch, D., and Wissler, R.W. (1976) 'Experimental atherosclerosis in rabbits fed cholesterol-free diets. V. Comparison of peanut, corn, butter and coconut oils', Exp. Molec. Pathol. 24, 375-391.
15. Kritchevsky, D., Davidson, L.M., Weight, M., Kriek, N.P.J., and duPlessis, J.P. (1982) 'Influence of native and randomized peanut oil on lipid metabolism and aortic sudanophilia in the vervet monkey', Atherosclerosis 42, 53-58.
16. Kritchevsky, D., Tepper, S.A., Vesselinovitch, D., and Wissler, R.W. (1983) 'Cholesterol vehicle in experimental atherosclerosis. XIII. Randomized peanut oil', Atherosclerosis 17, 225-243.
17. Kritchevsky, D., Tepper, S.A., Scott, D.A., Klurfeld, D.M., Vesselinovitch, D., and Wissler, R.W. (1981) 'Cholesterol vehicle in experimental atherosclerosis. 18. Comparison of North American, African and South American peanut oil', Atherosclerosis 38, 291-299.
18. Manganaro, F., Myher, J.J., Kuksis, A., and Kritchevsky, D. (1981) 'Acylglycerol structure of genetic varieties of peanut oils with varying atherogenic potential', Lipids 16, 508-517.
19. Kritchevsky, D., Tepper, S.A., Miller, J., Worthington, R.E., and Klurfeld, D.M. (1988) 'Cholesterol vehicle in experimental atherosclerosis. 19. Oleic acid-rich corn oil (Coker 77B)', Nutr. Rep. Int. 38, 853-857.
20. Kritchevsky, D. (1990) 'Trans unsaturated fat in nutrition and health', Lipids, in press.

24
Cholesterol-lowering action of diets rich in polyunsaturated fatty acids

A.C. BEYNEN

Department of Laboratory Animal Science, PO Box 80.166, 3508 TD Utrecht, The Netherlands

ABSTRACT. The hypothesis is advanced that the primary feature of the cholesterol-lowering action of dietary polyunsaturated fatty acids, when compared with saturated fatty acids, is inhibition of hepatic *de novo* cholesterol synthesis. This in turn causes an increase in the number of hepatic LDL receptors. Serum LDL cholesterol concentration will be reduced as a result of the combination of decreased formation and increased efficiency of catabolism of LDL.

1. INTRODUCTION

In general, the replacement of saturated by polyunsaturated fatty acids in the diet is the single most powerful intervention to lower plasma cholesterol levels in man. However, this statement needs qualification. Individual fatty acids exert different effects on serum cholesterol. Saturated fatty acids with either 12, 14 or 16 carbon atoms are considered hypercholesterolemic. Recent studies suggest that diets rich in the monounsaturated fatty acid, oleic acid, are as effective in reducing serum cholesterol as diets rich in the polyunsaturated fatty acid, linoleic acid (Mensink and Katan, 1989), while high oleic acid diets lower serum cholesterol to the same extent as do diets rich in stearic acid (Bonanome and Grundy, 1988). This could imply that as to cholesterol lowering it is immaterial whether C12-C16 saturated fatty acids are replaced by either linoleic, oleic or stearic acid.

This communication focusses on the hypocholesterolemic effect of linoleic acid when compared with saturated fatty acids. Specifically, the question is addressed how fats rich in linoleic acid lower serum cholesterol. We have proposed earlier that the cholesterol-lowering action of linoleic acid is related to preferential oxidation of this fatty acid by the liver (Beynen and Katan, 1985). At this moment, I feel that the observed inhibition of *de novo* cholesterol synthesis after the ingestion of fats rich in linoleic acid could be the key to their hypocholesterolemic effect.

2. FAT TYPE AND SERUM CHOLESTEROL

Table 1 summarizes the results of studies in which the effect of increased intakes of linoleic acid on serum total and low density lipoprotein (LDL) cholesterol concentrations were measured. It is assumed that in these studies the increased consumption of polyunsaturated (P) fatty acids was effected at the expense of saturated (S) fatty acids while monounsaturated fatty acids were kept constant. However, since various authors reported the dietary P/S ratio's but not the fatty acid composition of the experimental diets, this assumption may not be correct. It cannot be excluded that P/S ratio's were raised by lowering the intake of saturated fatty acids at the expense of monounsaturated fatty acids. As stressed above, such a change in dietary fatty acid composition will also lead to cholesterol lowering.

It is clear that increasing the consumption of polyunsaturated fatty acids results in a decrease in LDL cholesterol (Table 1). Some of the experimental diets had extremely high P/S ratio's which cannot, or only laboriously, be accommodated into a natural mixed solid diet. A dietary P/S ratio of 1.0 is the ratio generally recommended to the general public.

TABLE 1. Effect of increased proportions of polyunsaturated fatty acids in the diet on serum total and LDL cholesterol at a constant total fat intake in controlled experiments in man

		P/S ratio of diet		Change in serum cholesterol (%)	
Reference	n	Low	High	Total	LDL
Weisweiler *et al.*, 1985	22	0.2	1.0	-11	-13
Kuusi *et al.*, 1985	39/39	0.4	0.9	- 8	- 9
Schwandt *et al.*, 1982	30	0.3	1.0	-11	-14
Jackson *et al.*, 1984	6	0.4	1.0	- 6	- 9
Jones *et al.*, 1987	15/16	0.3	1.0	- 3	
Brussaard *et al.*, 1980	14/15	0.2	1.7	-10	-15
Katan *et al.*, 1988	47	0.2	1.9	-16	-21
Vessby *et al.*, 1980	30	0.2	2.0	-12	- 8
Schaefer *et al.*, 1981	11	0.2	2.0	-11	- 9
Zanni *et al.*, 1987	19	0.6	2.1	-12	-14
Chait *et al.*, 1974	23	0.2	2.4	-16	-10
Fisher *et al.*, 1983	9	0.1	2.7	-32	-36
Harris *et al.*, 1983	7	0.5	3.4	- 9	- 9
Shepherd *et al.*, 1980	8	0.3	4.0	-23	-22
Becker *et al.*, 1983	12	0.2	4.4	- 8	-13
Mattson and Grundy, 1985	12	0.2	6.5	-16	18
Vega *et al.*, 1982	10	0.2	6.5	-25	-26
Turner *et al.*, 1981	15	0.2	8.0	-16	-19

3. FAT TYPE AND CHOLESTEROL METABOLISM

Tables 2 and 3 show that the type of dietary fat influences various aspects of cholesterol metabolism in hamsters and rats. Hepatic cholesterol synthesis was reduced markedly in animals fed safflower oil (P/S = 11.8), which is rich in linoleic acid, when compared with coconut fat (P/S = 0.03), which is rich in saturated fatty acids. Inhibition of cholesterol synthesis may cause an increase of the number of hepatic LDL receptors as has been shown for compounds that inhibit cholesterol synthesis at the level of 3-hydroxy-3-methylglutaryl (HMG) CoA reductase (Brown and Goldstein, 1986). Indeed, it was demonstrated that the feeding of safflower oil produced an increase in hepatic receptor-dependent uptake of LDL (Tables 2 and 3).

TABLE 2. In-vivo cholesterol metabolism of hamsters fed cholesterol-enriched (0.12 %, w/w) diets containing either hydrogenated coconut fat (20 %) or safflower oil for 30 days

	Dietary fat type	
	Coconut fat	Safflower oil
Plasma cholesterol (mmol/l)	15.6 ± 0.9	5.2 ± 0.4
LDL cholesterol (mmol/l)	4.5 ± 0.3	1.8 ± 0.2
Hepatic cholesteryl esters (μmol/g)	10.8 ± 1.5	20.1 ± 1.5
Hepatic cholesterol synthesis (nmol/h/g)	20 ± 1	15 ± 1
Hepatic receptor-dependent LDL clearance rate (μl/h/g)	5 ± 2	42 ± 6

Means ± SE; n = 6. After Spady and Dietschy (1985).

TABLE 3. In-vivo cholesterol metabolism of rats fed diets containing either hydrogenated coconut fat (20 %, w/w) or safflower oil for 30 days

	Dietary fat type	
	Coconut fat	Safflower oil
Plasma cholesterol (mmol/l)	2.0 ± 0.1	1.5 ± 0.1
LDL cholesterol (mmol/l)	0.5 ± 0.1	0.3 ± 0.0
Hepatic cholesteryl esters (μmol/g)	0.8 ± 0.0	2.0 ± 0.2
Hepatic cholesterol synthesis (μmol/h/g)	1.9 ± 0.2	1.1 ± 0.3
Hepatic LDL receptor activity (% control)	100	133
LDL cholesterol production (% control)	100	77

Means ± SE; n = 6. After Ventura *et al.* (1989).

Depressed *de novo* cholesterol synthesis should theoretically be associated with a reduced synthesis of lipoprotein cholesterol. Table 3 shows that such an association was substantiated experimentally. In rats fed safflower oil, LDL cholesterol synthesis was decreased significantly when compared with their counterparts fed coconut fat. In humans similar effects have been observed. Table 4 documents that on diets with high P/S ratio's, LDL synthesis was decreased. The rate of synthesis of the precursor of LDL apoprotein B, that is VLDL apoprotein B, was also reduced when subjects went from a low to a high P/S diet (41.7 ± 12.2 versus 28.9 ± 8.9, means ± SD, n = 4; Cortese *et al.*, 1983).

TABLE 4. Effect of dietary P/S ratio on apoLDL synthesis in human subjects

		Dietary P/S ratio	
Authors	n	Low	High
		ApoLDL synthesis (mg/kg/d)	
Shepherd *et al.* (1980)	8	11.5 ± 1.9	10.9 ± 1.7
Turner *et al.* (1981)	7	11.5 ± 0.6	10.5 ± 1.0
	8	15.4 ± 2.1	12.7 ± 2.2
Cortese *et al.* (1983)	3	15.3 ± 0.8	11.8 ± 2.3

Means ± SD.

Thus it would appear that fats rich in linoleic acid lower serum LDL cholesterol by a combination of inhibition of LDL synthesis and increased efficiency of hepatic LDL catabolism. Eventually, a new steady state will be reached at which LDL production, which is depressed, equals LDL catabolism. At this new steady state after feeding polyunsaturated fatty acids, the absolute amount of LDL cholesterol taken up by the cells via the receptor-dependent and by the receptor-independent pathway should be decreased. Thus the net effect of the decreased LDL concentration and increased number of receptors should be a decreased catabolism of LDL.

4. CHOLESTEROL SYNTHESIS AS TARGET FOR POLYUNSATURATED FATS

If the primary feature of the cholesterol-lowering action of polyunsaturated fats is inhibition of cholesterol synthesis, how then is this effect brought about? Possibly, it is related to the observed increase in hepatic concentrations of cholesteryl esters after the feeding of polyunsaturated fats (Tables 2 and 3). This phenomenon might be related to a differential promotion of cholesterol esterification, implying that polyunsaturated fatty acids are preferentially chanelled into this pathway. Increased hepatic concentrations of esterified cholesterol may be associated with increased concentrations of free cholesterol.

Indeed, free cholesterol levels were found to be slightly increased in rats fed safflower oil when compared with coconut fat (Ventura *et al.*, 1989). Hepatic free cholesterol probably is the metabolic active form that downregulates cholesterol synthesis through lowering of the activity of HMG CoA reductase. *De novo* synthesized cholesterol might specifically influence LDL receptor synthesis. A decreased production of cholesterol is invariably correlated with an increased synthesis of LDL receptors (Brown and Goldstein, 1986).

Thus at steady state, cholesterol synthesis may be depressed in subjects consuming diets rich in polyunsaturated fats. In other words, polyunsaturated fats lower cholesterol turnover. This would imply that in subjects ingesting polyunsaturated fats the fecal excretion of neutral steroids and bile acids should be lower than in subjects on diets rich in saturated fatty acids. However, such a difference has not been demonstrated. In fact, studies in which the fecal excretion of steroids was determined, have not provided conclusive results (Brussaard *et al.*, 1983). Possibly, this relates to sources of noise such as variation of defecation frequency and bias due to analytical difficulty of separating plant sterols from cholesterol metabolites.

6. REFERENCES

Becker, N., Illingworth, D.R., Alaupovic, P., Connor, W.E. and Sundberg, E.E. (1983). Effects of saturated, monounsaturated, and w-6 polyunsaturated fatty acids on plasma lipids, lipoproteins, and apoproteins in humans. Am. J. Clin. Nutr. 37, 355-360.

Beynen, A.C. and Katan, M.B. (1985). Why do polyunsaturated fatty acids lower serum cholesterol? Am. J. Clin. Nutr. 42, 560-563.

Bonanome, A. and Grundy, S.M. (1988). Effect of dietary stearic acid on plasma cholesterol and lipoprotein levels. N. Engl. J. Med. 318, 1244-1248.

Brown, M.S. and Goldstein, J.L. (1986). A receptor-mediated pathway for cholesterol homeostasis. Science 232, 34-47.

Brussaard, J.H., Dallinga-Thie, G., Groot, P.H.E. and Katan, M.B. (1980). Effects of amount and type of dietary fat on serum lipids, lipoproteins and apolipoproteins in man. A controlled 8-week trial. Atherosclerosis 36, 515-527.

Brussaard, J.H., Katan, M.B. and Hautvast, J.G.A.J. (1983). Faecal excretion of bile acids and neutral steroids on diets differing in type and amount of dietary fat in young healthy persons. Eur. J. Clin. Invest. 13, 115-122.

Chait, A., Onitiri, A., Nicoll, A., Rabaya, E., Davies, J. and Lewis, B. (1974). Reduction of serum triglyceride levels by polyunsaturated fat. Studies on the mode of action and on very low density lipoprotein composition. Atherosclerosis 20, 347-364.

Cortese, C., Levy, Y., Janus, E.D., Turner, P.R., Rao, S.N., Miller, N.E. and Lewis, B. (1983). Modes of action of lipid-lowering diets in man: studies of apolipoprotein B kinetics in relation to fat consumption and dietary fatty acid composition. Eur. J. Clin.

Invest. 13, 79-85.

Fisher, E.A., Blum, C.B., Zannis, V.I. and Breslow, J.L. (1983). Independent effects of dietary saturated fat and cholesterol on plasma lipids, lipoproteins, and apolipoprotein E. J. Lipid Res. 24, 1039-1048.

Harris, W.S., Connor, W.E. and McMurry, M.P. (1983). The comparative reduction of the plasma lipids and lipoproteins by dietary polyunsaturated fats: salmon oil versus vegetable oils. Metabolism 32, 179-184.

Jackson, R.L., Kashyap, M.L., Barnhart, R.L., Allen, C., Hogg, E. and Glueck, C.J. (1984). Influence of polyunsaturated and saturated fats on plasma lipids and lipoproteins in man. Am. J. Clin. Nutr. 39, 589-597.

Jones, D.Y., Judd, J.T., Taylor, P.R., Campbell, W.S. and Nair, P.P. (1987). Influence of caloric distribution and saturation of dietary fat on plasma lipids in premenopausal women. Am. J. Clin. Nutr. 45, 1451-1456.

Katan, M.B., Berns, M.A.M., Glatz, F.J.C., Knuiman, J.T., Nobels, A. and De Vries, J.H.M. (1988). Congruence of individual responsiveness to dietary cholesterol and to saturated fat in man. J. Lipid Res. 29, 883-892.

Kuusi, T., Ehnholm, C., Huttunen, J.K., Kostiainen, E., Pietinen, P., Leino, U., Uusitalo, U., Nikkari, T., Iacono, J.M. and Puska, P. (1985). Concentration and composition of serum lipoproteins during a low-fat diet at two levels of polyunsaturated fat. J. Lipid Res. 26, 360-367.

Mattson, F.H. and Grundy, S.M. (1985). Comparison of effects of dietary saturated, monounsaturated, and polyunsaturated fatty acids on plasma lipids and lipoproteins in man. J. Lipid Res. 26, 194-202.

Mensink, R.P. and Katan, M.B. (1989). Effect of a diet enriched with monounsaturated or polyunsaturated fatty acids on levels of low-density and high-density lipoprotein cholesterol in healthy women and men. N. Eng. J. Med. 321, 436-441.

Schaefer, E.J., Levy, R.I., Ernst, N.D., Van Sant, F.D. and Brewer Jr, H.B. (1981). The effects of low cholesterol, high polyunsaturated fat, and low fat diets on plasma lipid and lipoprotein cholesterol levels in normal and hypercholesterolemic subjects. Am. J. Clin. Nutr. 34, 1758-1763.

Schwandt, P., Janetschek, P. and Weisweiler, P. (1982). High density lipoproteins unaffected by dietary fat modification. Atherosclerosis 44, 9-17.

Shepherd, J., Packard, C.J., Grundy, S.M., Yeshurun, D., Gotto Jr, A.M. and Taunton, O.D. (1980). Effects of saturated and polyunsaturated fat diets on the chemical composition and metabolism of low density lipoproteins in man. J. Lipid Res. 21, 91-99.

Spady, D.K. and Dietschy, J.M. (1985). Dietary saturated triacylglycerols suppress hepatic low density lipoprotein receptor activity in the hamster. Proc. Natl. Acad. Sci. USA 82, 4526-4530.

Turner, J.D., Le, N.-A. and Brown, W.V. (1981). Effect of changing dietary fat saturation on low-density lipoprotein metabolism in man.

Am. J. Physiol. 241, E57-E63.
Vega, G.L., Groszek, E., Wolf, R. and Grundy, S.M. (1982). Influence of polyunsaturated fats on composition of plasma lipoproteins and apolipoproteins. J. Lipid Res. 23, 811-822.
Ventura, M.A., Woollet, L.A., and Spady, D.K. (1989). Dietary fish oil stimulates hepatic low density lipoprotein transport in the rat. J. Clin. Invest. 84, 528-537.
Vessby, B., Gustafsson, I.-B., Boberg, J., Karlström, B., Lithell, H. and Werner, I. (1980). Substituting polyunsaturated for saturated fat as a single change in a Swedish diet: effects on serum lipoprotein metabolism and glucose tolerance in patients with hyperlipoproteinaemia. Eur. J. Clin. Invest. 10, 193-202.
Weisweiler, P., Janetschek, P. and Schwandt, P. (1985). Influence of polyunsaturated fats and fat restriction on serum lipoproteins in humans. Metabolism 34, 83-87.
Zanni, E.E., Zannis, V.I., Blum, C.B., Herbert, P.N. and Breslow, J.L. (1987). Effect of egg cholesterol and dietary fats on plasma lipids, lipoproteins, and apoproteins of normal women consuming natural diets. J. Lipid Res. 28, 518-527.

25
Receptor-mediated catabolism of LDL in rabbits fed cholesterol-free, semipurified diets containing casein or soy protein: a time-course study

S. SAMMAN, P. KHOSLA and K.K. CARROLL

Department of Biochemistry, University of Western Ontario, London, Ontario N6A 5C1, Canada

ABSTRACT. Rabbits were fed semipurified diets containing casein or soy protein for 4 weeks. Increases in low density lipoprotein (LDL) cholesterol and protein were apparent within the first two weeks that the diets were fed and the changes were considerably greater in the rabbits fed casein. Receptor-mediated LDL apolipoprotein B (apo B) fractional catabolic rate (FCR) was decreased within 5 days of feeding the casein diet, prior to any significant change in plasma cholesterol. These studies indicate that down regulation of LDL receptors in vivo precedes the elevation in plasma cholesterol level induced by a casein diet.

1. INTRODUCTION

When fed to rabbits as part of a low-fat, cholesterol-free, semipurified diet, casein induces a marked hypercholesterolemia. This can be prevented if the casein is replaced by isolated soy protein (Carroll, 1982). The excess serum cholesterol is carried mainly in the atherogenic LDL fraction (Hrabek-Smith & Carroll, 1987), but dietary casein also affects other components in all lipoprotein fractions (Terpstra et al, 1981).

Recent experiments in our laboratory have shown that the LDL pool is higher in rabbits fed casein than in their soy protein-fed counterparts (Khosla et al. 1989a; Samman et al. 1989). The increased pool size is due to a reduced FCR and increased production of LDL, particularly from very low density lipoprotein (VLDL)-independent pathways (Khosla et al. 1989a). Subsequent studies have shown that the reduced FCR is primarily due to down-regulation of LDL receptors (Khosla et al, 1989b).

To obtain further information on the mechanism responsible, the early stages of the effects of dietary casein on lipoprotein levels and metabolism were investigated.

2. MATERIALS AND METHODS

2.1. Animals and diets

Male New Zealand White rabbits (aged 6-8 weeks, weighing approximately 1.5 kg) were obtained from Reimen's Fur Ranches (Guelph, Ontario). Following one week of adaptation, rabbits were fed the casein or soy protein diets for 4 weeks. The composition of the semipurified diets has been described previously (Roberts et al. 1981). The diets were provided ad libitum and the rabbits had free access to water.

2.2. Study 1

Blood samples from fasted animals were collected at the beginning (week -1) and end (week 0) of the week of adaptation and weekly thereafter. VLDL ($d < 1.006$ g/ml), LDL ($1.006 < d < 1.063$) and high density lipoprotein (HDL, $1.063 < d < 1.21$) were isolated by sequential ultracentrifugation. Serum and lipoprotein cholesterol, and lipoprotein protein were determined as described previously (Roberts et al. 1981).

2.3. Study 2

All rabbits were adapted onto the soy protein diet and maintained on it for 2 weeks. Groups of rabbits (3-4 animals per group) were switched to the casein diet, which was fed for 5, 10 or 25 days.

LDL ($1.019 < d < 1.063$ g/ml) was isolated from the plasma of Chow-fed donor rabbits by 2 spin sequential ultracentrifugation. The LDL was divided into two aliquots. One aliquot was labeled with ^{125}I and the other with ^{131}I (Amersham, Oakville, Ontario). The ^{125}I-LDL was then reductively methylated by the procedure of Weisgraber et al. (1978).

Each rabbit was injected simultaneously with each tracer via the marginal ear vein. Eight blood samples were collected at timed intervals over 50h post-injection and plasma apo B radioactivity was determined (Yamada et al, 1986).

The plasma apo B radioactivity decay curves were resolved and analyzed by the procedure of Matthews

(1957). The FCR for the native ^{131}I-LDL and the methylated ^{125}I-LDL were calculated. The former represents the sum of both receptor-dependent and receptor-independent catabolism, whereas the latter represents receptor-independent catabolism. The difference therefore is a measure of receptor-dependent catabolism.

Statistical analyses were carried out using Student's unpaired t-test, or a one-factorial ANOVA.

3. RESULTS

3.1. Study 1

Both groups gained weight throughout the study period. As in previous studies, the rabbits fed casein became markedly hypercholesterolemic compared to rabbits fed soy protein (Table 1). For the rabbits fed casein, there was an increase in serum cholesterol following the week of adaptation (greater than two-fold). As of week 1 of the study, the serum cholesterol levels in the casein-fed rabbits were significantly higher than their soy protein-fed counterparts.

TABLE 1. Serum cholesterol (mg/dl) levels in rabbits fed diets containing casein or soy protein.

TIME (weeks)	DIET	
	CASEIN	SOY PROTEIN
-1	37 ± 5	34 ± 5
0	48 ± 8	30 ± 5
1	111 ± 12*	50 ± 6
2	187 ± 17*	66 ± 8
3	237 ± 20*	60 ± 7
4	267 ± 18*	57 ± 6

Each value is the mean±SEM of 8 rabbits except for the values at week -1 which are the means of n=4. Values bearing a symbol in the casein group are significantly higher than the corresponding values in the soy protein group as determined by Student's t test ($P < 0.05$).

Figures 1a and 1b show the changes in lipoprotein cholesterol and protein during the course of Study 1. For the rabbits fed casein (Figure 1a), LDL cholesterol more than doubled during the adaptation period followed by a somewhat slower increase during weeks 2-4. Differences were significant ($P < 0.05$) at weeks 1, 3 and 4. VLDL and HDL cholesterol rose slowly throughout the course of feeding casein but the percentage increase were much less than for LDL. The rise in VLDL cholesterol was significant ($P < 0.05$) at weeks 3 and 4. LDL protein levels began to rise during the adaptation period and rose steeply in the first week therafter. During weeks 1-4, LDL protein levels did not change significantly. By the end of week 2, HDL protein levels had dropped almost 2-fold.

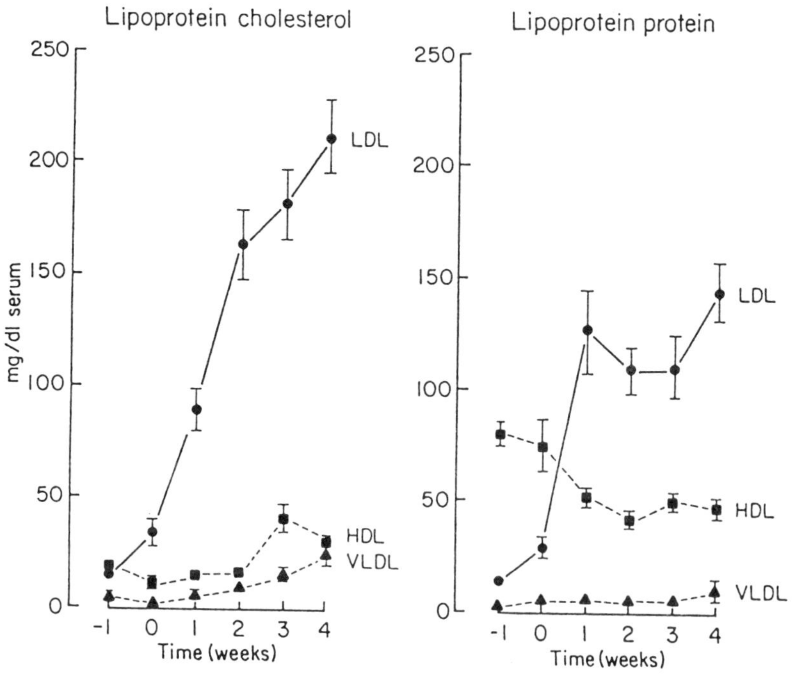

FIGURE 1A. Time course of the changes in lipoprotein cholesterol and protein in rabbits fed diets containing casein.

The rabbits fed soy protein (Figure 1b) showed

similar trends although the absolute levels of lipoprotein cholesterol and protein were much lower than in the corresponding group fed casein.

At the outset of the study, HDL was the principal transporter of lipoprotein cholesterol (week -1). However, from the earliest time that the semipurified diets were fed (adaptation period) LDL became the principal transporter of lipoprotein cholesterol (week 0) irrespective of the type of dietary protein.

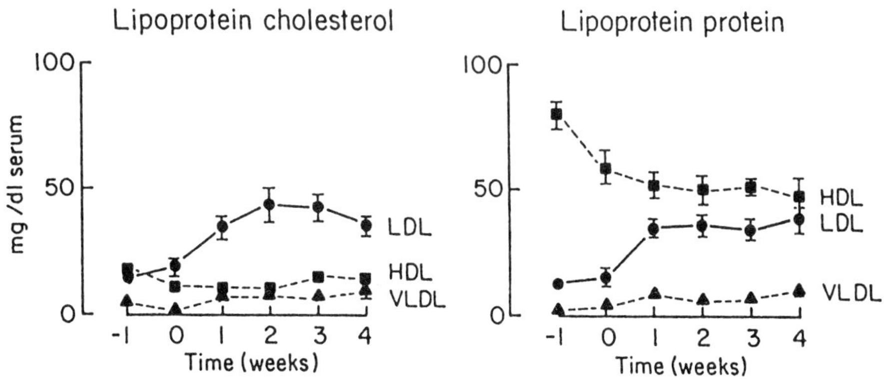

FIGURE 1B. Time course of the changes in lipoprotein cholesterol and protein in rabbits fed diets containing soy protein.

3.3. Study 2

Figure 2 shows the plasma cholesterol concentrations and receptor-dependent LDL apo B FCR in groups of rabbits transferred from the soy protein diet (day 0) to the casein diet for 5, 10 and 25 days. With the exception of the rabbits fed casein for 5 days, all other groups of rabbits fed the casein diet were significantly hypercholesterolemic in comparison to the rabbits fed soy protein. Both total and receptor-dependent FCR in casein-fed rabbits for each time period were significantly lower than the values observed in rabbits fed soy protein ($P < 0.001$). No significant difference was observed in receptor-independent FCR.

4. DISCUSSION

These results show that changes in LDL protein and cholesterol occurred within the first week that the rabbits were fed the semipurified diets. The results of the kinetic studies showed that the FCR of LDL decreased in casein-fed rabbits. From the differential uptake of the native and methylated LDL, it appears that the decrease in FCR in animals fed casein is due to a decrease in the receptor-dependent catabolism, compared to that in rabbits fed soy protein.

In vitro studies by Chao et al (1982) showed that hepatic LDL receptor activity was reduced in rabbits fed a wheat-starch casein diet in comparison to Chow-fed rabbits (Kita et al, 1981). The in vivo studies described in this report are supported by these in vitro findings. However, our results show that it is specifically the protein component of the cholesterol-free semipurified casein diet which causes impaired receptor-dependent catabolism in comparison to the semipurified soy protein diet.

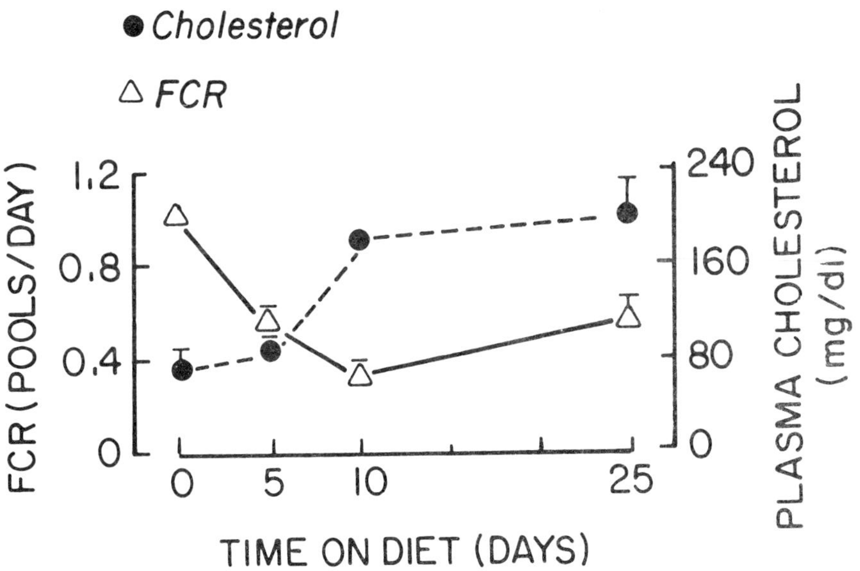

FIGURE 2. Plasma cholesterol (mg/dl) and receptor-dependent LDL apo B FCR (pools/d) in rabbits fed casein diet for 5, 10 and 25 days.

The decrease in receptor-mediated LDL apo B FCR is

apparent within 5 days of switching rabbits from the soy protein to the casein diet, and precedes the increase in plasma cholesterol concentrations. Hence, it can be concluded that casein-induced hypercholesterolemia is a consequence of decreased LDL receptor activity. The rapidity of this effect suggests that casein has the ability to inhibit LDL receptor status directly or indirectly. In contrast, it has been shown that soy protein has the ability to stimulate LDL receptor activity in human subjects consuming a soy protein diet (Lovati et al, 1987).

It is not clear how dietary proteins exert their effects on cholesterol metabolism. However, the ability to affect LDL receptors rapidly may involve the action of some dietary amino acid(s) or peptide(s) with hormonal-like behaviour (Redgrave, 1984).

(Supported by grants from the Heart and Stroke Foundation of Ontario and Protein Technologies Inc., St. Louis, MO., U.S.A. K.K. Carroll is a Career Investigator of the Medical Research Council of Canada).

5. REFERENCES

Carroll, K.K. (1982) Hypercholesterolemia and atherosclerosis: Effects of dietary protein, Fed. Proc. 41, 2792-2796.

Chao, Y.S., Yamin, T.T. and Alberts, A.W. (1982) Effect of cholestyramine on LDL binding sites to liver membranes from rabbits with endogenous hypercholesterolemia induced by a wheat-starch casein diet, J. Biol. Chem, 257, 3623-3627.

Hrabek-Smith, J.M. and Carroll, K.K. (1987) A comparative study of serum lipoproteins in rabbits fed a natural ingredient or low-fat, cholesterol-free, semipurified diets containing casein or isolated soy protein, Biochem. Cell Biol. 65, 610-616.

Khosla, P., Samman, S., Carroll, K.K., and Huff, M.W. (1989a) Turnover of ^{125}I-VLDL and ^{131}I-LDL apolipoprotein B in rabbits fed diets containing casein or soy protein, Biochem. Biophys. Acta, 1002, 157-163.

Khosla, P., Samman, S. and Carroll, K.K. (1989b) Receptor-mediated catabolism of LDL in rabbits fed casein or soy protein. FASEB J. 3, A957.

Kita, T., Brown, M.S., Watanabe, Y. and Goldstein, J.K. (1981) Deficiency of low density lipoprotein receptors on liver and adrenal gland of the WHHL rabbit, an animal model of familial hypercholesterolemia, Proc. Natl. Acad. Sci. USA., 78, 2268-2272.

Lovati M.R., Manzoni C., Canvavesi A. et al. (1987) Soybean protein diet increases low density lipoprotein receptor activity in mononuclear cells from hyperrcholesterolemic patients, J. Clin. Invest., 80, 1498-1502.

Matthews, C.M.E. (1957) The theory of tracer experiments with ^{131}I-labelled plasma proteins, Phys, Med. Biol., 2, 36-53.

Redgrave T.G. (1984) Dietary proteins and atherosclerosis, Atherosclerosis, 52, 349-351.

Roberts D.C.K., Stalmach M.E., Khalil M.W., Hutchinson J.C. and Carroll, K.K. (1981) Effects of dietary proteins on composition and turnover of apoproteins in plasma lipoproteins of rabbits, Can. J. Biochem, 56, 642-647.

Samman, S., Khosla, P. and Carroll, K.K. (1989) Effects of dietary casein and soy protein on metabolism of radiolabelled low density apolipoprotein B in rabits, Lipids, 24, 169-172.

Terpstra, A.H.M., Harkes, L. and Van Der Veen, F.H. (1981) The effect of different proportions of casein in semipurified diets on the concentration of serum cholesterol and the lipoprotein composition in rabbits. Lipids, 16, 114-119.

Weisgraber, K.H., Innerarity, T.L. and Mahley, R.W. (1978) Role of the lysine residues in high affinity binding to cell surface receptors on human fibroblasts, J.Biol. Chem., 253, 9053-9062.

Yamada, N., Shames, D.M., Stoudemire, J.B. and Havel, R.J. (1986) Metabolism of lipoproteins containing apolipoprotein B-100 in blood plasma of rabbits: heterogenity related to the presence of apolipoprotein E, Proc. Natl. Acad. Sci. USA, 83, 3479-3483.

26

The effects of monounsaturated fatty acids on serum lipoprotien levels in healthy adult volunteers

R.P. MENSINK and M.B. KATAN

Department of Human Nutrition, Agricultural University, PO Box 8129, 6700 EV Wageningen, The Netherlands

ABSTRACT

The effects of monounsaturated fatty acids on serum lipids were studied in healthy women and men in two separate well-controlled dietary studies. In the first study it was shown that replacement of saturated fatty acids by either monounsaturated fatty acids or carbohydrates caused similar changes in serum total and LDL cholesterol levels. The HDL cholesterol level, however, was significantly lower on the diet high in carbohydrates. In the second study it was found that replacement of saturated fatty acids by a mixture of monounsaturated and polyunsaturated fatty acids caused similar serum lipid levels as replacement with polyunsaturated fatty acids alone.

It is concluded that replacement of saturated fats by oils rich in monounsaturated fatty acids might be an attractive option for optimizing serum lipid levels.

INTRODUCTION

Twenty to thirty years ago Keys and coworkers [1] and Hegsted and coworkers [2] carried out series of well-controlled dietary studies in healthy men in order to relate changes in serum total cholesterol levels - the classical risk factor for coronary heart disease [3] - to changes in the intake of different classes of fatty acids. Both groups of investigators found that, relative to carbohydrates, saturated fat increased the level of cholesterol, while polyunsaturated fat lowered it. Gram by gram, the elevating effect of saturated fatty acids was twice as high as the lowering effect of polyunsaturated fatty acids. If monounsaturated fat was exchanged for carbohydrates the level of serum total cholesterol did not change. Effects of the different fatty acids on the cholesterol concentration in the different lipoproteins were not defined in these studies [1,2]. These effects are important, as the different lipoproteins have opposite effects on the risk for coronary heart disease. Low-density lipoprotein (LDL) cholesterol is atherogenic [4], while high-density lipoprotein (HDL) cholesterol might protect against coronary heart disease [5]. It has been stated that polyunsaturated fatty acids, currently used to decrease the level of serum total cholesterol, decrease HDL cholesterol as well [6]. Less information is available about the effects of monounsaturated fatty acids on the distribution of cholesterol over the various lipoproteins.

Here we summarize the results of two controlled dietary studies in healthy women and men on the effect of monounsaturated fatty acids on LDL and HDL cholesterol levels. Monounsaturated fatty acids were compared with carbohydrates in the first study [7], and with polyunsaturated fatty acids in the second study [8].

METHODS

Subjects and design

The subjects were mainly young healthy normolipidaemic students; their ages ranged from 18 to 59 years.

In both studies all subjects first consumed for 17 days a control diet high in saturated fatty acids. They were then randomly divided over two groups in such a way that both groups had the same number of males and females. For the next 36 days both groups received one of two test diets. Diets consisted of mixed solid foods and menus were changed daily. All foodstuffs were weighed out to the participant individually and supplied according to each person's energy needs. Body-weights were checked twice a week and energy intake adjusted when necessary.

Two fasting blood samples were obtained at the end of the control period and two or three samples at the end of the test period. At the end of the study serum was analysed for total serum and HDL cholesterol, and triglycerides. LDL cholesterol was calculated using the Friedewald equation [9].

Dietary composition

Experiment I:
Monounsaturates vs carbohydrates

Forty-eight healthy men and women first consumed for 17 days a diet high in saturated fat (20.0 percent of energy intake) and total fat (38.0 percent). Twenty-four of the subjects then consumed for 36 days an olive-oil-rich diet (24.0 percent from monounsaturated fat, 40.6 percent from total fat) and the other twenty-four a high-carbohydrate, high-fibre diet (22.1 percent from total fat). The amounts of protein (12-14 percent), polyunsaturated fat (4-5 percent) and cholesterol (31-35 mg/MJ) were similar in all three diets.

Experiment II:
Monounsaturates vs polyunsaturates

Fifty-eight healthy men and women first consumed for 17 days a diet high in saturated fat (19.3 percent of energy intake from saturated fat, 11.5 percent from monounsaturated fat, and 4.6 percent from polyunsaturated fat). For the next 36 days, they received a diet with the same fat content but enriched with olive oil and sunflower oil (12.9 percent of energy intake from saturated fat, 15.1 percent from monounsaturated fat, and 7.9 percent from polyunsaturated fat) or with sunflower oil alone (12.6 percent of energy intake from saturated fat, 10.8 percent from monounsaturated fat, and 12.7 percent from polyunsaturated fat). The amounts of protein (13 percent), carbohydrates (48-49 percent) and cholesterol (33-35 mg/MJ) were similar in all three diets.

Statistical analysis

The response to the test diet was calculated per subject as the percent change from the end of the control period to the end of the test period. A two-sided t-test was used to examine the difference in responses between the two diet groups [10].

RESULTS

Experiment I

Monounsaturates vs carbohydrates

The level of total serum cholesterol fell on both diets to the same extent. The level of LDL cholesterol fell by 13.7% (0.44 mmol per litre [17 mg per decilitre]) in subjects on the olive-oil-rich diet, which was not significantly different from the decrease of 9.5% (0.36 mmol per litre [14 mg per decilitre]) in subjects consuming the high-carbohydrate, high-fibre diet. The level of HDL cholesterol rose by 3.4% (0.03 mmol per litre [1 mg per decilitre]) in the olive oil group but decreased by 14.6% (0.20 mmol per litre [7 mg per decilitre]) in the carbohydrate group. The difference in change in HDL cholesterol between the diet groups was highly significant ($P<0.001$; 95 percent confidence interval for difference between diet groups, 12.0 to 24.0 percent). The ratio of HDL to LDL cholesterol increased by 21.6% in the subjects on the olive-oil-rich diet, while this ratio decreased by 2.8% in the subjects on the high-carbohydrate diet ($P<0.001$; 95 percent confidence interval for difference, 14.9 to 33.8 percent).

Average body weight fell by 1.0 kg (range -2.5 to +1.3 kg) in the olive oil group and by 0.5 kg (range -2.3 to +1.6 kg) in the carbohydrate group.

TABLE 1. Experiment I: effects of the olive-oil and the high-carbohydrate, high-fibre diet on serum lipid concentrations*

	Olive oil group (N=24)	Carbohydrate group (N=24)
Total cholesterol (mmol/L)		
Control period	5.05 ± 0.72	5.10 ± 0.95
Test period	4.59 ± 0.68	4.61 ± 0.89
Percent change	-8.9 ± 8.6	-9.5 ± 9.7
95% confidence interval	-4.7 to 5.9	
LDL cholesterol (mmol/L)		
Control period	3.16 ± 0.65	3.27 ± 0.81
Test period	2.72 ± 0.65	2.91 ± 0.69
Percent change	-13.7 ± 11.8	-10.6 ± 12.3
95% confidence interval	-10.1 to 3.9	
HDL cholesterol (mmol/L)		
Control period	1.47 ± 0.39	1.42 ± 0.35
Test period	1.50 ± 0.34	1.22 ± 0.31
Percent change+	3.4 ± 11.8	-14.6 ± 8.6
95% confidence interval	12.0 to 24.0	
HDL/LDL cholesterol ratio		
Control period	0.49 ± 0.20	0.46 ± 0.16
Test period	0.59 ± 0.22	0.44 ± 0.15
Percent change+	21.6 ± 17.4	-2.8 ± 15.0
95% confidence interval	14.9 to 33.8	

* Values are mean ± SD.
\+ Responses to the two diets significantly different: P<0.001

Experiment II:
Monounsaturates vs polyunsaturates

Total serum cholesterol levels fell by 14.1% (0.72 mmol per litre [28 mg per decilitre]) on the monounsaturated-fat diet, which was more than the fall of 9.7% (0.51 mmol per litre [20 mg per decilitre]) on the polyunsaturated-fat diet (95% confidence interval for difference, -8.6 to -0.3 percent). LDL cholesterol levels fell by 17.9% (0.59 mmol per litre [23 mg per decilitre]) on the monounsaturated-fat diet and by 12.9% (0.45 mmol per litre [17 mg per decilitre]) on the polyunsaturated-fat diet (95% confidence interval for difference: -9.9 to 0.0 percent). The responses of the level of HDL cholesterol and of the ratio of HDL to LDL cholesterol were not significantly different between the two diet groups.

Average body weight increased by 0.2 kg (range -3.2 to +2.4 kg) in the monounsaturated-fat group and by 0.2 kg (range -1.8 to +2.2 kg) in the polyunsaturated-fat group.

TABLE 2. Experiment II: effects of the monounsaturated-fat and the polyunsaturated-fat diets on serum lipid concentrations*

	Monounsaturated-fat group (N=29)	Polyunsaturated-fat group (N=29)
Total cholesterol (mmol/L)		
Control period	5.14 ± 0.88	5.11 ± 0.73
Test period	4.42 ± 0.89	4.60 ± 0.67
Percent change+	-14.1 ± 7.4	-9.7 ± 8.3
95% confidence interval	-8.6 to -0.3	
LDL cholesterol (mmol/L)		
Control period	3.30 ± 0.75	3.33 ± 0.68
Test period	2.71 ± 0.67	2.87 ± 0.60
Percent change+	-17.9 ± 7.7	-12.9 ± 10.9
95% confidence interval	-9.9 to 0.0	
HDL cholesterol (mmol/L)		
Control period	1.38 ± 0.32	1.41 ± 0.34
Test period	1.28 ± 0.32	1.35 ± 0.38
Percent change	-6.9 ± 13.8	-3.4 ± 10.9
95% confidence interval	-10.0 to 3.0	
HDL/LDL cholesterol ratio		
Control period	0.44 ± 0.15	0.44 ± 0.14
Test period	0.49 ± 0.15	0.50 ± 0.19
Percent change	14.0 ± 17.9	11.9 ± 14.2
95% confidence interval	-6.4 to 18.0	

* Values are mean ± SD
\+ Responses to the two diets significantly different: $P<0.05$

DISCUSSION

Experiment I:
Monounsaturates vs carbohydrates

In full agreement with the experiments of Keys et al [1] and Hegsted et al [2] this study showed that in healthy subjects replacement of saturated fatty acids by either monounsaturated fatty acids or complex carbohydrates lowered serum total cholesterol levels to the same extent. However, the diet high in monounsaturates selectively lowered LDL cholesterol levels, while the diet high in carbohydrates lowered both LDL and HDL cholesterol. As a result the HDL to LDL cholesterol ratio was higher on the olive oil diet than on the carbohydrate diet (Table 1). These observations are in agreement with the results of Grundy [11], who compared the effects of two high-fat liquid formula diets, rich in either saturated or monounsaturated fatty acids, and one low-fat liquid formula diet, rich in dextrose, on serum lipoproteins in middle-aged subjects. Grundy [11] showed that replacement of 21 percent of energy from monounsaturated fatty acids by carbohydrates increased the level of LDL cholesterol by 8 percent or 0.28 mmol per litre and decreased the level of HDL cholesterol by 18 percent or 0.18 mmol per litre. The diet high in monounsaturated fatty acids did not decrease HDL cholesterol concentrations relative to the diet high in saturated fatty acids. Both the study of Grundy [11] and our own results indicate that (i) the level of LDL cholesterol can be lowered without affecting the level of HDL cholesterol (ii) the level of total fat in the diet is positively related to the level of HDL cholesterol. The latter observation is supported by an epidemiological study of schoolboys from 13 different countries: a strong positive correlation was found between the group mean values of total fat intake and of HDL cholesterol [12].

Experiment II:
Monounsaturates vs polyunsaturates

According to Keys' equation [1] polyunsaturated fatty acids are superior to monounsaturated fatty acids for lowering serum total cholesterol levels. It has been suggested, however, that part of this effect is due to a lowering of the level of HDL cholesterol [13]. We tested this in healthy subjects who were fed mixed solid diets under strict dietary control. The amount of linoleic acid in the monounsaturated-fat diet amounted to 7.9 percent and in the polyunsaturated-fat diet to 12.7 percent of total daily energy intake, while the level of saturated fatty acids and cholesterol was the same in the two diets. We did not find lower serum total and LDL cholesterol levels on the polyunsaturated-fat diet (Table 2). These results are in disagreement with numerous [1, 2] - but not all [14] - previous trials.

The polyunsaturated-fat diet did not reduce HDL cholesterol levels to a greater extent than the monunsaturated-fat diet. This finding is in contrast with the results of Mattson and Grundy [14], who found that at a level of 28 percent of energy dietary linoleic acid lowered HDL cholesterol when compared with dietary monounsaturates. The level of linoleic acid employed, however, was unrealistically high. Diets with less extreme levels of polyunsaturated fatty acids had no effect on HDL cholesterol in most controlled trials [15].

Conclusions

Our studies have shown that, as far as lipoprotein levels are concerned, monounsaturated fatty acids might be helpful for the prevention of coronary heart disease. The first study showed that lipoproteins were more favourable on a diet rich in monounsaturated fatty acids than on a diet rich in complex carbohydrates. The second study suggested that replacing saturated fatty acids by a mixture of monounsaturated and polyunsaturated fatty acids caused the same favourable change in serum lipoproteins as replacement by polyunsaturated fatty acids alone. Although this last finding conflicts with many other data [1,2], these two studies do indicate that oils rich in monounsaturated fatty acids might be useful in the treatment of hypercholesterolaemia, provided that the intake is low enough to avoid increases in body weight.

ACKNOWLEDGEMENTS

We thank the volunteers for their cooperation and interest and the technical and dietary staff of the department for their assistance.

Our research was supported by grants from the Commission of the European Communities, the Netherlands Nutrition Foundation, the Netherlands Heart Foundation (grant D-87002), and the Netherlands Ministry of Welfare, Public Health, and Culture.

REFERENCES

1. Keys A, Anderson JT, Grande F. Serum cholesterol response to changes in the diet. IV. Particular saturated fatty acids in the diet. Metabolism 1965;14:776-787.
2. Hegsted DM, McGandy RB, Myers ML, Stare FJ. Quantitative effects of dietary fat on serum cholesterol in man. Am J Clin Nutr 1965;17:281-295.
3. Keys A, ed. Coronary Heart Disease in Seven Countries. Circulation 1970;41:suppl 1.
4. The Lipids Research Clinics Coronary Primary Prevention Trial Results. II. Therelationship of reduction in incidence of coronary heart disease to cholesterol lowering. JAMA 1984;251:365-374.
5. Schaefer EJ. Clinical, biochemical and genetic features in familial disorders of high density lipoproteins deficiency. Arteriosclerosis 1984;4:303-322.
6. Vega GL, Groszek E, Wolf R, Grundy SM. Influence of polyunsaturated fats on composition of plasma lipoproteins. J Lipid Res 1982;23:811-822.
7. Mensink RP, Katan MB. Effect of monounsaturated fatty acids versus complex carbohydrates on high-density lipoproteins in healthy men and women. Lancet 1987;i:122-125.
8. Mensink RP, Katan MB. Effect of a diet enriched with monounsaturated or polyunsaturated fatty acids on levels of low-density and high-density cholesterol in healthy women and men. N Engl J Med;321:436-441.
9. Friedewald WT, Levy RI, Fredrickson DS. Estimation of the concentration of low-density lipoprotein cholesterol in plasma without use of the preparative ultracentrifugation. Clin Chem 1972;18: 499-502.
10. Snedecor GW, Cochran WG. Statistical methods. 7th ed. Ames: Iowa State University Press, 1980.
11. Grundy SM. Comparison of monounsaturated fatty acids and carbohydrates for lowering plasma cholesterol. New Engl J Med 1986;314:745-748.

12. West CE, Sullivan DR, Katan, MB, Halferkamps IL, van der Torre HW. Boys from populations with high carbohydrate intake have higher fasting triglycerides than boys from populations with high fat intake. Am J Epidemiol, in press.
13. Vessby B, Boberg J, Gustafsson IB, Karlström B, Lithell H, Östlund-Lindquist AM. Reduction of high density lipoprotein cholesterol and apolipoprotein A-I concentrations by a lipid-lowering diet. Atherosclerosis 1980;35:21-7.
14. Mattson FH, Grundy SM. Comparison of effects of dietary saturated, monounsaturated, and polyunsaturated fatty acids on plasma lipids and lipoproteins in man. J Lipid Res 1985; 26:194-202.
15. Beynen AC, Katan MB. In: Vergroesen AJ, Crawford MA, eds. The role of fats in human nutrition. Impact of dietary cholesterol and fatty acids on serum lipids and lipoproteins in man. London: Academic Press Limited, 1989:238-54

27
Olive oil in nutrition and in prevention

C. DAL PALU', A. PAGNAN* and A. BONANOME**
**Clinica Medica I, University of Padova, Italy*
*** Patologia Speciale Medica, University of Padova, Italy*

Olive oil is one of the vegetable oils with the highest content of oleic acid (18:1), the major monounsaturated fatty acid. The nutritional role of monounsaturated fatty acids has been reevaluated in the recent years, when it has become clear that the substitution of saturated fatty acids for monounsaturated fatty acids induces a significant lowering of plasma cholesterol levels. Indeed, for a long time the leading opinion was that, contrary to polyunsaturated fatty acids, monounsaturates did not have a hypocholesterolemic effect (1,2). The epidemiological observations of the Seven Countries Study (3) however supported the opposite thesis, that is that diets rich in oleic acid have a cholesterol lowering effect. This was evident in the populations of the Mediterranean countries, whose diet is rich in oleic acid, due to the high consumption of olive oil. These populations have lower levels of plasma cholesterol as compared with the North American and North European populations, who consume much higher amounts of saturated fats with their diets.

Mattson and Grundy (4) were the first ones to demonstrate that monounsaturated fatty acids are equivalent to polyunsaturates for lowering plasma LDL cholesterol. These authors studied a group of normal volunteers who were admitted to a metabolic ward where they consumed diets rich in palmitic acid (16:0), oleic acid, and linoleic acid (18:2). Plasma levels of total and LDL cholesterol were equally lowered by both diets rich in unsaturated fatty acids. Further, the diet rich in monounsaturates did not lower plasma HDL cholesterol, which was reduced by the diet high in polyunsaturated fatty acids.

Other investigators have shown that polyunsaturated fatty

acids tend to reduce plasma HDL cholesterol (5). More recently, however, Mensink and Katan, besides confirming that diets rich in oleic acid lower LDL cholesterol in plasma as much as those rich in linoleic acid, have reported a slight decrease of plasma levels of HDL cholesterol with both these types of dietary regimen.

The cholesterol lowering potential of diets rich in mono= unsaturated fatty acids has also been compared with that of low fat, high carbohydrate diets, such as those that are tipical of orienatl countries, whose populations are known to have low levels of plasma cholesterol (7,8,9). Grundy (7) reported that these high monounsaturated fat diets and low fat diets induce similar changes of plasma LDL cholesterol levels. Also in this study, however, whereas the high intake of oleic acid did not lower plasma HDL cholesterol, the low fat diet significantly dcreased the plasma concentration of this lipid fraction. Furthermore, the high intake of carbohydrates was probably responsible for a raise of plasma triglyceride levels. Thus, although it is still questioned whether the hypertryglyceridemic effect of dietary carbohydrates is a transient phenomenon, the diet rich in monounsaturates showed more "advantageous" changes of the lipid profile from the viewpoint of the cardiovascular risk. These observations have been confirmed by other studies (8,9).

Diets enriched in oleic acid have been recently proposed by Garg et al. (10) for the treatment of non insulin dependent diabetes mellitus. These patients are generally advised to assume low fat diets, rich in complex carbohydrates and fiber. The rationale for this dietary approach is to improve glycemic control and to lower plasma LDL cholesterol levels. A high carbohydrate intake, however, mey not be optimal since, as it has been mentioned, it may also raise plasma triglycerides and lower plasma HDL cholesterol. The aforementioned study (10) indeed showed that a better lipid profile and and lower 24 hour levels of plasma glucose could be obtained with the diet rich in monounsaturates. One question that is still open is whether patients may gain weight more easily when they consume a higher intake of fat. Thus, more investigations are certainly needed to determine what diet can be recommended as the most suitable for patients with non insulin dependent diabetes mellitus.

The mechanism by which oleic acid lowers plasma cholesterol is probably the enhancement of LDL receptors and, consequently, a more efficient plasma clearance of LDL particles. Experimental data favor this hypothesis (11), although no lipoprotein kinetic studies performed in humans are available. Also, it is not known whether this is a direct effect of oleic acid but, more likely, it is the consequence of the substitution of saturated fatty acids in the diet.

The consumption of diets high in saturated fatty acids has been also related to higher levels of blood pressure (12). In accordance, the substitution of saturates with polyunsaturates has been reported to induce a hypotensive effect (12,13). Recently, Pagnan et al. (14) reported that the substitution of saturated fatty acids for monounsaturated fatty acids can also lead a significant, although small, lowering of blood pressure.

It has been speculated that dietary fatty acids might affect blood pressure levels by inducing changes in the cation transp= ort systems located on cell membranes (15). The fatty acid composition of cell memmbranes is known to change coherently with changes in the intake of dietary fat. A higher degree of unsaturationleads to a higher fluidity of membranes, which might affect the ion transport systems that have been implicated in the regulation of blood pressure (15,16,17).

In conclusion, diets rich in monounsaturated fats such as olive oil induce favourable metabolic effects which might be important for the prevention of cardiovascular disease.

REFERENCES

1. Keys A., anderson JT, Grande F. (1957). Prediction of serum cholesterol responses to changes in fat in the diet. Lancet, ii, 959-966.

2. Hegsted DM, McGandy RB, Myers ML, Stare FJ. (1965). Quantitative effects of dietary fat on serum cholesterol in man. Am.J.Clin.Nutr., 17, 281-295.

3. Keys A, ed. (1970). Coronary heart disease in seven coun= tries. Circulation, 41 (Suppl 1), 1-211.

4. Mattson FH, Grundy SM. (1985). Comparison of dietary satura= ted, monounsaturated and polyunsaturated fatty acids on plasma lipids and lipoproteins in man. J.Lipid Res., 26, 194-202.

5. Shepherd J, Packard CJ, Patsch JR, Gotto AM Jr;, Taunton OD.

(1978). Effects of dietary polyunsaturated and saturated fat on the properties of high density lipoprotein and the metabolism of apolipoprotein A-I. J.Clin.Invest., 60, 1582-1592.
6. Mensink RP, Katan MB. (1989). Effect of a diet enriched with monounsaturated or polyunsaturated fatty acids on levels of low density and high density lipoprotein cholesterol in healthy women and men. N.Engl.J.Med., 321, 436-441.
7. Grundy SM. (1986). Comparison of monounsaturated fatty acids and carbohydrates for plasma cholesterol lowering. N.Engl.J.Med. 314, 745-748.
8. Mensink RP, Katan MB. (1987). Effect of monounsaturated fatty acids versus complex carbohydrates on high-density lipo= proteins in healthy men and women. Lancet, 1, 122-125.
9. Grundy SM, Nix D, Whelan MF, Franklin L. (1986). Comparison of three cholesterol lowering diets in normolipidemic men. JAMA, 256, 2351-2355.
10. Garg A, Bonanome A, Grundy SM, Zhang ZJ, Unger RH. (1988). Comparison of high carbohydrate diet with high monounsaturated fat diet in patients with non insulin dependent diabetes melli= tus. N.Engl.J.Med., 319, 829-834.
11. Spady DK, Dietschy J. (1985). dietary saturated triglyce= rides suppress hepatic low density lipoprotein receptors in the hamster. Proc.Natl.acad.sci.USA, 82, 4526-4530.
12. Puska P, Iacono JM, nissinen A, et al. (1983). Controlled randomised trial of the effect of dietary fat on blood pressure. Lancet, 1, 1-5.
13. Iacono JM, Dougherty RM, Puska P. Reduction of blood pressu re associated with dietary polyunsaturated fat. Hypertension (1982), 4, 34-42.
14. Pagnan A, ambrosio A, Baggio G, et al. (1986). Changes in lipid pattern and blood pressure after substitution of separable fats with olive oil or sunflower oil in the diet: feasibility and efficacy in normolipidemic families (The Cittadella study). Giorn. Arteriosclerosi, 3, 180-181.
15. Pagnan A, Corrocher R, Ambrosio GB, et al. (1989). Effects of an olive oil enriched diet on erythrocyte membrane lipid composition and cation transport systems. Clinical Science, 76, 87-93.
16. Popp-Snijders C, Schouten JA, Van Der Meer J, Van Der Veen EA. (1986). Fatty fish induced changes in membrane lipid

composition and viscosity of human erythrocyte suspensions. Scand.J.Lab.Invest., 46, 253-258.

17. Canessa M, Spalvins A, Adragna N, Falkner B. (1984). Red cell sodium countertransport and cotransport in normotensive and hypertensive blacks. Hypertension, 6, 344-351.

ATHERSCLEROSIS, COMPUTER HANDLING STUDIES AND MATHEMATICAL MODELLING

28 Some methods for medical image processing using supercomputers

I. GALLIGANI

Department of Mathematics, University of Bologna, Italy

ABSTRACT. In the field of Medical Image Processing (MIP) many computing tools must be at our disposal. They concern with the resolution of problems of Pattern Recognition, Scene Analysis, Image Restoration and Image Reconstruction from Projections. Accurate solutions to many of these problems may be obtained by using supercomputers. In this note we present some MIP «special» interactive systems and some methods for image restoration problems ideally suited for implementation on a multiprocessor vector computer.

1. INTRODUCTION

Medical Image Processing (MIP) is an indispensable tool in medical diagnosis. It needs extremely interactive software systems. In particular, many «special purpose» interactive systems must be at our disposal; indeed, they provide an environment within which a wide variety of fundamental operations for the treatment of the images may be easily realized. These «special» systems are implemented on graphical workstations with a local high computational capability; sometimes, these workstations are connected with a supercomputer, as CRAY X-MP, for the execution of «elaborate programs».

At the *Laboratory of Numerical Analysis* of the University of Bologna two «special» systems for the analysis of various numerical methods and the simulation of different data collections in Computerized Tomography and for the elaboration of colposcopic maps have been developed [6], [7], [8], [9].

It is well known that the «effectiveness» of a «special» system is dependent on the range of the mathematical capabilities of the system. The advent of high-performance vector computers, such as the CRAY X-MP, is having a profound effect on this mathematical software. This is true, in particular, for algorithms and software for the image reconstruction from projections problem and for the image restoration problem.

In this paper, we present some of our work on the development of algorithms and software for the image restoration problem which are designed to be effective when used on multi-vector computers.

2. METHODS FOR IMAGE RESTORATION

Given an ideal image f(x y) and the corresponding degraded image g(x y), we will assume that g and f are related by

$$g(x\ y) = \int h(x\ y\ x'y')\ f(x'y')dx'dy + e(x\ y) \tag{1}$$

where h(x y x'y') is the point-spread-function and e(x y) the random noise that may be present in the output image. If we discretize equation (1), we obtain the following system of linear equations

$$\mathbf{g} = \mathrm{H}\ \mathbf{f} + \mathbf{e} \tag{2}$$

in which the dimension of the point-spread-function is quite large. For a low resolution image of 512x512 pixels, H takes on a size 262144x262144, which is difficult to operate upon in the computer; obviously storage alone is a monumental task.

The image restoration problem (1) is an ill-conditioned problem and H is a matrix with an ill-determined numerical rank. A well known and highly regarded method for dealing with such problems is the *method of regularization* by Phillips and Tikhonov.

When the point-spread-function is «space-invariant» this method is very attractive in terms of speed and storage requirements. We use the fast Fourier transform (FFT) algorithm to determine the regularized solution of (2). A Fortran program for a vector implementation on CRAY X-MP of this method has been developed [4], [5]. Also in the case in which the point-spread-funcion is «separable» the method of regularization may be implemented on a vector computer efficiently (limited amount of storage space and small computer time) by using the preconditioned conjugate gradient algorithm for determining the regularized solution of (2). In well defined conditions, polynomial preconditioning is a convenient choice [2].

The advent of multivector computers makes tractable the general case in which the point-spread-function has no specific form. Indeed, a natural approach to solve the problem (1) on these multiprocessing computing systems is based on the domain decomposition principle. The basic idea is to decompose the domain into subdomains and restore the image-patch in each subdomain separately so that the continuity is preserved across subdomains interfaces. In this case, we are concerned with an image-patch restoration problem in which some equality constraints are imposed on the image. That is, in each subdomain one must solve a medium-size equality constrained quadratic programming problem with no special structure [3]:

$$\text{minimize} \quad \frac{1}{2}\,\mathbf{w}^T A\mathbf{w} - \mathbf{w}^T\mathbf{r}$$

$$\text{subject to } E^T\mathbf{w} - \mathbf{s} = 0$$

The solution of this problem is obtained by the method of multipliers combined with the preconditioned conjugate gradient algorithm. This method is well suitable for a multiprocessor system. A Fortran program for a parallel implementaion on CRAY X-MP with CMIC$ microtasking directives of this method has been developed [3].

3. REFERENCES

[1] Andrews H.C., Hunt B.R. (1977) *Digital Image Restoration.* Prentice-Hall Inc., Englewood Cliff, N.J.

[2] Galligani I., Ruggiero V., Zama F. (1979) «A Polynomial Preconditioner for the Conjugate Gradient Method on Vector Computers». *Atti Accad. Scienze Istituto di Bologna XIV*, 6.

[3] Galligani I., Ruggiero V., Zama F. (1989) «Solution of the equality-constrained image restoration problem on a vector computer». *Proceedings of the International Conference on Parallel Computing 1989* (G.R. Joubert, D.J. Evans & F.J. Peters, eds.) Elsevier Science Publ., Amsterdam.

[4] Bacchelli Montefusco L., Guerrini C. (1989) «A Note on the Parameter Choice of Tikhonov Regularization in Image Restoration». *Atti Accad. Scienze Istituto di Bologna XIV*, 6.

[5] Guerrini C. (1989) «An Algorithm for Image Restoration» (submitted for publication).

[6] Guerrini C. (1989) «An Interactive Graphic system for Image Reconstruction from Projections». *Atti Accad. Scienze Istituto di Bologna XIV*, 6.

[7] Guerrini C., Spaletta G. (1989) «An Image Reconstruction Algorithm in Tomography: A version for the CRAY X-MP Vector Computer». (to appear in *Computer Graphics*).

[8] Guerrini C., Pagni G. (1985) «Metodi per l'Elaborazione di Immagini Termografiche». *Atti Accad. Scienze Istituto di Bologna XIV*, 2.

[9] Guerrini C., Trallo F., Costa S. (1989) «Elaboration of Colposcopic Maps by Means of an Interactive Graphic System» (to appear in *Medical Informations*).

29
A diffusion-governed model related to atheroma deposition

M. NICHELATTI[1], G. PALLOTTI[2] and P. PETTAZZONI[2]

[1]*Pierrel Pharmaceuticals, via Bisceglie 96, I-20152 Milan;* [2]*Department of Physics, University of Bologna, via Irnerio 46, I-40126 Bologna, Italy*

ABSTRACT. A mathematical model is presented in order to simulate the development of the atheromatic plaque from a phenomenological point of view. The model utilizes some geometrical factors involved in the flow of the lipoproteins into blood vessels. Following the assumptions and the mathematical treatment, the model may be useful in order to evaluate the probability bounded to sedimentation of a given molecule on the atheroma.

1. INTRODUCTION

The mathematical models applied to atherosclerosis seem give some useful indications about the possible development of the plaque, as recently demonstred by Descovich and co-authors (1987, 1989), who examined the atheroma growth utilizing the stochastic processes theory applied to the lipoproteins sedimentation on the arterial wall.

The model here presented also describes the plaque growth utilizing a stochastic approach but considering the capture of the involved molecules as the result of an active caption done by the atheroma. The description of the system is phenomenological and is subject to some geometrical limitations and to some physical assumptions.

We shall suppose all particles involved in the atheroma sedimentation be equal by size and main properties; the kinetics of the aggregation will be carried out by means of the Smoluchowski's treatment as described by Risken (1989) and Gardiner (1985).

2. MODEL

Let us consider the lipid particles traveling into blood stream, let us also assume the atheroma deposed on the arterial wall having a semispherical form: we shall suppose three co-ordinate axes centered in the atheroma and a "critical" distance for which all particles passing near to the plaque are captured and also sedimented on the atheroma itself.

From the above assumptions we shall deduce that all collisions are reactive and that no potential barriers are involved in the model.
The whole phenomenon will also depend on the diffusion kinetics of the particles considered in the system, and the evolution of the atheroma size will be determined by the number of collapsed particles and therefore by the critical distance R and by the number of particles passing through the artery in the time unit.
The time evolution of the system will be determined in the configuration space by the Fokker - Planck equation

$$\frac{\partial P(r,t)}{\partial t} = D \cdot \nabla^2 P(r,t) \tag{1}$$

where P(r,t) represents the probability density function, r is the distance between atheroma and particle, t is the time, D the diffusion coefficient and ∇^2 is the Laplacian del squared operator.
Equation (1) is 'restricted' to the configuration space, and hence does not take into account the velocities of the particles; in facts at relatively high viscosity values the velocities of the particles are rapidly relaxing towards equilibrium distribution, and hence to diffusion.
The boundary conditions are

$$P(r,0) = 1, \quad \forall\ r > R \tag{2a}$$

$$P(r,t) = 0, \quad r = R, \quad \forall\ t \tag{2b}$$

We can suppose a 'cloud' of lipoproteins flowing across the surface determined by the critical distance R; the flow will also follow the usual Fick's law, so that we shall calculate the flow of the particles towards the atheroma as follows:

$$\dot{F} = 2\Pi R^2 D \cdot C_P \left. \frac{\partial P(r,t)}{\partial t} \right|_R \tag{3}$$

in which $\dot{F}$ represents the particles flow and C_P the lipoprotein concentration.
Solving equation (1) also considering the boundary conditions (2a) and (2b) we get

$$P(r,t) = \frac{r - R}{r} + \frac{2R}{r[\Pi]^{1/2}} \int_0^{(r-R)/2[Dt]^{1/2}} \exp[- x^2]\ dx \tag{4}$$

and therefore if we substitute the calculated value of P(r,t) in equation (3), we obtain the explicit equation of the particles flow, written as

$$\dot{F} = 2\pi RD \cdot C_P + \frac{2\pi R^2 D \cdot C_P}{[\pi Dt]^{\frac{1}{2}}} \qquad (5)$$

3. DISCUSSION AND CONCLUSIONS

The graph of $\dot{F}$, qualitatively obtained by computer simulation, shows a behavior mainly similar to the curve obtained by Descovich and co-authors: the first step of sedimentation proceeds rapidly; the process becomes successively becomes more slower, and after the sedimentation tends to the asymptotic value $2\pi RD \cdot C_P$, reached after a time equal to infinity.

The whole system behaves as a series of chemical reactions between particles of different rank, following the scheme $X_i + X_j \rightarrow X_{i+j}$, for all positive integer values of i and j.

The rate constant will be given by

$$K_{ij} = 4\pi R_{ij} D + R_{ij} \frac{4\pi D}{[\pi Dt]^{\frac{1}{2}}} \qquad (6)$$

under condition of spherical symmetry.

The kinetic equation for the considered sequence of reactions is

$$\frac{dc_i}{dt} = \frac{1}{2} \sum_{m+n=i} c_m c_n K_{mn} - c_i \sum_{j=1}^{\infty} c_j K_{ij} \qquad (7)$$

The model contains some approximations and assumptions 'a priori', in particular from the biological viewpoint; equally, we think, it may be an useful new starting point for the theoretical investigations about the development of the atheromatic plaque.

The fact that two different mathematical models (this one and the model by Descovich and co-authors) can give similar qualitative results and findings (even if the models are starting from completely different assumptions) seems of particular relevance.

A difference between models is given by the fact that we did not consider the possibility of a complete obstruction of the interested artery, whereas in the other model this evenience has been taken into account. This was due to our considerations about the relatively small radius of the plaque with respect to the cross - section of the artery, at least during the first steps of the atheroma growth.

4. ACKNOWLEDGEMENTS

This work was supported by the 60% grants of the Italian Ministery of Public Education (Ministero della Pubblica Istruzione).

REFERENCES

Descovich, G.C., Gaddi, A., Pallotti, G., Pettazzoni, P., and Slawomirski, M.R. (1987) 'A Stochastic Process Approach to the Development of atheroma', Med. Hypotheses 23, 277.

Descovich, G.C., Gaddi, A., Nichelatti, M., Pallotti, G., Pettazzoni, P., and Slawomirski, M.R. (1989) 'Variance Analysis of the Atheromatic Sedimentation as a Stochastic Process', Clinica e Laboratorio 13, 5.

Gardiner, C.W. (1985) Handbook of Stochastic Methods, II Ed., Springer Verlag, Berlin.

Risken, H. (1989) The Fokker - Planck Equation, II Ed., Springer Verlag, Berlin.

30
Mathematical model: interpolation and simulation

A. DORMI, G.L. MAGRI, G. MANNINO and G.C. DESCOVICH

Chair of Geriatrics, Atherosclerosis Center, University of Bologna, via Massarenti 9, 40138 Bologna, Italy

ABSTRACT The application of most advanced mathematical models to epidemiology may prove useful and make it possible to test some methods of modern medicine.
In our experience, applied to the Brisighella Study, interpolation suggested the cut off point of 237 mg/dl of plasma cholesterol level to define cardiovascular high-risk population.
Simulation applied to the prevention of coronary fatal new events suggested the most powerful efficacy of a whole population intervention strategy over a high-risk intervention strategy.

Introduction

With the evolution of modern medicine interest is shifting towards prevention through community action strategies, and research also now tends to be based on different methods of studying pathologic phenomena. Clinical epidemiology, from a description of events and applying statistical tests, is now oriented towards mathematical models of the occurrence of an event in the attempt to discriminate possible etiopathogenetic links. Hence the need of having models available. Multiple Logistic Functions have been used for some time to study the "weight" of some parameters in the occurrence of an event. This "weight" indicates whether a certain parameter is either a risk or a protective factor in the occurrence of that event.
In recent years, in line with the international literature, we observed that the main cardiovascular risk factors are the following: age, sex, smoking, systolic pressure, blood cholesterol levels. Physical exercise is a protective factor. Based on these findings, more sophisticated models were applied: <u>INTERPOLATION</u> and <u>SIMULATION</u>.
Interpolation proves useful to identify cut off points where the risk curve peaks; using the acquired knowledge on risk factors, the main objective of our research is the standardization of the most suitable action strategies and the identification of parametric levels to enact prevention. Interpolation can suggest the best levels at which action should be started.
Once this has been determined, or tried to be determined, the simulation of a change in the level of risk factors

becomes important to verify changes in the calculated theoretical risk.

Materials and methods

Mathematical models have been applied to the population enrolled in the Brisighella Study. This study started in 1972 with the aim of obtaining epidemiological data on the main cardiovascular (CVD) risk factors, and 2939 subjects (1491 males and 1448 females aged 14-84) were recruited.
This observational longitudinal survey continued with four-year follow up controls until 1984 and then became the Brisighella Project: an interventional trial.
Multiple Logistic Function was calculated according to Walker and Duncan; interpolation was calculated according to spline function; simulation was performed calculating the variations of theoretical risk for coronary heart disease (CHD) deaths in "high-risk" populations (total cholesterol >239 mg/dl as the Consensus Conferences affirm) and in the whole population.

calculated theoretical risk with high significance parameters: age (a), total plasma cholesterol (tc), systolic blood pressure (sbp).

$$p = \frac{1}{1+\exp-[K+x(a)*c(a)+x(tc)*c(tc)+x(sbp)*c(sbp)]}$$

K=MLF constant, x=value, c=MLF coefficient

Interpolation was applied only to the male sample since CVD deaths were too few in the females.

Results

Multiple Logistic Function showed the significance of some parameters to predict cardiovascular diseases and coronary heart disease.
Age, total plasma cholesterol, systolic blood pressure and smoking emerged as the main risk factors; physical activity was a protective factor.
Total plasma cholesterol levels of the entire population and of cardiovascular events were interpolated and the two curves showed a point of shift at 237 mg/dl (fig.1). Over this value the interpolation of CVD cholesterol levels showed a fast raising; this cut off point may be considered the "high CVD risk" cholesterol level in our population.

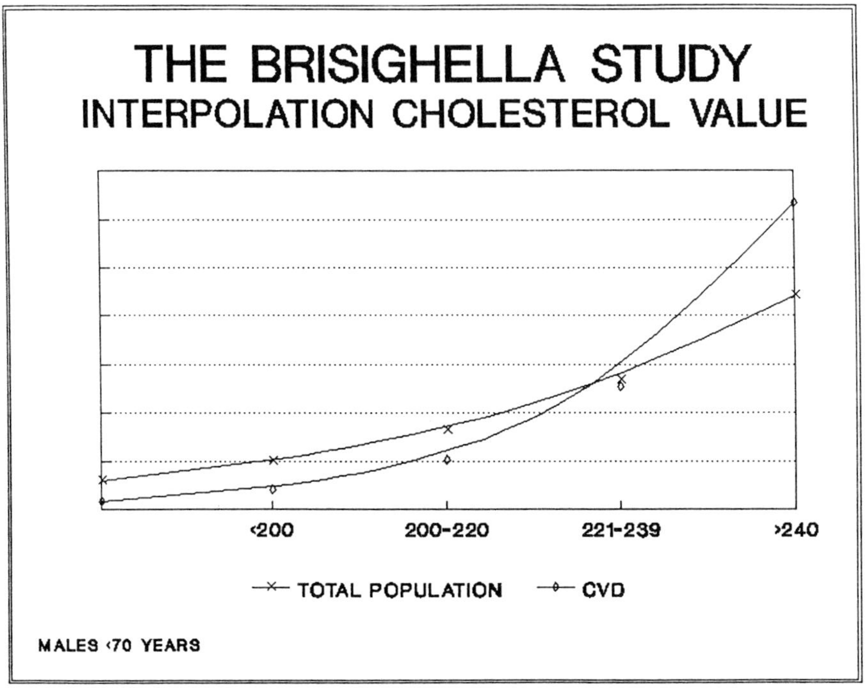
THE BRISIGHELLA STUDY
INTERPOLATION CHOLESTEROL VALUE
<200
200-220
221-239
>240
TOTAL POPULATION
CVD
MALES <70 YEARS

Fig.1

The simulation study was applied to the calculated theoretical risk for fatal CHD events.
In each subject a decrease of 5% of total plasma cholesterol and of systolic blood pressure was calculated.
This intervention caused a theoretical decrease of -1 (arbitrarily fixed) in high risk males, -14 in high risk females and -7 in all; in the whole population it caused a decrease of -10 in males, -80 in females and -44 in all. This example explains a high risk/whole population ratio of efficacy of 1/10 in males, 1/6 in females, 1/7 in all.

Discussion

Interpolation underlines a cholesterol value which may represent, in our population, the cut off point to isolate the "high-risk" population. Our purpose (237 mg/dl) is near to what the Consensus Conferences indicate (240 mg/dl). This result is similar to what was observed in other main trials (MRFIT etc.).
Our simulation affirms the most beneficial effect of population strategy over high-risk strategy; to choose one intervention does not exclude the other but whole populations must be preferred.
Mathematical models are very impressive but it must be remembered that man, the most perfect and imperfect inhabitant of the world, stands between mathematics and medicine.

Suggested references

Rao C.R. (1952): Advanced Statistical Methods in Biometric Research. J. Wiley & Sons, New York.

Walker S.H., Duncan D.B. (1967): Estimation of the probability of an event as a function of several independent variables. Biometrika, 54, 167.

Alexandrov A.D., Kolmogorov A.N., Lavrentev M.A. (1984): Mathematics: its Content, Methods, and Meanings. II edition. The MIT Press, Cambridge, Massachussets.

31
Limits of mathematical models in biology and medicine

P.G. NANNI, G. CASTELLANI, P. PETTAZZONI, G. PALLOTTI and C. PALLOTTI

Department of Physics, University of Bologna, via Irnerio 46, 40126 Bologna, Italy

ABSTRACT. Starting from analysis of the possible interaction between the medical user and the machine, the authors examine the limits of mathematical models in biology and medicine considering the complexity of the operations requested to human operator for medical image processing.

1. Introduction

The attempts of reconstructing the human decisional process are born with the first computers in the fascinating prospective to create an artificial intelligence in order to simulate step by step the logical human scheme [1].

Schematically, the decisional process of physician can be divided in three parts: the clinical experience, the data elaboration, the diagnosis. Each of these aspects can be simulated by the computer: experience is substituted by a *data bank of knowledge*, which obviously must be as large as possible; the data elaboration becomes reconstructed and simulated through a series of algorithms, that have to be brought to a logical conclusion (diagnosis).

Currently we have realised that the results provided by this kind of approach are certainly inferior to the expected hopes, for the following reasons. Primarily it seems to be a macroscopic error of prospective: too much trust was given to the quantitative data,.as if the physician education could be defined as a summation of only quantitative elements to suitable for a simple transfer to a computer. The main problem, which in the years was easily resolved, seemed to be the memory implement of the computer. Besides the excessive optimism inherent in this presumption implied equally an acritical attitude in the collection of data which in great quantity was surveyed with great simplification. This brought to a broad but higly unreadable storage of data bank. But the *clinical* education represents the results of a filtering process tied to the moment in which a new data is collected, to the previous experience, to the different weight given to the information that is memorized in a critical personal manner [2,3]. At present this kind of information is not, available for a computer.

There exists, furthermore, another critical difference between human argumentation and the algorithms which allow to get to a computerized diagnosis. Whilst the human mind proceeds in parallel, processing contemporally more information tied in an illegible manner, the computer can today only work in series strictly sequential mechanism.

2. Mathematical Models

The analogue and digital computers are an excellent aid in mathematical models, even if it is appropriate to make a few fundamental distinctions in order to evaluate which are the problems involved in the mathematical models of the biological phenomenon and how they have to be approached.

In the first place it is important to make a distinction, which is not simply formal, but substantial. We shall define two different types of mathematical models: direct and indirect models. Mathematical models are taken into consideration every time any phenomenon has to de explained and any time one has to investigate a quantity which varies as a function of an independent variable, for example, time. Using a Carthesian graph it is possible to show,in a roughly way, the mathematical law which desribes the process under examination.

Let us look into the difference between direct and indirect mathematical models. The task of direct models is to determine in which way a variable changes its values when varies a related independent quantity. Considering the indirect models these mathematical tools are very suitable for a wide anlysis of sistems under examination. But now an interdisciplinary collaboration is needed because the final goal depends on the scientific background of the committed researchers. The final aim is the reason that a given phenomenon occurs and develops with a given procedure that can be temporal and/or graphical, in any case dependent on certain variables.

The digital and analogue computers are of extreme interest and use in the analysis of data and in checking the development of the study in giving a confirmation of what had been proposed. At the origin of this paper is a constructive critic needed to get, on the basis of the data know, the general law of the system taken into examination.

3. Image Analysis

Clinical examination methods [4,5] have, in the last few years, made available a large number and a wide variety of images that are playing an ever more important role in the field of medical diagnostics. In addition to straightforward photography and to cytology and hystology, some techniques that are able to produce medical images are nuclear scintigraphy, X-ray radiography, echography and ultrasound, thermography and computerized axial tomography. Regardless of the way in which they were obtained, all bioimages have two predominant characteristics:

- high diagnostic information content;

- presence of disturbance, distortions and noise which reduce the quality of the image to a greater or lesser extent and, hence, diminish the possibility of accessing the information contained therein.

It is therefore useful, and sometimes indispensable, to adopt suitable preprocessing techniques that increase image interpretation. A first type of computer intervention is needed that of improving image quality so as to allow an easier extraction of the information [6,7]. In these applicatons, the computer is, in general, limited to the task of converting in images which, because of the way they are formed, cannot be immediately interpreted by man, into much easily observable images; any evaluation or interpretation of these images is, however, left to man.

A second type of operation, on the contrary, regards the extraction and possibly the interpretation of the information contained in the images so as to supply the human operator with wider and/or better diagnostic directions, up to reach a complete automation of the diagnosis.

The possibility of improving on, or, at least, matching man's performance in interpreting the information content of images for diagnostic purposes has been the subject of a great deal of intense research over the last few decades. This interest can be justified, on the one hand, by the desire for man to be freed from the need to carry out long and tiresome examinations of the large number of images that are obtained from mass-screening, and, on the other hand, by the need to standardize evaluation criteria so as to obtain greater objectivity in diagnostic judgements. The results that have so far been obtained are of considerable interest and have, in some cases, led to the routine utilization of particular methods and cumputerized techniques.

However, in the commercial personal computer based systems that are currently available, interaction with the operator is generally required and determined by a series of extremely rigid procedures, that are very often extraneous to the daily practice of laboratories; furthermore, the functions of the program are quite specialized and the user is often required to perform image preanalysis operations that are generally long, tiresome and, in any case, computationally cumbersome and not always adequate. In many cases, on the other hand, methods requiring a less rigid user interaction are suitably implementable only on computers of a certain size and consistent cost. In our opinion, both these factors have seriously limited the diffusion of these new diagnostic aids in the past and continue to do so at the present time. Their diffusion would, however, be facilitated by the availability of workstations possessing robust and versatile application programs that could be adapted to the wide variety of biological situations and analytical requirements ecountered.

4. Discussion and Conclusios

It is easy to check what great disappointment is brought when one tries to ask to to simulate with the computer what the machine cannot intrinsically give. Artificial intelligence is today something different to human intelligence, even if in our opinion the former will have an incredible development.

Therefore it has been necessary to change the attitude of those who thought they could resolve the question putting the computer at the doctor's place. The computer cannot substitute the man'mind but it is to a versatile and poverfull integrator of plans decisional activity.

Another error is traceable in the attempt of creating a computer as universal as possible. It is technically possible to store information regarding all the medical patterns, due to the fact that the computer's memory is expandable. However, a lot of informations are not feasible if one take into account that the increase of knowledge in medical-biological field reduplicates in a very short time. Moreover, the informations before the transfer to the data bank of knowledge, must be filtered critically, analized and correlated each other. The most part of time required for this is necessary for structuring and hierarchizing each information before the memory storage.

Lastly, it is important to emphasize the psychological aspect, the more a system increases the more it moves away from the medical-biological operator whose only feeling with the working machine is the keyboard, An intelligent operator refuse abruptly such a system, because the alternative is the total and acritical acceptance.

Thus, the use of analogue and digital computers in the bio-medical field presumes that there is a supervision on the part of someone who knows the progress of the natural process.

At present an investigator can try to use with some changes mathematical laws belonging to general evolution of the activities mankind (for instance economics) or explaining the physical behaviour of solid matter or real fluids.

But the biological compartements, the various organ, the different function and also the human body as a whole, show a high variability in the structure and behaviour that still now is not possible to describe correctly.

The enormous amount of images of medical interest daily produced by the modern investigation tools used for diagnostic purposes, makes the use of automatic means more and more necessary for their processing. One of the goals of such mean is that executing those routine tasks, often time consuming and boring, or not suited man, that allow to extract from the image quantitative information useful to formulate a diagnosis. Their use, however, is trongly often conditioned by the limited ability to handle complex situation in a fully automated way. Therfore, it is often necessary to resort to some kind of user interaction, that however, to be accepted by the user, should not be entangling.

References

1. Perkins W.J. (1977) "Biomedical Computing". Pitman Medical. New York.
2. Geddes L.A., Baker L.E. (1975) "Applied Biomedical Instrumentation". John Wiley and Sons, New York.
3. Swets J.A. (1964) "Signal Detection and Recognition by Human Observers". John Wiley and Sons, New York.
4. Lusted L.B. (1968) "Introduction to Medical Decision Making". Charles C. Thomas, Springfield, London.
5. Huber E.J. (1974) "A program to train physicians' assistants in diagnostic radiology". Appl. Radiol. 3, 31-52.
6. Pavlidis T. (1977) "Structural Pattern Recognition". Springer Verlag, Berlin.
7. Pavlidis T. (1979) "Filling Algorithms for Raster Graphics". Computer Graphics and Image Processing, 10,126-141.

32
The application of Markov process approach for the description of atherosclerotic phenomena

M.R. SLAWOMIRSKI

Instytut Gornictwa Naftowego i Gazownictwa, Ul. Lubicz 25A, PL-31-503 Krakow, Poland

ABSTRACT The study presents the mathematical model of particle sedimentation referred to the lipoprotein deposition in atherosclerotic disease. The theory enables us to determine the expected value of population of particles deposited on the wall of an artery at each time, i.e. to predict the development of disease in future. Certain aspects of atherosclerosis, e.g. its regresion and progression periods are theoretically explained by means of fluctuations.

1. PHENOMENOLOGICAL APPROACH TO ATHEROGENESIS

It is almost commonly assumed that atherogenesis is the result of interaction of lipoproteins with artery wall cells. The epidemiological studies present atherosclerosis as slowly evolving proliferative process modified by many biochemical, enviromental and genetic factors the knowledge of which is still incomplete.

Pathologists often condider the influence of the risk factors on pathogenesis. High amount of cholesterol in blood, smoking and high blood pressure are often regarded as significant elements in atherogenesis but the mechanism of their action is unclear. It is often assumed that risk factors may facilitate lipid deposition on the wall of an artery. There exist various concepts explaining particular aspects of atherogenesis but the main role of lipoprotein infiltration is widely confirmed.

Consequently, we may consider the molecular aspect of lipoprotein deposition on the wall of an artery. We shall regard the interaction of lipid particle with the wall of an artery as the sedimentation-like process. This approach is typically phenomenological because the reason of the phenomenon and its biological and biochemical aspects are not considered.

2. STOCHASTIC PROCESS MODEL

The number of lipid particles which may be sedimented on the wall of an artery is relatively great. In this study we assume that lipid particles are almost identical, i.e. it is impossible to distinguish a given particle from another. Taking into account that the sedimentation of a given particle instead of another is random we may consider the phenomenon of deposition of lipid particles form the standpoint of the theory of probability.

The probability that the genuine number of deposited particles is n at time t will be denoted by $\mathbb{P}\{N=n,t\}$. The number of particles n_0 deposited at initial time $t=0$ will be regarded as known.

Since the amount of sedimented particles at a given time moment is random therefore we may regard it as the random variable. Taking into account that the random variable N achieves different expected values at various time moments we may conclude that the development of population of sedimented particles should be regarded as the stochastic process bearing in mind that the considered process is a time-dependent function the image of which is the set of random variables.

If the population of sedimented lipid particles is n at time t the following options are possible at time $t+\Delta t$:

i. number of sedimented particles is increased by one in time interval Δt ,
ii. number of sedimented particles is increased more than one in time interval Δt ,
iii. number of sedimented particles remains unchanged in time interval Δt .

When time interval Δt is small we may assume that the probability of increase of the number of deposited particles by one in Δt period is proportional to the magnitude of Δt , i.e. we may write :

$$\mathbb{P}\{N=n+1,t+\Delta t\,|\,N=n,t\} = Q(n)\;\Delta t \tag{1}$$

where $Q(n)$ is intensity function independent of Δt and generally dependent on n . Symbol | denotes here conditional proportionality sign.

According to the rules of the probability calculus the probability of sedimentation of two particles in Δt period is the product of probabilities of sedimentation of each of them, i.e.:

$$\mathbb{P}\{N=n+2,t+\Delta t\,|\,N=n,t\} = Q^2(n)\;(\Delta t)^2 \tag{2}$$

Taking into account that the magnitude of Δt is small, the square of Δt is much smaller, and the probability of sedimentation of more than one particle in Δt may be neglected in comparison to the probability of sedimentation of one particle, i.e. we may write :

$$\mathbb{P}\{N>n+1, t+\Delta t \mid N=n, t\} \cong o(\Delta t) \tag{3}$$

where $o(\Delta t)$ is a small value.

Let us now consider the situation when at time $t+\Delta t$ the number of deposited particles is n . Then the population of particles at time t would be $n-1$ if one particle was sedimented in Δt or n if sedimentation has not occurred in this period. Consequently, according to the following formula on the total probability

$$\mathbb{P}\{A\} = \sum_{j} \mathbb{P}\{A \mid B_j\} \, \mathbb{P}\{B_j\} \tag{4}$$

the probability that the number of deposited particles is n at time $t+\Delta t$ may be expressed as :

$$\mathbb{P}\{N=n, t+\Delta t\} = Q(n-1)\,\Delta t\, \mathbb{P}\{N=n-1, t\} + [1-Q(n)]\, \mathbb{P}\{N=n, t\} \tag{5}$$

Equation (5) may easily be transformed to the form of the difference quotient :

$$\frac{\mathbb{P}\{N=n, t+\Delta t\} - \mathbb{P}\{N=n, t\}}{\Delta t} = -\,Q(n)\, \mathbb{P}\{N=n, t\} + Q(n-1)\, \mathbb{P}\{N=n-1, t\} \tag{6}$$

When interval Δt tends to zero, formula (6) leads to the following system of ordinary differential equations :

$$\left\{ \frac{d\, \mathbb{P}\{N=n, t\}}{d\ t} = -\,Q(n)\, \mathbb{P}\{N=n, t\} + Q(n-1)\, \mathbb{P}\{N=n-1, t\} \right\}_{n=1,2,\dots} \tag{7}$$

In this system the intensity function $Q(n)$ must explicitly be defined. Since the flow rate of blood which contains suspended lipoproteins depends strongly on the cross-section of an artery therefore we shall assume the following form of the intensity function

$$Q(n) = (m - n)\,\lambda \tag{8}$$

where m is the number of sedimented particles necessary to cover the entire cross-section of the artery, and λ is a constant value independent of m , n, t . Substituting expression (8) into equation (7) we obtain :

$$\left\{ \frac{d\,\mathbb{P}\{N=n,t\}}{dt} = -(m-n)\,\lambda\,\mathbb{P}\{N=n,t\} + (m-n+1)\,\lambda\,\mathbb{P}\{N=n-1,t\} \right\}_{n=1,2,\ldots} \tag{9}$$

3. EXPECTED VALUE

The system of differential equations written above may be solved applying the generating function defined by :

$$\Psi(s,t) = \sum_{n=0}^{\infty} s^n\,\mathbb{P}\{N=n,t\} \tag{10}$$

Since it has been assumed that at time $t = 0$ the population of sedimented particles was n_0 therefore we receive the following initial condition for Ψ function :

$$\Psi(s,t)\big|_{t=0} = s^{n_0} \tag{11}$$

The multiplication of each of equations (9) by s^n and addition corresponding sides of equations together gives :

$$\sum_{n=0}^{\infty}\left[s^n \frac{d\,\mathbb{P}\{N=n,t\}}{dt} \right] = -\sum_{n=0}^{\infty}\left[s^n\,(m-n)\,\lambda\,\mathbb{P}\{N=n,t\} \right] + \sum_{n=0}^{\infty}\left[s^n\,(m-n+1)\,\lambda\,\mathbb{P}\{N=n-1,t\} \right] \tag{12}$$

Bearing in mind formula (10) equation (12) may be expressed by means of the Ψ function in the following manner :

$$\frac{\partial\,\Psi(s,t)}{\partial\,t} + \lambda\,s\,(s-1)\,\frac{\partial\,\Psi(s,t)}{\partial\,s} = m\,\lambda\,(s-1)\,\Psi(s,t) \tag{13}$$

The solution of partial differential equation (13) with initial condition (11) is :

$$\Psi(s,t) = s^m \left[1 + \frac{1-s}{s}\exp(-\lambda\,t) \right]^{m-n_0} \tag{14}$$

The knowledge of the generating function $\Psi(s,t)$ enables us to determine time changes of the expected value and standard deviation of the considered stochastic process.

The expected value is defined by the following well known formula :

$$\mathbb{E}\{N(t)\} = \sum_{n=0}^{\omega} n \, \mathbb{P}\{N=n, t\} \tag{15}$$

The right hand side of this formula may easily be expressed by means of the generating function :

$$\mathbb{E}\{N(t)\} = \left. \frac{\partial \, \Psi(s,t)}{\partial \, s} \right|_{s=1} \tag{16}$$

The substitution of formula (14) into (16) gives finally :

$$\mathbb{E}\{N(t)\} = n_o + (m - n_o) \exp(-\lambda \; t) \tag{17}$$

The exponental function $\mathbb{E}\{N(t)\}$ has been graphically presented in Fig.1. It may be seen that the considered function after starting from the initial value n_o increases progressively in time, and finally tends to the asymptotic value m. The considered asymptotic value corresponds often to the situation when the entire cross-section of an artery is occupied by sedimented lipoproteins, and the flow of blood though the artery is impossible.

4. PREDICTION OF DEVELOPMENT OF ATHEROSCLEROTIC DISEASE

The expected value determines the most probable population of sedimented lipoprotein particles on the wall of an artery. Since the development of atherosclerotic disease depends on the amount of sedimented lipoproteins the expected value determines the most probable advance of the disease.

When λ and m parameters are known, it is possible to predict the most probable advance of disease in future because according to formula (17) the expected value is the explicit function of time. The considered function may easily be presented in the form of graph or table.

If the computations show that the most probable development of atherosclerosis in time is too quick, it is necessary to apply special treatment of a patient, e.g. decrease the amount of lipoproteins contained in blood. The magnitude of λ parameter and even m parameter is then reduced, and the expected value of population of sedimented particles increases much more slowly in time in comparison to the case when patient would not be subjected to the treatment (cf. Fig. 1).

Note that the expected value defines only the most probable development of sedimentation of lipid particles in time. In the real process the genuine population of

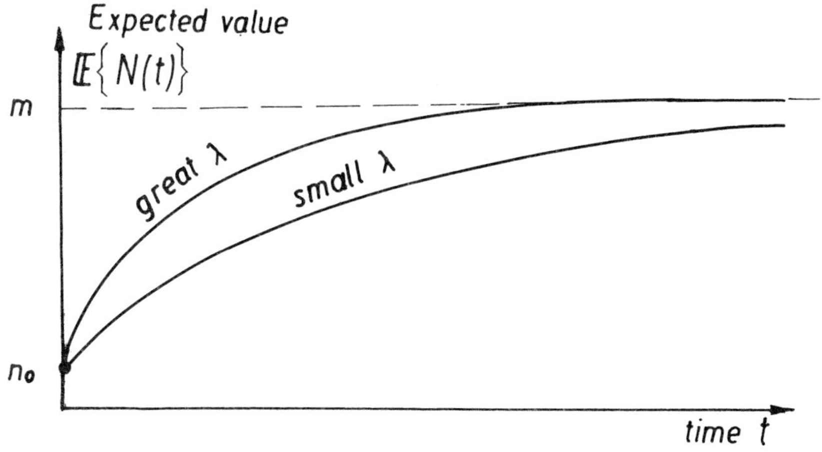

FIG. 1

The dependence of expected value of population of sedimented particles on time

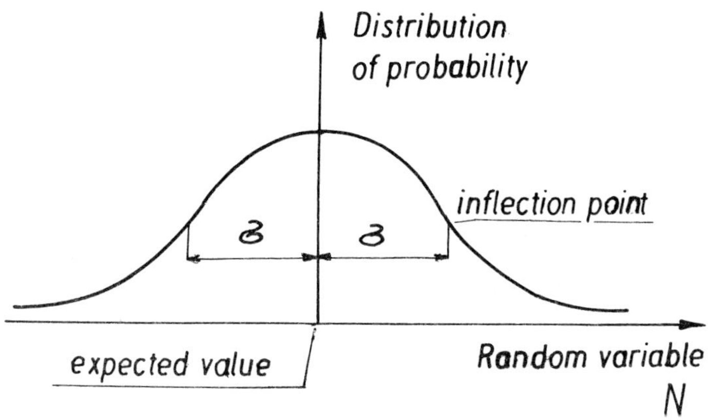

FIG. 2

The distribution of density of probability for population of sedimented particles at a given time moment deposited particles is equal to the expected value in rare cases only but it oscillates in the vicinity of the expected value. The considered deviations from the expected value are called fluctuations, and the probability of their arrival decreases strongly with their magnitude (cf. Fig.2).

The zone of probable disturbances from the expected value may be evaluated by means of the standard deviation σ which may be determined from the theory of probability applying the technique presented in Appendix.

The existence of theoretically predicted fluctuations explains certain aspect of the development of athero-sclerosis. Although the disease is generally progressive the periodical remissions may often be observed because they correspond to the fluctuations with respect to the expected value.

5. IDENTIFICATION OF λ AND m PARAMETERS

It has been written above that when λ and m parameters are known we are able to predict time-changes of the expected value which determines the development of the disease. Unfortunately, the considered parameters are not versatile, and they are typical of a given patient. It has been ob-served that for certain families the advance of the disease is very similar for individual persons but the confirmation of the hypothesis concerning the co-relation of λ and m parameters for various patients requires many investiga-tions. Consequently, it is necessary to determine the considered parameters for each patient.

The determination of λ and m parameters may be per-formed basing on the observation of development of disease during certain period of time. When the genuine population of sedimented particles at time moments $t_1, t_2, \ldots, t_I$ was $n_1, n_2, \ldots, n_I$ then the expected value function may be ob-tained applying the last square method. The function $\mathbb{E}\{N(t)\}$ given by formula (17) is now the function of time t and unknown elements λ, m, and therefore it will be de-noted here by $E(\lambda, m, t)$.

According to the idea of the last squares method the considered λ and m parameters should be appointed in such a manner that the sum of squares of distances between $E(\lambda, m, t)$ function and $n_1, n_2, \ldots, n_I$ values would achieve a minimal magnitude. Consequently, we obtain the following condition for the determination of λ and m :

$$\sum_{i=1}^{I} \left[E(\lambda, m, t_i) - n_i \right]^2 = \text{mimimum} \qquad (18)$$

Introducing a new function $\mathcal{J}(\lambda,m)$ defined by :

$$\mathcal{J}(\lambda,m) = \sum_{i=1}^{I} \left[E(\lambda,m,t_i) - n_i \right]^2 \tag{19}$$

we may reduce the problem to the determination of minimum of $\mathcal{J}(\lambda,m)$ function of two variables λ, m .

The conditions necessary for a minimum of $\mathcal{J}(\lambda,m)$ are:

$$\frac{\partial \mathcal{J}(\lambda,m)}{\partial \lambda} = 0 \tag{20}$$

$$\frac{\partial \mathcal{J}(\lambda,m)}{\partial m} = 0 \tag{21}$$

Conditions (20),(21) constitute the system of equations the solution of which gives 7alues λ_*, m_* . Moreover if at point (λ_*, m_*) we have

$$\frac{\partial^2 \mathcal{J}(\lambda,m)}{\partial \lambda^2} > 0 \tag{22}$$

and

$$\frac{\partial^2 \mathcal{J}(\lambda,m)}{\partial \lambda^2} \frac{\partial^2 \mathcal{J}(\lambda,m)}{\partial m^2} - \left[\frac{\partial^2 \mathcal{J}(\lambda,m)}{\partial\lambda \, \partial m} \right]^2 > 0 \tag{23}$$

then the considered point is the minimal point of $\mathcal{J}(\lambda,m)$ function. Quantities λ_*, m_* may then be accepted as parameters λ, m in expected value function $\mathbb{E}\{N(t)\}$ given by formula (17).

The practical realization of the identification process outlined above is complicated owing to non-linearity of the system of equations (20),(21). We may apply here the Newton-Raphson iteration technique but the convergence of this method depends strongly on the appointment of a starting point.

Moreover, during the indentification process we have to introduce additional restrictions referring to λ and m parameters, (e.g. λ and m must be positive). These conditions may be involved in the identification procedure by means of the Lagrange multipliers method but it introduces additional complication of the problem.

The problem of identification of λ and m parameters may also be solved applying non-linear programming technique. The considered method requires the experience in programing and the application of computers.

APPENDIX

Determination of standard deviation of the stochastic process

The standard deviation is defined as the square root of the variance of stochastic process:

$$\sigma = \sqrt{\mathrm{Var}\{N(t)\}} \tag{24}$$

Bearing in mind that the variance is expressed as the difference of the second moment and the square of the first moment of the stochastic process we have :

$$\mathrm{Var}\{N(t)\} = \mathbb{E}\{N^2(t)\} - [\mathbb{E}\{N(t)\}]^2 \tag{25}$$

or

$$\mathrm{Var}\{N(t)\} = \sum_{n=0}^{\infty} \left[n^2 \, \mathbb{P}\{N=n,t\}\right] - \left[\sum_{n=0}^{\infty} n \, \mathbb{P}\{N=n,t\}\right]^2 \tag{26}$$

Expressing the terms in the right hand side of this equation by means of the generating function we obtain :

$$\mathrm{Var}\{N(t)\} = \left.\frac{\partial^2 \Psi(s,t)}{\partial s^2}\right|_{s=1} + \left.\frac{\partial \Psi(s,t)}{\partial s}\right|_{s=1} - \left[\left.\frac{\partial \Psi(s,t)}{\partial s}\right|_{s=1}\right]^2 . \tag{27}$$

The substitution of solution (14) into formula (21) gives:

$$\mathrm{Var}\{N(t)\} = (m - n_o)\,[1 - \exp(-\lambda t)]\,\exp(-\lambda t) \tag{28}$$

It may be seen from formulae (24),(28) that the probability of fluctuation is equal to zero at the initial time moment $t = 0$, afterwards increases in time up to the maximum value, and finally tends to zero when the expected value tends to asymptotic quantity m .

REFERENCES

1. *Atherosclerosis and Cardiovascular Disease*, edited by S. Lenzi and G.C. Descovich (1984), MTP Press, Hingham.
2. Descovich G.C., Gaddi A, Pallotti G., Pettazzoni P., Sławomirski M.R. (1987) *A Stochastic Process Approach to the Development of Atheroma*, Medical Hypotheses **23**, 277-285.
3. Finkelstein L. (1979) *Mathematical Modelling of Dynamic Biological Systems*, Oregon Research Studies, Fores Grove.
4. Hoel P.G., Port S.C., Stone C.H.J. (1972) *Introduction to Stochastic Processes*, Houghton Miffin, Boston.
5. Lee K.T. (1985) *Atherosclerosis*, Annals of The New York Academy of Sciences, vol. 454.
6. Malinow R.M., Blaton V. (1984) *Regression of Atherosclerotic Lessions*, Atheroslerosis **4**, 292.
7. Sławomirski M.R. *Mathematical Modelling of Sedimentation*, 3rd European Symposium on Mechanics of Biological Tissues, Bagni di Lucca, Italy, April 1988.
8. Sławomirski M.R., Bollini D., Pallotti G., Pettazzoni P., Zannoli R., Descovich G., Gaddi A. *A Mathematical Model of Atheroma Sedimentation*, 5th International Conference on Mechanics in Medicine and Biology, Bologna, 1-5 July 1986.
9. Sławomirski M. R., Coli L., Stefoni S., Bonomini V., Pallotti G., Pettazzoni P. (1987) *Accelerated Arteriosclerosis in Dialysis Patients*, Automedica **9**, No 1-3.
10. Slawomirski M.R., Pallotti G. (1984) *A Probabilistic Approach to the Sedimentation*, Ingegneria - Rivista di scienza e tecnica, No. 1/2, p. 14.
11. Sławomirski M.R., Trzaska A. *A Stochastic and Numerical Approach to the Colmatage Phenomenon*, European Mechanics Colloquium 144 "Mechanics of Sedimentation and Fluidised Beds", Wien, Austria, 14-16 September 1981.
12. Sławomirski M.R., Trzaska A. (1986) *The Sedimentation of Solid Particles during the Flow of Suspension in a Long Channel*, in W. Bechteler (ed.) *Transport of Suspended Solids in Open Channels*, Balkema, Rotterdam - Boston.
13. Wissler R.W. (1979) *The Emerging Cellular Pathobiology of Atheroslerosis*, Artery **5**, 409.
14. Wissler R.W. (1981) *Principles of the Pathogenesis of Atherosclerosis*, in E. Braunvald (ed.) *A Textbook of Cardiovascular Medicine*, Saunders, Philadelphia.

33

Utility and limits of a Markov birth process in the study and simulation of the atheroma evolution

M. NICHELATTI[1], G. PALLOTTI[2], P. PETTAZZONI[2], A. GADDI[3], G.C. DESCOVICH[3] and M.R. SLAWOMIRSKI[4]

[1]Pierrel Pharmaceuticals, via Bisceglie 96, I-20152, Milan; [2]Department of Physics and [3]Chair of Geriatrics and Atherosclerosis Center, University of Bologna, Italy; [4]Department of Mathematical Modelling, Polish Petroleum Institute, Krakow, Poland

ABSTRACT. The paper analyzes the time evolution of the atheromatic plaque utilizing a Markov birth process to phenomenologically investigate the different steps of the arterial obstruction. A particular relevance is assigned to the variance analysis of the whole phenomenon, in which the regression of the lesion is also theoretically defined.

1. INTRODUCTION

The stochastic processes theory has been recently utilized as a method to qualitatively evaluate the growth of the atheroma. Descovich and coauthors (1987, 1989) have demonstred that the sedimentation of the lipid particles may be regarded as a random phenomenon, governed by probabilistic laws, and that the evolution of the whole system may be simulated by a Markov birth process.

The curve representing the number of the sedimented particles as funtion of the time elapsed seems correspond to the physiopatological evidences. Moreover, a variance analysis was successively carried out in order to evaluate the possible fluctuations of the number of sedimented particles, i.e. the possible theoretical explanation of the atheroma regression, in particular in the youngers, as well as the stabilization of the lesion in the old patients.

The model does not consider, at present, the antagonist removal mechanism for lipid particles, even if the phenomenon may be generalized, giving a global outlook of the patological events related to atherosclerosis.

2. MATERIALS AND METHODS

Following the definition of a Markov process, as given by Reichl (1980), we shall assume that many factors involved in the sedimentation are to

be enclosed in the definition of the sedimentation parameter λ.
This last may be considered as the efficiency of the plaque in the capture of the particles circulating into blood stream, and therefore the λ parameter contains the 'history' of the process until the time in which the observation is done.
Since the variance of the process is equal to the difference between the second moment and the squared first moment of the process, we obtain

$$\mathrm{Var}[N(t)] = \left.\frac{\partial^2\Psi}{\partial s^2}\right|_{s=1} + \left.\frac{\partial\Psi}{\partial s}\right|_{s=1} - \left\{\left.\frac{\partial\Psi}{\partial s}\right|_{s=1}\right\}^2 \tag{1}$$

from which the standard deviation was calculated as follows:

$$\sigma = \left[(m - n_0)\ (1 - \exp[-\lambda t])\ \exp[-\lambda t]\ \right]^{\frac{1}{2}} \tag{2}$$

where m is the number of sedimented particles covering the entire cross section of the artery, n_0 is the number of initially sedimented particles and t is the time elapsed.
The standard deviation was studied as function of time and λ parameter in order to better investigate the nature of the heteroscedasticity of the variance: if we put $n=m-n_0$ we obtain

$$\frac{\partial\sigma(\lambda,t)}{\partial t} = \frac{2\lambda n\ \exp[-2\lambda t] - \lambda n\ \exp[-\lambda t]}{2[n\ \exp[-\lambda t](1 - \exp[-\lambda t])]^{\frac{1}{2}}} \tag{3}$$

$$\frac{\partial\sigma(\lambda,t)}{\partial \lambda} = \frac{2tn\ \exp[-2\lambda t] - tn\ \exp[-\lambda t]}{2[n\ \exp[-\lambda t](1 - \exp[-\lambda t])]^{\frac{1}{2}}} \tag{4}$$

Since the derivatives of the standard deviation are simultaneously equal to zero only if $\lambda = t = 0$, and if $\lambda t = \ln 2$, we get, for the standard deviation a locus of critical points corresponding to the positive branch of the hyperbola $\lambda t = \ln 2$.
The above findings enable us to define a maximum value for the standard deviation (σ_M) equal to $[n]^{\frac{1}{2}}/2$ when the sedimentation parameter λ times t is equal to ln 2 for all positive values of t and λ .
By computer simulation we calculated the different curves of standard deviation at various values of the sedimentation parameter; the simulation has been carried out utilizing an arbitrary time scale. The results are given in table I.
We observe that the maximum value of standard deviation does not depend on the λ value, and does not depend (in particular) on the number of

λ	σ_M	t
0.1	2.73861279...	6.93144531...
.0.3	2.73861279...	2.31054688...
0.5	2.73861279...	1.38632813...
0.7	2.73861279...	0.99023437...
0.9	2.73861279...	0.77011718...

Table I. The maximum value of standard deviation is given for different arbitrary values of λ . The time necessary to standard deviation to reach the maximum is given on the column on the right h. s. The time scale is also arbitrary.

circulating lipoproteins, i.e. their concentration into blood stream.

3. DISCUSSION

We observe that the number $n = m - n_0$ is the only parameter affecting the size of σ_M ; this fact implies some considerations.

The size of n depends on the n_0 value, i.e. the smaller is n_0, the greater is n; in facts m is a fixed parameter, which depends only by the artery.

From the above considerations we obtain easily a theoretical justification of the great importance of the 'prevention' concept: an earlier correction of the risk factors as well as a change in the life style are of great importance, since we are acting on a system in which the value of n_0 is probably small, and therefore the size of the plaque may be subject to relatively great variations.

This fact can be considered also if we take into account the possibility of a removal mechanism for the yet sedimented particles. The relatively great variability of the size of the plaque is to be intended as a concrete possibility to have (under certain conditions) a regression of the atheromatic lesion.

Our model considers only a deposition phenomenon, without any removal mechanism, but the concept of prevention is easily applicable if we beare in mind that a great variability into atheroma size can indicate the possibility that the number of effectively sedimented particles reach their lower-limit value.

A generalization of the model as well their imporovement with experimen tal data is actually in progress.

Of particular relevance seems the evaluation of the sedimentation parameter as well as the possibility to influence the size: the lower is λ the longer is the time necessary for standard deviation to reach the maximum, and hence the time interval in which the atheroma may be subject to relatively great modifications is large.

4. CONCLUSIONS

The stochastic process approach is an useful and fruitful method to investigate the evolution and the possible modifications of the size of the atheromatic plaque.

The model is surely subject to some modifications and ameliorations, but actually, too, gives us some important indications about the theoretical evolution of the disease.

The 'mathematical' demonstration of the relevant role possibly played by the prevention suggests that the model started from right main hypotheses, and the actual findings we evolved seem also mainly correct.

A particular relevance is, following our opinion, to be assigned to the variance analysis of the phenomenon: the possibility of an atheroma regression can be taken into account also in order to plan a drug therapy avoiding drug overfeeding and utilizing the pharmacological approach maximizing the probability of successful results.

5. AKNOWLEDGEMENTS

This work was supported by the 60% grants of the Italian Ministery of Public Education (Ministero della Pubblica Istruzione).

REFERENCES

Descovich, G.C., Gaddi, A., Pallotti, G., Pettazzoni, P., and Slawomirski, M.R. (1987) 'A Stochastic Process Approach to the Development of Atheroma', Med. Hypotheses 23, 277.

Descovich, G.C., Gaddi, A., Nichelatti, M., Pallotti, G., Pettazzoni, P., and Slawomirski, M.R. (1989) 'Variance Analysis of the Atheromatic Sedimentation as a Stochastic Process', Clinica e Laboratorio 13, 5.

Reichl, L.E., (1980) A Modern Course in Statistical Physics, University of Texas Press, Austin.

NEW PERSPECTIVES IN THE TREATMENT OF HYPERCHOLESTEROLAEMIA AND THE PREVENTION OF ATHEROSCLEROSIS

34

Modification of lipoproteins in the intimal extracellular compartment that can contribute to atherogenesis

G. CAMEJO, E. HURT-CAMEJO, O. WIKLUND, G. FAGER and G. BONDJERS

Wallenberg Laboratory for Cardiovascular Research, Sahlgren's Hospital, University of Gothenburg, Gothenburg S-413 45, Sweden

ABSTRACT. In a normal artery, most of the apoB lipoproteins that cross the endothelium return to the arterial lumen. During lesion development, in the other hand, takes place a continuous extracellular immobilization and cellular uptake of apoB-lipoproteins. Both process appear to be initiated by modifications in physical and chemical lipoprotein parameters which occur in the extracellular compartment of the intima. In human and animal arterial intima, chondroitin sulfate-rich proteoglycans (CSPG) have been identified and characterized that specifically interact with low density lipoproteins (LDL) through arginine, lysine-rich regions of the apoB-100. During this association, the structure of apoB-100 surface segments in LDL is modified. The modification of these regions increased the binding and internalization of LDL by cultured human macrophages and smooth muscle cells causing lipid accumulation. The increased uptake of LDL does not down regulate the binding and internalization. It is postulated that the exaggerated occurrence of similar processes may be one of the contributing factors to atherosclerotic lesion development.

1. Introduction

In normal regions of human arteries there is only a slow and increase in the intima-media cholesterol content with age [1]. However, in atherosclerotic lesions there is a rapid focal accumulation of cholesterol and cholesterol esters [2]. The source of these lipids are mostly apoB-lipoproteins from plasma that are deposited extracellularly and also taken up by specially monocyte-derived macrophages and smooth muscle cells. One of the challenging research subjects on atherosclerosis is to delineate the molecular and cellular basis of the changes responsible for this focal alteration. Obviously, the presence of elevated levels of apoB-lipoproteins in plasma is an important contributor
because it will lead to a higher equilibrium level of lipoprotein particles in the normal intima and in lesions [3]. However, lipoprotein concentrations can not explain the focality of their accumulation or the presence of lesions in subjects with near to "normal" levels of plasma lipids. It is apparent that the balance and

outcome of localized cellular and molecular events which take place in the endothelium and intima, in response to stimuli associated with lipopoprotein ingress and residence modulate wether an artery ages normally or initiates an atherogenic process.

The lipoproteins which are extractable from normal and atherosclerotic extracellular regions of arteries are present in different stages of processing and association with macromolecular intima components [4,5]. Whereas those taken up by macrophages and smooth muscle cells are rapidly degraded and probably only their cholesterol molecules could be recognized as originating from lipoproteins since all other degradation products equilibrate rapidly with those of cells and the interstitial fluid [3]. The alterations suffered by apoB-lipoproteins can include a whole spectrum; from changes in protein conformation and lipid composition to chemical modifications as: protein fragmentation, side chain modification, lipid hydrolysis and phase segregation [6] There is not a sharp line separating the above changes and probably one leads to another. Accumulating evidence indicates that oxidative alterations, mediated by endothelial cells and macrophages, their secreted products as superoxide ions ($O_2{\cdot}-$) and hydroxyl radicals ($HO{\cdot}-$), and unsaturated fatty acid radicals originated in the cell membranes or in the lipoprotein lipids, can cause the mentioned chemical modifications of apoB-lipoprotein. Steinberg and collaborators have recently carefully reviewed this topic [7].

There are other changes of apoB-lipoproteins that apparently are associated with less drastic alterations than those induced by oxidative processes. These are related to specific and unspecific associations with macromolecules of the extracellular matrix as collagen, elastin, and proteoglycans, which are the most abundant elements in the almost acellular normal intima. Low density lipoprotein binding to collagen, and elastin leads to lipid transfer but its consequences for the lipoprotein structure have not been studied in detail [8].

The mammalian intima contains appreciable amounts of sulfated proteoglycans as chondroitin, dermatan and heparan. Heparan appears to be confined to cell surfaces, whereas chondroitin, dermatan and hyaluronic acid form a tridimensional mesh that interconnects cells, elastic fibers and collagen [8]. Although not all functions of proteoglycans are known, they contribute to the visco-elastic properties of the intima by immobilizing water. In addition, due to their high negative charge density and gel- exclusion properties probably provide a matrix support for maintaining gradients of macromolecules and metabolites in the extracellular compartment. Wight has published a comprehensive review on this subject [9]. One of the properties of arterial chondroitin sulfate proteoglycans (CSPG) is that they form soluble and insoluble complexes with apoB-lipoproteins. The existence of such complexes in human atherosclerotic lesions have been well documented [5,8,9,10,11]. However, the effect on the lipoprotein particle is just beginning to be studied. In the present article we will discuss recent evidence which suggest that proteoglycan-induced modifications of LDL may be important contributors to extracellular lipoprotein retention and to an increased uptake by macrophages and smooth muscle cells; two processes closely associated with atherogenesis.

2. Molecular basis for the association LDL-proteoglycan

The association of apoB-lipoprotein with arterial proteoglycans is mediated by ionic interactions between the negatively-charged sulfate groups of the CSPG and positive arginine and lysine-rich regions in the surface of the LDL particle. With the purpose of identifying some of the apoB-100 regions that may bind CSPG, apoB-100 peptide segments, 11 to 29 amino acids long, with high probability to reside in the surface of LDL were synthesized based in the apoB-100 consensus sequence peptides for the arterial CSPG was tested with the use of frontal elution affinity chromatography and competition experiments [14]. Three potential proteoglycan-binding segments of apoB-100 were identified and a minimal proteoglycan-recognizing sequence was established within the peptide region that shows the greatest affinity for CSPG. TABLE 1 presents the sequence, charge, hydrophilicity and affinity for the arterial CSPG of these peptides.

TABLE 1. Sequence and properties of synthetic apoB-100 peptides that bind to arterial chondroitin sulfate proteoglycans (CSPG).

Peptide	apoB segment	sequence (a)	Hydrophil. (b)	Kd (uM)
P-1	4230-4254	++ + - +- + +- LRKHKLIDVSMYRELLKDLSKEA OH OH	3.4	86
P-2	3359-3377	+ +++ + + RLTRKRGLKLATALSLSNK OH OH OHOH	7.3	63
P-22	3359-3367	+ +++ + RLTRKRGLK OH	6.0	86
P-11	2106-2121	+ +-+ ++ RQVSHAKEKLTALTKK OH OH OH	18.7	82

(a) The sequence in one letter code also indicates the position of the charged amino acid side chains and those with hydroxyls (Arg(R) and Lys(K)(+), Asp(D) and Glu(E) (-), Ser(S) and Thr(T) (OH).
(b) Hydrophylicity calculated according to Parker, Guo and Hodges (ref 15)

It can be observed that peptides P-1, P-2 and P-11, share the properties of being highly hydrophilic (polar) and having an excess of positive charges. The presence of hydroxylated side chains increase the polarity and this also increases the probability that in the intact LDL particle these segments reside in its surface. The sequence in peptide P-2, which is the one with highest affinity for

CSPG, was used to search for a minimal recognition sequence. Peptide P-22 was found to be the shortest to have an affinity comparable to P-2. Peptides shorter than P-22 had an appreciable lower dissociation constant (Kd) and inhibitory capacity of the interaction between LDL and CSPG.

Peptides P-1 and P-11 are contained within longer segments that have been previously identified by Hiroshe et al.[16] and Weisgraber and Rall [17] as heparin binding sites and therefore they represent sulfated glycosaminoglycan binding-regions. Furthermore, the shorter peptide P-22 (and P-2) contains one of the consensus sequence proposed recently by Cardin and Weintraub [18] as one of the attaching regions found in many glycosaminoglycan-binding proteins.

There are several properties of arterial proteoglycans and glycosaminoglycans that also modulate their association with apoB-lipoproteins. The kind of glycosaminoglycan chain and the molecular weigh appear to be important determinants of the affinity for LDL [19] In our hands, chondroitin sulfate proteoglycans rich in the 6-sulfate isomer appear to have the highest reactivity within those isolated from human arteries [8,20]. Alves and Mourao [21] working with human glycosaminoglycans reached a similar conclusion. It is interesting to mention that in experimental lesions of swine and rabbits chondroitin-6-sulfates become the more prominent proteoglycans [22,23].

3. Modifications induced in LDL by the association with arterial proteoglycans

Probably the main cause of the focal accumulation of apoB-lipoproteins during atherogenesis is the association with arterial proteoglycans [8-10]. Possible, several factors concur for the formation of such extracellular apoB deposits. One of them could be the increased biosynthesis of extracellular matrix which takes place when smooth muscle cells shift from the quiescent state to the biosynthetic state in early atherogenesis [9]. This may be accompanied by localized alterations of proteoglycan structure that may increase its apo-lipoprotein complexing capacity [24]. Other possibility is that modifications in gel exclusion properties of the extracellular matrix could lead to large focal concentrations of apoB-lipoproteins increasing their tendency to self-association or binding to proteoglycans [8,10].

Once LDL-proteoglycan associations are formed, changes in the lipid organization have been detected with the use of low angle X-ray scattering. These alterations may eventually lead to lipid phase segregation in irreversible LDL-CSPG complexes [25]. A process perhaps related to the presence of extracellular lipid droplets and to apoB-containing aggregates that are different from plasma lipoproteins [2,4,5].

We found that after complexing LDL in reversible aggregates with arterial proteoglycans, the redissolved lipoprotein, although retaining its monomeric size and charge, showed alterations in the surface arrengement of the protein. These alterations were manifested in a different pattern of tryptic peptides produced during controlled

hydrolysis [26].
Because surface-located, trypsin sensitive, apoB-100 regions are probably also involved in proteoglycan-binding and LDL receptor-binding these alterations may have effects on the subsequent interactions with intimal cells [2, 26].

4. Potentially atherogenic consequences of proteoglycan-induced modifications of apoB-lipoproteins

One of the possible effects of formation of reversible and irreversible associations between apoB-lipoproteins and arterial proteoglycans may result in a reduced clearance of the lipoproteins from the intima. This may potentiate oxidative changes, as suggested by Steinberg and collaborators [7]. Another effect, probably mediated by alterations of apoB-100 surface structure, is the increased cellular uptake of insoluble LDL-glycosaminoglycan complexes [27]. We have found that soluble, monomeric LDL (LDL-PG), pre-treated with human arterial CSPG, is taken up more avidly by human monocyte-derived macrophages (HMDM)[26] and smooth muscle cells (HSMC) [28]. In HMDM incubated with LDL-PG there is a several fold increase of cholesterol, cholesterol esters, triglycerides and phospholipids that is associated with the conversion to "foam cells". TABLE 2. presents results obtained after incubation of HMDM arterial smooth muscle cells and receptor negative fifroblasts LDL pre-treated with arterial CSPG and native LDL.

TABLE 2. Effect of incubation of human monocyte derived macrophages (HMDM), human smooth muscle cells (HSMC), human receptor positive (HFB(+)) and human receptor negative fibroblasts (HFB(-)) with ^{125}I-Tyramine cellobiose LDL pretreated with human arterial CSPG (LDL-PG) and with non CSPG treated labeled LDL (native LDL)

Cell type	Lipoprotein added ug/ml		Lipoprotein uptake ug/mg cell prot.
HMDM	native LDL	20	5.2
"	"	100	10.0
"	LDL-PG	20	9.0
"	"	100	17.6
HSMC	native LDL	20	4.5
"	"	80	7.0
"	LDL-PG	20	5.5
"	"	80	8.2
HFB(+)	native LDL	20	18.0
"	"	60	21.0
"	LDL-PG	20	25.0
"	"	60	32.4
HFB(-)	native LDL	20	1.0
	"	60	1.5
"	LDL-PG	20	2.5
"	"	60	6.0

The cells were pre-incubated for 24 hours in lipoprotein deficient serum and then incubated for 6 hors with ^{125}I-tyramine cellobiose-labeled native or proteoglycan-treated LDL. The cells where then washed, and cell associated radioactivity evaluated.

The results indicate that soluble proteoglycan-treated LDL (LDL-PG) was taken up more efficiently by human macrophages, sooth muscle cells and fibroblasts. The data from the receptor-negative fibroblasts suggest that most of the LDL-PG is internalized via the high affinity-LDL receptor. Competition experiments with the HMDM also suggest this. However, although the cells are internalising efficiently LDL-PG this does not down regulate the receptor expression or the HMG-CoA-reductase activity (data not shown). A phenomenon that may be responsible for the transformation of macrophages into foam cells.

Although most of the results discussed have been obtained with LDL-proteoglycan complexes, Recently, Bihari-Varga, Kostner and Col. [29] have found that Lp(a) can form complexes with arterial proteoglycans and this complexes were taken up more avidly by macrophages than native Lp(a). Elevated levels of Lp(a) have been shown to be strongly associated with clinical manifestations of atherosclerosis, and it may also contribute to extracellular and cellular accumulation during atherogenesis.

5. Conclusions

In vivo and in vitro results indicate that proteoglycans of the arterial intima form soluble and insoluble complexes with apoB lipoprotein, specially LDL. Some of the molecular structures involved in such interactions have been identified. In vitro experiments have provided clues about the consequences for LDL structure of their association with arterial proteoglycans and experiments with different cultured cells suggest that the modifications caused may be responsible for formation of foam cells. Therefore proteoglycan-induced modifications of apoB-lipoproteins may contribute both to their focal extracellular accumulation and to formation of foam cells, two basic processes during atherogenesis.

References

1. Katz, S.S. (1982) The lipids of grossly normal human aortic intima from birth to old age, J. Biol. Chem., 25
6, 12275-12280.
2. Small, D.M. (1988) Progression and regression of atherosclerotic lesions. Insights from lipid physical biochemistry, Arteriosclerosis, 8, 103-129.
3. Lindén, T., Bondjers, G., Fager, G., Olofsson, S-O, and Wiklund, O. (1989) Apolipoprotein B in human aortic biopsies in relation to serum lipids and lipoproteins, Atherosclerosis, 77, 159-166.
4. Hollander, W. Paddock, J. and Colombo, M. (1979) Lipoproteins in human atherosclerotic vessels. I. Biochemical properties of arterial low density lipoproteins, very low density lipoproteins and high

density lipoproteins, Exp. Mol. Pathol., 30, 144-171.
5. Camejo, G., Hurt, E. and Romano, M. (1985) Properties of lipoprotein complexes isolated by affinity chromatography from human aorta, Biomed. Bichim. Acta, 44, 389-401.
6. Jurgens, G., Hoff, H.F., Chisolm III, G.M., Esterbauer, H. (1987) Modification of human serum low density lipoprotein by oxidation-Characterization and phatophysiological implications, Chem. Phys. Lipids, 45, 315-336.
7. Steinberg, D., Parthasarathy S., Carew, T., Khoo, J.C. and Witzum J.L. (1989) Beyond cholesterol. Modifications of low density lipoprotein that increase its atherogenicity, New Engl. J. Med., 320, 915-924.
8. Camejo, G. (1982) The interaction of lipids and lipoproteins with the intercellular matrix of arterial tissue: its possible role in atherogenesis, Adv. Lipid Res., 19, 1-53.
9. Wight, T., (1989) Cell biology of arterial proteoglycans, Arteriosclerosis, 9, 1-20.
10. Berenson, G.S, Radhakrishnamurthy, B., Srinivasan, S.R., Vijayagopal, P., Dalferes, E.R. and Sharma, C. (1984) Carbohydrate-protein macromolecules and arterial wall integrity-A role in atherogenesis, Exp. Mol. Pathol., 41, 267-287.
11. Völker, W., Schmidt, A. and Buddecke, E. (1989) Cytochemical changes in a human arterial proteoglycan related to atherosclerosis, Atherosclerosis, 77, 117-130.
12. Yang, C-Y., Gu, Z-W., Weng, S-A., Chen, S-H., Pownal, H.J., Sharp, P.M., Liu, S-W., Li, W-H., Gotto, A.M. and Chan, L. (1989) Structure of apolipoprotein B-100 of human low density lipoproteins, Arteriosclerosis 9, 96-108.
13. Olofsson, S-O., Bjursell, G., Boström, K., Carlsson, P., Elovson, J., Protter, A., Reuben, M.A. and Bondjers, G. (1987) Apolipoprotein B: structure, biosynthesis and role in the apolipoprtein assembly process, Atherosclerosis, 68, 1-17.
14. Camejo, G., Olofsson, S-O., Lopez, F., Carlsson, P. and Bondjers, G. (1988) Identification of apoB-100 segments mediating the interaction of low density lipoproteins with arterial proteoglycans, Arteriosclerosis, 8, 368-377.
15.Parker, J.M., Guo, D. and Hodges R.S. (1986) New hydrophilicity scale derived from high-performance chromatography peptide retention date: correlation of predicted surface residues with antigenicity and X-ray derived accesible sites, Biochemistry, 86, 5425-5432.
16. Hiroshe, N., Blanckenship, D.T.,Krivanek, M., Jackson, R.L. and Cardin A.D. (1987) Isolation and characterization of four heparin-binding cyanogen bromide peptides of human apolipoprotein B, Biochemistry, 26, 5505-5512.
17. Weisgraber, K.H. and Rall, S.C. (1987) Human apolipoprotein B-100 heparin-binding sites, J. Biol. Chem., 262, 11097-11103.
18. Cardin, A.D. and Weintraub, H.R. (1989) Molecular modeling of protein-glycosaminoglycan interactions, Arteriosclerosis, 9, 21-32.
19. Srinivasan, S.R., Vijayagopal, P., Eberle, K., Dalferes, E.R., Radhakrishnamurthy, R. and Berenson, G. (1988) Low density lipoprotein binding affinity of arterial wall isomeric chondroitin

sulfate proteoglycans, Atherosclerosis, 72, 1-9.
20. Camejo, G., Ponce, E., Lopez, F., Starosta, E., Hurt, E. and Romano, M. (1983) Partial structure of the active moiety of a lipoprotein complexing proteoglycan from human aorta. Atherosclerosis, 49,241-254.
21. Alves, C.S. and Mourao, P.A. (1989)Interaction of high molecular weight chondroitin sulfate from human aorta with plasma low density lipoproteis, Atherosclerosis, 73, 113-124.
22. Hoff, H.F. and Wagner W.D. (1986) Plasma low density lipoprotein accumulation in aortas of hypercholesterolemic swine correlates with modifications in aortic glycosaminoglycan composition, Atherosclerosis, 61, 231-236.
23. Alavi, M.Z. and Moore, S. (1987) Proteoglycan composition of rabbit arterial wall under conditions of experimentally induced atherosclerosis, Atherosclerosis, 63,65-74.
24. Edwards, I.J. and Wagner, W.D. (1988) Distinct synthetic and structural characteristics of proteoglycans produced by cultured artery smooth muscle cells of atherosclerosis-susceptible pigeons, J. Biol. Chem., 263, 9612-9620.
25. Mateu, L., Avila, E. M., Camejo, G., León, V. and Liscano, V. (1984) The structural stability of low-density lipoprotein. A kinetic X-ray scattering study of its interaction with arterial proteoglycans, Biochim. Biophys. Acta, 795, 525-534.
26. Hurt, E. and Camejo, G. (1987) Effect of arterial proteoglycans on the interaction of LDL with human monocyte-derived macrophages, Atherosclerosis, 67, 115-126.
27. Vijayagopal, P., Srinivasan, S.R., Jones, K.M., Radhakrishnamurthy, B. and Berenson, G.S. (1988) Metabolism of low density lipoprotein-proteoglycan complex by macrophages: further evidence for a receptor pathway, Biochim. Biophys. Acta, 960, 210-219.
28. Bondjers, G., Camejo, G., Fager, G., Olovsson, S-O. and Wiklund, O. (1988) "Functional interrelationships between the smmoth muscle and macrophage cell populations of the atherosclerotic plaque", in C. Dal Palù and R. Ross (eds), Hypertension and Atherosclerosis, Exerpta Medica, Amsterdam, pp.75-86.
29. Bihari- Varga, M., Gruber, E., Rotheneder, M. Zechner, R. and Kostner, G. (1988) Interaction of of lipoprotein Lp(a) and low density lipoprotein with glycosaminoglycans from human aorta, Arteriosclerosis, 8, 851-857.

LDL APHERESIS: EFFICACY VERSUS ETHICAL AND SOCIAL ASPECTS

35
LDL apheresis: current situation in Japan

T. YASUGI

Nihon University, School of Medicine, Second Department of Internal Medicine, 30-1 Ohotaniguchi, Uemachi Itabashiku, Tokyo, Japan

ABSTRACT. LDL apheresis using dextran sulfate cellulose beads has been recognized as the best therapeutics for severe familial hypercholesterolemia. It was approved for commercial distribution by Japanese government in 1986. Since 1986, more than 15,000 treatments have been done on about 600 patients. Most of these patients had coronary disease and whose total cholesterol level could not be kept under 250 mg/dl on drug therapy. Although the therapy does not have long history yet, the beneficial effects of LDL apheresis such as reduction of xanthoma and Achilles tendon thickness, alleviation of angina pectoris and prevention and regression of coronary atherosclerosis have been reported. No serious complication has been reported.

Today there is no doubt that high cholesterol levels are strongly linked to an increased risk of coronary heart disease. In 1987, we discussed and decided the definition of hyperlipidemia at the consensus conference of Japan Atherosclerosis Society(Table 1). In this definition, case of more than 220 mg/dl of total cholesterol is hyperlipidemia and the person who has more than 220 mg/dl of total cholesterol should be under some treatment for hyperlipidemia. For hyperlipidemia, dietary therapy should be tried at first and the second is drug therapy. However, sometimes diet and drug therapies do not have so good efficiency for sever familial hypercholesterolemia. LDL apheresis has gained considerable attention in recent year as the best therapeutics for severe familial hypercholesterolemia in Japan. Here we report the current situation of LDL apheresis in Japan.

1. Liposorber System for LDL Apheresis

1.1. Automated Column Regenerating Unit System

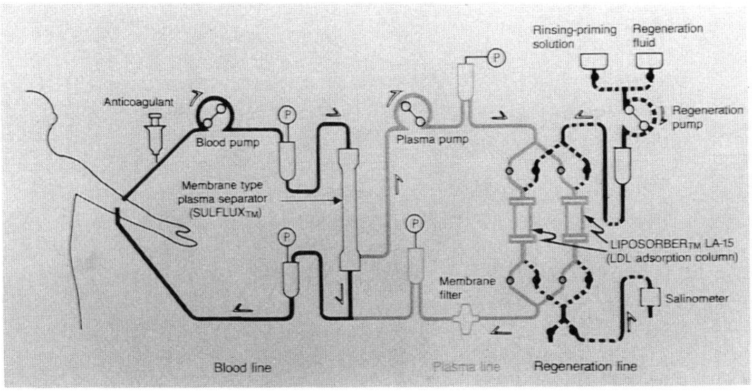

Figure 1. Automated column regenerating unit system for LDL apheresis

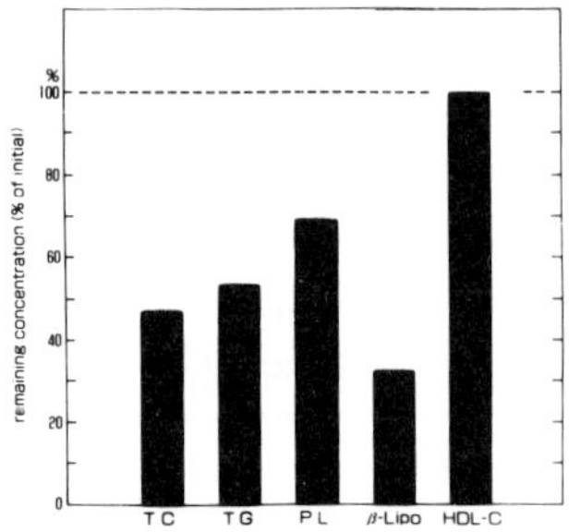

Figure 2. Adsorption of lipids with dextran sulfate cellulose beads (in vitro)

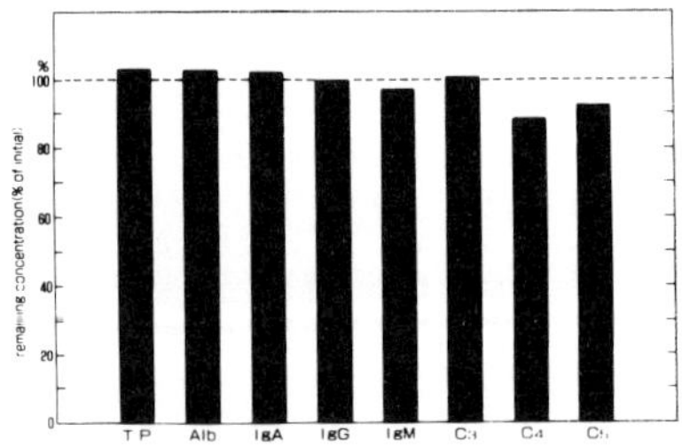

Figure 3. Adsorption of plasma proteins with dextran sulfate cellulose beads (in vitro)

Table 1. Definition of hyperlipidemia

TOTAL SERUM CHOLESTEROL	>220 mg/dl
SERUM TRIGLYSERIDE	>150 mg/dl
HDL-CHOLESTEROL	< 40 mg/dl

Table 2. Changes in plasma lipids and apoprotein immediately after 2,500 ml plasmapheresis

	Plasma Exchange	Double Filtration 30 nm*	Double Filtration 40 nm*	DSC Column† (LA-40)	*P* Value Double Filtration v DSC Column‡
Number of treatments	2	5	4	9	
Total cholesterol	44.7	37.0 ± 9.9	36.5 ± 7.5	44.9 ± 5.9	NS
VLDL-cholesterol	30.0	25.0 ± 23.7	22.1 ± 2.7	16.6 ± 13.4	NS
IDL-cholesterol	24.7	28.6 ± 6.0	33.7 ± 6.0	27.8 ± 10.7	NS
LDL-cholesterol	37.0	35.4 ± 9.7	30.8 ± 1.6	40.8 ± 6.2	NS
HDL-cholesterol	30.9	55.2 ± 14.5	60.8 ± 5.7	97.6 ± 3.0	<.001
Apoproteins§					
A-I	37.9	56.9 ± 11.4	71.7 ± 9.9	86.9 ± 6.5	<.001
A-II	57.7	60.1 ± 5.9	67.2 ± 12.6	88.1 ± 11.0	<.001
B	26.3	34.8 ± 8.7	38.2 ± 12.7	37.5 ± 5.9	NS
C-II	56.0	43.4 ± 14.1	44.1 ± 13.3	49.1 ± 13.1	NS
C-III	50.0	46.0 ± 7.7	45.3 ± 11.8	48.9 ± 12.4	NS
E	50.0	25.0 ± 23.7	35.2 ± 10.0	39.3 ± 16.0	NS

*Average pore diameter of the second filter membrane
†Mean ± SD values are expressed as the percentage of preplasmapheresis levels
‡Paired t test
§Apoproteins were [illegible] Metabolism 36:419 [illegible]

A membrane type hollow fiber plasma separator(Sulflux FS-05,Kanegafuchi Chemical Industry, Osaka, Japan) and 2 small LDL adsorption columns(Liposorber LA-15, Kanegafuchi Chemical Industry, Osaka, Japan) are used in Liposorber system for LDL apheresis.1 Separated plasma by the plasma separator goes through the LDL adsorption column and returns to the body with hemocyte. LDL in plasma is absorbed by the LDL adsorption column. Figure 1 shows an automated column regenerating unit system. Before LDL adsorption capacity of the first column is came up to a saturation, the plasma line is changed to the other column automatically. While the second column is used as an adsorbent, the first column is rinsed and activated. Therefore, any quantity of LDL can be removed from plasma by the 2 columns system. Total extracorporeal volume is 350-400 ml.

1.2. Selectivity of LDL Removal

The LDL adsorption column is filled up with the dextran sulfate cellulose beads. The dextran sulfate is covalently linked to cellulose beads. The beads has high affinity for apoprotein B-100 which is the structural protein of LDL. Figure 2 and 3 show a selective efficiency of the beads. Total cholesterol, triglyceride, phospholipides and -lipoprotein are absorbed. HDL cholesterol is not absorbed by the beads. The other components of blood such as albumin, immunoglobulin and complements are little changed. Table 2 shows the results of comparison of selectivity of LDL removal by plasma exchange, double filtration and Liposorber system (DSC Column) reported by Dr.Homma. Liposorber system reduced LDL but not HDL cholesterol while plasma exchange and double filtration reduced LDL and HDL cholesterol. These indicate that the dextran sulfate cellulose column has high selectivity of LDL removal and absorbs almost only apolipoprotein B containing lipoproteins.

2. Clinical Results

Liposober system for LDL apheresis was approved for commercial distribution by Japanese government in 1986. Since 1986, more than 15,000 treatments have been performed on about 600 patients in Japan and many beneficial effects of LDL apheresis have been reported.

2.1. Reduction of Achilles Tendon Thickness

In figure 4, the reduction of Achilles tendon thickness in 28 years old female with heterozygous familial hypercholesterolemia was shown. The total cholesterol level was more than 400 mg/dl before treatment and it was maintained around 150 mg/dl for 1 year by LDL apheresis and drug therapy. Both left and right Achilles tendon thickness were reduced from 20 mm to 17 mm.

2.2. Alleviation of angina pectoris

The clinical effects of long term reduction of plasma cholesterol on Achilles tendon thickness, skin xanthoma, electrocardiogram, frequency of angina pectoris were reported by Dr.Sinomiya. In all patiens treated by LDL apheresis more than 10 times, alleviation of angina pectoris were observed and there was no case of change for worse. Table 3 shows alleviation of angina pectoris by LDL apheresis in 48 years old woman with 3 VD reported by Dr.Yosida. Before the treatment, total cholesterol level was more than 450 mg/dl and ST depression had been observed within 2 minutes in electrocardiogram after ergonometer loading. But one year later, ST depression could not be observed within 6 minutes.

Many investigations of improvement on angina pectoris have been reported. This is one of these reports. We would say there is no doubt that reduction of xanthoma and Achilles tendon thickness and alleviation of angina pectoris will be possible by LDL apheresis, even if in case of sever familial hypercholesterolemia.

2.3. Prevention and of coronary atherosclerosis

Table 3 shows the effects of active cholesterol reduction on severe coronary atherosclerosis reported by Dr.Tatami. Group 1 was none treatment group and had very high cholesterol level. Group 2 was drug therapy group. Group 3 was LDL apheresis group. Cholesterol level of group 3 was reduced from 320 mg/dl to 142 mg/dl. Progression of coronary atherosclerosis which were shown as Coronary Atherosclerosis Index (CAI) were prevented only in the group 3 in which cholesterol level was controlled by LDL apheresis.

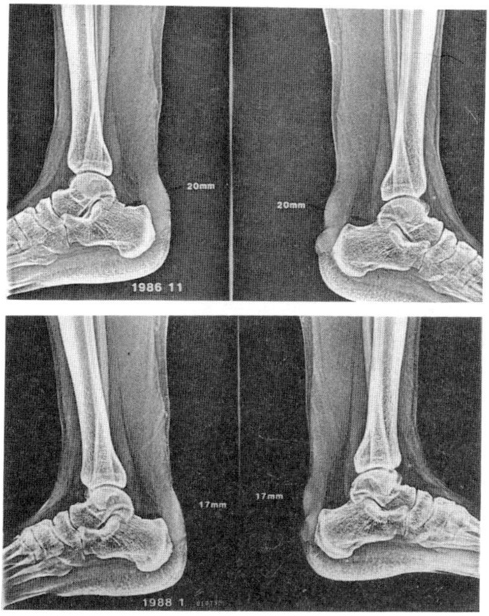

Figure 4. Reduction of Achilles tendon thickness

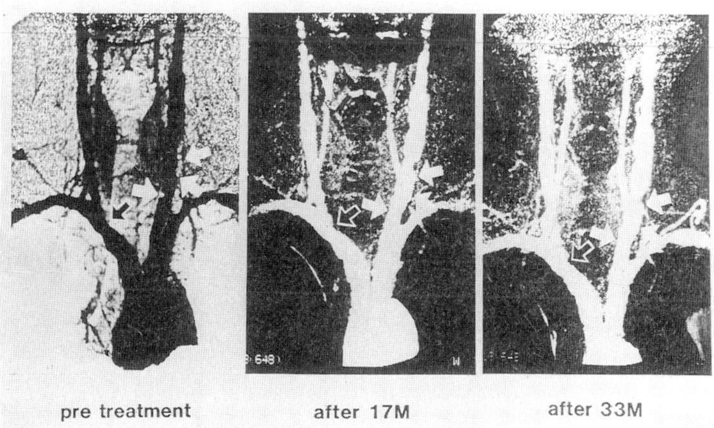

Figure 5. Digital subtraction angiography in heterozygous familial hypercholesterolemic 28 years old female.

TABLE 3. Improvement on symptoms by LDL apheresis

	PRE	1 YEAR	2 YEARS
ANGINA PECTORIS	+	−	−
ELECTROCARDIOGRAM	ST(+)	ST(−)	ST(−)
MASTER DOUBLE TEST	N.D.	NEGATIVE	NEGATIVE
ERGOMETER (ST)	2 MIN.	6 MIN.	N.D.
XANTHOMA	++	+	+
ACHILLES TENDON (LEFT/RIGHT)	14mm 16mm	13mm 15mm	13mm 11mm

From J Therap Vol 70, No 11, 2265, 1988 (M Sinoi et al)

TABLE 4. Effects of active cholesterol reduction on severe coronary atherosclerosis

	Age (Year)	Treatment period (month)	Morbided branches (No. of branches)	Serum cholesterol (mg/dl)	Serum Trigriceride (mg/dl)	CAI
Group I	60±2	23±3	2.4±0.1	266± 7 ·257± 6	149±17 ·130±15	23±2 ·27±2*
Group II	56±3	24±2	2.2±0.1	292±14 ·185±16	140±20 ·123±16	20±3 ·22±4
Group III	64±4	19±2	2.6±0.2	320±19 ·142± 5	125±20 · 87±17	23±4 ·23±5

Group I : Non-treatment
Group II : Drug therapy
Group III : Drug therapy and LDL Apheresis

*P 0.05 Mean · SEM

Tatami, R., Maizuru Kyosai Hp, Japan

In addition to this report, there are many reports respecting prevention. These reports suggest that coronary atherosclerosis would be prevented if cholesterol level was kept under 180 mg/dl.

2.4. Regression

Figure 5 shows pictures of digital subtraction angiography in 28 year old female. Cholesterol level was above 420 mg/dl before treatment and it was kept under 150 mg/dl by LDL apheresis, twice a month, with drug therapy such as cholestyramin and probucol during treatment. Moth-eaten was progressed all over the arterial wall. Regressions were observed in the left common carotid artery(white allow). A newly formed shadow(black allow) in brachiocepharic artery was not progressed any more. Subjective complains such as vertigo, losing consciousness and chest pain were completely disappeared.

In addition to this report, recently, some cases of regression of coronary artery stenosis have been reported. Regression of coronary atherosclerosis will be possible under active cholesterol reduction by LDL apheresis.

Conclusions

LDL apheresis has been performed on about 600 patients in Japan and most of the patients suffered coronary heart diseases and whose cholesterol level could not be kept under 250 mg/dl on drug therapy. There is no doubt that LDL apheresis is effective and safe for long term treatment of familial hypercholesterolemic patients and it is expected that LDL apheresis is indicated for secondary prevention of ischemic heart disease after coronary artery bypass graft or percutaneus transluminal coronary angioplasty.

In this moment, a question may be arisen, "How low total cholesterol level should be kept?" There is no sufficient data to settle it yet. However it is a view widely supported by most experts in this field that cholesterol level should be controlled under 180 mg/dl for prevention and under 150 mg/dl for regression of coronary atherosclerosis.

The efficiency of LDL apheresis is enough to evaluate and there is no problem around LDL apheresis in relation to ethical and social aspects in Japan.

References

H. Mabuchi, I. Michishita, M. Takeda, H. Fujita, J. Koizumi, R. Takeda, S. Takeda and M. Oonishi (1987) "A new low density lipoprotein apheresis system using two dextran sulfate cellulose columns in an automated column regenerating unit (LDL continuous apheresis)", Atherosclerosis 68, 19-25.

R. Tatami (1988) "Effects of active cholesterol reduction for coronary atherosclerosis", J. Therap. 70, 2269-2276.

M. Shinomiya, Y. Saito, S. Yoshida (1988) "Clinical evaluation of LDL apheresis", J. Therap. 70, 2263-2268.

Y. Homma, T. Tanimoto, Y. Mikami, S. Watanabe, H. Nomoto, G. Araki (1985) "A comparison in the selective removal of low density lipoprotein of double filtration and dextran sulfate cellulose column plasmapheresis", Therapeutic plasmapheresis (V) 321-324.

36

The effect of LDL-apheresis on some hemostatic parameters in homozygous familial hypercholesterolemia

G. DI MINNO, A.M. CERBONE, M. MARGAGLIONE, F. CIRILLO, G. VECCHIONE, O. RUSSO, N. SCARPATO, C. FALCO, A. GNASSO, M. MANCINI and A. POSTIGLIONE

Istituto di Medicina Interna e Malattie Dismetaboliche and Cattedra di Immunoematologia, II Policlinico, Università degli Studi di Napoli, Italy

ABSTRACT

Some selected parameters of hemostasis that are currently thought to play a major role in thrombogenesis were evaluated in 5 patients homozygous for familial hypercholesterolemia (FH) before and 7 and 14 days after a single LDL-apheresis. The sensitivity of platelets to threshold concentrations of ADP was normal and it was not affected by LDL-apheresis. On the other hand, the sensitivity to arachidonic acid or collagen was abnormally high and this enhanced sensitivity was unchanged 7 and 14 days after the apheresis. Monocyte pro-coagulant activity (PCA) was normal before the apheresis and its values were little affected by the procedure. Likewise, the levels of plasminogen activator inhibitor (PAI) as well as the release by vessel walls of tissue plasminogen activator (tPA) the major phisiological activator of fibrinolysis were functionally and antigenically normal before as well as 7 and 14 days after the apheresis. We conclude that the ability of LDL-apheresis to reduce the tendency to thrombosis of these patients is not associated with changes in these major parameters of hemostasis.

INTRODUCTION.

It is well established that patients with homozygous familial hypercholesterolemia [FH] have an abnormally high tendency to thrombosis and that thrombosis is a major complication as well as a critical determinant of atherosclerosis. In addition, current evidence suggests that an hypercoagulable state may be involved in the thrombotic tendency of some patients[2]. Abnormalities of t-PA, PAI as well as the aggregation of platelets and the expression of the pro-coagulant activity of monocytes may play a role in causing a hypercoa lable state, are known to be afected in vitro by the add :ion of LDL-cholesterol and are often abnormal in patients prone to arterial thrombosis[3]. The combined data were taken to suggest that cholesterol, expecially LDL-cholesterol, is involved in the thrombotic tendency of FH patients. LDL-apheresis has been shown to reduce the tendency to thrombosis of these patients and, few years ago, it has been shown that LDL-apheresis by dextrane sulphate adsorption was able to remove 50-60% of total as well as LDL-cholesterol in FH patients, and that cholesterol reverted to basal values within 2 weeks[4]. We thought that it could be important to determine the role of LDL-cholesterol on the hemostatic abnormalities described in these patients and whether the reported beneficial effects of LDL-apheresis on the tendency to thrombosis of FH patients involved changes in major hemostatic mechanisms.

Patients, Materials and Methods.

Human melanoma tPA was obtained from Dr. D. Collen, Centre for Thrombosis and Vascular Research, Belgium.Factor VII IX and X-deficient plasmas were from General Diagnostics, Warner Lambert, Morris Plains NJ. Sterile, pyrogen-free water was used to prepare the reagents and was passed throug a 0.2µm millipore filter. Plastic sterile disposable tubes, pipettes, petri dishes (60 mm ⌀) and syringes were from Falcon Labware Division (Becton-Dickinson Co., Oxnard, CA). EDTA (Carlo Erba, Milano, Italy) was used as a 100 mM stock solution (pH adjusted to 7.4 with NaOH). ADP (adenosine diphosphate) Hepes, human albumin, were from Sigma Chemical Co. ST. Lous, MO. ADP was dissolved in distilled water and stored at -20 C in small aliquots; Hepes was prepared as a 1 M stock solution and stored at 4 C. Antibiotic-antimycotic mixture contained 10,000 U/ml penicillin, 10,000 µg/ml streptomycin and 25 µg/ml fungizone and was obtained from Gibco Glascow, Scotland. Collagen was from Hormon-Chemie and arachidonic acid from Nu Check Prep Inc Elysian Mo. and it was diluted in 0.1 M sodium carbonate. Percoll was from Pharmacia Fine Chemicals, Uppsala, Sweden and Lymphoprep (1.077 density) from Nyegaard, Oslo, Norway. E. Coli 0111 LPS, W was from Difco Laboratories, Detroit Mi.

Plasma LDL-apheresis LDL-apheresis was carried out according to Yokoyama et al[4] with some modifications. Sterile, disposable materials were used throughout the procedure. Two distinct pumps were employed to settle the rate of blood and plasma flow. Maximum rate of the flows was 60 and 20 ml/min respectively. A 2,000 Units bolus of unfractionated heparin in ACD (Acid Citrate Dextrose) was injected into the system at the beginning of the procedure. Then the anticoagulant was employed throughout the apheresis at the rate of 20 Units/min. LDL-apheresis was perfomed in line. A polysulphone hollow fiber filter (Sulflux FS 05,Kanegafuchi Chem. Ind.

Osaka, Japan) with an average pore size of 0.2 µm and an effective surface area of 0.5 m^2 was used to separate plasma from cellular components of blood. Selective removal of plasma LDL was carried out passing the cell-free plasma alternatively through one of two 150 ml column of cellulose beads of dextrane sulphate (Liposorber LA-15, Kanegafuchi). Then, the eluate of the dextrane sulphate column and the cell-rich fraction were reinfused into the patient. In each case and for each patient, the system was pre-equilibrated with saline and then with a Ringer-lactate solution.

Protocol of the study

The study was carried out on 5 patients [2 males, 3 females] 14-26 yrs old, homozygous for familial hypercholesterolemia. Diagnosis of the homozygous state was based upon plasma cholesterol above 500 mg/dl with LDL-cholesterol levels consistently above 450 mg/dl, marked hypercholesterolemia in both parents, appearance of xanthomata in the first decade of life and, in 3 of them, receptor-deficiency in skin fibroblast cultures. For each patient and for matched controls, platelet aggregation in response to threshold concentrations of ADP, collagen and arachidonic acid as well as the pro-coagulant activity of monocytes were determined biologically.In contrast tPA and PAI, the major determinants of fibrinolysis were determined both antigenically. In FH patients, these studies were carried out immediately before LDL-apheresis and 7 and 14 days after it.The decision to determine these parameters before and 7 and 14 days after the apheresis was based on preliminary observations in which it was found that seven days after the apheresis, values of total and LDL-cholesterol were still 30% lower than before the apheresis and 14 days were required to restore pre-apheresis values. Thus we thought that this was a good opportunity to evaluate the hemostatic parameters selected.

Isolation of Cells

Preparation of platelet-rich plasma was performed according to standard procedures, while isolation and suspension of mononuclear cells was carried as described by Boyum[5].

Platelet aggregation

Platelet aggregation was quantified by employing the threshold aggregating concentrations. Treshold aggregating concentration was defined as the lowest concentration of an aggregating agent that when added to platelet-rich plasma, causes 50% light transmittance within 3 min.

Assay for PCA

The capacity of mononuclear phagocytes to produce PCA was determined as described by Montemurro et al[6] and expressed as arbitrary units by comparison of the clotting times obtained in the presence of the stimulated cells with the values of a standard curve of rabbit thromboplastin.

Assay of plasma fibrinolytic activity

The biological activity of tPA and PAI were determined immunologically as well as functionally according to previously described methods[7-10].

Results and Discussion

Based on the definition of the treshold aggregating concentration given above, it is clear that the lower the threshold, the higher the sensitivity of platelets to the agent.In the past years, we and others have found that platelets from FH patients have a low threshold, which means a high sensitivity to several aggregating agents such as collagen and arachidonic acid. This is in agreement with some in vitro studies that have shown that addition of cholesterol to normal platelets makes these cells hyperreactive to aggregating agents. As expected, platelets from the patients were hyperreactive to collagen and arachidonic acid ($p<0.05$). However, reduction of plasma cholesterol by LDL-apheresis did not suffice to correct the hyperaggregable state of these patients.

It is well established that monocytes may express a pro-coagulant activity [PCA]. Under resting conditions i.e. in the absence of any stimulation, the levels of this activity are between 4.4 and 19 U/10^5 in monocytes from control subjects and similar values were found in monocytes from FH patients before and 7 and 14 days after LDL-apheresis. Following incubation with E. Coli lipopolysaccharide, the ability of monocytes to form this activity increases dramatically, the PCA of normals ranging between 220 and 400 U/10^5, and in vitro pre-treament of the cells with LDL-cholesterol decreases such activity. Before the apheresis, when plasma LDL-cholesterol levels are very high, the PCA activity of stimulated monocytes from the patients was found to be within normal ranges, a finding at variance with the results of in vitro studies. On the other hand the procedure little affected the expression of this activity, normal values of PCA being found at 7 and 14 days after the apheresis. In addition since at 14 days the plasma LDL-cholesterol were almost comparable to pre-apheresis levels, as were the PCA values of monocytes from the patients, the

data suggest that the role of cholesterol on this activity remains to be fully understood.
PAI is the principal inhibitor of fibrinolysis and high levels of this protein have been found in patients with premature myocardial infarction. Normal levels of this inhibitor were found in FH patients and they were not affected by the apheresis as determined functionally as well as immunologically.
tPA, the key protein of the fibrinolytic system, is released from the vessel wall, and stasis is currently thought to be the an effective stimulus for the release. After stasis, vessel walls from control subjects release 15-20 ng/ml of tPA. The release from the vessels of FH patients was comparable and it was little affected by the apheresis. When evaluated in the absence of stasis, plasma levels of tPA refer to basal levels of this protein and, in control subjects, these values are between 1 and 7 ng/ml. Those of FH patients were well within these ranges and comparable results were found 7 and 14 days after the apheresis. This observation was further analyzed. tPA was isolated in the euglobulin fraction and its ability to cause lysis of fibrin plates was determined. This biological study confirmed and the pre-stasis and post-stasis observations.
In summary we have found that LDL-apheresis does not affect the abnormally high aggregation of platelets from FH patients, that monocyte-procoagulant activity is normal in FH and that it is not affected by the LDL-apheresis, and that tPA and PAI levels normal in FH patients before and after removal of LDL-cholesterol by the procedure. Thus it appears that the ability of this procedure to reduce the thrombotic tendency of these patients little involves the hemostatic parameters reported above. Based on the results, we also believe that in vitro data obtained incubating cholesterol with hemostatically active cells should be extrapolated with caution to explain the thrombotic tendency of FH patients.

REFERENCES

1) Goldstein, J.L., Brown,M.S., Familial hypercholesterolemia: A genetic defect in the low density lipoprotein receptor. New Engl. J. Med. 294:1386-1390,1976

2)Di Minno G, Mancini M. Measuring Plasma Fibrinogen to Predict Stroke and Myocardial Infarction. Arteriosclerosis 1989, in Press

3) Di Minno G, Cerbone AM. The Antithrombotic Potential of the Vessel Wall. Evidence From Studies on Patients Prone to Venous Thrombosis. Haematologica, 73, 75-78, 1988

4) Yokoyama, S., Hayashi, R., Kikkava, T., Tani, N., Takada, S., Hatanaka, K., Yamamoto, A., Specific sorbent of apolipoprotein B-containing lipoproteins for plasmapheresis: characterization and experimental use in hypercholesterolemic rabbits. Arteriosclerosis 4:276-282,1984

5) Boyum A 1976. Isolation of Lymphocytes, Granulocytes and Macrophages. Scand J. Immunol (Suppl)5: 9-15

6) Montemurro P, A Lattanzio, G. Chetta, L. Lupo, L. Caputi-Lambrenghi, M. Rubino, D. Giordano and N. Semeraro, 1985. Increased in vitro and in Vivo Generation of Pro-coagulanrt Activity (Tissue Factor) by Mononuclear Phagocytes after Intralipid Infusion in Rabbits. Blood, 65, 1391-1395.

7)Declerck PJ, Alessi MC, Verstreken M, Kruithof EKO, Juhan-Vague I, Collen D: Measurement of Plasminogen Activator Inhibitor 1 in Biological Fluids with a Murine Monoclonal Antibody-Based Enzyme-Linked Immunosorbent Assay. Blood 71, 220-225, 1988.

8)Colucci M, Paramo JA, Collen D. Generation in Plasma of a Fast-Acting Inhibitor of Plasminogen Activatoe in Response to Endotoxin Stimulation. J. Clin. Invest. 75, 818-824, 1985

9) Holvoet P, Cleemput H, Collen D: Assay of Human Tissue-Type Plasminogen Activator (tPA) With an Enzyme-Linked Immunosorbent Assay (ELISA) Based on Three Murine Monoclonal Antibodies to tPA. Thrombos. Haemostas. 54, 684-687, 1985.

10) Rijken DC, Collen D. Purification and Characterization of the Plasminogen Activator Secreted by Human Melanoma Cells in Culture. J. Biol. Chem. 256, 7035-7041, 1981.

DEVELOPMENTS IN LIPOPROTEIN AND APOPROTEIN RESEARCH

37
Regulation of VLDL metabolism by cellular receptors

E. SEHAYEK and S. EISENBERG

Hadassah University Hospital, Department of Internal Medicine B, PO Box 12000, il-91120 Jerusalem, Israel

Introduction

The triglyceride-rich lipoproteins chylomicrons and very low density (VLDL) lipoproteins serve to transport triglycerides of exogenous (dietary) and endogenous origin from the intestine and the liver to sites of storage and utilization (1). The lipoprotein lipase, situated at surfaces of endothelial cells, regulates triglyceride hydrolysis and uptake of free fatty acids by tissues. Lipase action results in depletion of core-triglycerides of the two lipoproteins; concomitantly and in coordination with triglyceride hydrolysis, redundant lipid and apoprotein molecules are excluded from the surface of the lipolyzed lipoproteins and are metabolized in HDL (2,3). This sequence of metabolic events causes conversion of large, triglyceride-rich particles, to small triglyceride-depleted lipoproteins. The fate of the triglyceride-depleted particles is in part similar and in part different for chylomicrons and VLDL. Lipolyzed chylomicrons are all transformed to remnant particles that are rapidly and completely cleared from the bloodstream, predominantly by interacting with receptors in liver cells. Some VLDL particles also become remnants and are removed from the plasma by a mechanism possibly identical to that responsible for the catabolism of chylomicron remnants. Other VLDL particles, however, continue to interact with lipases along the delipidation cascade and finally are converted to LDL. VLDL-derived LDL particles are in fact the main, if not the only source of LDL in humans and experimental animals (1,2). Therefore, regulation of VLDL remnants clearance is an exceedingly important mechanism that determines plasma LDL levels. For example, in some experimental animals (e.g. rats), low LDL levels are explained mainly by an avid process of VLDL-remnants catabolism by the liver (4,5). In humans, however, most LDL is derived from the VLDL->LDL cascade.

The mechanism(s) and receptors responsible for VLDL remnant uptake are yet unclear. While functional apo E molecules, E-3 or E-4, are absolutely necessary (6), neither the characteristics of the remnant particles nor the receptors involved with the remnant clearance process are known. Since apo E is a normal protein constituent of both chylomicrons and VLDL, a lipase-induced alteration of the particles must take place to properly express the apo E molecules on the surface of remnant particles. The nature of this alteration is unknown. In addition, while apo E containing lipoproteins interact avidly with LDL receptors, evidence from humans and rabbits that lack LDL receptor indicate that another, or an additional pathway must play a critical role in the process of remnant clearance (7).

In recent years, studies have been initiated in our laboratory with the aim of elucidating the determinants responsible for VLDL and VLDL remnant interactions with cells (8-11). These studies are summarized here.

Results

The initial study was carried out with VLDL density subfractions (I, II and III) and IDL isolated from the plasma of normolipidemic human subjects (8,9). Only subjects with apo E profile E 3/3 or E 4/3 were included. Binding, uptake and degradation of the lipoproteins after iodination were determined in upregulated human skin fibroblasts and compared to LDL. VLDL metabolic rates were extremely low and IDL, about one-half that of LDL, although all the VLDL populations and the IDL contained 2-3 molecules of apo E per particle. Because apo E was shown to be the ligand for IDL:cell interaction, it was decided to add exogenous, recombinant or plasmatic apo E-3 to the lipoprotein-cell system. A dramatic effect was observed. VLDL metabolism has increased by many-folds and IDL metabolism doubled. By using gel chromatography and agarose columns, association of appreciable amounts of the exogenous apo E-3 with the VLDL and IDL was demonstrated. Proteolytic degradation of these apo E-3 enriched lipoproteins approached that of LDL. Yet, in spite of association of 5-10 molecules of apo E-3 with the various VLDL populations and 3-6 molecules with IDL, protein degradation has not been higher than LDL.

These initial observations raise several important questions related to the physiology of VLDL/IDL cell interactions. <u>First</u>, the amount of apo E-3 associated with the lipoprotein particles is a rate-limiting for their cellular metabolism. The concentration of apo E in human plasma is perhaps less than optimal. <u>Second</u>, it appears that only a fraction of the apo E-3 present at the surface of VLDL and IDL is expressed in receptor binding assays. For some lipoproteins, e.g., VLDL-I, that fraction may not exceed 10-20% of the calculated capacity to interact with the cells. <u>Third</u>, although exogenous apo E-3 increases cell metabolism of plasma VLDL and IDL appreciably, the resulting catabolic rates are similar to those of LDL, a lipoprotein devoid of apo E. Thus, further alteration of the lipoprotein particle is necessary for expression of remnant properties. Four, it is possible that receptors other than the LDL receptor are involved with the remnant removal process. These questions were further studied by us.

The amount of apo E-3 and the specificity of this protein for uptake and degradation of VLDL and IDL by cells was determined in fibroblasts from normal subjects and from patients that lack functional LDL receptors (homozygous familial hypercholesterolemia). Optimal uptake and degradation of apo E-3 enriched lipoproteins occurred at apo E-3: lipoprotein-protein ratio of 4:10. Further increase of apo E-3 concentration either has not changed the cell metabolism of VLDL and IDL or was inhibitory, presumably because of competition between unassociated apo E-3 and the lipoproteins for binding to the receptor. Apo E-3 was ineffective in receptor-negative fibroblasts and apo E-2 was relatively ineffective in both cell lines. Thus, the effects of apo E-3 were specific for the functional form of the protein, were saturable and were dependent on the presence of receptors on the fibroblasts.

Next, the behavior of VLDL and IDL obtained from patients with hypertriglyceridemia (HTG) was investigated (10). Since HTG-VLDL differs in structure and composition from normal (N)- VLDL (12) it was hoped that its basal and/or apo E-3 stimulated metabolism would also differ. After centrifugation, HTG-VLDLs exhibit metabolic activities (binding, association and degradation) that are 3-5 folds higher than N-VLDL. These activities, however, were about one-tenth those of LDL. Addition of exogenous apo E-3 increased the activities of both N- and HTG-VLDL by many folds. Yet, a difference between N- and HTG-VLDL was still observed. This was especially pronounced for HTG-VLDL-I although the two preparations were optimally supplemented with exogenous apo E-3. The observation that the basal activity of HTG-VLDL is higher than N-VLDL can be explained by ability of HTG-lipoproteins to retain more apo E than N-lipoproteins during centrifugation. This hypothesis, however, fails to explain the higher ability of HTG-VLDL than N-VLDL to express apo E-3 in cell metabolism experiments when apo E-3 is provided in optimal concentration. Thus, we must conclude that HTG-VLDL must either associate more apo E-3 molecules or express the associated apo E-3 molecules better than N-VLDL. In an attempt to further understand this altered behavior of HTG-VLDL we have also studied VLDL from the same HTG- subjects after the initiation of triglyceride lowering therapy (with bezafibrate, BZ). BZ-VLDL behaved normally. Comparing the composition of the VLDLs to their uptake and degradation data, an interesting observation emerged. For all nine preparations studied (VLDL-I, II and II from N-, HTG- and BZ- subjects) a strong and significant relationship was found between the cell metabolism values and the cholesteryl ester to protein ratio. Whether the cholesteryl ester molecules have a direct effect on VLDL metabolism or on another structural-compositional abnormality that is related to the cholesteryl ester content of the lipoprotein is responsible for this phenomenon, is unknown.

Interaction between apo E-3 and other apolipoprotein - especially apo C - has been reported by Windler et al., to delay clearance of chylomicron remnants in the perfused rat liver (13,14). To explore the possibility that apolipoproteins may also affect the interaction of VLDL with the LDL receptor, we studied the effects of most human plasma soluble apolipoprotein (C-I, C-II, C-III-1, C-III-2, A-I and A-II) on VLDL and IDL cell interactions with the LDL receptors in cultured fibroblasts. Apo C-I, C-II, C-III-1 and C-III-2 were purified from human plasma VLDL by gel filtration on Sephadex followed by ion exchange chromatography on DEAE. Apo A-I and apo A-II were purified from human plasma HDL by filtration on Sephadex columns in the presence of mercaptoethanol. All four apo C preparations had strong inhibitory effect on the apo E-3 stimulated binding, association and degradation of normal and HTG-VLDL. Apo A-I and apo A-II in contrast had no effect on either the basal or apo E-3 stimulated cell metabolism of VLDL. Neither apo C proteins nor apo A proteins had any effect on LDL cell interaction. Thus, the inhibitory effect of apo C proteins on VLDL cell interaction could not be due to competition for binding to the receptor. The inhibitory effect of apo C therefore must reflect a direct action at the VLDL surface. To investigate this effect further, possible competition between apo C and apo E for binding on to the VLDL surface was determined. Both apo E-3 and apo C alone were found to associate well with VLDL particles. When the two apoproteins were incubated together with VLDL, both associated with the lipoprotein. Thus, it appears that specific interactions between apo C and apo E occur at the VLDL surface and that such interactions reduce considerably the affinity of the apo C, apo E-3 particles towards the fibroblast LDL receptor.

The studies described above have elucidated the major determinants that regulate the interactions of VLDL and IDL with the LDL receptor. In addition to availability of optimal concentration of apo E-3, the investigations clearly demonstrated the influence of lipoprotein structure and composition on the apo E-3 dependent cell metabolism of apo B-100 lipoproteins and the inhibitory effects of the C apoproteins. It can be concluded that several factors determine the extent of uptake and degradation of VLDL and IDL by the receptor. These are the concentration of apo E-3, the ability of apo E-3 to associate with the lipoproteins, the expression of apo E-3 epitopes that participate in the receptor binding process and the presence of other apoproteins predominantly apo C molecules. Even under optimal conditions, however, it was impossible to induce metabolic activities for VLDL and IDL that are considerably higher than those observed with LDL. Noteworthy, such high activities are an absolute requirement for significant regulation of LDL formation along the VLDL->IDL->LDL cascade. For example, affinities of VLDL or IDL that are 5-10 folds higher than LDL are necessary for being responsible for clearance of 50% of the VLDL particle prior to being converted to LDL.

This consideration prompted us to search for an additional, apo E-3 specific binding site in cells of hepatic origin that would be responsible for uptake and degradation of remnant particles.

The study was carried out with hepG-2 cultures that are composed of cells grown from human hepatoma tissue. The cells are minimally modified and express most if not all activities related to lipid and lipoprotein metabolism. These include synthesis of lipids and apolipoproteins, secretion of lipoprotein particles, synthesis of enzymes such as hepatic lipase and LCAT, formation and secretion of bile acids and expression of the LDL receptor activity and of the newly described LDL receptor related protein (LRP) (15).

The initial experiments with hepG-2 cells were carried out with IDL and investigated the capacity of IDL and apo E-3 enriched IDL to bind to cellular receptors (9). IDL, IDL+E-3 and LDL all exhibit capacities to displace bound ^{125}I-LDL from the cells proportionately to their affinity towards LDL- receptors. When tested for their ability to displace bound ^{125}I-IDL, the IDL preparations have clearly exhibited higher capacity than LDL, indicating that an apo E-3 specific binding site for IDL, distinctly different from the LDL-receptor is also present. The behavior of the apo E-3 specific binding site in metabolic pathways was investigated with VLDL and VLDL+E-3 (11). Comparing hepG-2 cultures to fibroblasts, several important observations were made. Significant uptake and degradation of VLDL not enriched with apo E-3 was found only in hepG-2 cultures. In the two cell types, a pronounced response was seen when the VLDL was supplemented with exogenous apo E-3. The cell metabolism of apo E-3 rich VLDL was more than LDL in the hepG-2 cells, and less than LDL in the fibroblast cultures. In both cell types, apo E-2 was ineffective indicating the high degree of specificity of the cell receptors to apo E isoforms. Competition of apo E-3 enriched VLDL metabolism was investigated with excess of unlabeled LDL and unlabeled VLDL+E. Both effectively reduced VLDL metabolism in fibroblasts but LDL was relatively ineffective (50% or less than VLDL+E) in hepG-2 cultures. In hepG-2 cultures, like in fibroblasts, apo C proteins exhibited a strong inhibitory effect on VLDL uptake and degradation either in the absence or presence of exogenous apo E-3.

These results indicate that hepG-2 cells contain a binding site specific for apo E-3 that is descernible from the LDL receptor and does not bind LDL. A hallmark of the biology of the LDL receptor is downregulation of receptor protein synthesis by LDL cholesterol (16). To determine whether similar regulation process affects the apo E-3 specific binding site in hepG-2 cultures, some of the experiments described above were repeated after cells (fibroblasts and hepG-2) were grown in the presence of high concentration of cholesterol. Downregulation of VLDL and VLDL+E metabolism was observed in fibroblasts to a degree similar to that of LDL. In hepG-2 cultures in contrast, VLDL and VLDL+E metabolism were depressed by only one-third to one-half of LDL metabolism. We thus concluded that the specific apo E-3 binding site is relatively, or absolutely insensitive to the cell cholesterol content.

Conclusions

The aim of the studies described above was to evaluate processes responsible for interactions of VLDL and IDL with receptors and to define the nature of the receptors that are responsible for the cellular uptake of the lipoproteins. It was expected that apolipoprotein E-3 plays an important role in this process and that the LDL-receptor is the main protein involved with cell catabolism of the lipoproteins. It was further speculated that regulation of VLDL/IDL cell interaction is complex and is affected by lipid and apoproteins other than apo B-100 and apo E. Studies were carried out with VLDL and IDL isolated from normal subjects and from patients with hypertriglyceridemia, all with E3/3 or 4/3 profiles. Cell metabolism experiments were conducted in cultured human fibroblasts and cultured human hepatomia cell line, hepG-2. Dependence of cell interaction of VLDL and IDL on presence of optimal concentrations of apo E-3 was clearly observed in the two cell types. To achieve optimal concentrations, however, it was necessary to supplement the lipoproteins with exogenous apo E-3. Of interest, recent studies in rabbits have shown a hypolipidemic effect after injection of exogenous apo E-3 (17,18). Exogenous apo E-3 associated with the lipoprotein particles and enhanced their cellular metabolism by many folds. This effect was specific for apo E-3 or E-4, not observed with apo E-2 (where an arginine->cysteine substitution occurred) (8) and was dependent on the presence of functional receptors at the cell surface. Yet, even when optimally enriched with apo E-3, neither VLDL nor IDL cell metabolism was much higher than LDL. Noteworthy, the apo E-3 enriched particles contained 4-8 molecules of apo E per particle and should have had a 4-8 higher affinity towards the LDL receptor as compared to LDL, a lipoprotein with only one binding site to the receptor on its apo B-100 moiety. These findings indicate that the expression of apo E-3 in biological systems is partial when the apoprotein is associated with triglyceride-rich lipoproteins. In fact, no more than 10-30% of the expected biological expression is observed.

Expression of the biological activity of apo E in VLDL and IDL could be changed by at least two mechanisms. The first was the cholesteryl ester content of the particle as demonstrated in the study of VLDL from hypertriglyceridemic subjects, and the second the content of apo C on the particles. HTG-VLDL has several structural-compositional abnormalities. It is therefore not certain that cholesteryl ester molecules themselves will alter the conformation of apo E at the lipoprotein surface. Yet, it is interesting to note that in recent experiments (not shown here) we found an effect of cholesteryl esters transferred to normal VLDL on the cell metabolism of the particle. Apo C molecules are abundant in large sized and less dense VLDL populations and are exchanged and transferred between VLDL and HDL (1,3). Inhibition of chylomicron remnant clearance by apo C has been demonstrated in the perfused rat liver (13,14). In the present study, a strong inhibitory effect of exogenous apo C on apo E-3 stimulated interaction of VLDL and IDL with LDL receptors was clearly observed. The mechanism of this phenomenon is not clear but it appears to reflect an apo C:apo E interaction at the lipoprotein surface. Whether specific transfer of apo C molecules from VLDL along the VLDL->LDL cascade will result in considerable increase of apo E dependent catabolism of lipolyzed VLDL is of course not known and should be determined in future studies.

The studies demonstrated that cells of liver origin (hepG-2) take up VLDL and IDL by both the LDL receptor pathway and an apo E specific binding site. Comparing the two binding sites, both are specific for the functional form of apo E, are insensitive to apo E-2, are inhibited by apo C and are competed by apo E-rich VLDL. The apo E-3 specific binding site, however, is not competed by LDL, recognizes apo E in intact particles (when the protein is not accessible to the LDL receptor) and is poorly or totally not sensitive to the cholesterol status of the cell. These properties signal the apo E-3 specific binding site as an outstanding candidate for remnant clearance processes, either of intestinal (chylomicron) or liver (VLDL) origin. As mentioned above, the recently described 500 Kd LDL receptor-related protein (15,19) possibly fulfils some of the characteristics of a remnant receptor. More studies, however, are necessary to confirm or rule out this possibility.

References

1. Eisenberg, S. & Levy, R.I. (1975) Lipoprotein metabolism, Adv. Lipid Res. 13, 1-89.
2. Eisenberg, S. (1983) Lipoprotein and lipoprotein metabolism. A dynamic evaluation of the plasma fat transport system, Klin. Wochenschr. 61, 119-132.
3. Eisenberg, S. (1984) High density lipoprotein metabolism (JLR Review), J. Lipid Res. 25, 1017-1058.
4. Eisenberg, S. & Rachmilewitz, D. (1973) Metabolism of rat plasma very low density lipoprotein. I. Circulation of the whole lipoprotein, Biochim. Biophys. Acta 326, 378-390.
5. Eisenberg, S. & Rachmilewitz, D. (1973) Metabolism of rat plasma very low density lipoprotein. II. Fate in circulation of apoprotein subunits, Biochim. Biophys. Acta 326, 391-405.
6. Mahley, R.W. & Angelin B. (1984) Type III hyperlipoproteinemia. Recent insights into the genetic defect of familial dysbetalipoproteinemia, Adv. Intern. Med. 29, 385-411.
7. Kita, T., Goldstein, J.L., Brown, M.S., Watanabe, Y., Hornick, C.A. & Havel, R.J. (1982) Hepatic uptake of chylomicron remnants in WHHL rabbits:A mechanism genetically distinct from the low density lipoprotein receptor, Proc. Natl. Acad. Sci. USA 79, 3623-3627.

8. Eisenberg, S., Friedman, G. & Vogel, T. (1988) Enhanced metabolism of normolipidemic human plasma very low density lipoprotein in cultured cells by exogenous apolipoprotein E-3, Arteriosclerosis, 8, 480-487.

9. Friedman, G., Eisenberg, S., Gavish, D., Vogel, T. & Marcel, I. (1987) Effects of exogenous apo E-3 on the cellular metabolism of human intermediate density lipoproteins, Arteriosclerosis, 7, 501a.

10. Eisenberg, S. & Sehayek, E. (1988) Effects of exogenous apo E-3 on cellular metabolism of hypertriglyceridemic (HTG) VLDL before and during bezafibrate (BZ) therapy. Comparison to normal (N) VLDL, Arteriosclerosis (Abs) 8, 560a.

11. Eisenberg, S., Sehayek, E. & Friedman, G. (1989) An apo E (ARG-158) specific binding site for human VLDL in cultured hepG-2 cells, Arteriosclerosis, 9, 731a.

12. Eisenberg, S., Gavish, D., Oschry, Y., Fainaru, M. & Deckelbaum, R.J. (1984) Abnormalities in very low, low and high density lipoproteins in hypertriglyceridemia. Reversal towards normal with bezafibrate treatment, J. Clin. Invest. 74, 470-482.

13. Windler, E., Chao, Y.-s. & Havel, R.J. (1980) Regulation of the hepatic uptake of triglyceride-rich lipoproteins in the rat, J. Biol. Chem. 255, 8303-8307.

14. Windler, E. & Havel R.J. (1985) Inhibitory effects of C apolipoproteins from rats and humans on the uptake of triglyceride-rich lipoproteins and their remnants by the perfused rat liver, J. Lipid Res. 26, 536- 565.

15. Herz, J., Hamann, U., Rogne, S., Myklebost, O., Gausepohl, H. & Stanley, K. (1988) Surface location and high affinity for calcium of a 500-kd liver membrane protein closely related to the LDL-receptor suggest a physiological role as lipoprotein receptor, EMBO J. 7, 4119-4127.

16. Brown, M.S. & Goldstein, J.L. (1986) A receptor-mediated pathway for cholesterol homeostasis, Science 232, 34-37.

17. Yamada, N., Shimano, H., Mokuno, H., Ishibashi, S., Gotohda, T., Kawakami, M., Watanabe, Y., Akanuma, Y., Murase, T. & Takaku, F. (1989) Increased clearance of plasma cholesterol after injection of apolipoprotein E into Watanabe heritable hyperlipidemic rabbits, Proc. Nat. Acad. Sci. USA 86, 665-669.

18. Mahley, R.W., Weisgraber, K.H., Hussain, M.M., Greenman, B., Fisher, M., Vogel, T. & Gorecki, M. (1989) Intravenous infusion of apolipoprotein E accelerates clearance of plasma lipoproteins in rabbits, J. Clin. Invest. 83, 2125-2130.

19. Kowal, R.C., Herz, J., Goldstein, J.L., Esser, V. & Brown, M.S. (1989) Low density lipoprotein receptor-related protein mediates uptake of cholesteryl esters derived from apoprotein E-enriched lipoproteins, Proc. Natl. Acad. Sci. USA 86, 5810-5814.

38
Current concepts in reverse cholesterol transport

G. GHISELLI, R. MUSANTI and A.M. GOTTO Jr.

Baylor College of Medicine and The Methodist Hospital, Department of Medicine, Houston, TX 77030, USA

Introduction

The term reverse cholesterol transport first introduced by Glomset (1), identifies a process where there is net flux of cholesterol from the peripheral tissues to the liver. Because the liver is the single organ capable of significant cholesterol elimination from the body via bile acids peripheral tissues must utilize this system for carrying excess cholesterol (both the newly synthesized and that derived from plasma) to the liver. Since the first inception of the idea it was held that circulating HDL were the plasma elements mainly implicated in reverse cholesterol transport. They would pick up cholesterol from extrahepatic cells through a process amplified by continous esterification of this cholesterol by lecithin cholesterol acyl transferase (LCAT), and final delivery to the liver. It has been within this conceptual framework that investigations on reverse cholesterol transport have developed in the last twenty years. The picture have become more complex with evidences for specific receptorial processes, protein(s) facilitating cholesteryl ester transfer between lipoproteins, and a number of other circulating putative tissue cholesterol acceptors/carriers in addition to HDL. The following is a brief account of the current status on reverse cholesterol transport research with some emphasis on the role of apolipoprotein A-IV (apoA-IV) which we have investigated more closely. The three main metabolic compartment composing the reverse cholesterol system, i.e. the peripheral tissue, the plasma compartment, and the liver, are discussed individually.

The peripheral tissue.

Key element for net cholesterol efflux from cells, is the presence at the exterior of an acceptor. Its characteristics would be such that a chemical potential is created allowing cholesterol to flow continously and irreversably outside the cell. Incubation of cells with the 1.21 g/dl ultracentrifuge infranate, increases in a dose and time dependent manner cholesterol efflux from cells (2). It is thus believed that lipoprotein deficient fraction (LDF) of plasma contains acceptors of cellular cholesterol. ApoA-IV in particular but also apoA-I, apoE, and probably others apolipoproteins are present in LDF and may form complexes with lipids (3-5). Fielding et al (6), immunoprecipitated apoA-I from plasmatic LDF and reported loss of cholesterol efflux-induced capability of the supernate suggesting the activity may reside in apoA-I or in a complex that contain it. Because of the elevated concentration of apoA-IV in human plasmatic LDF, attention has been paid to this apolipoprotein as well. We found (7) that apoA-IV in plasma LDF has kinetic properties distinct from those of the delipidated apolipoprotein, indirectly supporting the evidence that is complexed with lipids. Synthetic apoA-IV-phospholipid complexes have been shown to promote cholesterol efflux from cells (8). Moreover carefully investigating dynamic of cholesterol flux between cells and medium, it has been reached the conclusion that cholesterol efflux will be enhanced particularly if the acceptor is a small particle of high surface area per unit mass as in fact are LDF apoA-IV-lipid complexes (9). At present however there is no direct evidence that circulating LDF apoA-IV-phospholipid complexes are implicated in reverse cholesterol transport. This has been mainly because of the difficulty in isolating these complexes from plasma.

There is extensive literature demonstrating ability of HDL, particularly HDL3 - the smallest of the circulating HDL subfraction - to directly induce net cholesterol efflux from cells (10,11). Thus the conclusion has been drawn that mature circulating HDL may directly interact with peripheral tissues and become enriched with cholesterol. On the other hand, recently an alternative model through which cellular cholesterol may be conveyed to HDL has been postulated (12). Evidences were given for the presence in plasma of a series of apoA-I containing particles with prebeta mobility. When plasma is incubated with cells, these prebeta lipoproteins become enriched with free cholesterol. One particular species named LpA-I prebeta3, also contains LCAT, CETP (cholesteryl esters transfer protein), and apoD and is responsible for most of the esterification of efflued cellular cholesterol. Generated cholesteryl esters is the precursor of at least a major part of that found in HDL. Time course of these events is calculated to be in the order of minutes. Works like this underscore the need for caution in the interpretation of in vitro studies in which single isolated presumed components of reverse cholesterol transport, as opposed to whole plasma, are investigated.

Study on lipoprotein composition in peripheral lymph have given interesting informations on lipoprotein species actually interacting with cells in vivo. In peripheral lymph there is a larger proportion of HDL relative to VLDL and LDL than in plasma (13). Not a surprising finding given the limited permeability of large lipoprotein to the interstitium. Lymphatic HDL however appears to be rather different from those circulating in plasma. They are larger, mostly discoidal in shape and contain more unesterified cholesterol (14). Mayor apolipoproteins found are apoA-IV, apoE, and apoA-I. Cholesterol feeding to dogs increases concentration of apoA-IV and apoE in the discoidal unesterified cholesterol rich lymph lipoproteins (15). Whereas apoE is also synthesized extrahepatically and may be tissue derived, apoA-IV increase must be due to enhanced influx from plasma. Whether elevation of lymphatic cholesterol following cholesterol-enriched diet is secondary to increased plasmatic cholesterol infiltration, or rather reflects activated reverse cholesterol transport, is still not clear. The most convincing evidence gathered so far on an active role of lymphatic lipoproteins in promoting net cholesterol efflux from cells has been presented by Reichl et al (16). In their experiment labeled cholesterol was administered to human volonteers and cholesterol specific activity measured in plasma as well in lymphatic lipoproteins. At 9-10 months after injection unesterified cholesterol specific activity was higher in lymph lipoproteins than in plasma. This indicates that their cholesterol is not derived from plasma and thus must be originating from the tissue bathed by the lymph.

Much work has been carried out trying to shed light on the mechanism underlaying reverse cholesterol transport acceptor-cell interaction leading to net cholesterol efflux. Two differents thoughts have emerged. The first held that cholesterol efflux is a diffusive phenomenon. Its rate is a function of the cell type and both concentration and composition of the acceptor (17). At high concentration of the acceptor the rate limiting step for cholesterol efflux become desorption of cholesterol molecules from cell plasma membrane into the layer of unstirred water surrounding the cell. At low concentration of the acceptor, the limiting factor is the reduced frequency of collision between desorbed cholesterol and the acceptor. The second hypotesis (11), asserts that direct specific interaction between the cell and the cholesterol acceptor is taking place and in fact is a prerequisite for cholesterol efflux. This idea is based on evidences that binding site for cholesterol acceptor are expressed at the surface of the cell. By binding to a cell surface site, efflux process would be made very efficient because of physical contact between the cell and the cholesterol ecceptor. To our knowledge no conclusive experiments have been carried out to dismiss one of the two mechanisms as quantitatively unimportant. It is still possible that both mechanisms play a major role in reverse cholesterol transport.

HDL binding to different tissues has been demonstrated in various experimetal settings and a membrane binding protein has been identified by ligand blotting analysis (18). The protein recognizes apoA-I and apoA-II, the two major apolipoprotein constituents in HDL. In fibroblasts, apoA-IV-phospholipid complexes however bind with higher specificity and affinity than complexes containing apoA-I (19). Apparently the two apolipoproteins compete for the same binding site, but whereas apoA-I-phospholipid complexes are displaced by phospholipids and lipoproteins other than HDL, apoA-IV-phospholipid complexes are not. This may suggest that in peripheral cells apoA-IV mediated binding is favored. As for apoA-I, apoA-IV mediated binding is increased when cells are loaded with cholesterol. Obviously this is what would be expected if these apolipoproteins are to be involved in reverse cholesterol transport.

The plasma compartment

Importance of LCAT in promoting cholesterol efflux from cells is well documented. Although the rate of cholesterol diffusion in water phase is rather low, esterification further decreases it and prevent diffusion of cholesterol back to the tissues. Furthermore, removal of unesterified cholesterol from the lipoprotein surface creates a chemical potential warranting further net cholesterol efflux from cells. The essential role of LCAT has been clearly demonstrated in cell studies. When LCAT in the medium is inhibited or removed, cholesterol flux to the outside is taking place at the same rate, but is equivalent to the rate of influx. When LCAT is fully active, however, bulk of cholesterol efflux is associated with net cholesterol transport to the medium and there is esterification (20). In patients with LCAT deficiency red blood cells contains more cholesterol than in normal subjects (21). If LCAT-deficient patients receive a trasfusion of normal plasma, circulation lipoprotein colesteryl ester concentration increases and red blood cells cholesterol content decreases. This is consistent with the idea that functional LCAT is necessary to maintain appropiate cholesterol content in blood cells, and thus by extrapolation in every extrahepatic tissues.

As peripheral lymph contains little if nothing of LCAT activity, the bulk of the process must occur in plasma (14). ApoA-IV, apoA-I and apoE, all have been shown to be effective activators of LCAT. Thus lymphatic lipoprotein exiting the interstitium contain potent activators of cholesterol esterification. ApoE carring lipoproteins may be directly catabolized by the liver through the remnant receptor and this route of reverse cholesterol transport may be very significant (22). ApoA-IV containing lipoproteins also appear to be directly rapidly catabolized by the liver (19). We calculated (7) that in humans approximatly 200-300 mg in a day of cholesterol may be delivered to the liver by LDF apoA-IV lipoproteins. This represent up to 30% of the flux of cholesterol from slowly exchangeable body pools to the liver (23). The remaining of tissue derived cholesterol is trasported by HDL. In human plasma, however, HDL cholesteryl esters is partly transferred to both LDL and VLDL through the action of CETP (24). Thus cholesterol of tissue origin may ultimately reach the liver through uptake of these larger lipoproteins. This appears a less efficient route in reverse cholesterol transport as both VLDL and LDL may be catabolized also by extrahepatic tissues.

The liver site

There is no doubt that the liver is capable of major uptake of the lipoproteins carrying tissue derived cholesterol (25-27). There is also general agreement that liver express a number of binding site dedicated to uptake of these lipoproteins. These binding sites appears distributed on parenchymal as well as on non-parenchymal cells, including endothelial cells and Kupffer macrophage-type cells (28). Using synthetic apoA-I and apoA-IV phospholipid complexes it has been shown that both apolipoprotein may serve as molecular determinats for binding, although, as with fibroblasts, apoA-IV mediated binding appears more specific than that mediated by apoA-I (29). We found by ligand blot analysis that a microsomal membrane of 95,000 MW recognizes apoA-IV and apoA-I (30). This may be the plasma membrane protein specifically responsible for binding at the liver cells surface of the reverse cholesterol transport carriers. ApoA-IV and apoA-I share important structural similarities and this may be responsible for recognition by an identical cell surface binding protein (31). Elevated binding specificity of apoA-IV as opposite to that of apoA-I appears to have consequences for internalization of the associated lipids. Dvorin et al (31) found that rate of internalization of fluorescinated phospholipids complexed with apoA-IV far exceeds rate of internalization of the same when complexed with apoA-I, suggesting that apoA-IV is of significant importance for HDL lipid or more generally, peripheral tissue derived cholesterol uptake by the liver.

A mechanism whereby either HDL cholesteryl esters are selectively taken up by the liver or there is some apolipoprotein sparing, would be consistent with the kinetic evidence that there is dissimilarity between rate of uptake of HDL apolipoprotein and cholesteryl esters (25). Hepatic lipase has been postulated to play a sensitive role in HDL-liver interaction (33). The enzyme il likely located at the blood lining surface of hepatic endotelial cells. According to this hypothesis, the action of hepatic lipase on HDL would result in liver uptake of both unesterified and esterified cholesterol when surface phospholipids are hydrolyzed and lipoprotein surface shrink. Apolipoproteins may be lost during the process and return to circulation as regenerated reverse cholesterol transport acceptors. Evidence has been gathered that a retroendocytotic mechanism, i.e. involving whole lipoprotein particle uptake followed by cellular estrusion, may be of significance in HDL-liver interactions. Data in support of this idea are mainly derived from studies with macrophages (34). If HDL are in fact taken up by the liver in this way, may discarge cholesterol when inside the hepatocyte, but apolipoprotein moiety will be spared from degradation and return to circulation. Finally there is the possibility that only a specific subfraction of HDL is internalized and catabolized by the liver. HDL are indeed a mixture of heterogeneous lipoprotein populations with distinct metabolism and possibly physiological significance (35). Proof that there is preferential catabolism of specific HDL subfractions has been given showing that when HDL apoA-I and apoA-IV are individually radiolabeled, their catabolic rate is different (7,22). In addition, apoA-IV is preferentially catabolized by the liver, whereas apoA-I is mainly cleared by the kidney (19). In rat plasma an HDL subfraction enriched in apoA-IV has been isolated (5). The same subfraction may be present in human plasma (7). If HDL containing apoA-IV are preferentially taken up by the liver, one would see disparities in the disappearance of HDL cholesteryl ester and apoA-I.

Conclusions

Reverse cholesterol transport system appears much more complex than was initially realized. The number of potential acceptors/carriers of extrahepatic cholesterol circulating in plasma has increased beyond that was initially thought as new apolipoprotein entities have been discovered. In particular lipoproteins containing apoA-IV appear to play a major role, not only because this apolipoprotein mimic virtually all of the biological activities of apoA-I - once belived to be the only apolipoprotein involved in reverse cholesterol transport - but in fact its involvment in the process seems more specific. ApoA-IV is present in large amount in peripheral lymph lipoproteins and its concentration raises unlike that of apoA-I, following challange with a cholesterol enriched diet. Furthermore apoA-IV appears to be specifically recognized by both peripheral and hepatic cells, and cell recognition occurs at higher specificity than that for apoA-I. In many ways apoA-IV epitetomizes the ideal reverse cholesterol transport carrier. Small apoA-IV-phospholipid complexes circulating in plasma LDF may enter peripheral lymph and by interacting specifically with a cell surface binding site, induce net cholesterol efflux from extrahepatic tissues. The unesterified cholesterol-rich apoA-IV lipoprotein may exit the interstitium and become substrate for LCAT. The now cholesteryl esters-rich lipoproteins are then rapidly catabolized by the liver through a specific binding process. At present different data support this view. Yet further studies are needed to evaluate the significance of the apoA-IV-mediated process in the economy of whole body reverse cholesterol transport.

REFERENCES

1) Glomset J.A.: (1968) J. Lipid Res. 9:155-167

2) St. Clair R.W., and Leight, M.A.: (1983) J. Lipid Res. 24:183-193

3) Lefevre, M., and Roheim, P.S.: (1984) J. Lipid Res. 25:1603-1610

4) Otha T., Fidge N.H., and Nestel P.J.: (1984) J. Biol. Chem. 259:14888-14893

5) Dallinga-Thie G.M., Groot P.H.E., and van Tol A.: (1985) J. Lipid Res. 26:970-976

6) Fielding C.J., and Moser K.: (1982) J. Biol. Chem. 257:10955-10960

7) Ghiselli G., Krishnan S., Beigel Y., and Gotto A.M. jr.:

(1986) J. Lipid Res. 27:813-827

8) Stein O., Stein Y., Lefevre M., and Roheim P.S.: (1986) Biochim. Biophys. Acta 878:7-13

9) Bates S.R., and Rothblat G.H.: (1974) Biochim. Biophys. Acta 531:233-249

10) Stein O.J., Vanderhoek J., and Stein Y.: (1976) Biochim. Biophys. Acta 431:347-357

11) Oram J.F., Albers J.J., Cheung M.C., and Bierman E.L.: (1981) J. Biol. Chem. 256:8348-8356

12) Francone O.L., Gurakar A., and Fielding C.: (1989) J. Biol. Chem. 264:7066-7072

13) Sloop, C.H., Dory L., and Roheim P.S.: (1987) J. Lipid Res. 28:225-236

14) Sloop C.H., Dory L., Hamilton R., Krause B.R., and Roheim P.S.: (1983) J. Lipid Res. 24:1429-1440

15) Sloop C.H., Dory L., Krause B.R., Castle C., and Roheim P.S.: (1983) Atherosclerosis 49:9-21

16) Reichl D., Myant N.B., Rudra D.N., and Pflug J.J.: (1984) Atherosclerosis 53:297-308

17) Rothblat G.H., and Phillips M.C.: (1982) J. Biol. Chem. 257:4775-4782

18) Graham D.L., and Oram J.F.: (1987) J. Biol. Chem. 262:7439-7442

19) Ghiselli G., Crump W.L. III, Musanti R., Sherrill B.C., and Gotto A.M. jr.: Biochim. Biophys. Acta: in press

20) Fielding C.J., and Fielding P.E.: (1981) Proc. Natl. Acad. Sci. USA 78:3911-3914

21) Norum K.R., Berg T., Helgerud P., and Drevon C.A.: (1983) Physiol. Rev. 63:1343-1419

22) Pitas R.E., Innerarity T.L., and Mahley R.W.: (1980) J. Biol. Chem. 255:5454-5460

23) Lieberman S., and Samuel P.: (1982) In: Lipoprotein Kinetic and Modeling, Berman M., Grundy S.M., and Howard B.V., eds; Academic Press, N.Y., pp 332-336

24) Barter P.J., and Jones M.E.: (1980) J. Lipid Res.

21:238-249

25) Arbeeny C.M., Rifici A.V., and Eder H.A.: (1987) Biochim. Biophys. Acta 917:9-17

26) Sigurdsson G., Noel S.P., and Havel R.J.: (1979) J. Lipid Res. 20:316-324

27) Rinninger F., and Pittman R.C.: (1989) J. Biol. Chem. 264:6111-6118

28) van Berkel T.J.C., and van Tol A.: (1978) Biochim. Biophys. Acta 530:299-304

29) Ghiselli G., Crump, W.L.-III, and Gotto, M.A. jr.: (1986) Biochim. Biophys. Res. Comm. 139:122-128

30) Ghiselli G., Crump W.L. III., Musanti R., and Gotto A.M. jr.: Submitted for publication

31) Boguski M.S., Elshourbagy N.A., Taylor M.S., and Gordon J.L.: (1984) Proc. Natl. Acad. Sci. USA 81:5021-5025

32) Dvorin, E., Gorder, N.L., Benson, D.M., and Gotto, A.M., jr.: (1986) J. Biol. Chem. 261:15714-15718

33) Bamberger M., Lund-Katz S., Phillips M.C., and Rothblat G.H.: (1985) Biochemistry 24:3693-3701

34) Schmitz G., Robenek H., and Assmann G.: (1987) Atherosclerosis Rev. 16:95-107

35) Eisenberg S.: (1984) J. Lipid Res. 25:1017-1058

39
Regulation of hepatic lipoprotein biosynthesis by hormones

W. PATSCH, W. STROBL, N. GORDER, Y.C. LIN-LEE, A.M. GOTTO Jr. and J.R. PATSCH

Baylor College of Medicine, Mail Station A-601, 6565 Fannin, Houston, TX 77030, USA

ABSTRACT. To identify key regulatory processes of hepatic lipoprotein production, we studied the effects of hormonal perturbations on lipoprotein biosynthesis in the rat. Insulin administration to cultured hepatocytes inhibits the secretion of triglycerides, and apolipoproteins B and E, but does not alter secretory rates of apoproteins A-I and C-III. Net synthesis of apoB and E is not reduced by the hormone, but the rate of transport of apoB from the endoplasmic reticulum to the Golgi is diminished, and the association of apoB with triglyceride declines, resulting in reduced formation of nascent VLDL. Thus, intracellular transport of individual apoproteins is a specific process that can be selectively regulated by physiologic stimuli and that can affect net hepatic lipoprotein production. Thyroid hormones enhance hepatic net production of apoA-I in the rat. Twenty minutes after injection of a receptor saturating dose of T_3 into euthyroid rats, apoA-I gene transcription increases, reaches a maximum of 179% of control at 3.5 hours, and remains elevated for 48 hours. Levels of nuclear and cytoplasmic apoA-I mRNA increase at 1 hour and 2 hours, respectively, and exceed the levels expected from enhanced transcription more than twofold at 24 h. Daily administration of 35 ug T_3/100 g body weight s.c. for 1 week increases the abundance of nuclear and cytoplasmic apoA-I mRNA more than threefold, but reduces the transcription of the apoA-I gene to 42% of control injected animals. Thus, thyorid hormone rapidly stimulates apoA-I gene transcription, but posttranscriptional events enhancing the stability of nuclear apoA-I RNA contribute to the acute effect of T_3 on apoA-I mRNA levels. In chronic hyperthyroidism, stabilization of nuclear apoA-I RNA precursors is the principal mechanism for enhanced apoA-I gene expression and may cause feedback inhibition of apoA-I gene transcription. Our studies also imply that in euthyroid rats the majority of nuclear apoA-I mRNA precursors is degraded.

1. Introduction

Knowledge of the mechanisms determining hepatic lipoprotein biosynthesis is essential to our understanding of plasma lipoprotein transport. To identify rate limiting steps in the biosynthetic pathway of lipoproteins, we have used hormonal perturbations known or suspected to alter net hepatic lipoprotein production. We studied the effect of acute insulin administration in primary rat hepatocyte cultures. When compared to in vivo studies, this model system affords the advantage of determining effects of insulin without ambiguities caused by counterregulatory hormones or metabolites (1). We found that insulin acutely inhibits the secretion of triglycerides, apoB and apoE. While synthesis of apoB is not altered by the hormone, transport of apoB from the ER to the Golgi is reduced and the formation of nascent VLDL in the early secretory pathway is inhibited. Thyroid hormones have profound effects on hepatic lipid metabolism in that they increase fatty acid synthesis, fatty acid oxidation, and ketogenesis (2) . In rats, hepatic production of apoA-I and abundance of apoA-I mRNA abundance increases as a result of T_3 administration (3,4). To gain insight into the mechanism whereby T_3 stimulates apoA-I biosynthesis, we measured the effect of T_3 on apoA-I gene transcription rates and the abundance of nuclear and total cellular apoA-I mRNA abundance in rat liver. After a single receptor saturating dose of T_3, we found a rapid increase in apoA-I gene transcription followed by stabilization of nuclear apoA-I RNA precursors. In chronic hyperthyroidism, the stabilization of nuclear apoA-I RNA is maintained, while apoA-I transcription declines, perhaps, as a result of feedback inhibition.

2. Methods

Adult male Sprague-Dawley rats weighing 200-300 g were housed in a room with a 12-h light cycle. Hepatocyte cultures were prepared as described (1,5). ApoB, apoE, and apoA-I in media, cell homogenates, and subcellular fractions were determined by RIA (1,6). For pulse-chase labeling experiments, cultures were washed with leucine-free media prior to labeling with 1.0 mCi (4,5-^{3}H)-leucine in 2 ml leucine-free media for 5 min. Chase-medium contained 25 ug/ml leucine. Immunoprecipitation of labeled apoproteins A-I, B, E, and albumin in media and cell homogenates was performed with monospecific antisera in the presence of Triton X-100 (1%, g/v), desoxycholate (1%, g/v), benzamidine (1 mM), PMSF (0.3 mM) and leucine (5 mM). Immunoprecipitates were collected after the addition of protein A sepharose. Specificity of precipitation was established by using excess cold antigen. Immunoprecipitates were subjected to SDS gel electrophoresis (7). Radioactivity in gels was visualized by fluorography and quantified by counting the appropriate gel slices in a liquid scintillation counter. In subcellular fractionation experiments, a microsomal fraction was prepared by differential ultracentrifugation. The pellet containing the microsomes was suspended in 55% (w/w) sucrose and was overlayed in a SW40 centrifuge tube with 1.0 ml of 40%, 2.0 ml of 37.5% and 35%, and 1.5 ml of 30%, 25% and 20% sucrose solutions containing 1mM EDTA, 1 mM TrisHCL, pH 8.0. The gradient was spun at 32 000 rpm for 12 hours. One ml fractions were collected from the top of the tubes and membranes were pelleted by ultracentrifugation after dilution with 2 ml of 1 mM EDTA, 1 mM TrisHCl, pH 8.0. Pellets were resuspended in phosphate buffered saline, pH 7.6, containing 1% Triton X-100, homogenized by ultrasonication, and subjected to immunoprecipitation. Activities of glucose-6 phosphatase and galactosyltransferase were measured as marker enzymes (8,9).

To study effects of thyroid hormones on hepatic apoprotein biosynthesis, rats were injected with T_3, which was dissolved in 0.15 M NaCl, pH 11. Rats serving as injection controls received the alkaline saline only. Hypothyroidism was induced by feeding rat chow containing 0.1% propylthiouracil. T_3 was measured by radioimmunoassay. Total RNA was extracted from liver tissue by the guanidine hydrochloride method (10). The abundance of apoA-I, apoE, and albumin mRNA was determined by quantitative slot blotting (10). Northern transfer of RNA was performed according to Thomas (11). Liver cell nuclei were prepared by the method of Northeman (12). The DNA content in nuclei was measured fluorimetrically using salmon sperm DNA as a standard (13). Cell-free transcription was performed by the method of Birch et al. (14) as previously described (15). Under our conditions, transcription was DNA dependent, and 55% of total transcription was due to RNA polymerase II activity (15). The newly synthesized ^{32}P labeled transcripts were quantified by dot blot hybridization to an excess of plasmid containing apoA-I, apoE, or albumin cDNA inserts. Nonrecombinant plasmids were immobilized on nitrocellulose membranes to determine nonspecific hybridization. Hybridization efficiency was determined by using ^{3}H-labeled cRNAs, which were synthesized from the cDNA templates using DNA dependent RNA polymerase (16). Transcription rates are expressed in parts per million (ppm) and were calculated as described (15). Nuclear RNA was extracted by the method of Lamers et al. (17) and analyzed by Northern blotting and soft laser densitometry of autoradiograms.

3. Results and Discussion

3.1. Effect of Insulin on Hepatic Lipoprotein Biosynthesis

We have previously found that insulin administered to hepatocyte cultures inhibits the secretion of triglyceride, apoB and apoE (1). This inhibitory effect of the hormone was dose-dependent. The hormone did not alter the secretion of apoA-I, apoC-III and albumin. Cellular levels of apoB and apoE did not decrease. As a result, fractional accumulation rates of apoB and apoE, defined as apoprotein accumulation in media/hour/cellular apoprotein, declined from 0.15 + 0.04 to 0.08 + 0.03 and 0.37 + 0.13 to 0.20 + 0.05, respectively (mean

+ SD, $p < 0.01$, insulin vs. control). This suggested that the major effect of the hormone on net production of apoB and apoE was on cellular transport or secretion of these apoproteins rather than on synthesis of the proteins. In subsequent studies, we showed that the inhibitory effect of insulin on lipoprotein component secretion was mediated by the hormonal receptor on the cell surface (18). This conclusion was based on three lines of evidence: i) the activity of insulin analogs to inhibit lipoprotein component secretion was correlated with receptor affinity, ii) anti-insulin receptor IgG which inhibited binding of insulin mimicked the inhibitory effect of the hormone, and iii) reduction of surface receptor number was followed by reduced activity of insulin.

To validate the data of hormonal inhibilion which were based on measurements of apoprotein concentration in media and cellular homogenates by radioimmunoassay, apoproteins were immunoprecipitated after pulse chase labeling of cultures. Experimental cultures were exposed to insulin (800 uU/ml) for 4 h prior to pulse labeling for 5 minutes with tritiated leucine. Ten minutes after the chase with leucine-rich media, culture media and cellular homogenates were immunoprecipitated. At this time point, virtually no labeled apoproteins were found in media. In control cell homogenates, the percentage of total cellular radioactivity associated with apoB-48, apoE and apoA-I was 0.35, 1.10 and 0.18, respectively. The corresponding values in experimental cultures were similar (0.33, 1.15, and 0.2). Thus, insulin did not reduce the synthesis of any of the apoproteins studied. When immunoprecipitation was performed 90 min after the chase, the fraction of total radioactivity associated with apoB-100 and apoB-48 declined. In control cells, the ratio of media to cellular radioactivity was 0.88, 0.90, 1.15, and 1.54 for apoB-100, apoB-48, apoE and apoA-I, respectively. In insulinized cultures, these ratios decreased to 0,70, 0.66, and 0.85 for apoB-100, apoB-48, and apoE, respectively ($p < 0.05$). No change was observed for apoA-I. These results are consistent with the RIA data and indicate that insulin did not alter synthesis, but cellular transport and/or secretion (19). To distuingish between these possibilities, the distribution of newly synthesized apoproteins was determined in the secretory apparatus of control and insulinzed hepatocytes 90 minutes after pulse labeling. When compared with control cells, the proportion of tritiated apoB associated with fractions representing the rough endoplasmic reticulum was increased in insulinzed cells. This was a consistent finding in 3 separate experiments. Our studies suggest that the transport of apoB from the ER to the Golgi was decreased and that a fraction of apoB was degraded prior to reaching the Golgi. Thus, insulin may alter the early posttranslational processing of apoB which may be required for effective assembly of nascent VLDL in the ER. Alternatively, the hormone may affect the partitioning of triglyceride in the ER and reduce the amount of triglyceride available for interaction with apoB. Reduced association of apoB with triglycerides could result in decreased transport from the ER to the Golgi, since hydrophobic core lipids may be required for apoB to become competent for transport.

3.2. Effect of Thyroid Hormones on Apoprotein Gene Expression

To study the short term effect of thyroid hormones on hepatic apoprotein gene expression, we injected a single receptor saturating dose of 3 mg T_3/100 g body weight i.p. into euthyroid rats and followed the time course of gene transcription and abundance of nuclear and total cellular mRNA of apoA-I. ApoA-I mRNA synthesis, as determined by nuclear run-on assays, increased to 139% of controls at 20 min after T_3 injection, the earliest timepoint studied ($p < 0.05$), rose to 179% of controls at 3.5 hours, and remained significantly elevated for 48 h. At least three RNA species hybridized with the apoA-I cDNA on Northern blots of nuclear RNA. The rapid stimulation of apoA-I gene transcription was followed by an accumulation of the putative nuclear apoA-I mRNA precursors beginning 1 hour after the injection. The levels of nuclear apoA-I RNA continued to increase to 292% of control values at 24 h, even though apoA-I gene transcription had reached a plateu at 150-160% of control 6 h after the injection. No change in the proportions of nuclear apoA-I mRNA precursors was noted. Total cellular apoA-I mRNA was increased 2 hours after the injection and continued to rise to 298% of control levels at 24 hours. Transcription of the apoE gene was transiently increased to 153% of control at 20 min only, but then returned to baseline levels. The levels of nuclear apoE mRNA precursors increased 2 fold by 2 h after T_3 administration, but decreased thereafter to baseline levels. Total cellular mRNA abundance remained unaltered. Albumin gene transcription declined sharply to 15% of control 1 h after T_3, remained below baseline for 6 h, but returned to baseline at 24 h. The decreased rate of albumin mRNA synthesis was associated with a transient fall in nuclear and total cellular RNA. Control experiments showed that no such changes were observed by i.p. injection of the solvent only.

To determine the effect of chronic hyperthyroidism on apoA-I gene expression, euthyroid rats were injected daily with 35 ug T_3/100 g body weight for 7 days. This regimen increased plasma levels of T_3 and apoA-I to 430% and 184% of control, respectively. Total hepatocyte liver mRNA and nuclear apoA-I RNA increased to 286% and 278% of control, while transcription of the apoA-I gene was decreased to 42% of control ($p < 0.01$). No consistent effects on synthesis or abundance of apoE or albumin mRNA were observed in these rats (20).

These studies show that thyroid hormones rapidly induce transcription from the apoA-I gene. Increased transcription is the principal mechanism, whereby thyroid hormones enhance the expression of a number of genes (21). Transcriptional activation of the growth hormone gene may result from the binding of the nuclear T_3 receptor complex to cis acting sequences in the 5'flanking region of the gene (22). Such thyroid hormone responsive elements have been identified in transfection studies (23). The cis- and trans-acting elements involved in the expression of the rat apoA-I gene are incompletely understood, and thyroid hormone responsive elements have not been identified. However, the increase in transcriptional activity alone can not explain the increase of nuclear and total cellular apoA-I mRNA at 24 hours after hormone injection. Stabilization of nuclear apoA-I mRNA as suggested for the S14 gene transcripts (24) has to be implicated to explain our observations. Such stabilization may involve protection from or decreased activity of ribonucleases. Editing of ApoA-I gene transcripts could also play a role in stabilizing apoA-I mRNA precursors. There is precedence for such a hypothesis as thyroid hormones have been shown to increase apoB-48 production at the expense of apoB-100 by promoting the posttranscriptional insertion of a stop codon into apoB transcripts (25). In the chronic hyperthyroid rat, the enhanced apoA-I gene expression is solely due to posttranscriptional events because levels of nuclear apoA-I mRNA precursors remained threefold elevated, but transcriptional activity was decreased. The inverse relationship between apoA-I gene transcription and abundance of nuclear and cytoplasmic apoA-I mRNA is consistent with feedback inhibition of transcription. Studies of the molecular mechanisms explaining this scenario should enhance our knowledge of how eucaryotic gene expression can be regulated.

4. Acknowledgements

This work was supported by NIH Grant R01 HL 34457 and a fellowship (W.S.) made available through the Max Kade Foundation, Inc., New York.

5. References

1. Patsch, W., Franz, S., and Schonfeld, G. (1983) 'Role of insulin in lipoprotein secretion by cultured rat hepatocytes', J. Clin. Invest. 71, 1161 - 1174.
2. Heimberg, M., Olubadewo, J.O., and Wilcox, H.G. (1985) 'Plasma lipoproteins and regulation of hepatic metabolism of fatty acids in altered thyroid states', Endocrine Reviews 6, 590 - 607.
3. Wilcox, H.G., Keyes, W.G., Hale, T.A., Frank, R., Morgan, D.W., and Heimberg, M. (1982) 'Effects of triiodothyronine and propylthiouracil on plasma lipoproteins in male rats', J. Lipid Res. 23, 1159 - 1166.
4. Apostolopoulos, J.J., Howlett, G.J., and Fidge, N. (1987) 'Effects of dietary cholesterol and hypothyroidism on rat apolipoprotein YRNA metabolism', J. Lipid Res. 28, 642 - 648.
5. Yedgar, S., Weinstein, D.B., Patsch, W., Schonfeld, G., Casanada, F.E., and Steinberg, D. (1982) 'Viscosity of culture media as a regulator of synthesis and secretion of very low density lipoproteins by cultured hepatocytes', J. Biol. Chem. 257, 2188 - 2192.
6. Patsch, W., Tamai, T., and Schonfeld, G. (1983) 'Effect of fatty acids on lipid and apoprotein secretion and association in hepatocyte cultures', J. Clin. Invest. 72, 371 - 378.
7. Weber, K., and Osborn, M. (1969) 'The reliability of molecular weight determinations by dodecyl sulfate-polyacrylamide gel electrophoresis', J. Biol. Chem. 244, 4406 - 4412.

8. Rothman, J.E., and Fries, E. (1981) 'Transport of newly synthesized vesicular stomatitis viral glycoprotein to purified Golgi membranes', J. Cell Biol. 89, 162 - 168.
9. Aronson, N.N., Jr., and Touster, O. (1974) 'Isolation of rat liver plasma membrane fragments in isotonic sucrose', Methods Enzymol. 31,90 - 102.
10. Lin-Lee, Y.C., Kao, F.T., Cheung, P., and Chan, L. (1985) 'Apolipoprotein E gene mapping and expression: localization of the structural gene to human chromosome 19 and expression of apoE mRA in lipoprotein and non-lipoprotein-producing tissues', Biochemistry 24, 3751 - 3756.
11. Thomas, P. (1980) 'Hybridization of denatured RNA and small DNA fragments transferred to nitrocellulose', Proc. Natl. Acad. Sci. USA 77, 5201 - 5205.
12. Northemann, W., Heisig, M., Kunz, D., and Heinrich, P.C. (1985) 'Molecular cloning of cDNA sequences for rat $alpha_2$-macroglobulin and measurement of its transcription during experimental inflammation', J. Biol. Chem. 260, 6200 - 6205.
13. Kapuscinski, J., and Skoczylas, B. (1977) 'Simple and rapid fluorimetric method for DNA microassay', Anal. Biochem. 83, 252 - 257.
14. Birch, H.E., and Schreiber, G. (1986) 'Transcriptional regulation of plasma protein synthesis during inflammation', J. Biol. Chem. 261, 8077 - 8080.
15. Strobl, W., Gorder, N.L., Fienup, G.A., Lin-Lee, Y.C., Gotto, A.M., Jr., and Patsch, W. (1989) 'Effect of sucrose diet on apolipoprotein biosynthesis in rat liver: increase in apolipoprotein E gene transcription', J. Biol. Chem. 264, 1190 - 1194.
16. Roop, d.R., Nordstrom, J.L., Tsai, S., Tsai, M.J., and O'Malley, B.W. (1978) 'Transcription of structural and intervening sequences in the ovalbumin gene and identification of potential ovalbumin mRNA precursors. Cell 15, 671 - 685.
17. Lamers, W.H., Hanson, R.W., and Meisner, H.M. (1982) 'cAMP stimulates transcription of the gene for cytosolic phosphoenolpyruvate corboxykinase in rat liver nuclei', Proc. Natl. Acad. Sci. USA 79, 5137 - 5141.
18. Patsch, W., Gotto, A.M., Jr., and Patsch, J.R. (1986) 'Effects of insulin on lipoprotein secretion in rat hepatocyte cultures: the role of the insulin receptor', J. Biol. Chem. 261, 9603 - 9606.
19. Patsch, W., Lin-Lee, Y.C., Gotto, A.M., Jr., and Patsch, J.R. (1986) 'Hepatic lipoprotein biogenesis: the role of intracellular apolipoprotein transport', Arteriosclerosis 6, 536a.
20. Strobl, W., Gorder, N., Lin-Lee, Y.C., Fienup, G., Gotto, A.M., Jr., and Patsch, W. (1989) 'The role of thyroid hormone in hepatic Apolipoprotein A-I gene expression in the rat' Clin. Res. 37, 300a.
21. Samuels, H.H., Forman, B.M., Horowitz, Z.D., and Ye, Z.-S. (1988) 'Regulation of gene expression by thyroid hormone', J. Clin. Invest. 81, 957 - 967.
22. Nyborg, J.K., Nguyen, A.P., and Spindler, S.R. (1984)

'Relationship between thyroid and glucocorticoid hormone receptor occupancy, growth hormone gene transcription, and mRNA accumulation' J. Biol. Chem. 259, 12377 - 12381.

23. Glass, C.K., Franco, R., Weinberger, C., Albert, V., Evans, R., and Rosenfeld, M.G. (1987) 'A c-erb-A binding site in rat growth hormone gene mediates trans-activation by thyroid hormone. Nature 329, 738 - 741.
24. Narayan, P., and Towle, H.C. (1985) 'Stabilization of a specific nuclear mRNA precursor by thyroid hormone' Mol. Cell. Biol. 5, 2642 - 2646.
25. Davidson, N.O., Powell, L.M., Wallis, S.C., and Scott, J. (1988) 'Thyroid hormone modulates the introduction of a stop codon in rat liver apolipoprotein B messenger RNA' J. Biol. Chem. 263, 13482 - 13485.

40
Postprandial lipemia in patients with coronary artery disease

J.R. PATSCH, Th. HOPFERWIESER, W. PATSCH, H. DREXEL, V. MÜHLBERGER, E. KNAPP and H. BRAUNSTEINER

Department of Medicine, University of Innsbruck, Anichstrasse 35, 6020 Innsbruck, Austria

ABSTRACT. Conventional lipid parameters and the magnitude of postprandial lipemia following a standardized oral fat load were determined in 93 male patients, who underwent coronary arteriography and had fasting plasma triglyceride levels of less than 250 mg/dl. Compared were individuals with severe coronary artery disease (CAD) with controls. The subjects were divided into those with LDL-cholesterol below 175 mg/dl (group I) and those with LDL-cholesterol levels of over 175 mg/dl (group II). In the group I subjects fasting triglycerides and HDL_2 cholesterol were higher and lower, respectively, than in controls ($p = 0.02$). The magnitude of postprandial lipemia was higher in CAD cases than in controls ($p = 0.009$).

In group II neither conventional lipid parameters discriminated between cases and controls nor did the magnitude of postprandial lipemia. In individuals with normal LDL-cholesterol levels the fat load test discriminated between CAD cases and controls and added discriminative power.

1. INTRODUCTION

Plasma triglycerides have been associated with coronary artery disease (CAD) risk in several studies by univariate analysis (1-4) but in studies using multivariate analysis, triglycerides tend to lose their role as independent risk factor (5-8). This is caused chiefly by the fact that triglycerides are canceled out by HDL-cholesterol. HDL-cholesterol is an extremly powerful risk factor for CAD (9-11) and the magnitude of the negative association between HDL-cholesterol and CAD has been found to be at least as large as that of all other known risk factors for CAD (12). The mechanisms that underlie the negative association between HDL-cholesterol and CAD are not known. One possibility is the major role that HDL plays in reverse cholesterol transport (13). However, there exists no evidence to indicate that high HDL-cholesterol levels indeed reflect a very active reverse cholesterol transport conferring protection from CAD.

An alternative hypothesis regarding the role of HDL in CAD is based on the negative association between the levels of HDL-cholesterol and triglycerides (14,15). This association becomes even more pronounced when HDL levels, particularily these of HDL_2, are correlated with postprandial triglyceride levels (15, 16, 17). As mentioned above triglycerides are also a risk factor for CAD but in multivariate analyses, they are usually eliminated by HDL. This is not very surprising because the triglyceride levels show a greater variability so that single measurements appear not to be very reliable. At the contrary, HDL are quite constant so that single measurements are much more reliable than those of triglycerides.

The mechanisms by which the metabolisms of triglycerides and HDL are related are reasonably wellunderstood (18 - 21). Lipolysis of chylomicrons and VLDL provides surface components such as phospholipids, apolipoproteins and unesterified cholesterol which - with the help of lecithin: cholesterol acyltransferase (LCAT) - will lead to the formation of HDL-cholesteryl ester-rich HDL_2.

The cholesteryl esters transported by HDL can be transferred - with the help of lipidtransfer proteins (LTP) (22) - to apoB-containing lipoproteins such as chylomicrons and VLDL. The transfer of cholesteryl esters from HDL_2 to chylomicrons and VLDL is accompanied by a reciprocal transfer of triglycerides into HDL (19). The triglyceride-rich HDL fractions loose their triglycerides by the action of hepatic lipase under formation of triglyceride-depleted small HDL particles (19, 20).

A metabolic state where chylomicrons and VLDL are effectively lipolysed will provide a large supply of surface components allowing formation of the larger HDL_2. Effective chylomicron lipolysis will also prohibit chylomicron accumulation so that no triglyceride-rich HDL can be formed and thus, no HDL_2 is catabolized to HDL_3 by hepatic lipase.

The intimate relationship of the metabolism of chylomicrons and HDL and the demonstrated importance of chylomicron metabolism on HDL composition and levels suggest that triglycerides play an important potential role in CAD. The close association of triglycerides with the powerful risk factor HDL strongly suggests that triglycerides are important for the development of CAD in at least one of two ways: they could be atherogenic per se and this atherogenicity could be signaled by low HDL levels or they could be atherogenic by their ability to decrease the levels of the powerful risk factor HDL-cholesterol.

We have reported a strong inverse association between the magnitude of postprandial lipemia and the levels of HDL-cholesterol, particularly HDL_2 (15, 16). Because of this negative association it was resonable to investigate whether triglyceride metabolism as reflected in postprandial lipemia is able to discriminate between patients with CAD and controls; and whether postprandial lipemia can add discriminative power to established risk factors.

2. MATERIAL AND METHODS

2.1. Patients

Included were 93 male patients who underwent coronary arteriography and had fasting plasma triglycerides of less than 250 mg/dl. None of the subjects showed signs of diabetes, liver or kidney disease or thyroid dysfunction.

Coronary angiograms were taken at different projections according to the technique described by Judkins (23). Extent of CAD was estimated by visual interpretation of coronary cinearteriograms and based on reduction in luminal diameter as judged in multiple projections. Three angiographic patterns of dominance were recognized: right, left and balanced, depending on wether a posterior branch arose from the right coronary artery, the left circumflex artery, or both, respectively. Each coronary system was subdivided into 16 segments according to the pattern of dominance. Coronary score was obtained as the grand total of 16 scores each of which was derived by multiplying the score for a particular site with the degree of stenosis (24). As cases we selected patients with a CS of 50 and as controls we used individuals with a CS of 0.

The study subjects were subdivided on the basis of their LDL-cholesterol levels in a group with LDL-cholesterol below 175mg/dl (group I) and one with LDL-cholesterol over 175mg/dl (group II).

2.2. Analytical Procedures

Cholesterol, Triglycerides, HDL_2 and HDL_3-cholesterol, apolipoproteins A-I, A-II and B were quantified as described previously (15, 16). A standardized fatty meal as described previously was administered after a 14 hour overnight fast and blood samples were obtained for triglyceride analysis at 0, 2, 4, 6, and 8 hours, respectively (15).

3. RESULTS AND DISCUSSION

Group I (LDL-cholesterol below 175 mg/dl) consisted of 38 subjects, 13 cases and 25 controls. Group II (LDL-cholesterol over 175 mg/dl) consisted of 55 subjects, 38 cases and 17 controls. The distribution of cases and controls over these two groups clearly indicates that LDL-cholesterol was an important risk factor in our 93 subjects. Table 1 illustrates age and conventional lipid parameters in group I. Triglyceride concentrations were obtained on two occasions. Cases differed from controls in their fasting triglyceride levels (obtained at the first occasion) and their HDL_2-cholesterol levels. However, fasting TG-levels obtained on the second occasion failed to discriminate between cases and controls. The bottom line of Table 1 illustrates postprandial lipemia. The magnitude of postprandial lipemia was clearly and significantly larger in cases when compared to controls. Among all the parameters listed in Table1, postprandial lipemia discriminated strongest between cases and controls.

TABLE 1. Lipid parameters of cases and controls from Group I (LDL-Chol < 175)

	Cases (n=13) mean (SD)	Controls (n=25) mean (SD)	p
Age	56 (5)	51 (9)	N.S.
Cholesterol	228 (19)	218 (29)	N.S.
Triglycerides	129 (58)	90 (43)	.02
Triglycerides	129 (58)	98 (52)	N.S.
HDL-Cholesterol	47 (15)	56 (15)	N.S.
HDL2-Cholesterol	14 (6)	22 (12)	.02
HDL3-Cholesterol	34 (11)	33 (8)	N.S.
Apo A-I	136 (20)	143 (31)	N.S.
Apo A-II	47 (11)	41 (12)	N.S.
Apo B	82 (12)	74 (15)	N.S.
Postprandial Lipemia	981 (639)	531 (351)	.009

Table 2 gives an evaluation of postprandial triglyceride levels and their ability to discriminate between cases and controls. The first line gives the area under the triglyceride curve. Under the area are listed the fasting triglyceride levels followed by those obtained at 0, 2, 4, 6 and 8 hours after ingestion of the fatty test meal. While early time points are not useful for discrimination, later time points are: beginning with 6 hours postprandially, single triglyceride levels become discriminative with some of them equally powerful to the area under the triglyceride curve.

TABLE 2. Comparison of area under triglyceride curve with single triglyceride values between 0 and 8 hours after ingestion of test meal in group I subjects

	Triglycerides (mg/dl)		
Hour	Cases	Controls	p
Area	981	534	.009
0	129	98	.124
0	129	90	.021
2	173	157	.601
2-0	32	53	.277
4	308	231	.158
4-0	157	124	.413
6	350	201	.011
6-0	219	101	.008
8	234	130	.036
8-0	104	31	.045
(6+8):2	292	165	.014
(6+8):2-0	161	67	.010

The data presented in Table 2 suggest that late single triglyceride values in the course of the fat loading test may be equal or even superior to the area under the entire triglyceride curve in discriminating between cases and controls. Hence, the practicability of the fat load test may be greatly enhanced in that only one or two postprandial blood specimens per fat load test may be needed.

TABLE 3. Lipid parameters of cases and controls from Group II (LDL-Chol > 175)

	Cases (n=38)	Controls (n=17)	p
Age	54 (5)	52 (8)	N.S.
Cholesterol	283 (21)	293 (24)	N.S.
Triglycerides	133 (63)	132 (45)	N.S.
Triglycerides	133 (48)	132 (51)	N.S.
HDL-Cholesterol	45 (16)	48 (17)	N.S.
HDL_2-Cholesterol	13 (5)	14 (7)	N.S.
HDL_3-Cholesterol	32 (10)	36 (12)	N.S.
Apo A-I	130 (19)	131 (26)	N.S.
Apo A-II	45 (9)	45 (13)	N.S.
Apo B	101 (14)	101 (15)	N.S.
Postprandial Lipemia	971 (707)	780 (401)	N.S.

Table 3 illustrates lipid parameters of cases and controls in group II. In this group, cases and controls were not distinguished by any of the conventional lipid parameters; nor were they distinguished by the magnitude of postprandial lipemia (last line, Table 3).

Table 4 lists various fat load markers for group II. The area under the triglyceride curve did not discriminate between cases and controls but some single triglyceride values did. The triglyceride increase over the fasting value at 2 hours was lower in cases than in controls. At later postprandial time-points, however, triglyceride values were again higher in cases than they were in controls. Thus, for group II, some single time-points exhibited greater sensitivity in distinguishing cases from controls than the entire area under the triglycerid curve.

TABLE 4. Comparisons of various fat load markers

Group II (LDL-cholesterol > 175 mg/dl)
Triglycerides during Fat Load Test (mg/dl)

Hour	Cases	Controls	p
Area	971	780	.305
0	133	132	.909
0	133	132	.921
2	184	227	.058
2-0	50	95	.013
4	294	306	.750
4-0	161	175	.643
6	313	240	.118
6-0	180	109	.068
8	245	157	.072
8-0	112	25	.038
(6+8):2	279	198	.083
(6+8):2-0	146	67	.042

We conclude that the fat load test 1) discriminated between CAD cases and controls and 2) adds discriminative power were LDL-cholesterol levels are normal. With elevated LDL-cholesterol levels, the power of the fat load test is considerably weaker but some discrimination is maintained. Our results suggest that in the future some form an oral fat challenge may provide a useful tool to asses CAD risk.

REFERENCES

1.) Carlson, L.A., Böttiger, L.E. and Ahfeldt, P.E. (1979) "Risk factors for myocardial infarction in the Stockholm prospective study: a 14-year follow-up focussing on the role of plasma triglycerides and cholesterol", Acta Med Scand 206(5), 351-360.
2.) Brown, D.F. (1969) "Blood lipids and lipoproteins in atherogenesis", Am J Med 46(5), 691-704.
3.) Brunner, D., Altmann, S., Loebl K., et al (1977) "Serum cholesterol and triglycerides in patients suffering from ischemic heart disease and in healthy subjects", Atherosclerosis 28(2), 197-204.
4.) Carlson, L.A., Böttiger, L.E. (1972) "Ischemic heart disease in relationship to testing values of plasma triglycerides and cholesterol", Lancet 1, 865-868.
5.) Hulley, S.B., Rosenmann, R.H., Bawol, R.D., et al (1980) "Epidemiology as a guide to clinical decisions: the association between triglyceride and coronary heart disease" N Engl J Med 302(25), 1383-1389.
6.) Heyden, S., Heiss, G., Hames, C.G., et al (1980) "Fasting triglycerides as predictors of total and CHD mortality in Evans County, Georgia" J Chronic Dis 33(5), 275-282.
7.) Castelli, W.P., Doyle, J.T., Gordon, T., et al (1977) "HDL cholesterol and other lipids in coronary heart disease: the cooperative lipoprotein phenotyping study" Circulation 55(5), 767-772.
8.) Lewis, B., Chait, A., Oakley, C.M., et al (1974) "Serum lipoprotein abnormalities in patients with ischemic heart disease: comparisons with a control population" Brit Med J 3(5929), 489-493.
9.) Rhoads, G.G., Gulbrandsen, G.L. and Kagan, A. (1976) "Serum lipoproteins and coronary heart disease in a population study of Hawaii Japanese men" N Engl J Med 294, 293-298.
10.) Gordon, T., Castelli, W.P., Hjortland, M.C., Kannel, W.B. and Dawber, T.R. (1977) "High density lipoprotein as a protective factor against coronary heart disease" Am J Med 62, 707-714.
11.) Berg, K., Borresen, A.L. and Dahlen, G. (1976) "Serum-high-density-lipoprotein and atherosclerotic heart-disease" Lancet I, 499-501.
12.) Tyroler, H.A. (1980) "Epidemiology of plasma high-density lipoprotein cholesterol levels" Circulation 62(supplIV), IV-1-IV-3.
13.) Glomset, J.A. (1968) "The plasma lecithin: cholesterol acyl transferase reaction", J Lipid Res 9, 155
14.) Miller, G.J. and Miller, N.E. (1975) "Plasma-high-density lipoprotein concentration and development of ischaemic heart disease", Lancet i, 16-19.
15.) Patsch, J.R., Karlin, J.B., Scott, L.W. and Gotto, A.M., Jr (1983) "Inverse relationship between blood levels of high density lipoprotein subfraction 2 and magnitude of postprandial lipemia" Proc Natl Acad Sci (USA) 80, 1449-1435.
16.) Patsch, J.R., Prasad, S., Gotto, A.M., Jr. and Patsch, W (1987) " High Density Lipoprotein 2: Relationship of the Plasma Levels of this Lipoprotein Species to its Composition, to the

Magnitude of Postprandial Lipemia and to the Activities of Lipoprotein Lipase and Hepatic Lipase" J Clin Invest 80, 341-347.

17) Weintraub, M.S., Eisenberg, S. and Breslow, J.L. (1987) "Different patterns of postprandial lipoprotein metabolism in normals, type IIa, type III, and type IV hyperlipoproteinaemic individuals. Effect of treatment with cholestyramine and gemfibrozil" J Clin Invest 79, 1110-1119.

18.) Patsch, J.R., Gotto, A.M., Jr, Olivecrona, T., and Eisenberg, S. (1978) "Formation of high density lipoprotein2-like particles during lipolysis of very low density lipoproteins in vitro" Proc Natl Sci USA 75, 4519-4523.

19.) Patsch, J.R., Prasad, S., Gotto, A.M., Jr. and Bengtsson-Olivecrona (1984) "Postprandial Lipemia: A Key for the Conversion of HDL2 into HDL3 by Hepatic Lipase" J Clin Invest 74, 2017-2023.

20) Eisenberg, S. (1984) "High density lipoprotein metabolism" J Lipid Res 25, 1017-1058.

21.) Patsch, J.R., Gotto, A.M., Jr. (1987) "Metabolism of high density lipoproteins" Elsevier Science Publishers B.V., 221-259.

22.) Tall, A.R. (1986) "Plasma Lipid Transfer Proteins" J Lipid Res 27, 361-367.

23.) Judkins, M.P. (1967) "Selective coronary angiography, Part I: percutaneous transfemoral approach" Radiology 89, 815-819.

24.) Kaltenbach, M. (1980) "Röntgenanatomie und Nomenklatur, Quantifizierung und Dokumentation koronarangiographischer Befunde" in M. Kaltenbach, H. Roskam (eds.), vom Belastungs-EKG zur Koronarangiographie, Springer Verlag, Berlin

41
Lipid transport between plasma lipoproteins and cells: physicochemical regulation of lipid transfer rates and the secretion of very low density lipoproteins

H.J. POWNALL, R. HOMAN and J.B. MASSEY

Division of Atherosclerosis and Lipoprotein Research, Baylor College of Medicine and The Methodist Hospital, 6565 Fannin Street, MS A-601, Houston, TX 77030, USA

ABSTRACT. The transport of fatty acid has been studied *in vitro* and in cultured cells. The kinetics of transfer of fatty acids from albumin or lipid-protein complexes are dependent upon the chain length and unsaturation. The transport and metabolism of oleic and eicosapentaenoic acid (EPA) in HepG2 cells were compared. Equivalent fatty acid uptake and triglyceride (TG) formation were observed, but the formation of phospholipids from EPA was lower. Since it is known that phosphatidylcholine (PC) synthesis is obligatory for TG secretion, it is proposed that the inhibition of very low density lipoprotein secretion by EPA is linked to lower PC production.

Introduction

The plasma compartment contains a variety of lipid surfaces that may be divided among those that compose the plasma lipoproteins and those that form the plasma membranes of cells that are within or surround the plasma compartment. The destinations and the rates of transport of the molecules that are associated with albumin and plasma lipoproteins are a function of the microscopic character of each molecule and the more global behavior of the particle with which they are associated. This may be exemplified by the transport of fatty acids between albumin and cell membranes occurring on the time scale of seconds, whereas the lifetime of albumin in the plasma compartment is on the order of 10 days (Cohen et al., 1961). Similarly, the rate of removal of low density lipoproteins from plasma is about 0.5 per day (Berman et al., 1978), whereas the rates of transfer of cholesterol and many of the phospholipids by spontaneous or protein-mediated pathways are about 1 per hr (Phillips et al., 1987).

Two general pathways for the removal of the various components of mature lipoproteins from the plasma compartment can be cited. One of these is the receptor or non-receptor-mediated endocytosis of the entire lipoprotein particle by cells that line the vascular compartment; the other is the rate-limiting desorption of the sparingly-soluble components of lipoproteins into the surrounding aqueous compartment followed by diffusion-controlled insertion into the plasma membranes of cells. Hepatocytes are thought to be important in both processes and both the fate and the regulatory effect of molecules that enter cells by either of these routes remain important areas of research.

Recently, we have been interested in the transport of phospholipids and fatty acids among cell membranes and lipoproteins and the metabolic consequences of n-3 fatty acids on the production of glycerol lipids and very low density lipoproteins. Our recent research has focused on 1] in vitro fluorescence methods to quantify the kinetics of transport of fatty acids and phospholipids among albumin and model lipoproteins, 2] development of a quantitative model for prediction of lipid transfer rates, and 3] identification of the mechanism by which n-3 fatty acids inhibit the secretion of very low density lipoproteins.

Materials and Methods

Model reassembled lipoproteins were prepared according to the detergent removal method of Matz and Jonas (1982). Single bilayer vesicles of 1-palmitoyl-2-oleoyl phosphatidylcholine (POPC) were produced by ultrasonic irradiation. ApoA-I was isolated as previously described (Brewer et al., 1986). The kinetics of phospholipid transfer from reassembled high density lipoproteins to low density lipoproteins were performed according to the method of Ellsworth et al. (1982). The kinetics of fatty acid transfer were monitored according to the changes in the fluorescence of anthroyloxy-labeled albumin that are attendant to the binding of fatty acids. Fatty acid transfer to HepG2 cells was performed with radiolabeled glycerol or fatty acid precursors using standard tissue culture methods. Labeled lipids were quantified by high performance liquid chromatography (Homan and Pownall, 1989).

Results and Discussion

SPONTANEOUS LIPID TRANSFER

The rates of transfer of a number of physiologically important free fatty acids from various lipid and protein donors have been measured *in vitro*. These are summarized in Table 1, which shows that as the chain length of the fatty acid is increased, the rate of transfer decreases by a factor of about 20 for each methylene unit that is added. Similarly, the addition of each double bond to a fatty acid of a given chain length increases its transfer rate by a factor of 5. The rates of transfer of fatty acids from an albumin analog and from single bilayer vesicles of POPC are similar and can be predicted by the equation, $\log k_i = 0.55m - 0.57n + 10.26$, where k_i is the rate constant (sec^{-1}), and n and m are the number of carbons and double bonds in the acyl chain. The transfer of lysolecithin is slightly faster than that of the corresponding fatty acid.

TABLE 1. Summary of Kinetic Data for the Spontaneous Transfer of Fatty Acids and Lysolecithin*

Fatty acid	Donor	k, (30 deg, sec^{-1})	$t_{1/2}$, sec
Palmitic acid	POPC-SBV	17	0.04
	an-albumin	2.9	0.24
Stearic acid	POPC-SBV	0.78	0.90
	an-albumin	0.22	3.2
Behenic	POPC-SBV	0.0063	108.
Oleic acid	POPC-SBV	5.0	0.14
Lysopalmitoyl PC	POPC-SBV	20.	0.035

*POPC-SBV, single bilayer vesicles of POPC; An-albumin, anthraniloyl human serum albumin.

Table 2 contains similar data for the transfer of a homologous series of PCs between high density lipoproteins and acceptors that were composed of low density lipoproteins. Qualitatively, the effects of double bonds and chain length on the rates of transfer are similar to those observed with the fatty acids. Closer inspection, however, reveals that the contribution of each of these to the rates of transfer are substantially different. The contribution of chain length increment and the number of double bonds to the transfer rates of PCs is much smaller than that observed for the fatty acids. This is reflected in the equation derived from these data; i. e. $\log k_i = 5.52 + 0.19m - 0.23n$. Incremental changes in the rates of transfer of PCs are less than that of fatty acids as a function of the change in the number of double bonds or methylene units is that some of the hydrophobic surface area of the fatty acyl chains in the diacyl compounds such as PCs is shielded by the adjacent acyl chain so that neither of them express their full hydrophobic effect. It is interesting that the rates of transfer of PCs that contain very bulky fatty acyl chains do not fit this equation. We interpret this as being due to the extra bulk that is introduced by the extra kinks due to the double bonds.

TABLE 2. Rate Constants for the Spontaneous Transfer of PCs from Reassembled High Density Lipoproteins to Human Low Density Lipoproteins at 37 deg C

Lipid	k, (hr^{-1})
1-lauroyl-2-oleoyl PC	3.46
1-myristoyl-2-oleoyl PC	1.19
1-palmitoyl-2-oleoyl PC	0.41
1-palmitoyl-2-stearoyl PC	0.27
1-palmitoyl-2-linolenoyl PC	0.63
1-palmitoyl-2-linolenoyl PC	0.99
1-palmitoyl-2-eicosapentaenoyl PC	0.80
1-palmitoyl-2-docasahexaenoyl PC	0.42

FLUORESCENT LIPID TRANSFER AND METABOLISM

We have also measured the rates of transfer of fluorescent analogs of fatty acids and other lipids and identified a number of these that are good physiological analogs of natural lipids. The criteria for the selection of fluorescent fatty acids were that they 1] transferred from serum albumin to cells in culture (HepG2 and 3T3L1 adipocytes) at the same rates as some of the native fatty acids, 2], entered the same cellular pathways with rates that were similar to those of natural fatty acids, and 3] have absorption and emission properties that make them readily detectable by fluorescence methods with little or no photo-bleaching. Two fluorescent fatty acids satisfied these criteria were 8(pyrenyl) octanoic acid and 12(pyrenyl) dodecanoic acid; although these were the only pyrenyl fatty acids that we tested, we assume that similar homologues that have chain lengths between 8 and 12 are also suitable. Table 3 compares the rates of transfer of some pyrene-labeled fatty acids with those of some native lipids that are found in plasma; these data show that some of the pyrene-labeled lipids have spontaneous transfer rates that are similar to those of some of the native lipids.

Table 3 Spontaneous Transfer Rates of Pyrene-labeled Lipids

Transferred Lipid	Donor	k (30 deg)
12(pyrenyl)dodecanoic acid	POPC-SBV	0.22 sec^{-1}
	albumin	1.1 sec^{-1}
1-palmitoyl-2[9(1-pyrenyl)] nonanoyl PC	POPC-SBV	0.2 hr^{-1}
pyrene labeled cholesterol	POPC-SBV	0.4 min^{-1}

METABOLISM OF EICOSAPENTAENOIC ACID (EPA) IN HEPG2 CELLS

The cellular uptake and metabolism of oleic acid (OA) and EPA were compared in the hepatoma cell line, HepG2. The rates of entry of these two fatty acids into the cells were similar and they were saturable at about 0.3 mM (Figure 1 - Total). Using a high performance liquid chromatograph equipped with a radiolabel detector, the formation of glycerol lipids as a function of the dose of each fatty acid was followed by the incorporation of [^{3}H]glycerol. Similar amounts of TG were formed with both fatty acids; however, the amount of diglyceride (DG) that was formed from OA was much lower than that found with EPA and the formation of phosphatidylethanolamine (PE) and PC was much lower when OA was replaced by EPA in the incubation medium (Figure 1 - TG, DG, PE, PC). These results are consistent with a model of EPA metabolism in which the conversion of DGs that contain EPA to PE and PC is inhibited relative to that observed with OA.

The morphology of the HepG2 cells after incubation with OA and EPA and fixation with formaldehyde was inspected by digital imaging microscopy using differential interference contrast optics and fluorescence optics following the addition of the neutral lipid stain, Nile Red. Both techniques revealed that the appearance of the TG-rich particles formed by EPA was distinct from that found with OA incubations. In the former case the number of inclusions is smaller but their dimensions are much greater. This difference may be connected to the observation that there is less PC available to form the surface monolayer that surrounds inclusions of neutral lipids and keeps them dispersed in an aqueous environment.

These data are relevant to observations that have been made in cultured hepatocytes and in human subjects where addition of EPA to the culture medium or the diet, respectively, decreases the secretion of very low density lipoproteins. It has been reported in a number of laboratories that PC synthesis is obligatory to the secretion of very low density lipoproteins (Janero and Lane, 1983; Vance and Vance, 1985; Higgins and Fieldsend, 1987). Thus, the relative inhibition of PC synthesis by EPA affects an essential step in the assembly or secretion of very low density lipoproteins. The mechanism for this inhibition remains a matter of conjecture. PC synthesis may facilitate the translocation of apoB-100 from the cytoplasmic face of the endoplasmic reticulum to the lumen; PC might exert a detergent effect that solubilizes apoB-100 as it is transferred from the endoplasmic reticulum to the preformed TG-rich particle in the lumen of the endoplasmic reticulum; alternatively, PC might be needed to fill the space on the inner and outer leaflet of the endoplasmic reticulum that is vacated as it moves from its site of synthesis to the mature very low density lipoprotein particle. These hypotheses are now under investigation in our laboratory.

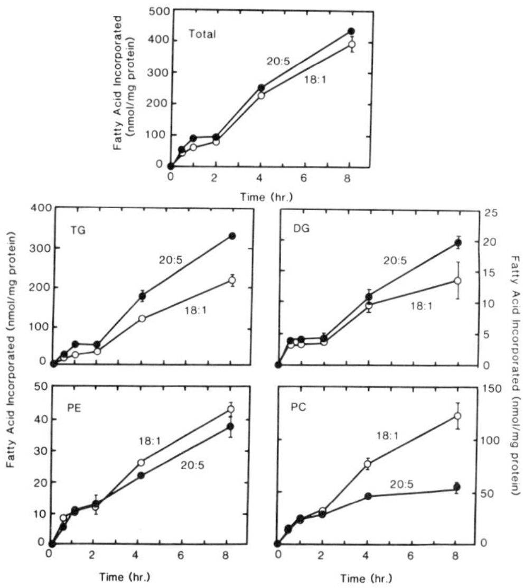

Figure 1: Effect of OA and EPA concentrations on the incorporation of [^{3}H]glycerol into cellular glycerolipids. HepG2 cells were incubated for 4 hr. in serum-free media containing [^{3}H]glycerol, and various concentrations of OA or EPA as shown. The fatty acids were complexed to albumin with 0.2 moles of fatty acid/mole of albumin. The bars represent the SEM except when it is less than the symbol size and none is shown.

References

Berman, M., Hall, M., Levy, R.J., Eisenberg, S., Bilheimer, D.W., Phair, R.D., and Goebel, R.H. (1978) "Metabolism of apoB and apoC lipoproteins in man", J. Lipid Res. 19, 38-56.

Brewer, H.B., Ronan, R., Meng, M., and Bishop, C. (1986) "Isolation and characterization of apolipoproteins A-I, A-II and A-IV", in Methods in Enzymology (J.P. Segrest and J.J. Albers, Eds.), Vol. 128, pp. 223-246.

Cohen, S., Freeman, T., McFarlane, A.S (1961) "Metabolism of 131-I labeled human albumin", Clin. Sci. 20, 161-1709.

Higgins, J.A., and Fieldsend, J.K. (1987) "Phosphatidylcholine synthesis for incorporation into membranes or for secretion as plasma lipoproteins by Golgi membranes of rat liver", J. Lipid Res. 28, 268-278.

Homan, R., and Pownall, H.J. (1989) "High performance liquid chromatographic analysis of acylated lipids containing pyrene fatty acids", Anal. Biochemistry 178, 166-171.

Janero, D.R., and Lane, M.D. (1983) "Sequential assembly of very low density lipoprotein apolipoproteins , triacylglycerol, and phosphoglycerides by the intact liver cell", 258, 14496-14504.

Matz, C.E., and Jonas, A. (1982) "Micellar complexes of human apolipoprotein A-I with phosphatidylcholines and cholesterol prepared from cholate-lipid dispersions", J. Biol. Chem. 257, 4546-4552.

Phillips, M.C., Johnson, W.J., and Rothblat, G.H. (1987) "Mechanisms and consequences of cellular cholesterol exchange and transfer," Biochim. Biophys. Acta 906, 223-276.

Vance, J.E., and Vance, D.E. (1985) "The role of phosphatidylcholine biosynthesis in the secretion of lipoproteins by hepatocytes", Can. J. Biochem. 63, 870-881.

THROMBOSIS AND ATHEROSCLEROSIS: CLINICAL INSIGHTS

42
Hypercholesterolemia and haemostatic function changes

A. STRANO, G. DAVÌ* and A. NOTARBARTOLO**

*Patologia Medica, II Università di Roma,*Ematologia, Università de Chieti,*
****Patologia Medica II, Università di Palermo, Italy*

PLATELET ACTIVATION AND LIPOPROTEINS

Patients with hypercholesterolemia have elevated levels of LDL and reduced plasma concentration of HDL.
Platelet activity in these subjects is also elevated and this is evident with regard to platelet adhesion, aggregation and serotonine release, plasma concentration of factor 4 and betathromboglobulin, availability of platelet factor 3, reduced life span and increased platelet turnover, increased circulating platelet aggregates and reduced whole blood bleeding time (1-5). Moreover, platelets from hypercholesterolemic patients give rise to increased formation of thromboxane (Tx) A_2 as well as to decreased sensitivity to PGI_2 (6,7).
Activation of the coagulation mechanism has also been noted (8,9).

The lipoproteins and platelets are important constituents of the blood that influence the atherosclerotic process. One accepted theory today regarding the pathogenesis of atherosclerosis is that of endothelial injury, which promotes local platelet activity, lipid accumulation and especially cholesterol accumulation at the site of the injury, which is thought to be mediated through the phagocytic action of adjacent macrophages (10). Endothelial injury, from wathever cause, results in platelets adhering to the area of denuded endothelium, having been attracted by the exposure of subendothelial collagen fibrils. Platelet adhesion could be accompanied by platelet activation. Many metabolically active substances are secreted during the activation process. Platelet-derived growth factor stimulates the proliferation of medial smooth muscle cells and promotes their invasion of the endothelial intima (11). Activated platelets have also been shown to release cholesterol which is taken up by smooth muscle cells and macrophages (12).
In hypercholesterolemic patients platelet-lipoprotein interactions are

associated with and possibly responsible for accelerating the atherosclerosis process. In fact, the development of the atherosclerotic lesion is affected by mitogens derived from platelets, macrophages and endothelium and by plasma lipids, which can generate such lesions and induce endothelial injury.

The observed changes in platelet activity in hypercholesterolemic patients are paralleled by the observation of raised levels of cholesterol and phospholipids in the platelets of these patients (13). This could be a result of membrane abnormality originating from the megakaryocyte in the bone marrow during platelet formation (14) or a consequence of the platelet-plasma lipoprotein interaction. Platelets have indeed been shown to possess specific LDL-receptors (15). The specificity of the LDL-binding sites is supported by the fact that both radioactively labeled and unlabeled lipoproteins interact with the platelets with the same apparent affinity. HDL has also been found to bind to the platelets (15). The binding of LDL and HDL was found to be independent of the state of platelet activation and was saturable. On incubating washed platelets with LDL, an increase in platelet cholesterol content is observed (16). Similarly, incubation of platelets with cholesterol-rich liposomes also results in an increase in platelet cholesterol (17). Fatty acid content of the platelet membrane qualitatively parallels that of the lipoprotein and a distinctly positive correlation has been found between cholesterol concentration as well as between the cholesterol:phospholipid ratio in the platelets and in LDL. Because of the inability of the platelets to take up cholesterol esters from the plasma lipoproteins, platelet-plasma interaction is limited to cholesterol exchange (18). The changes in the platelet membrane lipids and its fluidity appear in large measure to determine platelet responsiveness, since platelet activation is a membrane-associated phenomenon.

Incubation of physiologic concentrations of lipoproteins with platelets has been found to influence platelet function. Both LDL and VLDL result in enhanced platelet activation whereas HDL has the opposite effect (19). LDL results in increased in vitro platelet aggregation in response to ADP, epinephrine, collagen thrombin,and arachidonic acid and increased serotonin release in response to these aggregating agents, as well as in increased synthesis of TxA_2 (20).

The mechanisms underlying the observed effects of lipoproteins on platelet sensitivity to aggregating agents are not completely clear. The transfer of cholesterol and phospholipids from lipoprotein to platelet membrane could lead to changes in membrane fluidity and alterations in enzyme activity, such as that of adenylate cyclase (21). An increase in platelet cholesterol content has been described as resulting in enhanced activation of the arachidonate pathway (22). Platelet phospholipid uptake provides the precursors necessary for the synthesis of both platelet factors 3 and 4, which are important in the coagulation process. We have also to notice that VLDL and LDL obtained from hypercholeste rolemic patients enhanced platelet aggregation (23). Normal platelets incubated with hypercholesterolemic patient's plasma showed increased in vitro platelet aggregation and release as compared to the effects resulting from incubation of these same platelets with normolipidemic plasma (3). Conversely, incubation of platelets obtained from hypercholesterolemic subjects with normolipidemic plasma resulted in inhibition of the sensitivity of these platelets. The enhanced platelet sensitivity observed in the hypercholesterolemic patients remains even after removal of the platelets'plasma environment, such as after isolating the platelets by wshing procedures. This may suggest a defect in the mega karyocyte (14), but it does not exclude that plasma cholesterol affects platelet cholesterol content directly. The high cholesterol:protein ratio in the LDL and VLDL derived from hypercholesterolemic patients could contribute to the effect of the lipoproteins on platelet function. The quantitative composition of the apoproteins, such as the increased concentrations of apo C-III in the patients'VLDL as well as the high concentrations of apo B in both LDL and VLDL, may also be relevant (23).

It has recently been suggested that oxidatively modified lipoproteins circulating in plasma could contribute to atherosclerosis by promoting platelet reactions (24). As a result of increased lipid oxidation or a deficiency of pharmacological free radical scavengers such as vitamin E, LDLmay become oxidized during its circulation in plasma, causing it to became reactive to platelets. Although the functional implications of this are unclear, it could play an important role in modulating membrane receptors and other reactions important in platelet activation, including phosphatidylinositol turnover.

LIPID-LOWERING TREATMENT AND PLATELET FUNCTION

A real important question is if any therapeutic reduction in cholesterol levels is able to reduce platelet activity in hypercholesteromic patients.

Patients with IIa hyperlipoproteinemia have notable alterations in platelet lipid composition, with higher amounts of cholesterol and phospholipids (25). Cholesterol content and cholesterol/phospholipid molar ratio are important determinants of lipid membrane fluidity and their increase can reduce fluidity of cell membranes so affecting membrane-associated enzymes and receptors. Moreover platelets with higher cholesterol content are more sensitive to activating stimuli, with consequent enhanced aggregability, and produce increased amounts of TxA_2 (25). It has also been demonstrated an increase of arachidonate utilization by platelets via the lipoxygenase pathway (26), with augmented 12-Hete formation. Formation of lipoxygenase products contribute to the platelet hyperaggregability which is associated with the hyperlipidemic state (26).

Intralipid (solution containing soybean oil rich in linoleic acid, egg yolk lecithin and glycerol) infusion into humans caused reduction in platelet cholesterol content and elevation in platelet triglyceride and phospholipid; these changes were associated with reduced platelet aggregation in vitro (27). The reduction in platelet cholesterol content may result from net transfer of platelet membrane cholesterol to the lipid emulsion. The pattern of the changes in platelet free cholesterol content during and after the infusion followed that of platelet aggregation (27), suggesting that these two processes were associated.

Patients with homozygous familial hypercholesterolemia are often treated with plasmapheresis. As a consequence of this form of treatment, a fall in plasma cholesterol concentrations and a parallel drop in platelet activity has been demonstrated (28).

Recently, we have shown that administration of simvastatin (29) markedly reduced platelet aggregation and thromboxane formation induced by collagen and arachidonate in type IIa hypercholesterolemia. Maximum response was achieved at 4-8 weeks whereas lipid lowering effects were seen at 2 weeks. This finding seems to demonstrate that platelet changes cannot be explained by a direct effect of simvastatin on platelets, and that the antiplatelet response may therefore depend on platelet membrane lipid composition changes, particularly in the platelet cholesterol content of platelet membranes, following substantial reductions of total plasma cholesterol and LDL-cholesterol.

It has, also, been shown that cholestyramine treatment does not modify platelet hyperactivity and enhanced Tx formation, despite a 21% reduction in total plasma and LDL-cholesterol (30). Neverthless, cholestyramine treatment normalized platelet reactivity to prostacyclin (30).

The effect of simvastatin treatment on platelet reactivity and thromboxane synthesis may be explained by different changes induced on the lipid composition (phospholipid distribution and fatty acid patterns of individual glycerophospholipids) and cholesterol levels, total and individual phospholipid classes and arachidonate of platelet membranes from hypercholesterolemic subjects.

Therefore, we can conclude assuming that consistent reductions in LDL-cholesterol could induce a decrease in platelet hyperactivity and platelet eicosanoids production. These changes may play a role in the evolution of vascular diseases, particularly coronary heart disease, in hypercholesterolemic subjects.

REFERENCES

1. Carvalho A.C.A., Colman R.W., Lees R.S. (1974) 'Platelet function in hyperlipoproteinemia', N Engl J Med 290,434-437.
2. Colman R.W. (1978) 'Platelet function in hyperbetalipoproteinemia', Thromb Haemost 39,284-293.
3. Aviram M., Brook J.G. (1982) 'The effect of human plasma on platelet function in familial hypercholesterolemia', Thromb Res 26,101-109.
4. Corash L., Anderson J., Poindexter B.J. et al. (1981) 'Platelet function and survival in patients with severe hypercholesterolemia', Arteriosclerosis 1,443-448.
5. Tremoli E., Maderna P., Sirtori M. et al. (1979) 'Platelet aggregation and malondialdehyde formation in type IIa hypercholesterolemic patients', Haemostasis 8, 47-53.
6. Tremoli E., Folco G., Agardi E. et al. (1977) 'Platelet thromboxane and serum cholesterol', Lancet 1, 107 (letter).
7. Strano A., Davì G., Averna M. et al. (1982) 'Platelet sensitivity to prostacyclin and thromboxane production in hyperlipoproteinemia' Thromb Haemost 48,18-20.
8. Nordoy A., Brox J.H., Halme S. et al. (1983) 'Platelets and coagulation in patients with familial hypercholesterolemia' Acta Med Scand 213,129-135.
9. Shastri K.N., Carvalho A.C.A., Lees R.S. (1980) 'Platelet function and platelet lipid composition in the dyslipoproteinemias' J Lip Res 21,467-472.
10. Steinberg D. (1983) 'Lipoproteins and atherosclerosis: A look back and a look ahead' Arteriosclerosis 3, 283-301.
11. Raines E.W., Ross R. (1982) ' Platelet-derived growth factor' J Biol Chem 257, 5154-5176.

12. Kruth H.S. (1985) ' Platelet-mediated cholesterol accumulation in cultured aortic smooth muscle cells',Science 227,1243-1245.

13. Carvalho A.C.A., Lees R.S. (1980) ' Platelet intravascular coagulation and fibrinolysis in hyperlipidemias',Acta Med Scand 642, 101-112 (suppl.2).

14. Schick B.P., Schick P.K. (1985) ' The effect of hypercholesterolemia on guinea pig platelets , erythrocytes and megakaryocytes' Biochim Biophys Acta 833,291-302.

15. Aviram M., Brook J.G. (1983) 'Platelet interaction with high- and low-density lipoproteins' Atherosclerosis, 46, 259-268.

16. Aviram M., Brook J.G. (1981) 'Lipoprotein-platelet interaction: Effect on platelet cholesterol content and platelet function' Thromb Haemost 46,195 (abstr).

17. Shattil S.J., Anaya-Galindo R., Bennett J. et al. (1975) 'Platelet hypersensitivity induced by cholesterol incorporation' J Clin Invest 55,636-643.

18. Schick B.P., Schick P.K. (1985) 'Cholesterol exchange in platelets, erythrocytes and megakaryocytes', Biochim Biophys Acta 833,281-290.

19. Aviram M., Brook J.C. (1983) 'Characterization of the effect of plasma lipoprotein on platelet function in vitro', Haemostasis 13, 344-350.

20. Aviram M., Sirtori C.R., Colli S. et al. (1985) 'Plasma lipoproteins affect platelet malondialdehyde and thromboxane B_2 production', Biochem Med 34,29-36.

21. Ghiselli C., Sirtori C.R., Nicosia S. (1981) 'Effect of serum lipoproteins on adenylate cyclase activity of rat liver membranes' Biochem J 196,899-902.

22. Stuart M.J., Gerrard J.M., White J.G. (1980) 'Effect of cholesterol on production of thromboxane B_2 by platelets in vitro',N Engl J Med 302,610.

23. Viener A., Aviram M., Brook J.G. (1984) 'Abnormal plasma lipoprotein composition in hypercholesterolemic patients induces platelet activation', Eur J Clin Invest 14,207-213.

24. Ardlie N.G., Selley M.L., Simons L.A. (1989) 'Platelet activation by oxidatively modified low density lipoproteins',Atherosclerosis 76,117-124.

25. Prisco D.,Rogasi P.G., Paniccia R. et al. (1988) 'Altered lipid composition and thromboxane A_2 formation in platelets from patients affected by IIa hyperlipoproteinemia', Thromb Res 50,593-604.

26. Eynard A.R., Tremoli E., Caruso D. et al. (1985) ' Platelet formation of 12 Hete and Thromboxane B_2 is increased in type IIa hypercholesterolemic subjects', Atherosclerosis 60,61-66.

27. Aviram M., Deckelbaum R.J. (1989) 'Intralipid infusion into humans reduces in vitro platelet aggregation and alters platelet lipid composition', Metabolism 38,343-347.

28. Aviram M., Brook G. (1987) 'Platelet activation by plasma lipoproteins', Progress in Cardiovascular Diseases 30,61-72.

29. Davì G., Averna M., Novo S. et al. (1989) 'Effects of synvinolin on platelet aggregation and thromboxane B_2 synthesis in type IIa hypercholesterolemic patients' Atherosclerosis 79,79-83.

30. Löbel P.,Steinhagen-Thiesseu E., Scrör K. (1988) 'Cholestiramine treatment of type IIa hypercholesterolemia normalizes platelet reactivity against prostacyclin' Eur J Clin Invest 18,256-260.

43
Predictive value of fibrinogen in arterial thrombosis

P.M. MANNUCCI and D. MARI

Institute of Internal Medicine, A. Bianchi Bonomi Hemophilia and Thrombosis Center, University of Milan, Italy

ABSTRACT. In five large-scale prospective studies the predictive value of hemostasis parameters indicating the occurence of arterial thrombotic disease has been estimated in healthy individuals. Four studies have consistently found a statistically significant positive association between fibrinogen levels and arterial thrombotic disease. This relationship was closer than that for plasma cholesterol, indicating the important pathogenetic role played by alterations of the clotting system in arterial thrombotic disease.

After the successful identification of hypercholesterolemia as a risk factor for atherosclerosis, in the last few years epidemiologists have addressed attention to the problem of the predictive value of coagulation tests in arterial thrombotic diseases. In order to define a relationship of cause and effect between a laboratory test and a clinical event, several requirements must be fulfilled. First, there must be a statistically significant correlation between the clinical event and the alterations of the laboratory test. However, the existence of such a correlation is not sufficient to prove a relationship of cause and effect and to ascribe a predictive value to the laboratory test. It is also necessary to meet the following requirements:

a. adequate chronologic sequence (the alterations of the laboratory test should precede the clinical event);
b. presence of a biological gradient (the greater the alterations of the laboratory test, the more frequent the clinical event);
c. biological plausibility;
d. confirmation from intervention studies (pharmacological or

dietary interventions should favourably affect both the laboratory test and the clinical event).

This paper will review how epidemiological studies have first suggested the existence of a relationship between a plasma clotting factor (i.e., fibrinogen) and other well established risk factors for arterial thrombotic disease, and how prospective studies have subsequently demonstrated the predictive value of fibrinogen.

EPIDEMIOLOGICAL STUDIES

General epidemiological features of fibrinogen indicate that increased plasma levels of this clotting factor may play a role in the pathogenesis of arterial thrombotic diseases. Diabetes mellitus, obesity and age are associate with both increased risk of arterial thrombosis and increased plasma levels of fibrinogen(8). The relative risk of myocardial infarction or cerebral stroke increases with the estrogen dosage in women taking oral contraceptives (9); a very similar relationship also exists between estrogen dosage and plasma levels of fibrinogen (10). Recent studies show that hepatitis B surface antigen (HBsAg) carriers, who are at lower risk of cardiovascular mortality than the general population, have decreased plasma levels of fibrinogen (13). A trend towards rising fibrinogen levels associated with rising mortality rate is generally, although not consistently, seen in countries where arterial thrombotic diseases are endemic (14). Plasma fibrinogen levels are higher in smokers than in non-smokers(1). This would suggest that hyperfibrinogenemia is one of the possible mechanisms by which smoking increases the risk of arterial thrombotic diseases. When related to arterial thrombotic diseases, the interaction between age and fibrinogen is very similar to that between age and smoking (3).

PROSPECTIVE STUDIES

These preliminary data have led to the organization of large-scale prospective studies in order to evaluate whether clotting factors or other hemostatic parameters measured in apparently healthy individuals would predict the subsequent occurrence of arterial thrombotic disease.

Northwick Park Heart Study. Preliminary data of this study were published in 1980 (12) and showed a close relationship between plasma factor VII and fibrinogen levels and mortality rate from cardiovascular disease, chiefly coronary artery disease. The final report of the study confirmed the existence of such association (11). The study was carried out on 1511 white men aged from 40 to 64 years when first recruited, i.e., between 1972 and 1978. The mean duration of the follow-up was 10 years (range 7.3-13.5 years). The following laboratory tests were performed: plasma levels of factors V, VII, VIII, fibrinogen and antithrombin III, platelet count and platelet adhesion to glass bead columns. The end points considered were: total mortality, mortality from ischemic heart disease, nonfatal myocardial infarction and total episodes of ischemic heart disease. The mortality rate from all the causes was associated with higher plasma levels of fibrinogen and factor VII, but not with cholesterol levels or the other hemostatic parameters considered in the study. A statistically significant association between episodes of ischemic heart disease and plasma levels of factor VII and fibrinogen was stronger than for cholesterol levels within 5 years from the recruitment, although the latter relationship was, as expected, also found. Multivariate analysis showed that the increased risk due to factor VII and fibrinogen levels is independent from the influence of other known risk factors such as cholesterol levels, smoking and hypertension.

Hence, the Northwick Park Heart Study shows that:

i. increased plasma levels of fibrinogen (and factor VII) are associated with a risk of increased mortality rate both from all causes and coronary artery disease;
ii. the increased risk is independent from other risk factors;
iii. the increased risk of coronary artery disease due to high fibrinogen levels is greater than that due to hyperchlesterolemia (i.e. 84% against 43%).

Göteborg Study. In 1984 Wilhelmsen et al (19) published the results of a prospective study carried out on 792 men aged 54 years at the time of the recruitment. The study estimated the predictive value of the following hemostatic parameters: prothrombin and proconvertin (P&P) test (a modification of the prothrombin time), plasma fibrinogen, factor VIII and plasminogen as well as fibrinolytic activity on fibrin plates. The end points were represented by mortality rates due to ischemic heart disease, stroke or other causes. The study showed that there was significant association between plasma fibrinogen levels and the incidence of stroke and myocardial infarction. This association remained statistically significant only for stroke when the data were evaluated by multivariate analysis, which took into account the contribution of other risk factors (i.e., hypertension, smoking and hypercholesterolemia). In the case of stroke, the study also showed a synergistic effect between systolic blood pressure and hyperfibrinogenemia. A recent report has followed up this cohort of patients for a mean period of 18.5 years, confirming that increased plasma fibrinogen levels are highly correlated with the risk of stroke, other independent risk factors being increased blood pressure, obese abdomen and maternal history of stroke (18).

Leigh Study. In 1985 Stone and Thorpe (17) found an association between hyperfibrinogenemia and the incidence of coronary artery disease in a group of 297 men aged from 40 to 69 years; such association was stronger than for cholesterolemia, blood pressure or smoking. A synergism between hyperfibrinogenemia and hypertension was also found. Subjects whose plasma fibrinogen levels and systolic blood pressure values were comprised in the top distribution tertile had an incidence of coronary artery disease 12 times more elevated than those whose values fell in the bottom tertile.

Framingham Study. Kannel et al (6) have very recently reported a statistically significant association between hyperfibrinogenemia and incidence of cardiovascular disease in 1315 subjects of both sexes. The impact of fibrinogen level considered as a separate variable on cardiovascular disease was comparable with that of major risk factors such as blood pressure, hematocrit, obesity, cigarette smoking and diabetes mellitus. By multivariate analysis it was seen that fibrinogen level was still significantly and independently related to the incidence of cardiovascular disease in men, while such correlation was poorly significant in women.

Prospective Cardiovascular Münster Study (PROCAM). This study initiated in 1982 with goals similar to those of the Northwick Park Heart Study. The preliminary data from 1,674 of the recruited men (aged between 40 and 65 years) without history of myocardial infarction or stroke at entry were recently presented (2). Subjects who experienced events of coronary artery disease had higher plasma levels of factor VII and fibrinogen than subjects without such events. In subsequent analysis carried out recently in a larger number of individuals followed-up for a longer period, the relationship between high fibrinogen and coronary events reached statistical significance ($p < 0.02$), whereas that between factor VII and events did not hold true(J. van de Loo, personal communication, 1989). Hence, these data strengthen the importance of the predictive role of fibrinogen levels in ischemic heart disease.

In conclusion, five independent predictive studies have found a statistically significant association between hyperfibrinogenemia and arterial thrombotic disease. These data, together with those relative to factor VII from the Northwick Park Heart Study suggest an important pathogenetic role of clotting system alterations in the arterial thrombotic disease of the heart and brain. However, they are not sufficient to prove a relationship of cause and effect, since they only fulfil requirements a (adequate chronologic sequence) and b (presence of a biological gradient) among those listed above.

HYPERCOAGULABILITY AND THROMBOSIS

The next question to answer is that relative to requirement c, i.e., if it is biologically plausible that a relationship of cause and effect exists between high plasma levels of fibrinogen and arterial thrombotic disease. Hyperfibrinogenemia, being fibrinogen an acute-phase protein, may be caused by a wide variety of clinical conditions as well as environmental factors (e.g., smoking) and by genetic factors (5). Whatever its cause, hyperfibrinogenemia may predispose to thrombogenesis for at least four different reasons, i.e.:

i. fibrinogen and fibrin are important constituents of atheromas(16)

ii. in vivo platelet aggregation and blood viscosity are a function of plasma fibrinogen concentration (7, 15, 16);

iii. studies carried out on laboratory animals with experimentally induced thrombosis showed that the amount of fibrin formed in the thrombi is a function of the initial plasma fibrinogen concentration (4).

Thus, the aforementioned data demonstrate that it is biologically plausible that high levels of fibrinogen facilitate the occurrence of arterial thrombotic disease.

INTERVENTION STUDIES

The existence of a relationship of cause and effect between plasma levels of fibrinogen and arterial thrombotic disease needs ultimate confirmation from intervention studies (requirement d), which are not yet available. In theory, the reduction of plasma levels of fibrinogen should determine a reduction of the incidence of thrombotic episodes in at risk subjects. The reduction of plasma levels of fibrinogen seems to be difficult. Dietary modifications are not effective, while lowering effects of drugs or compounds such as stanazolol, ticlopidine pentoxifylline or fish oils need further confirmation.

CONCLUSIONS

The results of recent prospective studies (2,6,11, 17,18,19) ascribe a well defined epidemiological relevance to the concept of hypercoagulability. Increased plasma levels of factor VII and fibrinogen affect the natural history of stroke and coronary artery disease; thus, their measurement should be performed for evaluating the thrombotic risk. Unfortunately, the available methods do not justify their widespread utilization, being still far from adequate standardization. Further efforts in this direction are therefore needed.

REFERENCES

1 Balleisen, L., Bailey, J., Epping, P.H., Schulte, H., van de Loo, J. (1985). 'Epidemiological study on factor VII, factor VIII and fibrinogen in an industrial population. I. Baseline data on the relation to the age, gender, body weight, smoking, alcohol, pill using and menopause', Thrombos Haemost 54, 475.

2 Balleisen, L., Schulte, H., Assmann, G., Eppind, P.H., van de Loo, J. (1987). 'Coagulation factors and the progress of coronary heart disease', Lancet ii, 461.

3 Doll, R., Peto, R. (1976). 'Mortality in relation to smoking: 20 years' observation on male British doctors', Brit Med J ii, 1525.

4 Gurewich, V., Lipinski, B., Hyde E., (1976). 'The effect of the fibrinogen concentration and the leukocyte count on intravascular fibrin deposition from soluble fibrin monomer complexes', Thromb Haemost 36, 605.

5 Humphries, S.E., Cook, M., Dubowitz, M., Stirling, Y., Meade, T.W. (1987). 'Role of genetic variation at the fibrinogen locus in determination of plasma fibrinogen concentration', Lancet i, 1452.

6 Kannel, W.B., Wolf, P.A., Castelli, W.P., D'Agostino, R.B. (1987). 'Fibrinogen and risk of cardiovascular disease. The Framingham Study', J Amer Med Ass 258, 1183.

7 Lowe, G.D.O. (1985). 'Blood rheology in arterial disease', Clin

Sci 68, 419.

8 Meade, T.W. (1984). 'Clotting factors and ischemic heart disease: the epidemiological evidence', In: Meade T.W. (ed):Anticoagulants and myocardial infarction', J Wiley, Chichester p. 91.

9 Meade, T.W., Chakrabarti, R.R., Haines, A.P., North, W.R.S., Stirling, Y. (1977). 'Haemostatic, lipid and blood pressure profiles of women and oral contraceptives containing 30 or 50 ug oestrogens', Lancet ii, 948.

10 Meade, T.W., Greenberg, G., Thompson, S.G. (1980). 'Progestogens and cardiovascular reaction associated with oral contraceptives and a comparison of the safety of 50 and 30 ug oestrogen preparations', Brit Med J i, 157.

11 Meade, T.W., Mellows, S., Brozovic, M., Miller, S.G., Chakrabarti, R.R., North, W.R.S., Haines, A.P., Stirling, Y., Imeson, J.D., Thompson, S.G. (1986). 'Haemostatic function and ischemic heart disease: principal results of the Northwick Park Heart Study', Lancet i, 1050.

12 Meade, T.W., Stirling, Y., Thompson, S.G., Ajdukiewicz, A.B., Barbara, J.A.J., Chalmers, D.M. (1987). 'Carriers of hepatitis B surface antigen: possible association between low levels of clotting factors and protection against ischemic heart disease', Thrombos Res 45, 709.

13 Meade, T.W., Stirling, Y., Thompson, S.G., Vickers, M.V., Woolf, L., Ajdukiewicz, A.B., Stewart, C., Davidson, J.F., Walker, I.D., Douglas, A.S., Richardson I.M., Weir, R.D., Aromaa, A., Impivaara, O., Maatela, J., Hladovec, J. (1986). 'An international comparison of hemostatic variables in the study of ischemic heart disease', Int J Epidemiol 15, 331.

14 Meade, T.W., Vickers, M.V., Thompson, S.G., Seghatchian, M.J. (1985). 'The effect of physiological level of fibrinogen on platelet aggregation', Thrombos Res 38, 527.

15 Meade, T.W., Vickers, M.V., Thompson, S.G., Stirling, Y., Haines, A.P., Miller, G.J. (1985). 'Epidemiological characteristics of platelet aggregability', Brit Med J 290, 428.

16 Smith, E.B. (1985). 'Fibrinogen, fibrin and fibrin degradation products in relation to atherosclerosis', 15, 355.

17 Stone, M.C. and Thorpe, M.J. (1985). 'Plasma fibrinogen - a major coronary risk factor', J Roy Coll Gen Practit, 35, 565.

18 Welin, L, Svardsudd, K., Wilhelmens, L., Larsson, B., Tibblin G.(1987).'Analysis of risk factor for stroke in a cohort of men born in 1913', New Engl J Med 317, 522.

19 Wilhelmsen, L., Svardsudd, K., Korsan-Bengtssen, K., Larsson, B., Welin, L., Tibblin, G. (1984).'Fibrinogen as a risk for stroke and myocardial infarction', New Engl J Med 311, 501.

GLYCOSAMINOGLYCANS AND THEIR CLINICAL IMPLICATIONS

44

Glycosaminoglycans and the proliferation of arterial smooth muscle cells

R. TIOZZO, M.R. CINGI, D. REGGIANI and S. CALANDRA

Institute of General Pathology, University of Modena, via Campi 287, 41100 Modena, Italy

ABSTRACT.

Glycosaminoglycans (Gags) are highly negative charged sugar polymers. Heparin, heparan sulfate, dermatan sulfate and chondroitin sulfate are the most abundant Gags in many tissues. Their physiological role is not fully understood. Beside its anticoagulant activity, heparin has an inhibitory effect on the proliferation of arterial smooth muscle cells in vivo and in vitro. The anti-proliferative effect of heparin is also exerted on the other cells types of different origin. Heparin-like compounds (like Sulodexide and Low Molecular Weight Heparin) which have a reduced or negligible anti-coagulant activity were found to maintain an anti-proliferative effect similar to that of commercial heparin. The anti-proliferative activity is presumably related to the capacity of heparin and heparin-like compounds of binding several growth factors. It is conceivable that heparin-like compounds play a role in maintaining the physiological integrity of the arterial wall and in preventing the formation and progression of atherosclerotic lesions.

INTRODUCTION

Glycosaminoglycans (Gags), are long unbranched polysaccharide chains composed of repeating disaccharide units. Gags are negatively charged molecules because of the presence of sulfate and carboxyl groups. The negative charge may contribute to some biological properties of Gags by facilitating their interactions with other molecules. Gags, such as chondroitin sulfate, dermatan sulfate, keratan sulfate, heparan sulfate and heparin are present in nearly all mammalian tissues, especially in the connective tissue. One or more Gags chains can be covalently bound to extracellular proteins generating compounds called proteoglycans. Gags and proteoglycans are thought to play an important role in the extracellular matrix by influencing some basic biological processes like cell proliferation, cell recognition, cell differentiation etc (1). In this presentation I shall briefly review the biological effects of heparin and heparin-like compounds on the endothelial and the smooth muscle cells of the arterial wall.

Heparin is a linear, highly sulfated polysaccharide, consisting of alternating uronic acid (either L-iduronic or D-glucuronic) and D-glucosamine residues. Variantions in in the size of the polysaccharide chain, in the degree and distribution of sulfated groups make commercial heparins extremely heterogenous. Heparin is known for its anticoagulant, antithrombotic, lipolytic and fibrinolitic properties. More recently this spectrum of biological activities has been expanded to include a variety of functions related to the control of vascular growth and the activity and proliferation of cells present in the arterial wall.

Heparin has a great affinity for vascular endothelium; binding of heparin to endothelial cells has been shown after intravenous administration (2) and incubation of vessel fragments with heparin solutions (3). Commercial heparin and low molecular weight fragments derived from it bind to human endothelial monolayers in a specific and saturable manner. Other Gags, such as chondroitin sulfate, dermatan sulfate were not able to compete with heparin for binding (4). Cultured endothelial cells produce Gags having anti-coagulant activity (5) which is destroyed by treatment with heparinase. Interestingly this heparin-like molecule inhibits the proliferation of growth arrested arterial smooth muscle cells (6) thus suggesting a possible role " in vivo " of heparin like glycosaminoglycans in the regulation of the proliferation of arterial smooth muscle cells. Heparin contributes to maintain the normal negative charge of endothelial surface, and, in addition, it binds and presumably inactivates many substances (histamine, serotonin, angiotensin, endogenous and bacterial toxins and plasma low density lipoproteins) (7).

The first report concerning the effect of heparin on the proliferation of smooth muscle cells was published in 1977 when it was shown that the administration of heparin to rats reduced the smooth muscle cell proliferation produced by intimal denudation (8). Both anticoagulant active and anticoagulant inactive heparin significantly inhibited the growth of smooth muscle cells (9). In the last few years it was also reported that heparin inhibits the proliferation of arterial smooth muscle cells (10) and their migration (11) "in vitro". Recently it has been shown that heparin reduces the in vitro proliferation of other cell types (12). As previously pointed out commercial heparins are heterogeneous mixtures of highly sulfated glycosaminoglycans. This heterogeneity accounts for the large variations in the anti-proliferative property of these compounds. For this reason attempts have been made to obtain more homogeneous preparations of heparin or heparin-derived molecules with constant and reproducible anti-proliferative activity. The present study was aimed to ascertain whether some heparin-like compounds (such as Low Molecular Weight Heparin) and Sulodexide (a compound containing predominantly electrophoretically fast-moving heparin) can maintain the anti proliferative effect of commercial heparin.

MATERIALS AND METHODS

Sulfated Glycosaminoglycans added to the culture medium.

The following sulfated Gags were used in the present work:

1) commercial unfractionated heparin, M.W. 15 kD, 73 USP/mg, containing fast and slow moving heparins and dermatan sulfate.

2) Low Molecular Weight Heparin (OP/LMWH, Opocrin, Modena, Italy), M.W. 4-5 kD, 46 USP/mg, containing predominantly fast-moving heparin (12).

3) Sulodexide (SDX), M.W. 5-8 kD, 73 USP/mg, containing fast moving heparin (65%) and dermatan sulfate (35%) (12).

Heparin and SDX were extracted from pig duodenum. OP/LMWH was prepared by depolymerization of unfractionated heparin OP/LMWH and SDX show antithrombotic activity but are less effective than heparin as anticoagulant. These compounds were dissolved in water, sterilized by filtration and stored at 2°C until used.

Culture of arterial smooth muscle cells

The isolation and the culture of arterial smooth muscle

cells were carried out according to the procedure described by Tiozzo et al. (12).

Measurement of cell growth

The measurement of smooth muscle cells proliferation was carried out by cell count and 3H thymidine incorporation (12).

Heparin-Sepharose affinity chromatography

Fetal calf serum was diluted with 0.002M phosphate buffer to reduce NaCl concentration to 0.025M and applied to a (1 x 20 cm) heparin-Sepharose column (Pharmacia) previously equilibrated with the same buffer. The material was separated into three fractions by the stepwise addition of the following buffers: 0.002M phosphate and 0.025M NaCl (Fraction I, unbound material); 0.002M phosphate buffer and 0.150M NaCl (Fraction II) and 0.002M phosphate buffer and 0.250M NaCl (Fraction III). All operations were carried out at 4°C. Fraction I (94% of original FCS applied to the column), containing FCS depleted of heparin-binding factors was concentrated by filtration and used at 10% concentration in the incubation medium. The effect of this fraction on the growth of arterial smooth muscle cells was compared to that observed using 10% unfractionated fetal calf serum of the same batch, which had undergone the same manipulations as Fraction I except for the passage through the heparin-Sepharose column.

RESULTS

Heparin (100 ug/ml) reduced the in vitro proliferation of exponentially growing human arterial smooth muscle cells. Heparin produced 47% inhibition of cell proliferation on 4th day and 40% on 6th day in culture (Table 1). The proliferation of smooth muscle cells incubated in the presence of dermatan sulfate (100 ug/ml) was 6% and 9% lower than that found in the control cells on the 4th and 6th day of culture respectively (Table 1). SDX and OP/LMWH were equally effective in reducing the proliferation of human arterial smooth muscle cells (Table 2) after 4 and 6 days in culture. The anti-proliferative effect was detectable at a concentration as low as 5 ug/ml and was dose-dependent at least up to a concentration of 100 ug/ml. At a higher concentration (300 ug/ml), SDX and OP/LMWH produced a similar reduction of cell proliferation (48%-46% on the 4th day and 50%-45% on the 6th day of culture) (Table 2).

TABLE 1. Effect of heparin and dermatan sulfate on the in vitro proliferation of arterial smooth muscle cells.

	Days in culture 4	6
Control	100%	100%
Heparin (100ug/ml)	53%	60%
Dermatan S. (100 ug/ml)	94%	91%

The effect of these compounds was also tested on smooth muscle cells that had been growth arrested. Heparin, SDX and OP/LMWH produced the same inhibition found in exponentially growing cells at the 4th and 6th day in culture (Table 3).

TABLE 2. Effect of haparin-like compounds on the proliferation of arterial smooth muscle cells.

		Days in culture 4	6
Control		100%	100%
Sulodexide	(5 ug/ml)	82%	90%
"	(50 ")	64%	74%
"	(100 ")	55%	66%
"	(300 ")	52%	50%
OP/LMWH	(5 ")	79%	94%
"	(50 ")	72%	93%
"	(100 ")	55%	70%
"	(300 ")	54%	55%

TABLE 3. Effect of heparin and heparin-like compounds on the proliferation of growth arrested arterial smooth muscle cells.

		Days in culture 2	4	6
Control		100%	100%	100%
Heparin	(100 ug/ml)	70%	46%	52%
Sulodexide	(")	59%	64%	63%
OP/LMWH	(")	66%	71%	65%

The inhibition of cell proliferation induced by heparin and heparin-like compounds was found to be reversible (Fig. 1) (12).

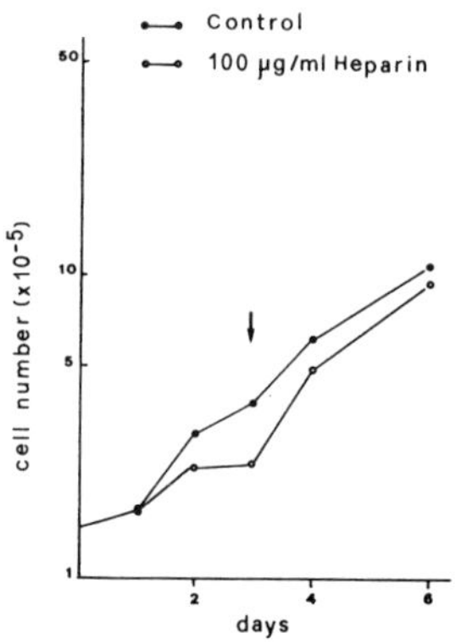

Figure 1. Reversal of the effect of heparin on the in vitro proliferation of human arterial smooth muscle cells.

The experiment illustrated in Figure 2 was designed to investigate whether the stage of culture growth plays a role in the response of cells to SDX and OP/LMWH. If these compounds were added at day 0, the degree of inhibition was as expected (50% inhibition at 3th day or 6th day respectively). If the compounds were added on the third day of culture their inhibitory effect was negligible. To test whether the effect of heparin-like compounds was due to the binding of growth factors present in fetal calf serum added to the culture medium, we applied fetal calf serum to a column of heparin-Sepharose and collected the unbound fraction (Fraction I) containing serum devoid of heparin-binding substances. When this fraction was added to the incubation medium, the incorporation of 3-H thymidine by arterial smooth muscle cells was much lower than that obtained with unfractionated fetal calf serum (Figure 3).

CONCLUSIONS

These studies suggest a possible physiological role for heparin as a regulator of the proliferation of smooth muscle cells in the arterial wall. Under physiological conditions heparin and heparin-like compounds would maintain smooth muscle cells in a quiescent state; on the other hand they would reduce the excessive proliferation which follows the intimal injury. Our findings also suggest that the anti-proliferative effect of heparin, could be due to its interaction with soluble growth factors present in serum.

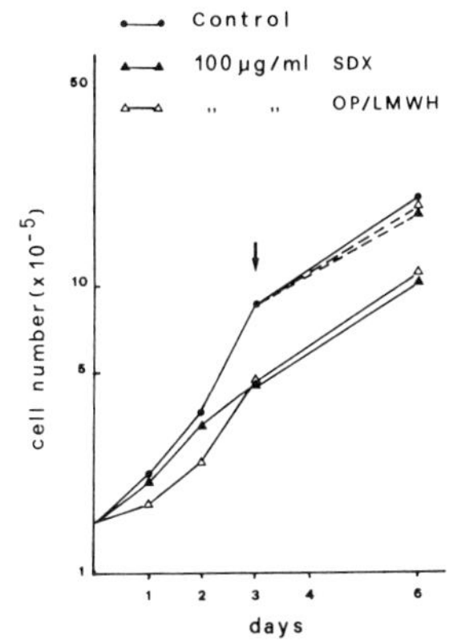

Figure 2. Effect of OP/LMWH and Sulodexide on different stage of in vitro proliferation of smooth muscle cells.

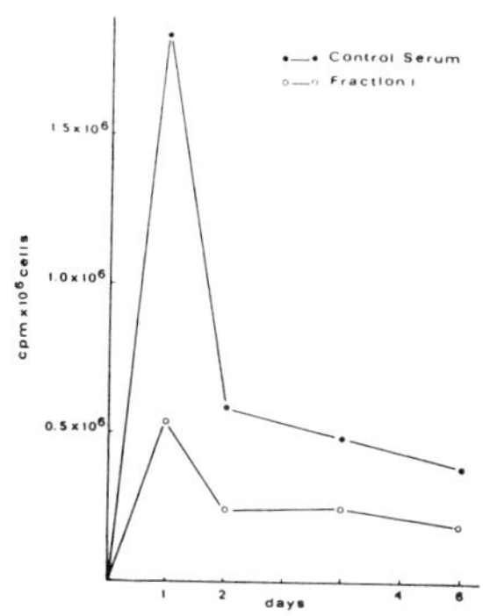

Figure 3. Effect of FCS depleted of heparin-binding factors on the 3H-thymidine incorporation by human arterial smooth muscle cells in vitro.

REFERENCES

1) Poole, A.R. (1986) 'Proteoglycans in health and disease: structure and functions', Biochem. J. 236, 1-14.
2) Heibert, L.M., and Jaques, L.B.(1976) 'The observation of heparin on endothelium after injection', Throm. Res. 8, 195-204.
3) Mahadoo, J., Heibert, L., and Jaques, L.B.(1978) 'Va

scular sequestration of heparin', Thromb. Res. 12, 79-9

4) Barzu, T., Van Rijin, J.L.M.L., Petitou, M., Molho, P. Tobelem, G., and Caen, J.P.(1986) 'Endothelial sites for heparin. Specificity and role in heparin neutralization', Biochem. J. 238, 847- 854.

5) Marcum, J.A., and Rosenberg, R.D., (1985) 'Heparinlike molecules with anticoagulant activity are synthesized by cultured endothelial cells', Biochem.Biophys. Res. Comm. 126, 365-372.

6) Castellot, J.J. Jr., Addonizio, M.L., Rosenberg, R., and Karnovsky, M.J. (1981) 'Cultured endothelial cells produce a heparinlike inhibitor of smooth muscle cells growth', J. Cell Biol. 90, 372-379.

7) Engelberg, H. (1984) 'Heparin and atherosclerosis process', Pharmacol. Rev. 36, 91-110.

8) Clowes, A.W., and Karnovsky, M.J. (1977) 'Suppression by heparin of smooth muscle cell proliferation in injured arteries', Nature 265, 625-626

9) Guyton, J.R., Rosenberg, R.D., Clowes, A.W., and Karnovsky, M.J. (1980) 'Inhibition of rat arterial smooth muscle cell proliferation by heparin. In vivo studies with anticoagulant and non-anticoagulant heparin', Circ. Res. 46, 625-634.

10) Hoover, R.L., Rosenberg, R.D., Hareing, W., and Karnovsky, M.J. (1980) 'Inhibition of rat smooth muscle cells proliferation by heparin. II in vitro studies', Circ. Res. 47, 578-583.

11) Majack, R.A., and Clowes, A.W. (1984) 'Inhibition of vascular smooth muscle cells migration by heparin-like glycosaminoglycans', J. Cell. Physiol. 118, 253-256.

12) Tiozzo, R., Cingi, M.R., Pietrangelo, A., Albertazzi, L., Calandra, S., and Milani, M.R. (1989) 'Effect of heparin-like compounds on the in vitro proliferation and protein synthesis of various cell types', Arzneim. Forsch. Drug. Res. 39, 15-20.

CALCIUM ANTAGONISTS AND ATHEROSCLEROSIS

45
Do calcium antagonists inhibit atherogenesis?

P. PAULETTO and G. SCANNAPIECO

Clinica Medica I, Università di Padova, Italy

ABSTRACT

In the last few years calcium antagonists have been reported to act as antiatherosclerotic agents independently from any modification of risk factors. Since these compounds have no adverse effect on plasma lipoproteins profile and are effective antihypertensives, they may represent first-line drugs in this field. However, contrasting results are reported in the literature on the antiatherogenic effect of calcium antagonists in experimental animals, and only preliminary data exist on the effect in humans. This paper summarizes the main in vivo and in vitro studies so far conducted in this field and focuses on the mechanisms by which calcium antagonists may exert their antiatherosclerotic action.

INTRODUCTION

From the chemical and pharmacological point of view, calcium antagonists represent a heterogeneous group of compounds. As a common feature , they are able to reduce the amount of Ca^{++} which enters the cells. These drugs are quite relevant in the clinical practice as they are effective in the treatment of different cardiovascular diseases including hypertension, ischaemic heart disease , and certain arrhythmias (1). Unlike many of the drugs commonly employed in this field , calcium antagonists as a group display only minor side effects and relatively few adverse effects. In particular, they have never been reported to worsen the plasma liporotein pattern in patients on long-term treatment. This makes calcium antagonists suitable for patients with overt or at risk for atherosclerosis. In addition , some experimental studies carried out in animals fed a cholesterol-enriched diet support the hypothesis that calcium antagonists are able to inhibit dietary-induced atherogenesis (2,3). On the other hand, some other studies do not confirm this effect (4,5).

This paper deals with the present knowledge on the antiatherogenic effect of different calcium antagonists and summarizes the main in vivo and in vitro studies so far conducted.

IN VIVO STUDIES

Nifedipine, nicardipine, flordipine, and isradipine

Nifedipine was the first calcium antagonist to be evaluated for antiatherosclerotic activity. Henry and Bentley (2) investigated the effects of nifedipine in 2% cholesterol-fed New Zealand white (NZW) rabbits. Treatment with orally administered nifedipine, at a dosage of 40 mg (20mg b.i.d.)/day/rabbit, was instituted concomitantly with the beginning of the cholesterol-enriched diet, and lasted 8 weeks. Very high levels of cholesterolemia were found in these animals (about 1900 mg/dl). Only a transient hypotensive effect was observed immediately after nifedipine administration. At the end of the study, although hypercholesterolemia was unaffected, a significant decrease in the extent of atherosclerotic lesions was found in the nifedipine-treated animals.

Since the dosage of nifedipine in the above mentioned study was about 10-fold that recommended for the treatment of hypertension, subsequent studies (4) were performed using much lower doses of the drug, similar to those employed in humans. In these studies,the cholesterol added to the diet was reduced to 0.25 % and the animals developed a cholesterolemia of about 400 mg/dl. As a result, the aortic surface involved with atherosclerotic lesions was only about 20 % in the control animals and nifedipine did not seem to have any effect on the extent of the aortic atherosclerotic lesions.

Another study by Stender et al. (5) failed to confirm that a high dosage of nifedipine could suppress atherogenesis. A remarkable difference between this study and the previous ones is that in this study the White Danish Country rabbit instead of the NZW was used. However, a further study carried out in Dutch-belted rabbits using high dosages of nifedipine or nicardipine (3) resulted in decreased atherogenesis with both drugs. Interestingly, nicardipine was reported to be effective in reducing plasma cholesterol levels in cholesterol-fed rats, with concomitant increase in HDL plasma levels (6). Another dihydropyridine derivative, flordipine, was shown to have no effect in preventing aortic sudanophlia of NZW rabbits fed a 1 % cholesterol diet for 10 weeks. In this study (7), animals were treated at dosages of 5, 15 or 45 mg/kg/day.

The existing studies have provided conflicting results also on the efficacy of nifedipine in reducing pre-exsisting atheromas. Overturf et al (8) induced moderate renovascular hypertension (one kidney- one clip) in NZW rabbits fed a 0.1 % cholesterol diet. Nifedipine administration (about 1 mg/day/rabbit) begun 5 weeks later, and resulted in normalization of blood pressure. However, nifedipine treatment did not revert aortic atherosclerosis. Thiery et al (9) found that nifedipine 40 mg/rabbit/day induced the regression of pre-exsisting atheromatous lesions in 1.5 % cholesterol-fed NZW rabbits after stopping the cholesterol diet with the beginning of the treatment. A similar study carried out by our group in 1 % cholesterol-fed NZW rabbits kept on cholesterol diet during nifedipine treatment, did not show any regression of atherosclerotic lesions. Nevertheless, the aortic smooth muscle cells (SMC) subpopulations involved with the atherogenic process were found to be markedly reduced in the media (10, 11, & in preparation). These results are consistent with a specific role of this calcium antagonist as: 1)inducer of SMC differentiation, and/or 2)blocker of cell proliferation of a SMC subpopulation present both in the plaque and in the underlying media which displays properties in common with SMC of foetal type. These observed changes at the cellular level helps explain why atherosclerosis can be prevented rather than reversed by nifedipine. It is worthwile noting that this finding fits very well with the results of the INTACT Study (12). This study, the only one so far conducted in humans, was designed to ascertain whether progression of coronary atherosclerosis could be reduced in patients with early or mild lesions. The 425 patients enrolled in the double-blind, placebo controlled trial were given nifedipine 80 mg/die for three years. In the actively treated patients, the coronary angiograms performed before and after the treatment period showed a 20 % reduction in newly formed lesions together with a significant reduction of lesions progression towards stenosis and occlusion.

Isradipine is another dihydropyridine derivative evaluated as an antiatherosclerotic agent (13). A low dosage of this calcium antagonist (1 mg/Kg/day) reduced by 44 % the arterial enroachment in a normocholesterolemic rat model of intimal hyperplasia. The result indicated that reduced progression of intimal lesions was achieved through changes in SMC migration and proliferation. Habib et al (14) also found that low doses of isradipine are able to prevent the development of atherosclerotic lesions in cholesterol-fed NZW rabbits. Moreover, impairment of endothelium-dependent relaxation and decreased aortic cholesterol content were observed.

Verapamil

The antiatherogenic effect of verapamil, a phenilalkylamine, was studied for the first time by Rouleau et al (15) in NZW rabbits using a protocol very similar to that of Henry and Bentley (2). Animals were kept on 0.5 % cholesterol diet and, due to scarce absorption of oral verapamil in rabbits, the daily dose administered was about 8 mg/Kg, far above the largest recommended dose for humans. Oral verapamil did not result in reduced atherogenesis; however, a significant reduction was found when parenteral verapamil was also administered. In a subsequent study (16), orally administered verapamil at doses of 40, 100, 400 mg/day resulted in reduced atherogenesis only in those animals which displayed appreciable serum levels of the drug. Surprisingly, the subcutaneous administration of the drug did not modify the development of atherosclerotic lesions even when verapimil was detectable in the serum.

Diltiazem, & combination drug studies with flunarizine or nicardipine

The antiatherogenic effect of diltiazem, a benzothiazepine derivative, was tested in cholesterol-fed Japanese white rabbits (17). Diltiazem (50 mg daily) administered intraperitoneally was reported to reduce the aortic atherosclerotic lesions in these rabbits. As in the case of nicardipine (6), reduced plasma levels of both total cholesterol and low-density lipoproteins were demonstrated. Diltiazem was also studied together with flunarizine (18), a piperazine derivative, according to a protocol very similar to that of Henry and Bentley (2). The thoracic aorta of animals treated with high doses of diltiazem showed a significant reduction in surface involved with atherosclerotic lesions. There was no effect on either the abdominal aorta or the intramural coronary arteries. Flunarizine did not suppress atherogenesis at any level. In another study (19), diltiazem (210 mg/day) or nicardipine (60 mg/day) treatment was instituted in Japanese white rabbits 2 weeks after the beginning of a cholesterol-enriched diet. Neither calcium antagonist was effective in reducing atherosclerosis.

IN VITRO STUDIES

Nifedipine, nilvadipine, and diltiazem.

The possibility that nifedipine may prevent atherogenesis and/or inhibit the progression of intimal lesions by interfering with the phenotypic modulation and proliferation of arterial SMC has been tested in studies carried out on SMC isolated from the arterial media (20). The results indicate that, in primary cultures, micromolar concentrations of nifedipine are able to slow down the transformation rate of SMC from a "contractile" to a "synthetic" phenotype. Moreover, in secondary cultures, nifedipine reduces PDGF- and serum- induced growth of SMC and inhibits DNA synthesis, as evaluated by [3H] -thymidine incorporation into the cells. Finally, nifedipine is able to lower the intracellular concentration of cyclic AMP (20). In another study (21) migration of SMC from explants was inhibited mainly by a new calcium antagonist, namely nilvadipine, and in decreasing order by nifedipine, verapamil and diltiazem. Schmitz et al (22,23) investigated the effects of nifedipine on cholesterol metabolism in cultured macrophages. In this study it was demonstrated that nifedipine induces an increase in the efflux of acetylated-LDL from macrophages independently of the presence of HDL in the culture medium. Thus, nifedipine seems to be able to directly and positively affect lipoprotein metabolism in macrophages.

On the whole, nifedipine and other dihydropiridine derivatives are thought to slow down SMC proliferation by: 1)

reducing cellular availability of calcium and possibly by interfering with the calcium-calmodulin complex, which plays a role in regulating cell proliferation; 2) decreasing intracellular cyclic AMP. In addition, nifedipine has been shown to modulate LDL metabolism by macrophages.

Verapamil

The in vitro cellular and metabolic effects of verapamil have been studied mainly by Stein et al. These Authors demonstrated that verapamil causes an increase in LDL uptake and degradation by bovine endothelial cells and human skin fibroblasts in culture (24), probably through an increase in the number of LDL receptors. In a subsequent study (25) the same Authors observed that verapamil markedly decreases DNA synthesis and cell proliferation in both rabbit SMC and human fibroblasts. This reduction was still evident even after adding cholesterol-rich serum (which usually induces cell proliferation) to the culture medium. Similar results were obtained by Orekhov et al. (26). These Authors observed that verapamil significantly reduces, in a dose-dependent manner, the in vitro proliferation of SMC isolated from human fatty streaks. In the same study, it has been shown that the addition of verapamil to the culture medium induces a reduction in collagen synthesis and in lipid content of SMC.

CONCLUSIONS

At the present time, general conclusions on the antiatherogenic effects of calcium antagonists cannot be drawn. The effects of each calcium antagonist should be individually defined according to the experimental setting, being the antiatherosclerotic action dependent not only on the chemical structure of the drug, but also on other factors: the dosage administered, the route of administration and the breed of rabbit or the animal species used. Another possible source of discrepancy among results obtained in the various studies is represented by the different methods used in assessing atherosclerotic lesions. In particular, most studies have been conducted by assessing the extent of aortic surfaces involved with sudanophilia. In our experience this surface measurement of atherosclerosis has a low reliabilty (27).

A very important issue is represented by the results obtained in humans after long-term treatment with nifedipine; at present, some clinical studies designed to define the antiatherogenic effect of other calcium antagonists in are in progress.

The in vitro studies have provided new insights to the possible mechanisms and levels of action of the different calcium antagonists. Based on the present knowledge, the possible mechanisms underlying the antiatherosclerotic action of calcium antagonists can be summarized as follows: 1) reduced cholesterol content of the aorta; 2) reduced endothelial permeability to cholesterol; 3) reduced collagen synthesis by SMC; 4) increased LDL uptake and degradation by both SMC and endothelial cells; 5) reduced SMC proliferation; 6) interference with SMC differentiation processes.

REFERENCES

1) Opie LH. Calcium antagonists. Mechanisms, therapeutic indications and reservations : a review. Quart J Med 1984 ; New Series LIII/209:1-16.

2) Henry PD, Bentley KI. Suppression of atherogenesis in cholesterol-fed rabbit treated with nifedipine. J Clin Invest 1981; 68:1366-1369.

3) Willis AL, Nagel B, Churchill V et al. Antiatherosclerotic effect of nicardipine and nifedipine in cholesterol-fed rabbits. Arteriosclerosis 1985; 5: 250-255.

4) Overturf ML, Smith SA. Failure of a high therapeutic dosage of nifedipine to suppress atherogenesis in cholesterol-fed rabbits. Arteriosclerosis 1982; 2: A408.

5) Stender S, Stender I, Nordestgaard B, Kjedsen K. No effect of nifedipine on atherogenesis in cholesterol-fed rabbits. Arteriosclerosis 1984; 4: 389-394.

6) Ohata I, Sakamoto N, Nagano K, Maeno H. Low density lipoprotein-lowering and high density lipoprotein-elevating effects of nicardipine in rats. Pharmacol 1984; 33: 2199-2205.

7) Kritchevsky D, Tepper SA, Klurfeld DM. Flordipine, a calcium channel blocker, which does not influence lipidemia or atherosclerosis in cholesterol-fed rabbits. Atherosclerosis 1988; 69: 89-92.

8) Overturf ML, Sybers H, Schaper J, Taegtmayer H. Hypertension and atherosclerosis in cholesterol-fed rabbits.II. One kidney-one clip Goldblatt hypertension treated with nifedipine. Atherosclerosis 1987; 66: 68-73.

9) Thiery J, Niedmann PD, Seidel D. The beneficial influence of nifedipine on the regression of the cholesterol-induced atherosclerosis in rabbits. Exptl Med 1987; 187: 359-376.

10)Pauletto P, Sartore S, Scannapieco G et al. Immunocytochemical analysis of myosin isoform distribution in the atherosclerotic lesions of cholesterol-fed rabbits. In: Hypertension and Atherosclerosis, C Dal Palu', R Ross, eds., Excerpta Medica, 1989: 107-112.

11) Pauletto P, Sartore S, Borrione A C et al. A nifedipine-sensitive smooth muscle cell subpopulation in the aortic media of hypercholesterolemic rabbit.X International Symposium on drugs affecting lipid metabolism .November 8-11, 1989 Houston, Texas. (abstract)

12) Lichtlen PB, Hugenholtz PG, Rafflenbeul W, Jost S, and the INTACT Study Group. Retardation of the progression of coronary artery disease in man by nifedipine; the international nifedipine trial on antiatherosclerotic therapy. in: Focus on Adalat.

Vancouver, April 30 - May 2, 1989 (abstract).
13) Handley DA, Van Valen RG, Melden MK, Saunders RN. Suppression of rat carotid lesion development by the calcium channel blocker PN-200-110. Am J Pathol 1986; 124: 88-93.
14) Habib JB, Bossaller C, Wells S. Preservation of endothelium-dependent vascular relaxation in Cholesterol-fed rabbits by treatment with calcium blocker PN-200-110. Circ Res 1986; 58: 305 309.
15) Rouleau JL, Parmley WW, Stevens J et al. Verapamil suppresses atherosclerosis in cholesterol-fed rabbits. J Am Coll Cardiol 1983; 1(6): 1453-1460.
16) Blumstein SL, Sievers R, Kidd P, Parmley WW. Mechanism of protection from atherosclerosis by verapamil in the cholesterol-fed rabbit. Am J Cardiol 1984; 54: 884-889.
17) Sugano M, Nakashima Y, Matsuchima T et al. Suppression of atherosclerosis in cholesterol-fed rabbits by diltiazem injections. Arteriosclerosis 1986; 6: 237-241.
18) Ginsberg R, Davis K, Bristow MR et al. Calcium antagonists suppress atherogenesis in aorta but not in the intramural coronary arteries of cholesterol-fed rabbits. Lab Invest 1983; 9:154-158.
19) Naito M, Kuzuya F, Asai K et al. Ineffectiveness of Ca^{++} antagonists nicardipine and diltiazem on experimental atherosclerosis in cholesterol-fed rabbits. Atherosclerosis 1984; 51: 343-344.
20) Nilsson J, Sjolund M, Palmerg L et al. The calcium antagonist nifedipine inhibits arterial smooth muscle cell proliferation. Atherosclerosis, 1985; 58: 109-122.
21) Nomoto A, Hirosumi J, Sekiguchi C et al. Antiatherogenic activity of FR34235 (Nilvadipine), a new potent calcium antagonist. Atherosclerosis, 1987; 64:255-261.
22) Schmitz G, Robenek H, Beuck M et al. Ca^{++} antagonist and ACAT inhibitors promote cholesterol efflux from macrophages by different mechanisms .I. Arteriosclerosis, 1988; 8:46-56
23) Robenek H and Schmitz G. Ca^{++} antagonist and ACAT inhibitors promote cholesterol efflux from macrophages by different mechanisms .II. Arteriosclerosis, 1988; 8: 57-67
24) Stein O, Leitersdorf E, Stein Y. Verapamil enhances receptor-mediated endocytosis of low-density lipoproteins by aortic cells.Arteriosclerosis, 1985; 5:35-44.
25)Stein O, Halperin G, Stein Y. Long-term effects of verapamil on aortic smooth muscle cells cultured in the presence of hypercholesterolemic serum. Arteriosclerosis, 1987; 7: 585-592.
26) Orekhov A, Tertov V, Khashimov K et al. Evidence of antiatherosclerotic action of verapimil from direct effects on arterial cells. Am J Cardiol 1987; 59: 495-496.
27) Pauletto P, Angelini A, Vescovo G et al. The surface measurement of aortic atherosclerosis: critical survey and comparison with histologic findings. Int J Cardiol 1985; 8: 361-373.

46

Atherosclerosis-related effects of verapamil, anipamil and other calcium antagonists studied on cell culture

A.N. OREKHOV, V.V. TERTOV, E.M. PIVOVAROVA, S.G. KOZLOV, A.A. LYAKISHEV and M. YA. RUDA

USSR Cardiology Research Center, 3rd Cherepkovskaya Street 15A,121552 Moscow, Russia

INTRODUCTION

It has been shown that calcium antagonists suppress experimental atherosclerosis in animals (1). Recently it was demonstrated that nifedipine and verapamil suppress the development of human coronary atherosclerosis and induce regression of atherosclerosis in patients (2,3). The mechanisms of antiatherogenic (preventive) and antiatherosclerotic (leading to regression) actions of calcium antagonists remain obscure.

We have recently reported that calcium antagonists elicit direct antiatherosclerotic effects on primary culture of human aortic cells reducing the intracellular lipid level, proliferative activity and synthesis of the extracelular matrix (4-8). Verapamil apperared to be the most potent agent; depending on antiatherosclerotic efficiency other drugs can be arranged as follows: nifedipine, darodipine, isradipine, diltiazem, thiapamil, gallopamil, nitredipine, felodipin, cinnarizine (7,8).

Here we report the results of testing a new calcium antagonist anipamil and compare its antiatherosclerotic action with that of verapamil. In addition, we have examined the effects of continuous calcium antagonist administration on the atherosclerosis-related properties of blood plasma.

MATERIALS AND METHODS

Anipamil, its enantiomers, (+)-anipamil and (−)-anipamil, as well as varapamil were obtained from Knoll AG (Ludwigshafen, West Germany). Nifedipine (Corinfar) for per os administration was purchased from Germed VEB Arzneimittenwerk (Dresden, East Germany).

Patients with coronary artery disease received per os 20 mg nifedipine and then blood was drawn and blood plasma was prepared as described previously (7).

Human aortic subendothelial intimal cells were isolated from autopsy material obtained within 2-3 hours after death. Cells were harvested by enzymatic digestion of atherosclerotic plaques with 0.15% collagenase for 3-4 hours, and seeded into 96-well culture plates. Intimal cells were cultivated for seven days in Medium 199, containing 10% fetal calf serum, glutamine, and antibiotics. The drugs' activity was evaluated by their impact on atherosclerotic indices such as incorporation of [^{3}H]thymidine into cellular DNA, intracellular lipid level and total protein synthesis. On the seventh day of cultivation, test agents were added together with labeled precoursors. Following extensive washing, atherosclerotic indices were determined 24 hours after the addition of the agents. Protocols for cell isolation and cultivation as well as technical details of the experiment are presented elsewhere (4,9).

Lipids were extracted from cells with a chloroform-methanol mixture (1:2, v/v) according to Bligh and Dyer (10). The total cholesterol content in the lipid extracts was determined using Boehringer Mannheim Monotest^R (Boehringer Mannheim GmbH, Mannheim, FRG). Phospholipids, triglycerides, free cholesterol and cholesteryl esters extracted from the cells were separated by TLC and measured by scanning densitometry as described elsewhere (9).

DNA synthesis was evaluated by the incorporation of [^{3}H]thymidine into acid-insoluble cell fraction as described earlier (4).

After incubation with 1 uCi/ml [4,5-^{3}H]leucine (135 Ci/mmol, Amersham International plc., England), the incubation medium and the cells suspended with rubber policeman were heated for 10 min at 80°C, and proteins were precipitated by 10% TCA. The precipitate was washed twice with a 5% TCA and twice with diethyl ether, dissolved with 0.5 N KOH and precipitated again by a 10% TCA. The precipitate was resuspended in a 5% TCA and its radioactivity was measured.

Differences between obtained data were evaluated by means of dispersion analysis with the use of a package of statistical BMDP programs (11).

RESULTS AND DISCUSSION

Earlier it has been shown that phospholipid, free cholesterol, cholesteryl ester and triglyceride contents in human aortic cells cultured from atherosclerotic plaque are considerably higher than in cells cultured from uninvolved intima (4,9). Incubation with anipamil, its enantiomers or verapamil for 24 h considerably reduced the intracellular content of esterified cholesterol, triglyceride and, to a lesser extent, free cholesterol; neither anipamil nor verapamil had any effect on the phospsholipid content (Table 1).

Table 1

Influence of calcium antagonists on atherosclerotic cellular parameters

Parameter	Drug effect, % of control			
	Anipamil	(+)-Anipamil	(-)-Anipamil	Verapamil
Cholesteryl esters	48±3*	42±5*	50±3*	49±5*
Triglycerides	32±4*	48±7*	43±4*	42±5*
Free cholesterol	74±6*	70±8*	73±5*	75±4*
Phospholipids	90±6	93±4	92±9	88±12
DNA synthesis	52±4*	57±3*	50±5*	49±8*
Protein synthesis	68±5*	64±4*	70±2*	62±3*

Drugs were used in concentration $3x10^{-5}$ M. Data of one out of tree representative experiments are shown.
*, Significant difference from the control ($p<0.05$).

Table 2

Effect of plasma obtained after nifedipine administration on cholesterol content in cultured cells

Patient, #	Cholesterol content, % of control		
	1-st day	7-th day	28-th day
1, prior	246±19	237±14	159±14**
1, 4 h after	154±13*	145±10*	112±7*
2, prior	185±17	140±11	131±8**
2, 4 h after	130±9*	101±6*	94±6*
3, prior	254±14	218±12	181±17**
3, 4 h after	178±7*	167±13*	130±10*
4, prior	367±26	342±27	327±28
4, 4 h after	285±19*	261±17*	248±16*

Blood was collected after an overnight fast prior and 4 h after nifedipine administration. Plasma was added to cultured human aortic cells, and the increase in intracellular cholesterol content was determined.
*, significant difference from the values obtained prior to nifedipine administration;
**, significant difference from the values obtained prior to nifedipine administration on the first day of treatment.

Enantiomers of anipamil, racemate and verapamil produced essentially similar effects on the proliferative activity of atherosclerotic cells and total protein synthesis (Table 1).

Thus, anipamil produced an antiatherosclerotic effect on cultured atherosclerotic cells: it reduced their lipid content, proliferative activity and total protein synthesis. Anipamil efficacy appeared to be similar to that of verapamil which is the most potent among calcium antagonists tested previously. In the light of recent data on antiatherogenic and antiatherosclerotic effects of verapamil and nifedipine elicited in humans and in experiental animals, one can suggest that anipamil is efficient not only in vitro but also in vivo.

In mentioned clinical investigations the optimal tactics of direct antiatherosclerotic therapy using calcium antagonists was not developed (2,3). Patients received relatively high doses of these drugs, however, there is no convictive evidence to suggest that such a treatment produces maximal antiatherogenic or antiatherosclerotic effects. Previously we have reported that blood plasma of patients who received calcium antagonists per os acquires an antiatherogenic potential (7). We believe that specific approach to the optimization of the therapy aimed at a direct antiatherosclerotic effect can be developed by analysing the patient's plasma for atherogenicity following administration of the therapeutic agent. As the first step in this direction, we have examined serum atherogenicity after a single administration of nifedipine and after long-term therapy.

Previously, we have shown that both serum and plasma of patients with angiographically documented coronary atherosclerosis are atherogenic, i.e. they induce cholesterol accumulation in cultured human aortic cells (12-15). Blood was collected prior and 4 h after nifedipine administration on day 1, on day 7 and on day 28 of continuous therapy (60 mg daily). On day 7, nifedipine lowered plasma atherogenicity just as effectively as on day 1 (Table 2). On day 28, in 3 out of 4 cases the atherogenicity of plasma obtained prior to the drug administration was lower than the initial atherogenicity at the beginning of the treatment. At the same time, in 2 out of 4 cases atherogenicity disappeared after nifedipine administration. Thus, long-term nifedipine therapy produces a beneficial effect on blood plasma: it lowers the initial atherogenicity, and causes more prominent antiatherogenic effect after the drug administration.

We hope that the control over the atherosclerosis-related properties of plasma obtained from patients after drug administration may be helpful in the optimization of direct antiatherogenic and antiatherosclerotic therapy.

REFERENCES

(1) Blumlein S.L., Sievers R., Kidd P., Parmley W.W. (1985). Modification of experimental atherosclerosis by calcium-channel blockers. Am J Cardiol, 55, 165B-171B.

(2) Kober G., Schneider W., Kaltenbach M. (1989). Can the progression of coronary sclerosis be influenced by calcium antagonists? J Cardiovasc Pharmacol, 13, S2-S6.

(3) Lichtlen P.R., Hugenholtz P.G., Rafflenbeul W., INTACT-group (1989). Possible protective effect of nifedipine against progression of atherosclerosis in man (INTACT-study). In: "4th International Symposium on Calcium Antagonists: Pharmacology and CLinical Research. Abstract Book", Florence (Italy), pp. 127-130.

(4) Orekhov A.N., Tertov V.V., Kudryashov S.A. et al. (1986). Primary culture of human aortic intima cells as a model for testing antiatherosclerotic drugs. Effects of cyclic AMP, prostaglandins, calcium antagonists, antioxidants, and lipid-lowering agents. Atherosclerosis, 60, 101-110.

(5) Orekhov A.N., Tertov V.V., Khashimov Kh.A. et al. (1986). Antiatherosclerotic effects of verapamil in primary culture of human aortic intimal cells. J Hypertension, 4, S153-S155.

(6) Orekhov A.N., Tertov V.V., Khashimov Kh.A. et al. (1987). Evidence of antiatherosclerotic action of verapamil from direct effects on arterial cells. Am J Cardiol, 59, 495-496.

(7) Orekhov A.N., Baldenkov G.N., Tertov V.V. et al. (1988). Cardiovascular drugs and atherosclerosis: effects of calcium antagonists, beta-blockers, and nitrates on atherosclerotic characteristics of human aortic cells. J Cardiovasc Pharmacol, 12, S66-S68.

(8) Baldenkov G.N., Akopov S.E., Li H.R., Orekhov A.N. (1988). Prostacyclin, thromboxane A_2 and calcium antagonists: effects on atherosclerotic characteristics of vascular cells. Biomed Biochim Acta, 47, S324-S327.

(9) Orekhov A.N., Tertov V.V., Novikov I.D. et al. (1985). Lipids in cells of atherosclerotic and uninvolved human aorta. I. Lipid composition of aortic tissue and enzyme isolated and cultured cells. Exp Mol Pathol, 42, 117-137.

(10) Bligh E.G., Dyer W.J. (1959). A rapid method of total lipid extraction and purification. Can J Biochem Physiol, 37, 911-917.

(11) Dixon W.J., Brown M.B. (1977). Biomedical Computer Programs. P-Series. University of California Press, Berkeley, pp. 185-198.

(12) Chazov E.I., Tertov V.V., Orekhov A.N. et al. (1986). Atherogenicity of blood serum from patients with coronary heart disease. Lancet, 2, 595-598.

(13) Orekhov A.N., Tertov V.V., Pokrovsky S.N. et al. (1988). Blood serum atherogenicity associated with coronary atherosclerosis. Evidence for nonlipid factor providing atherogenicity of low-density lipoproteins and an approach to its elimination. Circ Res, 62, 421-429.

(14) Chazov E.I., Orekhov A.N., Tertov V.V. et al. (1988). Atherogenicity of blood plasma from patients with coronary atherosclerosis and its correction. Atherosclerosis Rev, 17, 9-20.

(15) Tertov V.V., Orekhov A.N., Martsenyuk O.N. et al. (1989). Low density lipoproteins isolated from the blood of patients with coronary heart disease induce the accumulation of lipids in human aortic cells. Exp Mol Pathol, 50, 337-347.

47
Antiatherosclerotic effects of anipamil, verapamil and other calcium antagonists studied on cell culture

A.N. OREKHOV, V.V. TERTOV, S.G. KOZLOV, A.A. LYAKISHEV and M. YA. RUDA

USSR Cardiology Research Center, 3rd Cherepkovskaya Street 15A, 121552 Moscow, Russia

ABSTRACT. Calcium antagonists exhibit direct antiatherosclerotic action in primary culture of human aortic atherosclerotic cells by lowering intracellular lipid content, proliferative activity and synthesis of the extracellular matrix. Verapamil exhibited the highest efficacy in this respect. New calcium antagonist, anipamil, and its enantiomers have been tested in cell culture. At 10^{-6} M and higher concentrations, anipamil and its enantiomers produced considerable decrease in intracellular contents of cholesteryl esters, triglycerides and free cholesterol, suppressed cell proliferation and inhibited synthesis of the extracelular matrix. The efficacy of anipamil enantiomers and racemate was similar to that of verapamil. Blood plasma obtained from patients after administration of 80 mg verapamil or 20 mg nifedipin significantly lowered the cholesterol content of cultured cells. Blood plasma of most atherosclerotic patients possesses atherogenic properties, i.e. it is able to increase cholesterol content in cultured cells. Plasma atherogenicity manifested in culture decreased considerably or even disappeared after both nifedipine and verapamil administration. After 28 days of nifedipine therapy, plasma ahterogenenicity was lower compared with the initial value at the beginning of the treatment. These observations suggest that control of plasma atherogenicity after drug administration may provide an additional tool for optimization of direct antiatherogenic and antiatherosclerotic therapy.

1. INTRODUCTION

Calcium antagonists have found a wide application in the treatment of cardio-vascular diseases. It has been shown that they suppress experimental atherosclerosis in animals [1]. Both nifedipine and verapamil suppress the development of human coronary atherosclerosis, and verapamil even induces regression of atherosclerosis in patients [2,3]. The mechanisms of antiatherogenic (preventive) and antiatherosclerotic (leading to regression of atherosclerosis) actions of calcium antagonists remain obscure.

We have recently reported that calcium antagonists elicit direct antiatherosclerotic effects on primary culture of human aortic cells [4-8]. These agents reduced the intracellular lipid level, proliferative activity and synthesis of the extracelular matrix. Thus, calcium antagonists normalized the major manifestations of atherosclerosis at the cellular level. Verapamil appeared to be the most potent agent; depending on antiatherosclerotic efficacy other drugs can be arranged as follows: nifedipine, darodipine, isradipine, diltiazem, thiapamil, gallopamil, nitredipine, felodipin, cinnarizine [7,8]. After peroral administration of these drugs, the patients' sera acquire an antiatherosclerotic potential that can be revealed in cell culture [7]. Based on these observations, it can be concluded that calcium antagonists may exhibit an antiatherosclerotic action and induce regression of cellular manifestations of atherosclerosis not only in vitro but also in vivo.

Here we report the results of testing a new calcium antagonist, anipamil, and its enantiomers and compare its antiatherosclerotic action with that of verapamil. In addition, we have examined the effects of continuous calcium antagonist administration on the atherosclerosis-related properties of blood plasma.

2. MATERIALS AND METHODS

Anipamil, its enantiomers, (+)-anipamil and (-)-anipamil, as well as varapamil were obtained from Knoll AG (Ludwigshafen, West Germany). Verapamil (Finoptin) for per os administration was purchased from Orion Corporation Ltd. (Espoo, Finland), nifedipine (Corinfar) was obtained from Germed VEB Arzneimittelwerk (Dresden, East Germany).

TABLE 1. Influence of calcium antagonists on atherosclerotic cellular parameters

Parameter	Drug effect, % of control			
	Ani	(+)-Ani	(-)-Ani	Vera
Cholesteryl esters	48±3*	42±5*	50±3*	49±5*
Triglycerides	32±4*	48±7*	43±4*	42±5*
Free cholesterol	74±6*	70±8*	73±5*	75±4*
Phospholipids	90±6	93±4	92±9	88±12
DNA synthesis	52±4*	57±3*	50±5*	49±8*
Protein synthesis	68±5*	64±4*	70±2*	62±3*

Ani, anipamil; Vera, verapamil. Drugs were used in concentration 3×10^{-5} M. Data of 1 out of 3 representative experiments are shown. *, Significant difference from the control ($p<0.05$).

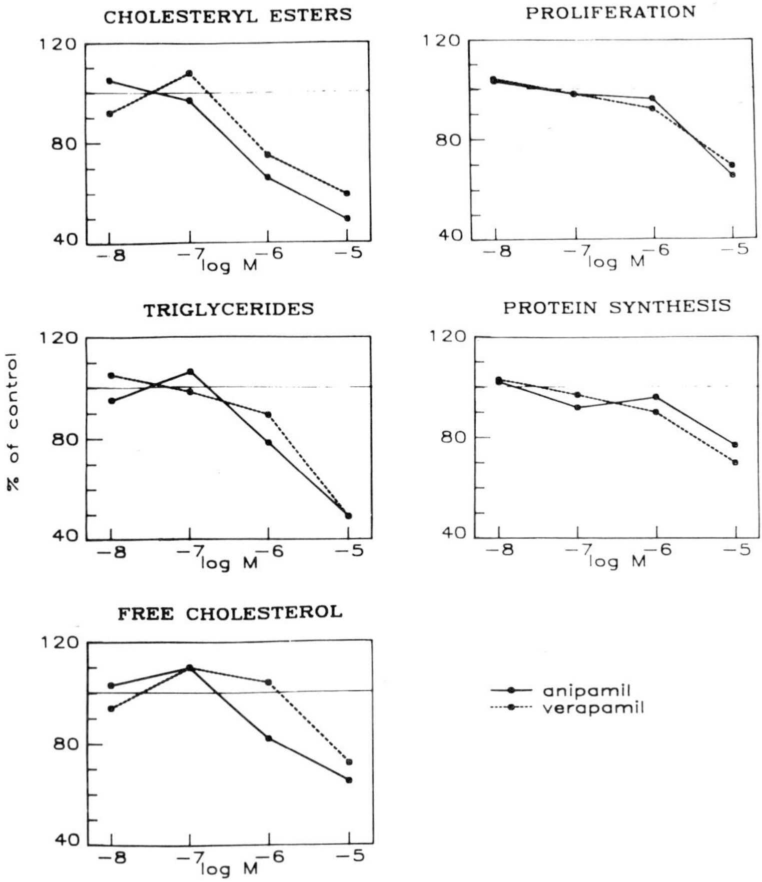

Figure 1. Dose-dependent effects of anipamil and verapamil on athero-sclerosis-related parameters of cultured human aortic cells.
Data of 1 out of 3 representative experiments are shown. Each point is the mean of three determinations.

The blood of coronary artery disease patients who received drugs for angina pectoris resulting from the angiographically documented coronary atherosclerosis was analysed. Patients' characteristics were described elsewhere [7]. Patients received per os 80 mg verapamil or 20 mg nifedi-pine, then blood was drawn and blood plasma was prepared as described previously [7].

Human aortic subendothelial intimal cells were isolated from autop-sy material obtained within 2-3 h after death. Cells were harvested by enzymatic digestion of atherosclerotic plaques with 0.15% collagenase for 3-4 h. and seeded into 96-well culture plates. Intimal cells were cultivated for seven days in Medium 199, containing 10% fetal calf serum, glutamine, and antibiotics. The drugs' activity was evaluated by their impact on atherosclerotic indices such as incorporation of [^{3}H]thymidine into cellular DNA, intracellular lipid level and total protein synthesis. On the seventh day of cultivation, test agents were added together with labeled precoursors. Following extensive washing, atherosclerotic indices were determined 24 h after the addition of the agents. Protocols for cell isolation and cultivation as well as technical details of the experiment are presented elsewhere [4,9].

Before lipid determination the cells were rinsed three times with phosphate buffered saline (PBS), treated with an 0.025% Trypsin-EDTA for 5 min, and washed with PBS 5 times (all reagents were from GIBCO Europe Ltd., Paisley, UK). The cells were removed from the substrate with an 0.25% Trypsin-EDTA and washed twice by centrifugation (200xg, 10 min). Lipids were extracted from cells with a chloroform-methanol mixture (1:2, v/v) according to Bligh and Dyer [10]. The total cholesterol content in the lipid extracts was determined using Boehringer Mannheim Monotest^R, Cholesterol CHOD-PAP Method (Cat. no. 236691, Boehringer Mannheim GmbH, Mannheim, FRG). Cholesterol stock standard (Stock no. 965-25, Sigma Chemical Company, St. Louis, MO) was used for standard preparation. Phospholipids, triglycerides, free cholesterol and cholesteryl esters extracted from the cells were separated by TLC and measured by scanning densitometry as described elsewhere [9].

DNA synthesis was evaluated by the incorporation of [^{3}H]thymidine into acid-insoluble cell fraction as described earlier [4].

After incubation with 1 uCi/ml [4,5-^{3}H]leucine (135 Ci/mmol, Amersham International plc., England), the incubation medium and the cells suspended with rubber policeman were heated for 10 min at 80°C, and proteins were precipitated by 10% TCA. The precipitate was washed twice with a 5% TCA and twice with diethyl ether, dissolved with 0.5 N KOH and precipitated again by a 10% TCA. The precipitate was resuspended in a 5% TCA and its radioactivity was measured.

Differences between obtained data were evaluated by means of dispersion analysis with the use of a package of statistical BMDP programs [11].

3. RESULTS AND DISCUSSION

3.1. In Vitro Effects of Anipamil

Earlier it has been shown that phospholipid, free cholesterol, cholesteryl ester and triglyceride contents in human aortic cells cultured from atherosclerotic plaque are considerably higher than in cells cultured from uninvolved intima [4,9]. Incubation with anipamil (10^{-6} M and higher concentrations) 24 h considerably reduced the intracellular content of esterified cholesterol; the efficacy of verapamil in this respect was somewhat lower (Fig. 1). Both anipamil and verapamil significantly decreased the intracellular triglyceride content and, to a lesser extent, free cholesterol content. Neither anipamil nor verapamil had any effect on the phospholipid content (data not shown).

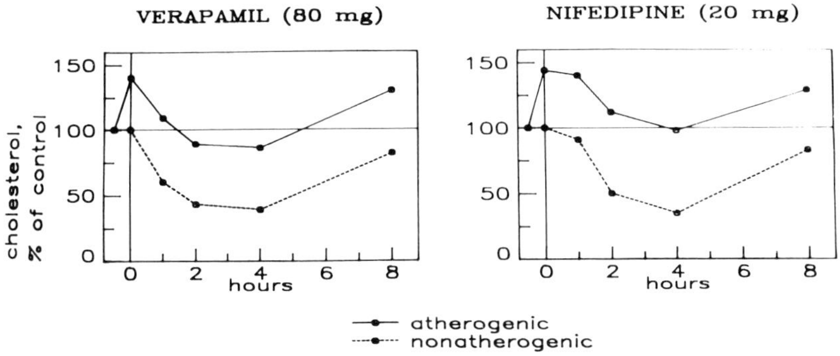

Figure 2. Effect of plasma obtained after administration of verapamil or nifedipine on cholesterol content in cultured atherosclerotic cells. Atherogenic (solid line) and non-atherogenic (broken line) blood was collected prior and 1, 2, 4 and 8 h after the drug administration. Plasma was added to cultured atherosclerotic cells. Intracellular cholesterol content was determined after a 24-h incubation and expressed as the percent of cholesterol content in cells cultured under standard conditions (control). Results of 1 out of 6 representative experiments are shown. Each point is the mean of 3 determinations.

Anipamil and verapamil produced essentially similar effects on the proliferative activity of atherosclerotic cells and total protein synthesis (Fig. 1). It should be mentioned that this effect was observed at 10^{-5} M anipamil concentration, while the effective concentration lowering the intracellular lipid level was 10^{-6} M.

Enantiomers of anipamil, racemate and verapamil produced similar antiatherosclerotic effects on cultured atherosclerotic cells (Table 1).

Thus, anipamil and its enentiomers produced an antiatherosclerotic effect on cultured atherosclerotic cells: they reduced cellular lipid content, proliferative activity and total protein synthesis. Anipamil efficacy appeared to be similar to that of verapamil which is the most potent among calcium antagonists tested previously. In the light of recent data on antiatherogenic and antiatherosclerotic effects of verapamil and nifedipine elicited in humans and in experiental animals, one can suggest that anipamil is efficient not only in vitro but also in vivo.

3.2. Ex Vivo Effects of Calcium Antagonists

In above mentioned clinical investigations the optimal tactics of direct antiatherosclerotic therapy using calcium antagonists was not developed [2,3]. Patients received relatively high doses of these drugs, however, there is no convictive evidence to suggest that such a treatment produces maximal antiatherogenic or antiatherosclerotic effects. Previously we have reported that blood plasma of patients who received calcium antagonists per os acquires an antiatherogenic potential [7]. We believe that specific approach to the optimization of the therapy aimed at a direct antiatherosclerotic effect can be developed by analysing the patient's plasma for atherogenicity following administration of the therapeutic agent. As the first step in this direction, we have examined serum atherogenicity after a single administration of verapamil and nifedipine and after long-term nifedipine therapy.

TABLE 2. Effect of plasma obtained from coronary heart disease patients after a single nifedipine administration on intracellular cholesterol content in cultured human aortic cells

Patient, #	Cholesterol content, % of control		
	1-st day	7-th day	28-th day
1, prior	246+19	237+14	159+14**
1, 4 h after	154+13*	145+10*	112+7*
2, prior	185+17	140+11	131+8**
2, 4 h after	130+9*	101+6*	94+6*
3, prior	254+14	218+12	181+17**
3, 4 h after	178+7*	167+13*	130+10*
4, prior	367+26	342+27	327+28
4, 4 h after	285+19*	261+17*	248+16*

Blood was collected after an overnight fast prior and 4 h after nifedipine administration. Plasma was added to cultured human aortic cells, and the increase in intracellular cholesterol content was determined. Cholesterol content was are expressed as percent of the control (63+4 ug/mg cell protein). *, significant differences from the values obtained prior to nifedipine administration; **, significant differences from the values obtained prior to nifedipine administration on the first day of treatment.

Blood plasma obtained 2 h after administration of verapamil (80 mg) or nifedipine (20 mg) was tested in culture of atherosclerotic cells. After a 24-h incubation, a considerable decrease in intracellular cholesterol content was observed (Fig. 2). Plasma obtained 4 h after the drug administration exhibited a higher antiatherosclerotic activity which disappered in 8 h.

Previously, we have shown that both serum and plasma of patients with angiographically documented coronary atherosclerosis are atherogenic, i.e. they induce cholesterol accumulation in cultured human aortic cells [12-15]. Fig. 2 illustrates an increase in intracellular cholesterol content after a 24-h incubation with atherogenic patient's plasma. Plasma atherogenicity lowered 2 h after nifedipine administration, and disappeared in 4 h. Verapamil reduced plasma atherogenicity 1 h after a single administration. In 2-4 h the atherogenicity disappeared and reappeared 8 h after administration of this agents. Thus, both nifedipine and verapamil produce not only antiatherosclerotic but also preventive antiatherogenic effect.

We have also studied the effect of long-term nifedipine therapy on plasma atherogenicity of patients with coronary atherosclerosis. Blood was collected prior and 4 h after nifedipine administration on day 1, on day 7 and on day 28 of continuous therapy (60 mg daily). On day 7, nifedipine lowered plasma atherogenicity just as effectively as on day 1 (Table 2). On day 28, in 3 out of 4 cases the atherogenicity of plasma obtained prior to the drug administration was lower than the initial atherogenicity at the beginning of the treatment. At the same time, in 2 out of 4 cases atherogenicity disappeared after nifedipine administration. Thus, long-term nifedipine therapy produces a beneficial effect on blood plasma: it lowers the initial atherogenicity, and causes more prominent antiatherogenic effect after the drug administration.

We hope that the control over the atherosclerosis-related properties of plasma obtained from patients after drug administration may be helpful in the optimization of direct antiatherogenic and antiatherosclerotic therapy.

4. REFERENCES

1. Blumlein, S.L., Sievers, R., Kidd, P. and Parmley, W.W. (1985) "Modification of experimental atherosclerosis by calcium-channel blockers", Am. J. Cardiol., 55, 165B-171B.
2. Kober, G., Schneider, W. and Kaltenbach, M. (1989) "Can the progression of coronary sclerosis be influenced by calcium antagonists?", J. Cardiovasc. Pharmacol., 13, S2-S6.
3. Lichtlen, P.R., Hugenholtz, P.G., Rafflenbeul, W. and INTACT-group (1989) "Possible protective effect of nifedipine against progression of atherosclerosis in man (INTACT-study)", in Abstract Book, 4th International Symposium on Calcium Antagonists: Pharmacology and CLinical Research, Florence (Italy), May 25-27, 1989, pp. 127-130
4. Orekhov, A.N., Tertov, V.V., Kudryashov, S.A., Khashimov, Kh.A. and Smirnov, V.N. (1986) "Primary culture of human aortic intima cells as a model for testing antiatherosclerotic drugs. Effects of cyclic AMP, prostaglandins, calcium antagonists, antioxidants, and lipid-lowering agents", Atherosclerosis, 60, 101-110.
5. Orekhov, A.N., Tertov, V.V., Khashimov, Kh.A., Kudryashov, S.A. and Smirnov, V.N. (1986) "Antiatherosclerotic effects of verapamil in primary culture of human aortic intimal cells", J. Hypertension, 4, S153-S155.

6. Orekhov, A.N., Tertov, V.V., Khashimov, Kh.A., Kudryashov, S.A. and Smirnov, V.N. (1987) "Evidence of antiatherosclerotic action of verapamil from direct effects on arterial cells", Am. J. Cardiol., 59, 495-496.
7. Orekhov, A.N., Baldenkov, G.N., Tertov, V.V., Li Hwa Ryong, Kozlov, S.G., Lyakishev, A.A., Tkachuk, V.A., Ruda, M.Ya. and Smirnov, V.N. (1988) "Cardiovascular drugs and atherosclerosis: effects of calcium antagonists, beta-blockers, and nitrates on atherosclerotic characteristics of human aortic cells", J. Cardiovasc. Pharmacol., 12, S66-S68.
8. Baldenkov, G.N., Akopov, S.E., Li, H.R. and Orekhov, A.N. (1988) "Prostacyclin, thromboxane A_2 and calcium antagonists: effects on atherosclerotic characteristics of vascular cells", Biomed. Biochim. Acta, 47, S324-S327.
9. Orekhov, A.N., Tertov, V.V., Novikov, I.D., Krushinsky, A.V., Andreeva, E.R., Lankin, V.Z. and Smirnov, V.N. (1985) "Lipids in cells of atherosclerotic and uninvolved human aorta. I. Lipid composition of aortic tissue and enzyme isolated and cultured cells", Exp. Mol. Pathol., 42, 117-137.
10. Bligh, E.G. and Dyer, W.J. (1959) "A rapid method of total lipid extraction and purification", Can. J. Biochem. Physiol., 37, 911-917.
11. Dixon, W.J. and Brown, M.B. (1977) Biomedical Computer Programs. P-Series, University of California Press, Berkeley, pp. 185-198.
12. Chazov, E.I., Tertov, V.V., Orekhov, A.N., Lyakishev, A.A., Perova, N.V., Kurdanov, Kh.A., Khashimov, Kh.A., Novikov, I.D. and Smirnov, V.N. (1986) "Atherogenicity of blood serum from patients with coronary heart disease", Lancet, 2, 595-598.
13. Orekhov, A.N., Tertov, V.V., Pokrovsky, S.N., Adamova, I.Yu., Martsenyuk, O.N., Lyakishev, A.A. and Smirnov, V.N. (1988) "Blood serum atherogenicity associated with coronary atherosclerosis. Evidence for nonlipid factor providing atherogenicity of low-density lipoproteins and an approach to its elimination", Circ. Res., 62, 421-429.
14. Chazov, E.I., Orekhov, A.N., Tertov, V.V., Pokrovsky, S.N., Adamova, I.Yu., Lyakishev, A.A., Gratsianski, N.A., Nechaev, A.S., Perova, N.V., Khashimov, Kh.A., Kurdanov, Kh.A., Kukharchuk, V.V. and Smirnov, V.N. (1988) "Atherogenicity of blood plasma from patients with coronary atherosclerosis and its correction", Atherosclerosis Rev., 17, 9-20.
15. Tertov, V.V., Orekhov, A.N., Martsenyuk, O.N., Perova, N.V. and Smirnov, V.N. (1989) "Low density lipoproteins isolated from the blood of patients with coronary heart disease induce the accumulation of lipids in human aortic cells", Exp. Mol. Pathol., 50, 337-347.

48
Can the progression of coronary heart disease be influenced by calcium antagonists?

W. SCHNEIDER, P. ROEBRUCK, G. KOBER, M. ALLE, N. REIFART, H.F. SPIES, P. SATTER and M. KALTENBACH

Divisions of Cardiology and Cardiothoracic Surgery, Johann Wolfgang Goethe-University, Theodor-Stern-Kai 7, 6000 Frankfurt a. M., Department of Medical Statistics, University of Heidelberg, Federal Republic of Germany

ABSTRACT. The experimental atherosclerosis in animals, preferentially induced by cholesterol-rich food, can be successfully suppressed by calcium channel blocking agents such as verapamil, nifedipin, nicardipin, and diltiazem.

The question whether calcium channel blockers can favourably influence atherosclerosis in humans remains a matter of debate. A few observational investigations in the past showed positive results of calcium channel blocker therapy in patients with angiographically proven coronary artery disease (CAD).

At present three prospective randomized clinical trials are under way (**INTACT**-study, **FIPS**-study, Study from the Montrael Heart Institute). Target variable is the severity of coronary atherosclerosis as assessed by angiography.

445 patients after coronary bypass surgery were included in the FIPS trial (**F**rankfurt **I**soptin **P**rogression **S**tudy) and randomly allocated to either verapamil 120 mg t.i.d. or placebo treatment. Extent of coronary atherosclerosis, assessed by sequential angiography 1 and 3 years after randomization, is expressed by scores with separate evaluation of non-bypassed vessels, segments distal to the peripheral bypass insertion, bypassed segments and grafts.
The 1-year follow-up was completed by 162 patients (Group A = 80 patients; group B = 82 patients). There was a homogeneous distribution in both groups for all clinical variables, graft patency rates [75 % (A) / 76 % (B)] and the incidence of clinical events (myocardial infarct, need for cardiac surgery or PTCA, cardiac death): 5 % in both groups. The overall progression of atherosclerosis was small.
The question whether calcium channel blockers can retard

progression of coronary atherosclerosis will be answered after completion and careful data evaluation of the aforementioned trials.

1. Introduction

With regard to the complex interaction between calcium and the development of atherosclerosis much interest was focussed in the last decade on calcium channel blocking agents as possible prophylactic and/or therapeutic drugs.

The following mechanisms of action of calcium channel blockers could form the basis for their therapeutic efficacy [1-5]:

a. Improvement of membrane function, especially protection of the endothelium. This protection could enhance the resistance of the endothelium to various noxious agents including a deleterious calcium influx into the cells.

b. Reduction of wall tension due to smooth muscle relaxation.

c. Slowing down of cell migration from the media into the subendothelium and retardation of smooth muscle and mononuclear cell proliferation.

d. Inhibition of the interaction between platelets and the endothelium.

e. Reduction in cellular uptake of LDL cholesterol and improvement of the intracellular lipid metabolism.

2. Experimental Data and Clinical studies

In a series of animal studies it could be convincingly shown in the past that atherosclerosis induced by cholesterol-rich diet alone or in combination with mechanical or electrical irritation of the vessel wall could be successfully suppressed by a broad variety of calcium channel blocking agents [2, 4, 6].
Effectiveness of calcium antagonist therapy was documented by a reduction of the area of atheromas in the large arteries, preferrably in the aorta.

Studies in cultured cells obtained from human atheromas revealed an inhibition of proliferation in the presence of verapamil [7].

Few retrospective studies on patients undergoing sequential angiography suggested beneficial effects of calcium channel blocking agents on the progression of coronary atherosclerosis [8, 9].

Stimulated by these data prospective trials were initiated.

At present 3 prospective trials are under way

1. The **INTACT** study (International Nifedipine Trial on Antiatherosclerotic Therapy) included 425 patients with coronary atherosclerosis who preferrably had early stages of the disease, i.e. it were mainly patients with 1- or 2-vessel disease of minor to moderate severity with well-preserved left ventricular function [1, 10, 11]. The patients received either nifedipine (80 mg daily) or placebo. Target variable was the severity of coronary artery disease as assessed by angiography. The follow-up period was 3 years. Progression of atherosclerosis was assessed by a computerized system (CAAS). The **INTACT** protocol was completed recently and first data will be available in near future. In preliminary communications the authors reported that nifedipine was able to significantly retard development of new stenoses (- 27 % as compared to placebo) while preexisting lesions were not influenced [12].

2. In 1987 the design of a study planned by the **Montreal Heart Institute** was published [13]. 383 patients with angiographically proven coronary artery disease should be entered in a prospective randomized trial (Table 1 a,b). These patients had to show clinical and angiographical parameters which suggested a high likelihood of progression of atherosclerosis. The patients were randomized to receive either nicardipine 90 mg daily or placebo. The follow-up period is designed to be 2 years. The evaluation of angiograms is performed by CAAS. Results are not yet available.

3. In the **FIPS-study** (**F**rankfurt **I**soptin **P**rogression **S**tudy) 445 patients were randomized immediately after coronary bypass surgery to either verapamil 120 mg t.i.d. or placebo. In these patients the severity of coronary atherosclerosis in different vascular regions as well as patency rates and morphological changes of the bypass grafts are investigated.
The follow-up period is 3 years. The protocol of the FIPS-study includes two repeat angiographies 1 and 3 years after randomization. Progression of atherosclerosis is assessed by calibrated measurements of stenoses. I.e. Diameters of stenoses and adjacent normal wall segments are measured with the help of a caliper after projection and magnifica-

tion of the angiography films to a screen.
In this study the coronary vessels are divided into 16 segments. A location factor is attributed to each segment depending on its functional importance. I.e. proximal segments (e.g. the left main artery) receive high figures, distal segments get low figures [14](Fig. 1).
Stenoses are then classified into 5 groups according to their severity.

Then for each segment of the coronary arteries which shows stenoses a score is obtained by multiplication of the stenosis factor with the location factor.

The segmental scores are then added up to give the sum score for an individual patient.

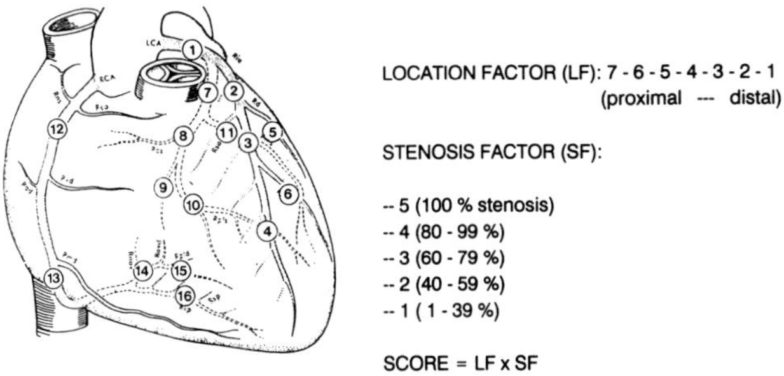

Fig. 1: Division of the coronary vessels into 16 segments: Segment 1: left main coronary artery; segments 2 - 6: LAD; segments 7 - 11: circumflex artery; segments 12 - 16: right coronary artery.
A location factor (LF)(1 - 7) and a stenosis factor (SF) are attributed to each stenosis with regard to the functional importance of the segment and the severity of the stenosis. A score is obtained by multiplication of the stenosis factor with the location factor.

The fact that the **FIPS**-study included patients after coronary bypass surgery made it necessary to differentiate between a core score and auxiliary scores.

The core score comprises non-bypassed segments or vessel portions distal to the peripheral graft insertion. Thus, the core score will represent vessel segments with a supposed natural course of the disease.

Auxiliary scores apply to bypassed segments and the grafts.

Randomization for this study was started in November 1984 and completed in July 1987. The final results wil be reported in August 1990.
207 out of 445 patients (46.5 %) dropped out of the study prior to the first repeat angiography (Table 2). The majority of these patients (73.4 %) left the study within the first 3 months after randomization without having started drug treatment.
It should be emphasized that the patients gave their consent to participation shortly after coronary artery bypass surgery. Events in the following course e.g. need for calcium channel blockers or a change in mind in the postoperative period was responsible for the high early dropout rate.
Beyond the first year the drop-out rates tended to zero. Thus, the number of patients available for final analysis 1990 will not differ significantly from the figures given here.
Additional 36 patients had to be excluded from the 1-year evaluation due to violations of the protocol. 40 patients refused repeat angiography at 1 year. However, the majority of them remained in the study to undergo the 3-year repeat angiography.
The data of 162 patients form the basis for the 1-year report.

Group A (n = 80) had received a total of 185 bypass grafts (mean: 2.31 grafts per patient). In group B (n = 82 patients) a total of 191 grafts (mean: 2.33 grafts per patient) was inserted (Fig. 2).

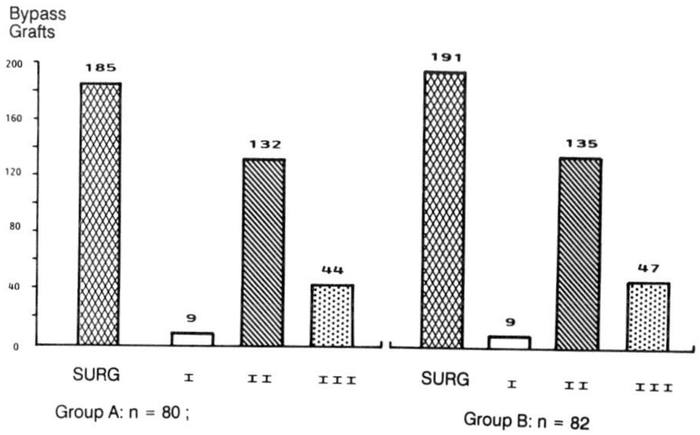

Fig. 2: Bypass patency 1 year after CABG. In group A (n = 80) 185 grafts were inserted, in group B (n = 82) 191 grafts.

I: Patent grafts with stenoses
II: Patent grafts
III: Closed grafts

At repeat angiography, the patency rates were 76 % in group A (141 grafts) and 75 % in group B (144 patent grafts) respectively. In each group 9 grafts showed luminal narrowings.

Overall progression of coronary artery disease in the first year was expectedly small, with no significant differences between both groups.

44 % of the patients of group A and 43 % of the patients in group B showed progression in at least one segment.

Progression in the first year after bypass surgery was not related to any risk factor (i.e. Hypertension, history of smoking, diabetes, hyperlipidemia).

3. Conclusions

a. The currently available experimental data support the view that calcium channel blocking agents are able to retard coronary atherosclerosis.

b. The beneficial pharmacological effects of calcium channel blocking agents on vessel walls comprise:

- Protection of the membranes (endothelium)
- Inhibition of platelet aggregation and liberation of PDGF
- Inhibition of proliferation and migration of smooth muscle cells and macrophages
- Inhibition of cellular calcium accumulation

c. The question of the clinical relevance of calcium channel blocker therapy for the development of human coronary atherosclerosis can be answered after termination of the prospective trials and careful evaluation of the angiographic data.

d. Preliminary data of one of the prospective trials suggest that calcium channel blockers may prevent formation of new stenoses rather than affect preexisting stenoses.

4. References

1. Hugenholtz, P.G., Lichtlen, P., Van der Giessen, W., Becker, A.E., Nayler, W.G., Fleckenstein, A. and Hülsmann, W.C. (1986) 'On a possible role for calcium antagonists in atherosclerosis. A personal view' Eur. Heart J. 7, 546-559

2. Betz, E., Hämmerle, H., Kling, D., Lenke, D., Müller, C.D. (1986) 'Wirkungen von Verapamil am Arteriosklerose-Modell' in: J. Rosenthal (ed.), Calcium-Antagonisten und Hypertonie - Aktueller Stand, Excerpta Medica Amsterdam, Hongkong, Princeton, Sydney, Tokyo, pp. 83-97

3. Henry, P.D. and Bentley, K.L. (1981) 'Suppression of atherogenesis in cholesterol-fed rabbits treated with nifedipine'. J. Clin. Invest. 68: 1366-1369

4. Nayler, W.G. (1988) 'Calcium antagonists and atherosclerosis'. in: W.G. Nayler (ed.), Calcium antagonists, Academic press, Harcourt Brace Jovanovich, Publ., London, San Diego, New York, Berkely, Boston, Sidney, Toronto, Tokyo, pp. 325-247

5. Stein, O., Leitersdorf, E. and Stein, Y. (1985) 'Verapamil enhances receptor-mediated endocytosis of low-density lipoproteins by aortic cells in culture' Arteriosclerosis 5, 35-44

6. Henry, P.D. (1985) 'Atherosclerosis, calcium, and calcium antagonists' Circulation 72, 456-459

7. Orekhov, A.N., Tertov, V.V., Khashimov, K.A., Kudryashov, S.S. and Smirnov, V.N. (1987) 'Evidence of antiatherosclerotic action of verapamil from direct effects on arterial cells' Am. J. Cardiol. 59, 495-496

8. Klein, W., Lufty, A. and Schreyer, H. (1983) 'Effect of long-term tretament with calcium blockers on human coronary atherosclerosis', in: A. Fleckenstein, K. Hashimoto, M. Hermann, A. Schwartz and L. Seipel (eds.), New Calcium Antagonists. Recent Developmewnts and Prospects. Gustav-Fischer-Verlag, Stuttgart, p. 183

9. Kober, G., Nickelsen, T., Jakobs, B. and Kaltenbach, M. (1986) 'Der Einfluß einer Langzeittherapie mit Calciumantagonisten auf die Entwicklung der stenosierenden Koronarsklerose' in: J. Rosenthal (ed.), Calcium-Antagonisten und Hypertonie - Aktueller Stand. Excerpta Medica Amsterdam, Hongkong, Princeton, Sydney, Tokyo, pp. 98-107

10. Jost, S., Deckers, J., Nellessen, U., Rafflenbeul, W., Hecker, H., Reiber, J.C.H., Lippolt, P., Hugenholtz, P.G., Lichtlen, P.R. and INTACT-Studiengruppe (1989) 'Computergestützte geometrische Meßtechnik in koronarangiographischen Intervallstudien: Ergebnisse bei Erstangiogrammen der INTACT-Studie' Z. Kardiol. 78, 23-32

11. Lichtlen, P.R., Nellessen, U., Rafflenbeul, W., Jost, S. and Hecker, H. (1987) 'International Nifedipine Trial on antiatherosclerotic therapy (INTACT)' Cardiovasc. Drugs and Ther. 1, 71-79

12. Lichtlen, P.R. (1989), quoted in: Fortschr. Med. 107, Suppl. 71, 5-8

13. Waters, D., Freedman, D., Lesperance, J., Theroux, P., Lemarbre, L., Kamm, B., Joyal, M., Dyrda, I., Gosselin, G., Hudow, G., Hache, M., Halloran, J. and Havel R.J. (1987) 'Design features of a controlled clinical trial to assess the effect of a calcium entry blocker upon the progression of coronary artery disease' Controlled Clin. Trials 8, 216-242

14. Kaltenbach, M. (1975) 'Quantitative Bewertung koronarographischer Befunde mit Hilfe eines Punktsystems (Score)' Z. Kardiol. 64, 597-606

ATHEROSCLEROSIS REGRESSION FROM A CLINICAL AND ANATOMO-PATHOLOGICAL STANDPOINT

49

A five year follow up of carotid atherosclerosis using B-mode imaging ultrasound

M. MERCURI, A. SUSTA, M.G. VEDOVELLI, G. BRUNETTI, G. LUPATTELLI, U. SENIN and A. VENTURA

2nd Department of Internal Medicine, University of Perugia, Policlinico Monteluce, 06100 Perugia, Italy

ABSTRACT. A high resolution, real-time scanner was used to follow up atherosclerotic carotid lesions in 95 subjects during five years. After a mean follow-up time of 45.7 months 77 new stenoses were imaged, 28 stenoses progressed of at least 10%; 10 stenoses regressed.

INTRODUCTION. Atherosclerosis is the most common direct cause of ischaemia. While infarction, due to thrombosis or artery-to-artery embolism, is usually a sudden phenomenon, atherosclerosis begins years before the development of clinical signs and symptoms; it progresses silently during the early stages. The haemodynamic inbalance; i.e. sudden thromboembolic occlusion and vasospasm, is the classic pathogenetic mechanism to explain necrosis at the site of ischemia, but the atherosclerotic source of emboli is most of the times located proximally to the occluded vessel. In cerebral ischaemic events, atherosclerosis of the bifurcation area, i.e. distal common carotid, carotid bifurcation, and internal carotid arteries, plays a key role. In 1984, a longitudinal research to investigate the etiology and natural history of carotid atherosclerosis using a B-mode Imaging ultrasound system was designed in order to generate hypothesis to be tested in population-based studies on atherosclerosis. We report here the results of an up to five year study period in 95 major stroke asymptomatic subjects affected by carotid bifurcation area atherosclerosis.

MATERIAL AND METHODS. Ninetyfive men and women, age range: 45-80 years, who had been recruited between January 1984 and December 1985, were followed up in an interval of time ranging between 6 and 12 months for at least 3 years (mean follow-up: 45.7 months). Subjects were referred to our clinic for a variety of reasons: TIA (28), Heart Diseases (15), Peripheral Artery Diseases (19) and/or major atherosclerotic risk factors (Hypertension -48, Hyperlipidemia -29, Diabetes -15); 44 of them had a smoking habit. The apparatus used was a high resolution, small-part, real-time scanner (Biosound Inc., Indianapolis IN, USA). The examinations were recorded by a 3/4" professional 'U-Matic' VCR. Reproducibility of measurements (target object separation, phantom vessel lumen, and simulated wall thickness) were checked periodically against an ultrasound phantom (RMI, UK). A videoprinter (Mitsubishi, Japan) provided hard copies of images both in real-time and during later evaluations.

A continuous Doppler and a computer-assisted spectrum analysis of the Doppler signal, were also used to confirm the diagnosis of occlusion when no discernible lumen was seen. The quality controls were regularly carried out by the registered Biosound technicians on a six month basis, or whenever necessary. Anterior, lateral, posterolateral, and transverse projection scans were performed. In order to detect lowreflecting plaques the Time Gain Control was kept initially high (6/10), then adjusted just at the point where the image degrades by noise artifacts. To indicate the exact seat of the lesions, carotid bifurcation was divided into four sites: common carotid (CCA), bifurcation (BIF), internal carotid (ICA), and external carotid (ECA) arteries. The vessel wall was also indicated as anterior, posterior, lateral and medial. The electronic marker pinpointed the stenosis on the videoscreen, and this was videotaped for later analysis together with the echographic images of the vessel wall. Carotid and peri-orbital Doppler tests supplemented these data to provide a comprehnsive vascular evaluation. The same procedure was used for all the checkups. The sonographer performed the subsequent evaluation looking for stenoses in their maximal point and clear view in each sites. Blind readings of videotapes and prints of the stenotic sites were carried out by two different readers. The severity of atherosclerotic lesions were measured by an indirect method; we used the "Stenosis" (S) of the vessel as our major "lesion" endpoint. The "Combined Mean Maximum Stenosis" (CMMS) was used as an indirect index of the extent and severity of carotid atherosclerosis for the right and left side. Our criteria of interpretation were as follows: 1. Maximum Arterial Stenosis (S) in each of the 6 (3 on the right and 3 on the left) sites. This was calculated using the following formula: S = (Dt - /Dr+K/)/ Dt %.
2. Combined Mean Maximum Stenosis (CMMS): CMMS = (S1+S2+S3 / 3) X 10. Stenosis was defined by comparing the images from different projections and choosing the one revealing its maximum point. Stenosis was considered changed (progressed or regressed) when a variation exceeding 10% of the previous measurement was found. The validation study is fully described in Senin et al. 1988 (1).

RESULTS. At the baseline examinations 224 carotid stenoses (113 on the right side and 111 on the left) were imaged by B-Mode ultrasound in 95 subjects. Forty-one stenoses were imaged on the common carotid arteries (CCA), 107 on the bifurcations (BIF), and 76 on the internal carotid arteries (ICA). In 140 sites stenoses were smaller than 35% of the vessel diameter (mean stenosis: 24.85%), in 66 between 35 and 50% (41.2%), and in 17 larger than 50% (75.12%). After a mean follow-up of 45.7 months, 77 new stenoses were imaged (+34.4%); 28 stenoses progressed of at least 10% (12.5%); 10 stenoses regressed (4.46%). Stenoses smaller than 35% had a mean progression of 5% (from 24.85 to 29.98); the one between 35 and 50% a mean regression of about 6% (41.2-35.32); those larger than 50% were almost unchanged (75.12-72.41). After 45.7 months stenoses had a mean regression of about 2% on CCA, a mean progression of about 2% on both BIF and ICA. When all the 95 subjects were included into the analysis the mean stenoses progressed on each of the three arterial segments. The progression was of about 2.5% on CCA, 4% on BIF, and 7% on ICA. The CMMS for the carotid bifurcation area, which is an indirect index of exent and severity of atherosclerosis, progressed in 95 subjects from

134.4 to 183.9 (+49.5) on the right side, and from 126.5 to 188.3 (+61.8) on the left side. CONCLUSION. Ninety-five subjects affected by atherosclerosis of the carotid bifurcation were followed up, for an average period of 47.5 months, using B-Mode imaging ultrasound. The carotid bifurcation area is particularly prone to atherosclerosis; the geometry of this arterial segment is the basis for haemodynamic conditions associated with plaque formation (2). A number for haemodynamic variables have been proposed to account for the selective distribution of plaques (3), i.e. wall shear stress, flow separation and stasis, oscillation of shear stress vectors, turbulence, and hypertension. Furthermore it is now evident that as plaques develope, a closely associated enlargement of the affected artery segment tends to limit the stenosing effect (4). It has been shown that when the coronary plaque involves the entire circumference of the vessel producing more than 40% stenosis, the artery is no longer able to enlarge sufficiently to prevent the narrowing of the lumen. However, different segments of the coronary tree respond differently to increasing plaque, and no similar data is avalaible to describe the behaviour of the carotid bifurcation. Furthermore progression and regression of atherosclerosis over the years is quite well-documented by serial angiography or echotomography of coronary, carotid and femoral arteries (5-7). Our data showed that maximum arterial stenosis of the carotid bifurcation area progressed in 95 atherosclerosis high risk subjects, the mean progression being between 2.5 and 7% according to the site (CCA, BIF, ICA). Furthermore after 45.7 months 77 new stenosis were imaged. This data was confirmed by the progression (ranging between 41.5 and 61.8) of the CMMS, which is an indirect index of severity and extent of atherosclerosis. However, the 224 stenoses detected at recruitment had a different behaviour; in fact the rate and direction of changes were different according to both the initial arterial stenosis and site. Our data suggests that the rate of progression was slower for stenoses ranging between 35 and 50% compared to the ones smaller than 35%. Furthermore, the direction of changes was negative on CCA, but positive on BIF and ICA. It suggests that CCA is more prone to compensatory onlargement compared to BIF and ICA. Finally the number of stenoses larger than 50% was insufficient to suggest any specific trend in that group. In conclusion our prospective investigation, using B-Mode imaging throws some light on an important area of the natural history of atherosclerosis; the compensatory enlargments of the arterial wall as an answer to the intimal development of the plaque should be more deeply investigated and considered. AKNWOLEDGEMENT. We wish to thank Simonetta Simonetti, MD, Giuseppe Valigi, MD, Alfredo Villa, MD for their technical assistance, and Dr. M.Rita Pignatelli for her assistance in the preparation of this manuscript.

REFERENCES.

1. Senin, U., Parnetti, L., Mercuri, M. et al.(1988) ' Evolutionary trends in carotid atherosclerotic plaques: results of a two year follow-up study using an ultrasound imaging system ', Angiology 5, 429.

2. Zarins, CK., Glagov, S.(1989) ' Artery wall pathology in atherosclerosis, in R.B. Rutherford (Ed), Vascular surgery, Philadelphia, p.178.

3. Caro, CG., Pedley, TJ., Schroter, RC. et al.(1978) The mechanics of the circulation, Oxford University Press, Oxford.
4. Glagow, S., Weisenberg, E., Zarins, CK., et al.(1987) 'Compensatory enlargement of human atherosclerotic coronary arteries', N.Engl.J. Med. 316, 1371.
5. Olsson, AG., Erickson,U., Helmius, G., et al. (1984) 'Regression of femoral atherosclerosis in humans', in M.R. Malinow and W.H. Blatons (Eds), Regression of atherosclerotic lesions, Plenum Press, New York, p.311.
6. Hennerici, M., Rautenberg, W., Trockel, U., et al.(1985) 'Spontaneous progression and regression of small carotid atheroma', Lancet 1,1415.
7. Brown, BG., Liin, JT., Kelsey, S., et al.(1989) 'Progression of coronary atherosclerosis in patients with probable familial hypercholesterolemia. Quantitative arteriographic assessment of patients in NHLBI type II study', Arteriosclerosis 9, 1-81.

50
Preliminary results of the program on the surgical control of the hyperlipidemias (POSCH)

H. BUCHWALD, C.T. CAMPOS and the POSCH Group

Department of Surgery, Box 290 UMHC, University of Minnesota, Minneapolis, MN 55455, USA

ABSTRACT. The Program on the Surgical Control of the Hyperlipidemias (POSCH) is a randomized, prospective, secondary intervention trial examining the effects of lipid modification on overall mortality and the course of atherosclerotic cardiovascular disease in 838 survivors of a single myocardial infarction. Partial ileal bypass, a surgical procedure developed at the University of Minnesota and introduced in 1963, was selected as the intervention modality in POSCH. Complete, five-year lipid results are available currently in 660 POSCH participants, 330 surgical patients and 330 control patients treated with the Phase II American Heart Association diet. Total plasma cholesterol was 24.3 ± 0.9 percent lower (mean ± SEM) and low density lipoprotein (LDL) cholesterol was 38.7 ± 1.2 percent lower in the surgical group when compared with the diet-treated controls five years following operation. High density lipoprotein (HDL) cholesterol was 6.9 ± 1.8 percent higher in the surgical patients. In a subgroup of 185 control and 190 surgical patients undergoing apolipoprotein and HDL subfraction analysis, apolipoprotein B-100 was significantly lower and apolipoprotein A-I and HDL subfraction 2 were significantly higher in the operated patients in comparison with the controls. Partial ileal bypass has induced marked, sustained, favorable lipid modification. Based on morbidity and mortality assumptions derived from epidemiologic analyses, these lipid alterations should result in significant reductions in atherosclerotic cardiovascular disease morbidity and mortality when the final POSCH morbidity and mortality experience is examined at the conclusion of the trial in July, 1990.

1. INTRODUCTION

The lipid (cholesterol)-atherosclerosis theory states that atherosclerosis is a disease of multiple causes in which altered lipid metabolism, particularly hypercholesterolemia, plays an integral role [1]. The causal relationship between cholesterol and atherosclerosis has been demonstrated clearly in experimental models and by epidemiologic analyses [2]. Conclusive evidence supporting the therapeutic arm of the lipid-atherosclerosis theory, namely that reducing elevated total plasma cholesterol and LDL cholesterol levels will decrease overall and atherosclerotic cardiovascular disease morbidity and mortality, remains elusive. The principal intervention trials to-date have demonstrated a reduction in coronary atherosclerosis progression assessed angiographically 3 and a decrease in atherosclerotic cardiovascular disease morbidity and mortality when multiple endpoints are combined for statistical examination [4,5]. However, lipid modification has not been demonstrated significantly to alter individual cardiovascular disease endpoints, and no significant overall survival benefit has been demonstrated [3-5].

The Program on the Surgical Control of the Hyperlipidemias (POSCH) is a randomized, prospective intervention trial examining whether the lipid modification achieved by partial ileal bypass has any beneficial effect on overall and atherosclerotic cardiovascular disease morbidity and mortality in survivors of a single myocardial infarction. Between 1975 and 1983, 838 patients were entered into this trial, with 417 randomized to the control group and 421 undergoing partial ileal bypass. Both groups received instruction in the Phase II American Heart Association diet limiting fat intake to 25 percent of daily calories and restricting daily cholesterol consumption to between 200 and 250 milligrams. As of October 1, 1988, complete five-year lipid results were available in 660 POSCH patients, 330 in the control group and 330 in the surgical group. These data are the basis of this report.

2. PARTIAL ILEAL BYPASS

Partial ileal bypass was developed and introduced for the management of hypercholesterolemia in 1963. Over 600 partial ileal bypass procedures have been performed in programs in the United States and abroad currently evaluating this method of lipid modification [6-8]. The operative procedure is illustrated in Figure 1.

Prior to surgery, intestinal preparation is undertaken, at least overnight, with a clear liquid diet, oral antibiotics, and cathartics. Under general anesthesia, the abdomen is entered through a right lower quadrant, transverse incision 2 cm below the umbilicus unless an additional procedure (e.g., cholecystectomy) is planned, in which case an upper transverse or a vertical midline incision is employed. The small bowel length is measured along the mesenteric border (1), allowing 25 cm for the duodenal length. The intestine is transected 200 cm proximal to the ileocecal valve or at a distance one-third the small bowel length from the ileocecal valve if the total length is greater than 600 cm (2). The distal end of the divided ileum is closed (3), and the proximal end is anastomosed, in end-to-side fashion, into the anterior taenia of the cecum approximately 6 cm above the inverted appendiceal stump (4,5). If present, the appendix is removed routinely. The closed end of the bypassed ileum is sutured to the anterior taenia of the cecum, between the anastomosis and the appendiceal stump, to prevent intussusception of this segment (6). The mesenteric defects are closed to prevent internal herniation. The abdomen is thoroughly irrigated with antibiotic-containing saline, is aspirated dry, and is closed using interrupted, non-absorbable sutures to complete the procedure.

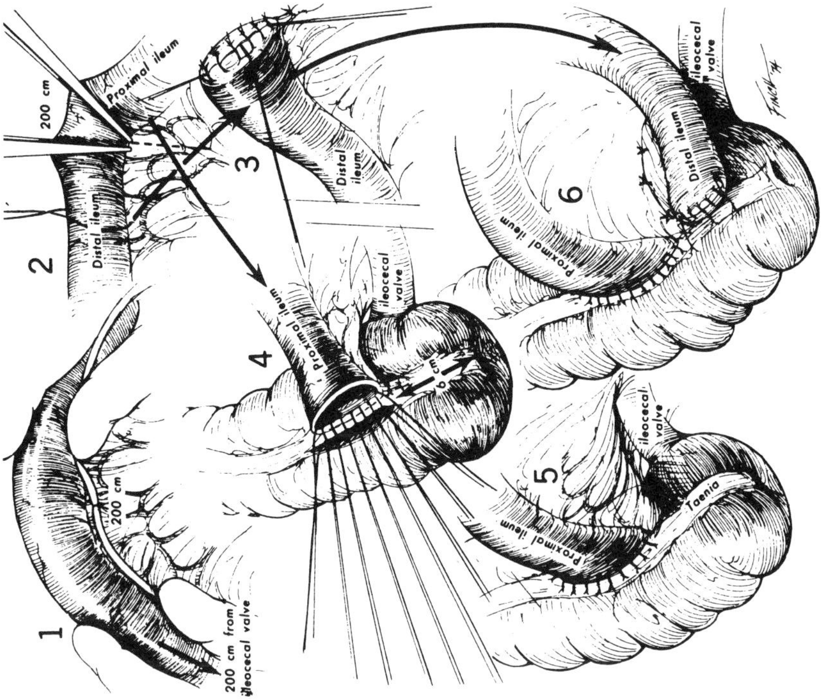

Figure 1. The partial ileal bypass procedure.

3. RESULTS

3.1 Baseline Characteristics

The control and surgical groups were well matched by randomization. Compared to the surgery group, a greater number of control patients had stopped cigarette smoking (187 versus 157, corrected X^2 = 5.38, p = 0.02), and the control group fasting glucose was slightly lower (96 ± 0.5 mg/dl versus 98 ± 0.6 mg/dl, p = 0.06). The majority of patients displayed the normal World Health Organization lipoprotein phenotype -- hypercholesterolemia was present; however, total plasma cholesterol did not exceed the 90th percentile or plasma triglycerides did not exceed the 95th percentile for age and sex required for assignment to a specific phenotype. Selected baseline characteristics are summarized in Table 1.

Table 1. Baseline characteristics of the 330 control and the 330 surgical patients

	Control	Surgery
Age (yrs)	50.8 ± 0.4	51.5 ± 0.4
Male	303 (92)	293 (89)
Caucasian	323 (98)	321 (97)
Systolic B.P. (mm Hg)	122 ± 0.8	121 ± 0.8
Diastolic B.P. (mm Hg)	79 ± 0.5	79 ± 0.5
Quetelet index (gm/cm^2)	2.7 ± 0.02	2.7 ± 0.02
Fasting glucose (mg/dl)	96 ± 0.5	98 ± 0.6
Cigarette smoking		
Never	42 (13)	45 (14)
Former	187 (57)	157 (48)
Current	101 (31)	128 (39)
Lipoprotein phenotype		
Normal	200 (61)	195 (59)
Type II-A	52 (16)	58 (18)
Type II-B	9 (3)	10 (3)
Type IV	69 (21)	67 (20)

Continuous data as mean ± SEM.
Values in parentheses are percentages.

3.2. Total Plasma Cholesterol, LDL Cholesterol, and HDL Cholesterol Results.

The lipid results in the 330 control and the 330 surgical patients are presented in Table 2.

Table 2. Total plasma cholesterol, LDL cholesterol, and HDL cholesterol results

		TC	LDL	HDL
Baseline	C	249.0 ± 1.7	176.8 ± 1.8	40.4 ± 0.5
	S	251.2 ± 1.9	179.3 ± 2.0	40.1 ± 0.5
3 months	C	248.0 ± 2.7	176.7 ± 2.5	40.9 ± 0.6
	S	166.9 ± 1.9*	95.3 ± 1.6*	42.2 ± 0.7+
1 year	C	244.7 ± 2.0	173.1 ± 2.1	40.1 ± 0.5
	S	175.1 ± 1.7*	99.8 ± 1.4*	43.1 ± 0.6*
2 years	C	243.8 ± 2.0+	173.8 ± 1.9	39.4 ± 0.5
	S	177.9 ± 1.8*	101.1 ± 1.4*	42.1 ± 0.6+
3 years	C	239.1 ± 1.8*	170.4 ± 1.9+	39.3 ± 0.5
	S	175.9 ± 1.7*	98.8 ± 1.4*	42.4 ± 0.6+
4 years	C	242.8 ± 1.9+	171.3 ± 1.9+	39.9 ± 0.5
	S	181.2 ± 1.8*	101.7 ± 1.5*	42.4 ± 0.5+
5 years	C	237.2 ± 1.9*	166.1 ± 1.9*	40.1 ± 0.5
	S	178.9 ± 1.8*	100.3 ± 1.5*	42.5 ± 0.6+

TC = total plasma cholesterol; C = Control; S = Surgery.
Values as mean ± SEM in mg/dl. + $p < 0.05$ versus baseline;
* $p < 0.002$ versus baseline.

Total plasma cholesterol levels were similar between the control and surgery groups at baseline. Three months following partial ileal bypass, total plasma cholesterol decreased significantly in the surgery group. This marked reduction from baseline was sustained over the five-year follow-up period. The control group total plasma cholesterol also fell significantly over the five-year follow-up period; however, this reduction was much smaller than that observed in the surgery group. Five years after operation, total plasma cholesterol was 24.3 ± 0.9% lower in the surgery group compared to the diet-treated control group.

LDL cholesterol levels were comparable between groups at baseline (Table 2). Three months following surgery, LDL cholesterol fell dramatically and remained significantly lower than baseline throughout five years of follow-up. LDL cholesterol also decreased after five years in the control group; however, not nearly to the extent observed in the surgical group. Compared to the control group, LDL cholesterol was 38.7 ± 1.2% lower in the surgical group five years after partial ileal bypass.

HDL cholesterol levels were nearly identical between groups at baseline (Table 2). Three months following partial ileal bypass, HDL cholesterol increased significantly from baseline. This increase from baseline was sustained throughout the follow-up period. In the control group, HDL cholesterol remained unchanged over time. Five years following surgery, HDL cholesterol was 6.9 ± 1.8% higher in the surgery group in comparison with the diet-treated controls.

3.3. Apolipoprotein and HDL Subfraction Results

After June of 1985, apolipoprotein and HDL subfraction analyses were performed on all POSCH patients presenting for routine follow-up. Apolipoprotein A-I, apolipoprotein B-100, HDL subfraction 2, and HDL subfraction 3 levels were available in the subgroup of 185 control and 190 surgical patients returning for five-year follow-up after June, 1985 (Table 3).

Table 3. Five-year apolipoprotein and HDL subfraction results

	Apolipoprotein A-I	Apolipoprotein B-100	HDL-2	HDL-3
Control	105.2 ± 1.5	124.5 ± 1.6	8.5 ± 0.4	31.4 ± 0.5
Surgery	120.8 ± 1.5*	91.5 ± 1.3*	11.3 ± 0.5*	31.6 ± 0.5

Values as mean ± SEM in mg/dl. * $p < 0.001$ Control versus Surgery.

A significantly lower apolipoprotein B-100 level and significantly higher apolipoprotein A-I and HDL subfraction 2 levels were observed in the surgery group in comparison with the diet-treated controls.

4. DISCUSSION

The five-year lipid results of the Program on the Surgical Control of the Hyperlipidemias confirm that partial ileal bypass leads to marked, obligatory total plasma cholesterol and LDL cholesterol reductions. HDL cholesterol increases slightly, but significantly, following operation and is nearly 7% higher in comparison to diet-treated controls five years after surgery. The maximal effect occurs within three months and is sustained, essentially unchanged, over five years. Decreased partial ileal bypass efficacy with small intestinal adaptation over time does not occur. Five years after surgery, apolipoprotein B-100 levels were significantly lower and apolipoprotein A-I and HDL-2 levels were significantly higher in comparison with diet-treated controls. Decreased apolipoprotein A-I and HDL subfraction 2 levels and increased apolipoprotein B-100 levels are correlated with greater atherosclerosis incidence and severity.

Partial ileal bypass leads to lipid modification through a two-fold drain on body cholesterol pools. A direct drain results from increased fecal loss of normally absorbed exogenous (dietary) and endogenous (biliary and intestinally-secreted) cholesterol. An indirect drain occurs as hepatic conversion of body cholesterol to bile salts increases to maintain the normal bile acid reservoir. Evaluation of cholesterol dynamics following partial ileal bypass has demonstrated a 60% reduction in intestinal cholesterol absorption and a 3.8-fold increase in total fecal steroid excretion with a 4.9-fold increase in bile acid and a 2.7-fold increase in neutral steriod losses. A compensatory 5.7-fold increase in the cholesterol synthesis rate occurs. One year after partial ileal bypass, the total exchangeable cholesterol pool is reduced by 33%, reflecting decreases in both the freely miscible (plasma, red blood cells, liver, and intestinal mucosa) and in the less freely miscible (fat stores, muscle, solid organs, and vessel walls) cholesterol pools [9,10].

Diarrhea is the most frequent side effect following partial ileal bypass. Generally, this is neither a significant nor a persistent problem. One year post-operatively, 86% of patients have fewer than five bowel movements per day without bowel-controlling medications. Further intestinal adaptation occurs with an increase in stool firmness and a further decrease in stool frequency [6]. Vitamin B_{12} absorption is severely impaired or lost following surgery. All patients receive 1,000 micrograms of vitamin B_{12} intramuscularly every six to eight weeks to prevent pernicious anemia. Calcium oxalate renal calculi occur more frequently following partial ileal bypass. Oral calcium supplementation, maintenance of adequate hydration, and restriction of dietary oxalate intake are recommended but have had minimal success in reducing the incidence of oxalate stones. The effect of urine alkalization using oral potassium citrate on kidney stone occurrence is currently undergoing evaluation. Excessive, foul-smelling flatus and the gas-bloat syndrome occur infrequently after partial ileal bypass. These symptoms generally improve with oral metronidazole therapy. It is important to distinguish partial ileal bypass from the more extensive jejunoileal bypass formerly employed for the treatment of morbid obesity. Partial ileal bypass does not induce weight loss, the electrolyte imbalances, the nutrient malabsorption, and the hepatic insufficiency occasionally observed after jejunoileal bypass [11].

Despite a lack of evidence demonstrating any beneficial effect of lipid modification on overall mortality, it has become standard medical practice to recommend cholesterol reduction in hypercholesterolemic patients. Dietary restriction of fat and cholesterol intake and pharmacologic alternatives have assumed a predominant role. The lipid modification accomplished by partial ileal bypass is significant and of a magnitude attainable only with high-dose, combination drug therapy or with maximal doses of a relatively new class of agents, the inhibitors of 3-hydroxy-3-methylglutaryl coenzyme A (HMG-CoA) reductase, whose long-term efficacy and side effect profile remain undefined.

Epidemiologic evidence from the Framingham Study [12] and from the Lipid Research Clinics - Coronary Primary Trial [4] suggests that a 2% reduction in cardiovascular mortality will be realized from each 1% reduction in total plasma cholesterol. Based on this assumption, marked reductions in atherosclerotic cardiovascular disease morbidity and mortality may be anticipated when the final morbidity, mortality, and serial angiographic results of the Program on the Surgical Control of the Hyperlipidemias are examined in July, 1990.

5. ACKNOWLEDGEMENTS

This work is supported by grant HL-15265 and by National Research Service Award HL-07586 (CTC) from the National Heart, Lung, and Blood Institute of the National Institutes of Health.

6. REFERENCES

1. Frantz, I.D. Jr. and Moore, R.B. (1969) 'The sterol hypothesis in atherogenesis', Am. J. Med., 46, 684-690.
2. Ross, R. (1986) 'The pathogenesis of atherosclerosis - an update', N. Engl. J. Med., 314, 488-500.
3. Blankenhorn, D.M., Nessim, S.A., Johnson, R.L., et al. (1987) 'Beneficial effects of combined colestipol-niacin therapy on coronary atherosclerosis and coronary venous bypass grafts', J.A.M.A., 257, 3233-3240.
4. Lipid Research Clinics Program. (1984) 'The Lipid Research Clinics Coronary Primary Prevention Trial results: I. Reduction in incidence of coronary heart disease', J.A.M.A., 251, 351-364.
5. Frick, M.H., Elo, M.O., Haapa, K., et al. (1987) 'Helsinki Heart Study: primary prevention trial with gemfibrozil in middle-aged men with dyslipidemia', N. Engl. J. Med., 317, 1237-1245.
6. Buchwald, H., Moore, R.B., Varco, R.L. (1974) 'Ten years clinical experience with partial ileal bypass in management of the hyperlipidemias', Ann. Surg., 180, 384-392.
7. Koivisto, P., Miettinen, T.A. (1984) 'Long-term effect of ileal bypass on lipoproteins in patients with familial hypercholesterolemia', Circulation, 70, 290-296.
8. Schouten, J.A., Beynen, A.C. (1986) 'Partial ileal bypass in the treatment of heterozygous familial hypercholesterolemia: a review', Artery, 13, 240-263.

9. Moore, R.B., Frantz, I.D. Jr., Buchwald, H. (1969) 'Changes in cholesterol pool size, turnover rate, and fecal bile acid and sterol excretion after partial ileal bypass in hypercholesterolemic patients', Surgery, 65, 98-108.
10. Buchwald, H., Moore, R.B., Varco, R.L. (1974) 'Surgical treatment of hyperlipidemia', Circulation, 49(suppl I), 1-37.
11. Buchwald, H., Moore, R.B., Varco, R.L. (1983) 'Partial ileal bypass for control of hyperlipidemia and atherosclerosis', in D.C. Sabiston, Jr. and F.C. Spencer (eds.), Gibbon's Surgery of the Chest, W.B. Saunders, Philadelphia, pp. 1515-1534.
12. Cornfield, J. (1962) 'Joint dependence of risk of coronary heart disease on serum cholesterol and systolic blood pressure: a discriminant function analysis', Fed. Proc. 21(suppl 11), 58-61.

51
The time course of atherosclerotic lesion regression in macaque monkeys

R.W. WISSLER and D. VESSELINOVITCH

Department of Pathology and The Specialized Center of Research in Atherosclerosis, University of Chicago, Chicago, IL 60637, USA

ABSTRACT. Nine two-year regression experiments, seven utilizing rhesus monkeys and two using cynomolgus monkeys, have been conducted. Induction of lesions was carried out with a mixture of coconut oil and butterfat in five experiments, and with peanut oil in four experiments, all with 2% cholesterol in the ration. The study plan consisted of one year of lesion induction and one year of intervention with diet alone or with diet plus serum lipid lowering drugs or with a combination of drugs.

In rhesus, a very low fat, low cholesterol diet reduced the advanced and intermediate raised lesions produced by coconut oil, butter, and cholesterol by about 2/3. The same diet combined with cholestyramine yielded an average lesion size reduction of 5/6, whereas the more fibrous peanut oil induced lesions were reduced by about the same proportion in surface area and were less reduced in thickness or in morphometrically measured microscopic lesion area.

Time interval studies using coconut oil and butter for lesion induction indicate that microscopic regression of lesion areas is very prompt, with about half occurring in the first four months and with almost 2/3 of the microscopically stainable lipid removed in the same time period. Gross lesion surface area and microscopic lesion thickness follow somewhat more slowly.

1. INTRODUCTION

The purpose of this manuscript is to report on some of the main results of four studies performed with rhesus and cynomologus monkeys in which the development and regression of the lesions of atherosclerosis were measured at intervals of four months. Two of these experiments utilized peanut oil as the main food fat for induction of the experimental atherosclerosis and in two of the studies a 1:1 mixture of coconut oil and butterfat was used to induce the lesions. In all four experiments the induction diet contained 2% cholesterol and was based on a special purina monkey chow compounded to our specifications by the special diets division of the Ralston Purina Company (Richmond, Indiana). Figure 1 shows the specific plan of the study in which it is evident that animals were autopsied at four month intervals during progression of the lesions and then at four month intervals during regression. In all instances the regression diet consisted of a low fat, low cholesterol prudent diet to which cholestyramine was added. Assessment of the extensiveness of lesion involvement in terms of surface area covered by grossly visible atheromatous changes at each of these intervals along with the microscopic evaluation of the amount of lipid in the lesion, the lesion thickness, and the area of the lesion in the three standard aortic samples which were studied, could all be utilized to construct curves which in general reflect the rate of progression and the rate of regression relative to these four types of lesion evaluations.

In this report, emphasis will be placed on the measurement of these end points in animals fed the two contrasting diets for induction (1) and on the differences that have been noted between the lesions in rhesus and cynomolgus monkeys during both induction and regression. As we have reported earlier, the cynomolgus monkeys are much more subject to atheroarteritis which results in concentric and transmural lesions, probably related to immune complexes in the serum.

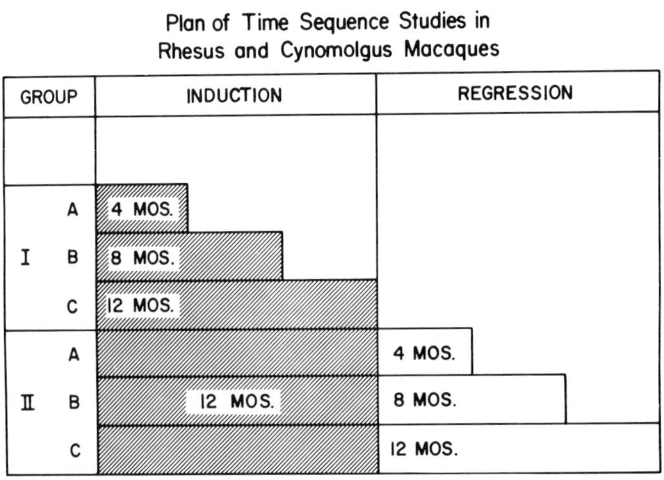

Figure 1. This diagram indicates the general plan of these four experiments. Small groups of animals, usually four to a group, were autopsied at intervals of four months during induction and then at four month intervals following the initiation of the lipid lowering regimen. This plan makes it possible to evaluate several features of the atherogenic process and the process of regression so that one can begin to evaluate the potential for successful regression of lesions in human trials.

2. MATERIALS AND METHODS

Experimental Animals

With few exceptions the macaque monkeys used in these studies were young adult male animals which had been fully conditioned to recommended ILAR laboratory conditions and AAALAC specified housing facilities in individual cages within the AJ Carlson Animal Resource Center at the University of Chicago. The animals were all captive, feral bred, and imported. None had overt or clinical laboratory signs of disease prior to the beginning of the study. They all had exhibited excellent appetites and activity. In general, each of the four studies involved twenty-four animals at intervals of four, eight, and twelve months and four, eight, and twelve months during regression. Since the animals were rather comparable in age and weight, the four animals studied at each time period were randomly distributed in a balanced manner so that each group contained monkeys showing about an equal range of weights and serum cholesterol values at the beginning of the study.

Rations and Feeding

The general formulation of the three major rations used in this investigation are given in table 1. As can be seen, all of the rations were based on a specially developed and quite uniform Purina Monkey Chow, which was formulated in a uniform manner throughout the entire experimental period and purchased by us in a pulverized condition with

TABLE 1.: DIET PREPARATION[a]
Expressed as Percentage of Wet Weight

Ingredients	Atherogenic diets (%)		Prudent diet (%)
Peanut oil	21.74	0.00	0.00
Butter oil	0.00	10.87	0.00
Coconut oil	0.00	10.87	0.00
Corn oil	0.00	0.00	18.00
Cholesterol	1.74	1.74	0.05
Vitamin mix	0.87	0.87	0.87
Gelatin	1.30	1.30	1.30
Monkey chow	61.31	61.31	47.61
Orange juice	13.04	13.04	13.04
Water	0.00	0.00	19.13
Total	100.00g	100.00g	100.00g
Cal/100g	482	482	389

[a]Pulverized primate ration with no animal fat added was obtained through the Purina Ralston Company

no animal products added. It was utilized as a basis for all of our experimental diets. To this chow were added the food fats to be used during the induction of atherosclerosis, in which the cholesterol had been dissolved during the preparation of the diet. A vitamin mix and extra ascorbic acid were also incorporated in each ration and the prepared diets were stored at -20° until they were removed for the daily feeding.

During regression all animals received a similar diet but with only a relatively small quantity of corn oil and much less cholesterol, plus 2.5% of cholestyramine which was incorporated into the diet and thoroughly mixed with the dry ingredients before the melted or liquid oils containing the disolved cholesterol were added. In general, the animals gained weight both during the progression and regression parts of the study and all maintained excellent food consumption during both parts of the experiment. No signs of ill health due to dietary inadequacies were observed at any time.

Blood Chemistry Including Lipid Values

All animals were bled at the beginning of each experiment and at intervals of four months during the lesion induction and regression. The baseline results and the values limited to the animals being studied at autopsy at each of these intervals are given in table 2. In addition, Chem-17 clinical chemical values were determined at the beginning, at the midpoint, and at the end of the study on all surviving animals. These results failed to reveal any significant abnormalities.

Aortic and Tissue Sampling

The aorta was sampled in a standardized way which has been described previously (2) and the various lesion components which were measured microscopically were based on quantitative values obtained from oil red O stained frozen sections of these standard samples. In addition, the gross intimal surface covered by lesions was estimated by two observers utilizing a modification of the method described by Howard et al. using a modified gross point counting technique (3).

Other Lesion Parameters Quantitated

In addition to the gross intimal surface covered by lesions, three measurements are included in this report, each of which was derived by study of the standard oil red O stained sections from the three sampling sites and quantitated by means of a computer assisted morphometric apparatus using a Leitz projecting microscope, a Hewlett-Packard digitzer plate, and a Hewlett-Packard microcomputer which has been previously described (4, 5). The measurements include intimal lesion area in microns^2 as judged on the fat stain, greatest intimal lesion thickness in microns as measured with this same computer assisted apparatus, and percentage of the lesion made up by oil red O positive staining similarly measured and computed.

TABLE 2: SERUM LIPIDS

	Baseline		Progression (Atherogenic Diets)						Regression (Prudent Diet)					
	Ch	Tg	Ch	Tg	Ch	Tg	Ch	Tg	Ch	Tg	Ch	Tg	Ch	Tg
	0 Weeks		4 Weeks		8 Weeks		12 Weeks		4 Weeks		8 Weeks		12 Weeks	
Peanut Oil Cholesterol														
CM-35	128	36	868	26	437	7	719	54	119	32	117	37	90	54
RH-37	131	33	529	8	494	6	419	3	137	14	124	39	146	34
Coconut Oil Butterfat Cholesterol														
CM-39	109	31	1296	74	948	87	1241	74	116	52	124	60	83	44
RH-38	143	38	968	36	938	34	931	90	235	43	402	37	488	100

Ch - Cholesterol mg%

Tg - Triglycerides mg%

3. RESULTS

Blood Lipid Chemistries

As is evident in table 2, all the groups, both cynomolgus and rhesus, started with average blood cholesterols and triglycerides at a similar basal level. These values increased gradually during the induction period with more increase noted in those animals receiving the coconut oil/butter ration as compared to those receiving the peanut oil ration. Furthermore, the cynomolgus monkeys showed a greater response to each diet than did the rhesus monkeys. All of these reactions to atherogenic regimens are similar to ones which we have observed previously (2, 6). The blood lipid responses to the low fat, low cholesterol rations which were started at the end of the year of induction were prompt and all in the same direction. In general, the drop in cholesterol and trigylcerides measured in the cynomologus and rhesus monkeys at four month intervals were marked by prompt decrease in serum cholesterol and relatively little change in triglycerides. Furthermore, the serum cholesterol decreases were similar in the cynomologus and rhesus monkeys. In each case the blood cholesterol values had declined to almost basal levels by the fourth month after the initiation of the low fat, low cholesterol and cholestyramine containing ration.

Lesion Response With Time

The four sets of data-derived curves reproduced in figure 2 reflect in broad strokes the major features of the response of the aortic plaques in these animals. In each instance a point in the graphs represents an

---

Figure 2. These groups of data-derived "best fit" curves document our experience in attempting to quantitate the development of atheromatous lesions and the regression of lesions with time.

It is evident that the results of these four experiments indicate there is less effective regression both grossly (intimal surface involved) and microscopically (especially lesion thickness) in the cynomolgus monkeys. These animals are consistently found to have circulating immune complexes in comparison to young adult male rhesus monkeys, which are free or almost free of these antigen-antibody/complement combinations. The curves also indicate that the limited regression is almost as prompt and effective in the fibrous atherosclerotic lesions of the monkeys fed the peanut oil diets as in the more lipid rich butter/coconut oil fed animals (note the similarities between the results of CM 35 and 39). The puzzling inhibited development of lesions (area and thickness) of the rhesus monkeys in experiment Rh 38 and the completion of the 12 month regression data are still receiving attention.

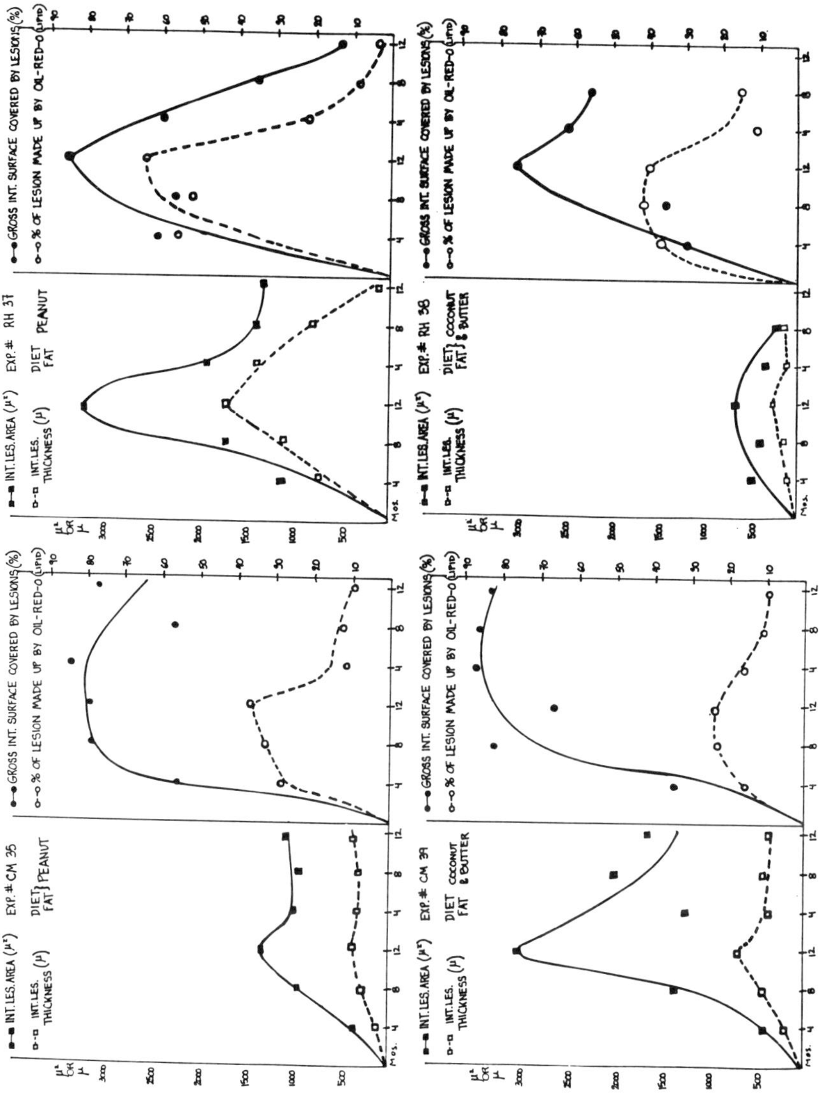
EXP. # CM 35
DIET FAT } PEANUT
INT. LES. AREA (μ²)
INT. LES. THICKNESS (μ)
GROSS INT. SURFACE COVERED BY LESIONS (%)
% OF LESION MADE UP BY OIL-RED-O (LIPID)
EXP. # RH 37
DIET FAT PEANUT
EXP. # CM 39
DIET COCONUT FAT & BUTTER
EXP. # RH 38
DIET FAT } COCONUT & BUTTER
MOS.

average of data obtained either from the point counting quantitation of the gross intimal surface involved by lesions or obtained from the microscopic oil red O stained sections from each of the three standard samples which were measured by means of the computer assisted micromorphometric digitized observations. These yielded data on microscopic intimal lesion area, on intimal lesion thickness, and on the percent of the lesion made up by oil red O positive staining in the lesion.

As can be seen from these data-derived curves, the cynomolgus monkeys responded much more actively in terms of intimal lesion area to the feeding of coconut oil and butter than to the peanut oil ration. Both of these diets produced a remarkably strong response by eight months in gross intimal surface covered by lesions and a lower response in terms of the percent of lesion made up by oil red O positive material. As can be seen, while the cynomolgus aortas' intimal lesion areas regressed to a considerable extent in four months, it was not very effective in the sense that the values never returned to near the base line. This was probably related to the inflammatory elements in the active lesions. Similarly, there was little evidence of regression of gross intimal surface covered by lesions in this species in contrast to the almost complete disappearance of the lipid. The rhesus monkeys, on the other hand, showed a particularly prompt and effective response of the lesions to the therapeutic regimen. This was true for those resulting from the feeding of the peanut oil as well as the coconut oil/butter ration. In fact, the intimal lesion thickness went back almost to the baseline, and the intimal lesion areas, while not as completely resolved, nevertheless demonstrated a remarkable regression response. The gross intimal surface covered by lesions also was much more completely reversed compared with the results obtained with cynomologus monkeys whether the original diet was peanut oil or coconut oil. The data for the coconut oil/butter ration is still incomplete, but there is ample indication of a prompt and effective decrease in gross intimal surface covered by lesions as well as the percent of the lesions made up by positive oil red O stained lipid.

These responses with time in relation to both progression and regression represent one of the first attempts to measure in quantitative terms the rates at which a number of important parameters of the atherosclerotic process may respond, both to atherogenic stimuli and to intervention by means of effective therapeutic regimens.

Obviously, this type of investigation can be extended so that more firmly established points can be derived and other lesion components can be included in the quantitative results. As of now, it appears that the size of the lesions and the amount of lipid are the most labile parts of the atherosclerotic process when the blood lipids are lowered during therapy. The gross intimal surface covered by lesions and intimal thickness are somewhat more resistant, especially when peanut oil is used as a part of the atherogenic stimulus and when the lesions have a relatively active inflammatory component as is consistly the case in the cynomolgus monkey atheroarteritis.

4. DISCUSSION

This study of the rate of development and the rate of regression of atherosclerosis in two species of macaque monkeys and in monkeys fed two types of atherogenic diet was designed to provide quantitative data. It is the first attempt we know of in which the influence of the type of atherosclerotic lesion induced is being related to the way in which several of the measures of atherosclerotic severity respond to a common therapeutic regimen. Although the study is preliminary in the sense that only a few animals were studied at each point during progression and regression, it is quite clear that there are certain trends that may help guide future therapeutic intervention trials.

Among the lesion variables which might be expected to influence the regression process many have called attention to the nature of the fully developed and frequently severe atherosclerotic plaque which sometimes contains abundant collagen and calcium. This study indicates that the collagenous lesions which are typical of the atherosclerotic process induced by peanut oil will indeed respond to therapy and that all of the measures which we followed including lesion area, thickness, gross intimal surface, and oil red O stained lipid were rather promply reversed in rhesus monkeys in which severe disease was produced by a diet containing peanut oil as the sole source of food fat. Furthermore, these peanut oil induced aortic lesions responded similarly in the cynomolgus monkeys when they were compared to the response of the coconut oil/butter induced lesions. Although the cynomolgus lesion responses were always sluggish, this appears to be related primarily to the inflammatory nature of the cynomolgus monkeys' lesions which in turn are probably related to the circulating immune complexes which are a part of the pathogenesis of the cynomolgus atheromatous disease (7, 8). Whatever the underlying cause it is quite evident that the advanced lesions in this species do not regress readily, a phenomenon which others have noted (9).

In summary, the variations in advanced atherosclerotic lesions which can be induced in the macaque models help to provide new information about the factors which may influence regression of this process. In this study the influence of the collagen content of the lesions and the presence of an atheroarteritic process have led to the general conclusion that the much more fibrous peanut oil induced lesions regress as readily as the very lipid rich coconut oil/butter induced lesions. On the other hand, the concentric transmural lesions which result from circulating immune complexes in hyperlipidemic cynomolgus monkeys are very resistant to regression as has been predicted (8).

ACKNOWLEDGMENTS: The authors are grateful for the editorial assistance provided by Gertrud Friedman, the expert word processing by Alexander Arguelles, and the photographic contributions by Gordon Bowie. The work was supported by the Specialized Center of Research in Atherosclerosis (HL- 15062) and much of the data was obtained with the support of HL-33740.

5. REFERENCES

1. Vesselinovitch, D., Wissler, R.W., Schaffner, T.J. and Borensztajn, J. (1980) The effects of various diets on atherogenesis in rhesus monkeys. Atherosclerosis 35, 198-207.

2. Vesselinovitch, D., Wissler, R.W., Hughes, R., and Borensztajn, J. (1976) Reversal of advanced atherosclerosis in rhesus monkeys. Atherosclerosis 23, 155-176.

3. Howard, C.F. Jr. (1979) Aortic atherosclerosis in normal and spontaneously diabetic Macaca nigra, Atherosclerosis 33, 479-493.

4. Wissler, R.W., Vesselinovitch, D., Schaffner, T.J. and Glagov, S. (1980) Quantitating rhesus monkey atherosclerosis progression and regression with time, in A.M. Gotto, Jr., L.C. Smith and B. Allen (eds.), Atherosclerosis V (Proc. Vth Int. Symp.), Springer-Verlag, New York, pp. 757-761.

5. Vesselinovitch, D., Wissler, R.W., and Schaffner, T. (1982) Quantitation of lesions during progression and regression of atherosclerosis in rhesus monkeys, in H. Naito (ed.), Nutrition and Heart Disease, S.P. Medical and Scientific Books, New York, pp. 121-149.

6. Wissler, R.W. and Vesselinovitch, D. (1984) Interaction of therapeutic diets and cholesterol-lowering drugs in regression studies in animals, in M.R. Malinow and V.H. Blaton (eds.), Regression of Atherosclerotic Lesions, Plenum, New York, pp. 21-41.

7. Wissler, R.W. and Vesselinovitch, D. (1983) Atherosclerosis - Relationship to coronary blood flow, Am. J. Cardiol. 52, 2A-7A.

8. Wissler, R.W., Vesselinovitch, D., Davis, H.R., Lambert, P.H. and Berkermeier, M. (1985) A new way to look at atherosclerotic involvement of the artery wall and the functional effects, Ann. N.Y. Acad. Sci. 454, 9-22.

9. Hollander, W., Kirkpatrick, B., Paddock, J., Colombo, M., Nagraj, S. and Prusty, S. (1979) Studies on the progression and regression of coronary and peripheral atherosclerosis in the cynomolgus monkey, Exp. Mol. Pathol., 30, 55-73.

52

Human atherosclerosis and inflammation. An immunocytochemical and ultrastructural investigation

G. PASQUINELLI and R. LASCHI

Institute of Clinical Electron Microscopy, University of Bologna, S. Orsola Hospital, via Massarenti 9, 40138 Bologna, Italy

ABSTRACT. The authors have performed light and electron microscopic studies of the distribution of various inflammatory cell types in human carotid and aortic atherosclerotic arterial lesions. In addition, some specimens have been studied immunocytochemically by using a panel of monoclonal antibodies. Fatty streaks were composed of subendothelial aggregates of foam cells mainly of monocyte-macrophage derivation. T-lymphocytes and smooth muscle cells were also observed. Uncomplicated fibrous-fatty plaques showed surface and subsurface accumulation of monocyte-macrophages and T-lymphocytes at the periphery of the lesion as well as just beneath the fibrous cap. Abdominal atherosclerotic aneurysms showed an inner plaque associated with a well-developed outer fibroinflammatory component. These observations suggest an active partecipation of inflammatory cells in the development of human atherosclerotic lesions. A better understanding of the role of inflammation in atherosclerosis may be potentially useful for prevention and therapy.

INTRODUCTION

Although the presence of "monocytoid cells" in the early atherosclerotic lesions of hypercholesterolemic rabbits was originally described by Duff et al. in 1958 (quoted in [6]), for many years was given to the presence and role of monocyte-macrophages and lymphocytes in both experimental and human atherosclerosis. At the beginning of the 80's, some authors have demonstrated that monocyte-macrophages are implicated in the onset of experimental atherosclerosis (for a review, see [5]). Most recently, Majno et al. [6] stated that "the beginnings of atherosclerosis have something in common with chronic inflammation". At present, inflammatory cells have been disclosed in the lesions of human atherosclerosis, i.e., fatty streaks [7], eccentric intimal thickenings [2], fibro-fatty plaques [3,4] as well as atherosclerotic abdominal aortic aneurysms (AAAs) [11].

To further investigate the importance of such inflammatory components in human atherosclerosis we have studied, by means of light, scanning and transmission electron microscopy as well as by immunocytochemistry, human carotid and aortic atherosclerotic lesions at different stages of evolution.

MATERIALS AND METHODS

Segments of carotid artery and aorta were obtained from the Institute of Vascular Surgery, S. Orsola Hospital, Bologna. Carotid endarterectomy specimens (from n = 41 patients) were collected as previously described [9]. AAAs (from n = 7 patients) were selected on the bases of their gross appearance, i.e., dense perianeurysmal fibrosis and thickening of the anterior and lateral aneurysm walls. A total of 65 specimens from 48 individuals (40 men, 8 women) were examined.

Light and electron microscopy.

A portion of all tissues were fixed by submersion in 2.5% buffered glutaraldehyde for 10 min. in the O.R. Samples for transmission electron microscopy (TEM) were additionally fixed with 2.5% glutaraldehyde in 0.1 M cacodylate buffer (pH 7.3) for 3 h, postfixed with 1% OsO_4 in the same buffer for 1 h, dehydrated in a graded series of alcohol and embedded in araldite. Semithin and thin sections were obtained with a Reichert OMU3 ultramicrotome. Semithin sections for light microscopy (LM) were stained with toluidine blue. Thin sections were counterstained with uranyl acetate and lead citrate and examined in a JEOL 100B transmission electron microscope. Samples for scanning electron microscopy (SEM) were fixed as above and after ethanol dehydration they were critical point dried, coated with gold and observed in a Philips 505 scanning electron microscope.

Immunohistochemistry.

A second portion of tissues were snap-frozen in liquid-nitrogen-cooled isopentane and stored in liquid nitrogen. Cryostat sections (6 µm) were cut, air-dried, and fixed in acetone. The sections were incubated with appropriate dilutions of the following monoclonal antibodies: anti-pan-B cell antibody DAKO-CD22, anti-pan-T cell antibody DAKO-CD3, anti-helper / inducer-T cell DAKO-CD4, anti-suppressor/cytotoxic-T cell DAKO-CD8, anti-macrophage DAKO-p150.95, anti-interleukin-2-receptor DAKO-IL2-R, anti-ki-1 antigen DAKO-Ber-H2 (Dakopatts). The labeling was revealed using the alkaline phosphatase monoclonal anti-alkaline phosphatase method (APAAP).

Immunoelectron microscopy.

Some specimens were fixed with 0.1% glutaraldehyde in phosphate buffered saline (pH 7.3) for 5 min at 4°C and then incubated with three distinct monoclonal antibodies: anti-pan-T cell antibody DAKO UCHL1, anti-macrophage DAKO-MAC 387, anti-ki-1 antigen DAKO-Ber-H2 (Dakopatts). After initial incubation, the specimens were incubated in a protein A-gold solution and successively fixed with 2.5% buffered glutaraldehyde for 3 h. The reaction was silver-enhanced by the IntenSEII silver enhancement kit (Ortho) using a devolpment time of 10 min. The specimens were dehydrated in ethanol and critical point dried. The specimens were then coated with a thin layer of evaporated carbon and examined in a Philips 505 scanning electron microscope with secondary and backscattered electron detectors.

RESULTS

Fatty streaks.

Fatty streaks were identified grossly as slightly raised minute yellow dots. These lesions, when examined by means of SEM, appeared as focal elevations of the vascular lumen due to the subendothelial accumulation of multiple layers of foam cells. Endothelial cells showing changes in cell shape and size continuously covered the lesion (Fig. 1). No significant adhesions of circulating leukocytes were observed. Foam cells were mainly oval in shape and showed lipid inclusions, lisosomal lipid bodies and cholesterol crystals in their cytoplasm (Fig. 2). In addition, a few spindle-shaped foam cells were present in correspondence with the inner elastic lamina. Lymphocytes were observed in discrete numbers particularly next to degenerating lipophages characterized by pyknotic nuclei and cytoplasmic autophagic vacuoles. In these areas cell debris and extracellular lipid deposits consisting of bizarrely-shaped cholesterol crystals were frequently encountered. Most of the lesional foam cells were immunostained with MAC 387. The non-reactive foam cells were located more deeply. Lymphocytes were characterized as T4 and T8 cells which were scattered among the foam cells. No particular difference was observed among the two lymphocytes subtypes.

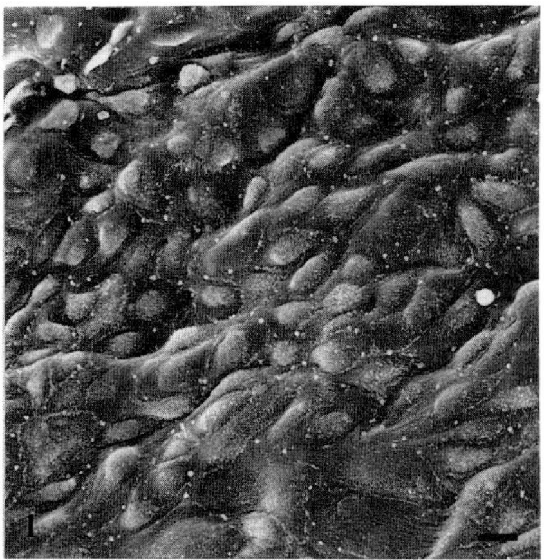

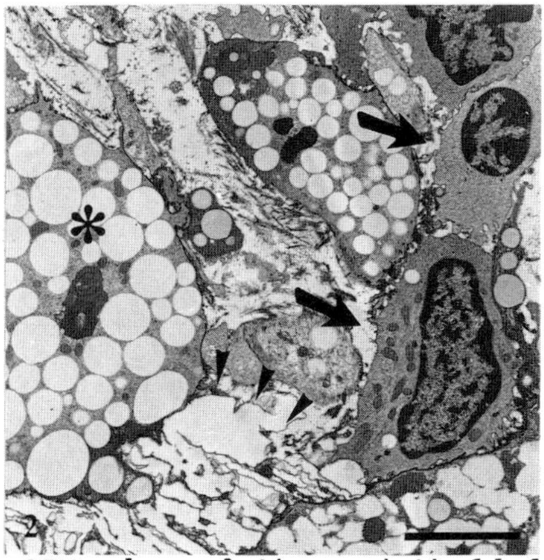

Fig. 1. Human fatty streak. SEM view of the endothelial cell layer. Bar = 10 µm.
Fig. 2. Human fatty streak. TEM shows foam cells (*) and lymphocytes (arrows). The arrowheads indicate some extra-cellular lipid deposits. Bar = 5 µm.

Fibrous-fatty plaques.

Fibrous-fatty plaques were characterized by a basal necrotic-lipid core bounded by an extensive fibrous cap. SEM observation revealed that the endothelial lining showed aspects of non-denuding injury. Endothelial cells presented as having an uneven orientation, focal loss of polarity and degenerative features. Adhesions of monocytes and lymphocytes were a common finding in plaques at the shoulder zone (Fig. 3). TEM in conjunction with immunocytochemistry revealed that a large portion of the cells within the lesion were lymphocytes and monocyte/macrophages. T lymphocytes were arranged as single cells and in clusters, especially in the cellular zone located beneath the fibrous cap. T cells were also observed in close association with macrophages, smooth muscle cells (Fig. 4) and mesenchymal cells. Positive populations of T4 and T8 cells were both recognized. Macrophages reacted with MAC 387. LM showed that many of the T cells were also activated which was demonstrated by their positivity for Ber-H2. Immuno-SEM showed that T lymphocytes may express the CD 30 antigen while still adhering to the endothelium.

Abdominal aortic aneurysms (AAAs).

Grossly, the AAAs were encased in a whitish dense fibrous tissue involving the aorta adventitia and the adjacent periadventitial tissues. The thickening was predominantly

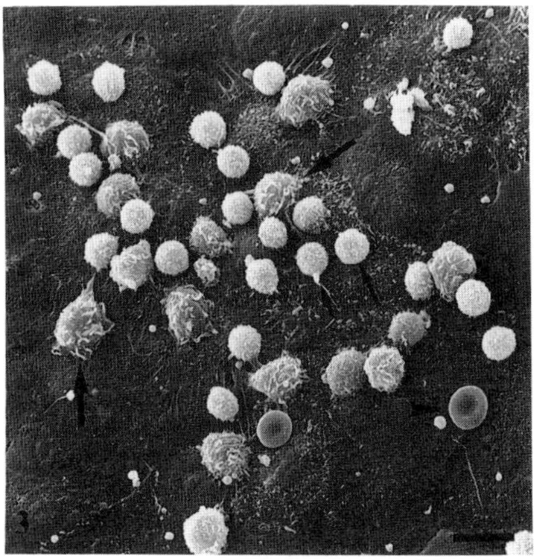

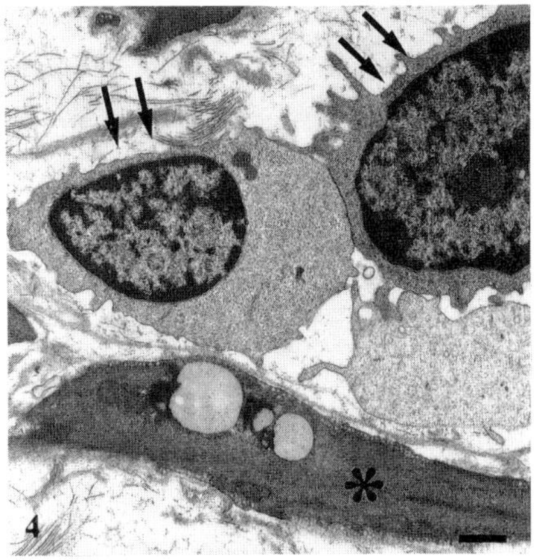

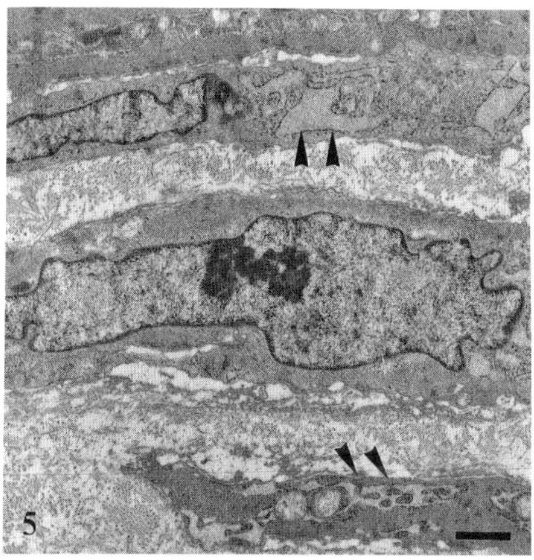

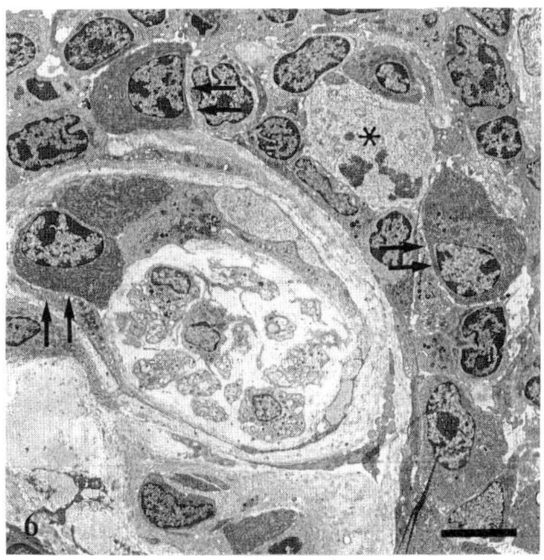

Fig. 3. Human fibrous-fatty plaque. SEM shows the adhesion of lymphocytes (small arrows) and monocytes (large arrows) to the endothelial cell layer. The arrowhead shows a red blood cell. Bar = 10 μm.

Fig. 4. Human fibrous-fatty plaque. TEM micrograph showing some lymphocytes (arrows) adjacent to a smooth muscle cell. Bar = 10 μm.

Fig. 5. Human abdominal atherosclerotic anuerysm. TEM view of the fibrous adventitial component. Fibrosis resulted from layers of smooth muscle cells with dilated cisternae of rough endoplasmic reticulum (arrowheads) and collagen fibers. Bar = 1 μm.

Fig. 6. Human abdominal atherosclerotic anuerysm. TEM of a follicular inflammatory aggregate. The arrows indicate some plasma cells. The asterisk marks a mitoses. Bar = 5 μm.

anterior and lateral and usually spared the posterior wall. In all cases there was evidence of intimal fibrosis and media involvement. The media was atrophic due to the lysis of elastic tissue and loss of smooth muscle cells. There was increased amounts of collagen tissue and cholesterol clefts were evident. The adventitia and periadventitial tissues were characterized by marked fibrosis associated with varying degrees of chronic inflammation. TEM showed fibrosis of hyperplastic smooth muscle cells having a synthetic phenotype (Fig. 5) admixed with collagen fibres and proteoglycan particles. Entrapment of nerves and fatty tissue as well as adventitial endarteritis and phlebitis were common features. The cellular infiltrate was composed of T4, T8, B lymphocytes, macrophages and plasma cells. T lymphocytes of helper phenotype predominated over suppressor cells. The inflammatory process presented a mixed pattern, i.e., diffuse/follicular. Nodular aggregates frequently showed well-developed germinal centers and were associated with hyperplastic vessels of the post-capillary venule type (Fig. 6). At the ultrastructural level, the plasma cell infiltrate was well defined and characterized by a dilated cisternae of rough endoplasmic reticulum containing synthetized amorphous-granular material. The pattern of positivity for Ber-H2 and IL2-R revealed that a conspicuous percentage of infiltrating macrophages was activated. A specific T4 lymphocytes and macrophage cell infiltration through the aortic media as well as adventitial vessels was observed.

DISCUSSION

In this study, the authors have demonstrated that T and B lymphocytes are present in the atherosclerotic lesions of surgically removed human carotid and aortic arteries. T4 and T8 cells were observed in carotid fatty streaks and fibrous-fatty plaques. In these latter lesion some of the T cells were activated as demonstrated by the CD 30 antigen expression. Activated T cells were detected while adhering to the endothelial cell layer as well as infiltrating into the subendothelial intimal space. These findings further support and extend the views of Munro et al. [7] and Jonasson et al. [4] who originally demonstrated the presence of T cells in human fatty streaks and atherosclerotic plaques by means of LM.

On the other hand both T and B lymphocytes were present in human atherosclerotic AAAs. The degree of lymphocyte infiltration varied significantly and was particularly remarkable in those cases associated with florid adventitial fibrosis. Most of the T cells were T4-positive therefore indicating a positive inducer/helper subtype. A small percentage of T4 cells were activated. It is interesting to note that B cells predominated and frequently aggregated in follicles with well-developed germinal centers. The plasma cell component was very prominent and seemed to be engaged in the local synthesis of antibodies. This antibody production, in turn, may result in immune complex formation and activation of the complement system whose importance in inducing complement-mediated cytotoxicity and antibody dependent cell-mediated cytotoxicity are already well known [12].

Another important feature is the frequent presence of lymphocyte infiltrates also containing monocyte/macrophages. It has been demonstrated that monocyte/macrophages are implicated in the onset of atherosclerosis in some animal models in which experimental atherosclerotic lesions were induced by hypercholesterolemic diets [8]. Numerous studies have sited the complex regulatory cooperation among T cells, B cells and monocyte/macrophages in the immune-response along with the potential implications concerning pathogenesis of a wide variety of human diseases [10]. Therefore, it is probable that analogous interactions occur in the atherosclerotic arterial lesions thus contributing to the development of arterial disease. This hypothesis may be further supported by the detection of activated macrophages and T lymphocytes in our studies. Activated inflammatory cells acquire numerous inducible functions, many of which may be significant in atherogenesis [8].

In summary, these observations suggest an active partecipation of inflammatory cells in the arterial lesions of human atherosclerosis. Cell-mediate immune responses as well as B-cell effector mechanisms seem to be operative in different stages of the disease. Atherosclerosis might involve an immune reaction against a lipid derived from the vessel lumen or against an antigen native to the arterial wall. However, the implication of viral antigens [1] or immune complex deposition can not be entirely ruled out. A better understanding of the role of inflammation in human disease may be potentially useful concerning prevention and therapy.

ACKNOWLEDGEMENTS

The authors gratefully acknowledge Prof. M. D'Addato (Institute of Vascular Surgery, University of Bologna) for providing the pathological specimens and Prof. S. Pileri (Institute of Haematology, University of Bologna) for supplying the monoclonal antibodies. We are also greatly indebted to Dr. P. Preda and Dr. M. Vici for their technical assistance.

REFERENCES

1. Cunningham, M.J., Pasternak, R.C. (1988) The potential role of viruses in the pathogenesis of atherosclerosis. Circulation 77, 964-966.
2. Emerson, E.E., Robertson, A.L. (1988) T lymphocytes in aortic and coronary intimas. Their potential role in atherogenesis. Am J Pathol 130, 369-376.
3. Gown, A.M., Tsukada, T., Ross, R. (1986) Human atherosclerosis. II. Immunocytochemical analysis of the cellular composition of human atherosclerotic lesions. Am J Pathol 125, 191-207.
4. Jonasson, L., Holm, J., Skalli, O., Bondjers, G., Hansson, G.K. (1986) Regional accumulations of T cells, macrophages, and smooth muscle cells in the human atherosclerotic plaque. Arteriosclerosis 6, 131-138.
5. Laschi, R., Pasquinelli, G., Versura, P., Bonvicini, F. (1989) "Scanning electron microscopy in clinics", in P. Motta (ed.), Cells and Tissues. A three dimensional approach by modern techniques in microscopy, Alan R. Liss, Inc., New York, pp. 605-621.
6. Majno, G., Joris, I., Zand, T. (1985) Atherosclerosis: new horizons. Hum Pathol 1, 3-5.
7. Munro, M.J., van der Walt, J.D., Munro, C.S., Chalmers, J.A.C., Cox, E.L. (1987) An immunohistochemical analysis of human aortic fatty streaks. Hum Pathol 18, 375-380.
8. Munro, M.J., Cotran, R.S. (1988) Biology of disease. The pathogenesis of atherosclerosis: atherogenesis and inflammation. Lab Invest 58, 249-261.
9. Pasquinelli, G., Cavazza, A., Preda, P., Stella, A., Cifiello, B.I., Gargiulo, M., D'Addato, M., Laschi, R. (1989) Endothelial injury in human atherosclerosis. Scanning Microscopy 3, in press.
10. Prud'homme, G.J., Parfrey, N.A. (1988) Biology of disease. Role of T helper lymphocytes in autoimmune diseases. Lab Invest 59, 158-172.
11. Sterpetti, A.V., Hunter, W.J., Feldhaus, R.J., Chasan, P., McNamara, M., Cisternino, S., Schultz, R.D. (1989) Inflammatory anuerysms of the abdominal aorta: incidence, pathologic, and etiologic considerations. J Vasc Surg 9, 643-650.
12. Stites, D.P., Stobo, J.D., Wells, J.V. (1987) Basic & Clinical Immunology, Appleton-Lange, Los Altos.

53

Carotid plaque volume measurement

F. ZACA', D. ROVINETTI, L. STEFFANON, M.S. BENASSI, T. BOMBARDINI, C. DE COLLIBUS, M. MOSCA and C.F. MANETTI

Istituto di Patologia Speciale Medica e Metodologia Clinica, Università degli Studi di Bologna, via Massarenti 9, 40138 Bologna BO, Italy

ABSTRACT

Calculation of the carotid atheromatous plaque volume is a more sophi = sticated procedure than one dimensional plaque measurement, percent ste nosis calculation and stenotic area determination.

Ultrasonography was employed in this study in order to investigate 16 ca rotid plaques which were excised at autopsy from pts (patients) wrose cause of death was "stroke" and 16 pts carotid plaques removed from li= ving pts before undergding TEA surgery.

The volume of the atheromatous carotid plaques was determined by echo = tomographically sectioning the plaque in both longitudinal and transver se planes and then summing the partial volumes of each section.

In order to calculate the partial volumes of each section the following formula was utilized: V = S x h

- where h (equivalent height) is the relationship between the Area (A) and the height b of the transverse section;
- S corresponds to the area of the longitudinal section of that point.

This specific diagnostic approach has proved to be extreamly valuble and strongly supported by percent differences observed in plaque volumes de termined echographicly and in those plaque volumes determined by means of measuring the volume of liquid displaced with submersion of the exci= sed carotid plaque in water. Percent differences were recorded on the order of +/- 10 %.

The investigation was able to be reproduced thanks to the employment of a mechanical system.

Determination of the atheromatous plaque volume is one means of studying the progression and regression of atherosclerotic lesions.

AIM OF THE STUDY

Is calculation of plaque volume significantly more accurate than percent stenosis determination of the same plaque.

Verification that the volume of atheromatous plaques can be obtained by means of ultrasonography and to exactly what degree these calculations are reliable.

MATERIALS

A VINGMED CFM 700 echography and a 7.5 Mhz automatic scanning probe with an oscillating piezoelectric transducer was used.

The scanning probe was attached directly to a mechanical system that enabled unrestricted movements in 3 directions as well as rotating on transverse and longitudinal axes. The scanning probe-mechanical system apparatus consisted of a wooden base, capable of being positioned at various angles +/- 90 % degrees. The base supported an arc that had flexible joints attached to arms which in turn supported the ultrasondic probe.

The mechanical system in the horizontal plane was equipped with a micrometer screw adjustment which operated in millimeters thus allowing very precise quantification of minute movements (mm and 1/10 mm).

Movements achieved by means of the joint-arms were measured in mm and/or degrees°.

After the joint arm movements were established, 2 blocking systems were used to immobilize the vertebro-cranial articulation of the pt being examined. One was applied to the chin the other positioned at the level of the parietal bones bilaterally.

This allowed the pt to be maintained in a fixed, if necessary, reprodeceable position, in order to accurately keep track of the reference scale setting at various times during the investigation.

The ability to measure minute movements in the horizontal plane was provided by the micrometer screw adjustment together with the associated reference scale. This particular set up allowed extreamly precise measurments of the plaque morphology being studied either "in vitro" or "in vivo" (length, height, distance between transversal sections).

Movements concerning the support of the ultrasonic probe are helpful in improving the echographic images. These images can also be checked for diagnostic accuracy and also be duplicated, if necessary, on follow-up exams provided the ultrasonic probe movements are identical. This particular arrangment allows long term assessment of atheromatous plaque "regression" or "progression".

In vitro studies of carotid atheromatous plaques removed at autopsy and plaques removed just after TEA surgery were carried out by placing the samples in a container felled with a known quantity of physiologic saline solution. The ultrasonographic probe was then immersed in the container of solution, the distal probe extremity was held a fixed distance from the specimen in orders to optimize the relative images.

Rotating the probe around its longitudinal axis creates short axis sections. The various scanning possibilities are infinite (Fig. 1).

METHOD

Echographic determination of atheromatous plaque volume is based on the following formula: $V = S * heq$; this is specific for irregular solid body volume determination. - S is the surface area of the longitudinal section; - heq is the equivalent height that corresponds to the relationship between A/b: A equials the surface area of the transverse section and b is the height of the same transverse section.

$V = S * heq$ in reality represents the partial volume delimited by one and of the plaque and the first transverse section or two contiguous

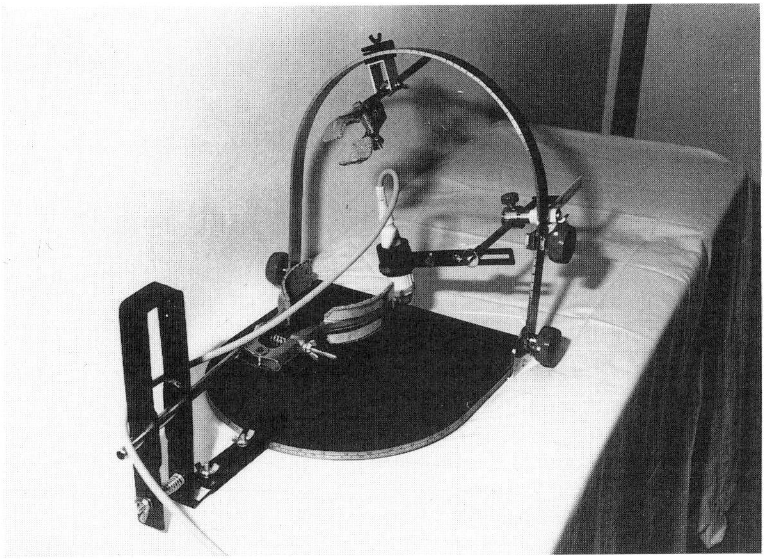

Fig. 1

transverse sections throught it.
Once the partial volumes are obtained they are added together; the end result equaling the total volume. (Fig. 2)

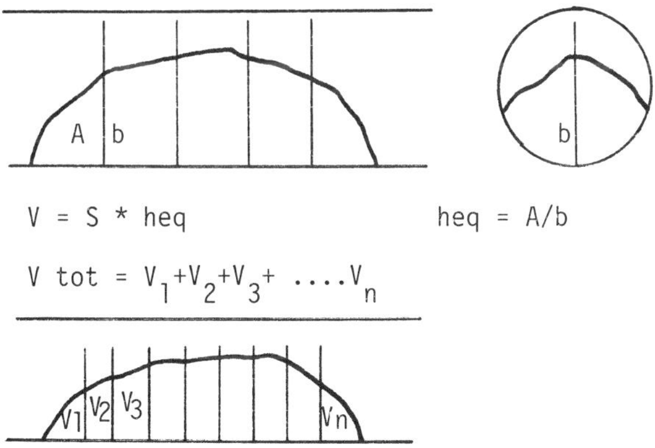

Fig. 2

Measurements were obtained as follows: once the atheromatous plaques were placed in the containers and once the pt was positioned, the ultra sonographic probe was then carefully positioned for a long-axis image echograph.

At this point in time the micrometer screw adjustment was used to more the probe parallel to the long-axis of the plaque in such a way that one extream of the corresponding echographic image coincided with a fixed reference scale visable on the monitor. The reference scale is positio= ned according to examiner preference (in this case a median vertical line that ran down the entire echographic field).
This procedure makes it possible to directly establish on the reference scale, a point that corresponds exactly to the atheromatous plaque.
Turning the micrometer screw adjustment moves the echographic image un= til the opposite ends of the plaque no longer corresponds with the refe rence scale on the monitor. Measurement of the probe movement (expres sed in mm and 1/10 mm) corresponds to the total lenght of the plaque which is real on the millimeter reference scale (the lenght of the pla= que is determined in order to have a reference value on which to base the successive measurements EG transverse scanning mm per mm).
Repeating this operation, the echographic images are frozen in corre = spondence with 1 mm movements of the ultrasonographic probe from one si de to the other. The height of each image (the distance between the in= ferior margine of the plaque and the point of intersection of the echo= graphic plaque surface with the median vertical reference line) corre = sponds to the value of b. Each mm movement allows precise monitoring of the varying heights of the plaque which are necessary in subdividing them into partial volumes. This particular method allows a more precise total volume determination.
Once the values of b are obtained (b1, b2, b3, ... bn) the ultrasono = graphic probe is rotated aroung its axis in order to obtain echographic short-axis images of the atheromatous plaque.
Scanning of the plaque, once again moving from one side to the other (using as reference the total lenght measurement initially determined for that plaque) the echographic images of the transverse sections are frozen in correspondence with 1 mm movements of the ultrasonographic probe.
Then the probe was repositioned again for long-axis imaging in order to make sure that the millimeter reference scale was calibrated correctly.
Numerical values of A (A1, A2, A3, ... An) and S (S1, S2, S3, ...Sn) were measured with the aid of an electronic pen and board (Digi Pad) having a resolution of 144 points per mm2, and an IBM PC-AT computer.
The total volumes of the plaques were then determined.
The echographic images obtained of the atheromatous plaque was determi= ned superiorly from the free surface and inferiorly from the echogenic line. The echogenic line is defined as that line passing between the media layer of the vessel and that portion involved in the atheromatous lesion (note that the plaque is a lesion involving the intima and the media without extending all the way through to the adventitia).
When the variation in echogenicity wasn't defined adeguately, the infe= rior limit of the plaque was obtained by drawing an imaginary line bet= ween the two extreams of the non-pathologic portion of the internal va= scular surface.
Once the carotid plaques were excised, either at autopsy or surgically, the actual volume was then determined by total immersion in physiologic saline solution. The real volume was then calculated by means of the

volume displacement of liquid theory.
Volume values obtained by means of echography were then confronted with those volume values obtained from the immersion method.
All calculations, echographic and immersion, obtained in this investigation were determined by two individual reaserchers and double checked.
16 atheromatous plaques obtained at autopsy and 16 plaques obtained from pts selected prior to undergoing TEA surgery. Smooth carotid plaques were eliminate from this study to avoid ambiguity.

RESULTS
This particular method of study proved to be effective and extreamly valuble.
All results were first compared to these obtained in the "in vitro" study, then checked with those results obtained in the "in vivo" study.

In vitro study
Volume data calculated echographically by two separate individual reaserchers was almost identical. The students T was 0,087.
The difference is not statistically significant. Comparing the volumes determined echographically and the volumes determined via the immersion technique, it was demonstrated that in 13 of the 16 plaques studied the percent difference was +/- 10 %.
In only 3 cases the percent difference was greater than 10 %.
In 2 cases the echographically determined volume was significantly inferior to the actual volume: these were 2 atheromatous plaques with actual volumes greater than 300 mm3.
In one particular case the echographically determined volume was inferior to the actual volume: the plaque had an actual volume of less than 100 mm3.

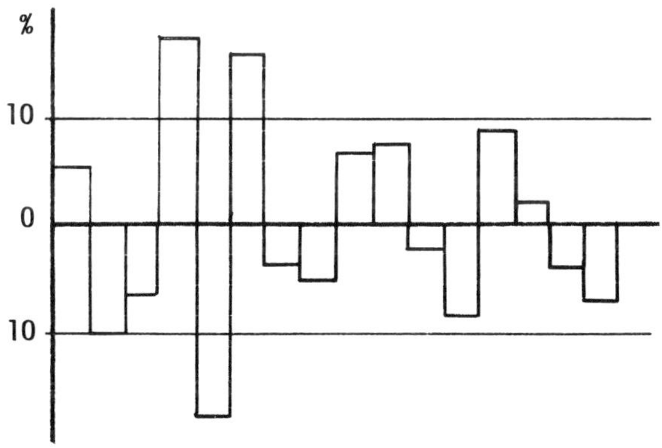

VEAP01	VLAP	%	VEAP01	VLAP	%
270	255	+5.8	260	245	+6.1
261	290	-10	203	187	+8.5
254	275	-7.6	198	204	-2.9
379*	320	+18.4	147	160	-8.1
75*	87	-13.6	137	125	+9.6
405*	345	+17.3	220	215	+2.3

278	290	-4.1	240	252	-4.7
237	250	-5.2	190	206	-7.7

In vivo study
Volume data calculated echographically by two individual researchers was almost identical. In this study the students T was - 0.505. The difference is not statistically significant. Comparing the volumes determined echographically and the volumes determined via immersion tec hnique it was demonstrated as in the "in vitro" study group of 16 pts, 13 cases had a percent difference of +/- 10 %. In 3 cases again, the percent difference was greater than 10 %.

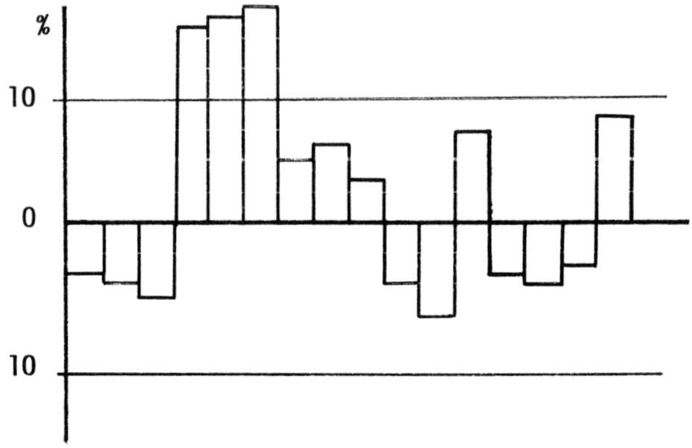

VECO1	VLC	%	VECO1	VLC	%
260	275	-5.4	295	250	+3.6
210	225	-6.6	228	245	-6.9
270	291	-7.2	145	160	-9.3
495*	420	+17.8	239	225	+6.2
460*	388	+18.5	275	294	-6.4
390*	327	+19.2	200	217	-7.8
290	275	+5.5	249	265	-6.0
270	288	+6.2	318	295	+7.7

In all three cases the actual volume of the atheromatous plaque was greater than 300 mm3.

DISCUSSION
Concerning the necessity to precisely examine carotid vascular stenosis, determination of the atheromatous plaque volumes seems to be the prefer= red means of approach with reguard to the percent stenosis method. On the other hand, the percent stenosis method is an index obtained by taking into consideration only the height of the plaque, while the volu me method is a three-dimensional assessment of the plaque. Therefore, volume determination of atheromatous plaques seems to be a more accura= te index in assessing the characteristics of solid bodies, in this ca = se being atherosclerotic lesions.

An important point to take into consideration is that 2 atheromatous plaques having identical heights but, echographically determined morphology being significantly different can cause different kinds of vascular obstruction in spite of having identical percent stenosis values.
In addition, this echographic study has brought to light many noteworthy characteristics concerning volume of atheromatous plaque investigation:
- the most significant differences were observed in comparison with echographically determined volume and volume determined via the immersion technique which demonstrated actual plaque volumes greater than 300 mm3 and less than 100 mm3.
However, plaques with large dimensions (volume > 300 mm3) are difficult to evaluate and for this reason tend to be over estimated in some cases. Some plaques on the contrary tend to be under estimated perhaps due to a "soft" echogenicity.
In concluding, it can be stated that atheromatous plaques having a regular profile and a homogeneous echogenicity would be the ideal lesions for echographic volume determination.
These lesions would also be optimal for follow-up regressive / progressive investigations.

REFERENCES

- ACKERMAN R.H., PRYOR D.S., TAVERAS J.M.: Evaluation of a real time ultrasound imaging sistem for the carotid artery. Stroke, 7: 2, 1976.
- BLACKSHEAR W.M., PHILLIPS D.J., HIRSH J.H., THIELE B.L., CHICOS P.M., WARD K.J., STANDNESS D.E.: Detection of carotid occlusive disease by ultrasonis imaging and pulsed doppler spectrum analysis. Surgery, 86: 968, 1979.
- BOMBARDINI T., ZACA' F.: Il doppler cardiaco - Dalle applicazioni cliniche alle indicazioni chirurgiche. Ed. L. Pozzi, Roma pp. 161-165,1988.
- BORGATTI E., DE FABRITIS A., SCONDOTTO G., AMATO A., CONTI E., FILIPPINI M.: Evolutività della lesione ateromasica carotidea valutata mediante ecotomografia. In: Angiologia '86. Ed. Moruzzi - Bologna, pp. 1319 -1326, 1986.
- COLTON T.: Statistica in medicina. Piccin Editore, Padova, 1979.
- COMEROTA A.J., CRANLEY J.J., COOKE S.E. (1981): Real-time B-mode carotid imaging in diagnosis of cerebrovascular disease. Surgery '85; 718 -729, 1981.
-COOPERBERG P.L., ROBERTSON W.D., FRY P., SWEENEY V.: "High resolution real time ultrasound of the carotid biforcation". J. Clin. Ultrasound. 7, 13, 1979.
- CURTI T., ZACA' F., TRIANNI M., CIFIELLO B.I., PEDRINI L., STELLA A., PALUMBO N., DESCOVICH G.C.: Utilizzazione del Duplex Scanner nella diagnostica della malattia delle carotidi extracraniche. "Ather. Cardiov. Dis.", 345, Ed. Compositori, Bologna, 1984.
- KATZ M.L., JONSON M., POMAJZL M.J., CAMAROTA A.J., AHRENSFIELD D., MAUDEL L., HAYDEN W., FOGARTY T.: The sensitivity of Real-Time B-mode carotid imaging in the detection of ulcerated plaques. Bruit, 8, 13,1983.
- LENZI S., DESCOVICH G.C.: Atherosclerosis and Cardiovascular Diseases. 449-453, HTP Press Limited. Lancaster England, 1984.
- NUZZACI G., BERTINI D., GORI F., STEFANI P., RIGHI D., PRATESI C.,

LUCENTE E., TONARELLI F., MANGONI N.: Valore e limiti del dupplex-scan= ner ad alta risoluzione in tempo reale nella diagnostica per immagini della malattia occlusiva della carotide extracranica. In: Diagnostica per immagini in patologia vascolare. Monduzzi Ed. Bologna, 1985.
- POURCELOT L.: Visualization des plaques atheromateuses par echotomo = grafic rapide. In: Circulation Cerebrale. André Bes-Gilles Geraud, Tou= louse, 1979.
- REILLY L.M., LUSBY R.J., HUGHES L., FERREL L.D., STONEY R.J., EHREN = FELD W.K.: Carotid plaque histology using Real-Time ultrasonography: clinical and therapeutic implications. Ann. J. Surg., 146, 188, 1983.
- SANDOK B.A., EVANS T.C.Jr., GREEN P.S.: Clinical evaluation of Real-Time ultrasonic B-Scan imaging of the carotid artery: A preliminary re= port. Stroke, 7, 3, 1976.
- WEBER G., TANGANELLI P.: Valutazione morfometrica pre-operatoria del grado di stenosi carotidea: studio di validazione delle immagini ecogra fiche. In: Diagnostica per immagini in patologia vascolare. Moruzzi Ed. Bologna, 1985.
- WOLVERSON M.K., BASHITI H.M., PETERSON G.J.: Ultrasonic tissue charac terization of atheromatous plaques using a high resolution Real-Time scanner. Ultrasound in Med. & Biol. 9, 599, 1983.
- ZANETTE E., BOZZAO L., BUTTICELLI C., MARITTINI A., PAPPATA' S., LEN= ZI G.L.: High resolution Real-Time B-Mode echotomography in the diagno= sis of extracranial carotid lesions. Comparison with traditional angio= graphy. Acta Neurochir. (Wien) 84, 43-47, 1987.

54

Humoral factors of direct influence on the formation and regression of atheromatous plaques

M. BIHARI-VARGA

Semmelweis Medical University, 2nd Pathology Department, Division of Biochemistry, Üllöi ut 93, H-1091 Budapest, Hungary

ABSTRACT. Changes in the concentration of two types of modified serum lipoproteins: peroxidated lipoproteins and Lp(a) with age, atherosclerosis and various risk factors for atherosclerosis were studied. Malondialdehyde level (an index of peroxidation) was significantly increased in the total serum and in the LDL fraction of atherosclerotic and of diabetic patients. The mean concentration of Lp(a) was significantly increased in patients with coronary heart disease or cerebrovascular disease; the elevation was more expressed when atherosclerosis was associated with type II hyperlipidemia or diabetes. In 40-60% of children with familial risk for atherosclerosis increased Lp(a) concentrations were measured as well. The mechanism of the pathogenicity of modified lipoproteins was successfully studied in cell culture experiments and by in vitro investigations. In the course of prevention/regression studies, plasma factors, interfering with the binding of LDL to arterial extracellular matrix were isolated; their physiological role has been investigated in model experiments.

INTRODUCTION

Epidemiological studies have established that the higher the plasma concentration of apo-B containing lipoproteins the greater the risk of atherosclerosis. Recently, numerous observations suggest that not only the concentration but also structural features of low-density lipoproteins (LDL) are important to the development of the disease. The properties and absolute amounts of modified LDL in the plasma of an individual might be due to genetic background, or initiated by interactions with blood components or vascular cells or macromolecules. In our previous studies [1,2] alterations in various properties of LDL were found to be important factors in the mechanism of arterial lipid deposition. These findings suggested that the early detection of modified LDL might be of great interest in the prevention of atherosclerosis and stimulated us to perform clinical epidemiological investigations. We measured the plasma concentration of peroxidated lipoproteins and of Lp(a) in atherosclerotic, in diabetic and in type II hyperlipemic patients and performed a screening study on children with familial risk for atherosclerosis. Our *in vitro* experiments aimed to clarify the mechanisms of the underlying pathological proccesses.

Studying the possibilities of the prevention or reversibility of LDL entrapment, natural compounds, interfering with the binding of LDL by proteoglycans (PG) or elastin were identified in human serum.

MATERIALS AND METHODS

A total of 508 patients between the age of 40 and 80 years, suffering from advanced ischaemic vascular disease (IVD) of varying localization (coronary, cerebral) and 158 children between the age of 2 and 15 years with familial risk for atherosclerosis were included into the studies, Selection criteria for adult patients were: 1. ischaemic heart disease (IHD) group (n=180), myocardial infarction at least 6 months prior to the investigation or typical anginal pains and ECG signs for myocardial ischaemia; 2. cerebrovascular disease (CVD) group (n=175), acute cerebrovascular accident with focal neurological signs in the case history at least 6 months prior to the investigation; 3. diabetes group, type 1 and type 2 diabetics (n=40 and 65, resp.), with or without angiopathic complications; 4. patients with type IIa and type IIb hyperlipidemia (n=21 and 27, resp.)

Selection criteria for the endangered children: a. IHD group, parents surviving myocardial infarction below the age of 45 years (n=47); b. CVD group, parents with hypertension and apoplexy, hypertonic children (n=52); c. diabetes group, diabetic families with angiopathic complications (n=47); d. multi-risk group, coexistence of 2 or 3 of the above risk factors in the family history (n=12).

Control groups were selected from age-, and sex-matched healthy individuals (n=283 and 102 for adults and for children, resp.)

Fractionation of serum lipoproteins and the isolation of the d> 1.24 g/ml protein fraction was carried out by ultracentrifugation.

Fibronectin was prepared from normal human plasma by affinity chromatography on gelatin Sepharose [3].

Arterial glycosaminoglycans (GAG) and PG were isolated from human aorta intima [4].

Malondialdehyde (MDA) level was measured as an index of peroxidation by the thiobarbituric acid (TBA) method according to Lee [5].

Lp(a) was quantitated by the Laurell technique according to Krempler et al. [6].

Elastase-type protease activity and pancreas elastase inhibitory capacity was measured by the method of Bieth [7].

The interaction between aortic GAG/PG and serum lipoproteins was studied as described in details previously [8].

RESULTS AND DISCUSSION

1. Peroxidated lipoproteins

It is now generally agreed that elevated concentration of lipid peroxides in serum might initiate atherogenesis and participate in its progression by causing chronic stress for endothelial cells and by reorienting arachidonic cascade towards intensified thromboxane synthesis. Reports concerning the correlation between the age of the individual and the lipid peroxide level in plasma are still contradictory. As reported previously [9[in our studies significant age-related increase could be demonstrated both in healthy individuals and in atherosclerotic patients. The elevation was mainly due to increased lipid peroxide level in the LDL fraction. Atherosclerotic patients had significantly higher lipid peroxide levels than the age-matched control subjects.

Lipid peroxidation by blood components, such as platelets, may be present in diabetes, since platelets from diabetic patients are known to show an increased sensitivity to aggregating agents, and MDA might be released in increased amounts from diabetic platelets inducing a chemical modification of LDL.

In our studies significantly increased MDA levels were found in the serum of diabetic patients (0.87 and 0.67 nmol/ml in diabetics and in control subjects, resp., $p < 0.05$). The elevation was of highest significance in diabetic patients with angiopathic complications (1.13 nmol/ml, $p \leq 0.01$ vs. control), suggesting that the link between atherosclerosis and diabetes may very well be related to lipoprotein abnormalities not only in the quantitative sense, but also in the qualitative sense. The increase of lipid peroxidation could mainly be attributed to the intensification of lipid peroxidation in the LDL fraction. In diabetic-atherosclerotic patients significant elevation of MDA content occurred in the HDL (HDL-3) fraction as well.

In order to throw more light on the mechanism of lipid peroxidation *in vitro* investigations were performed. The results of our studies on cell cultures support the assumption that endothelial cells play a role in the biologic generation of oxidized LP-s and that on the other hand oxidized LP-s have a metabolic effect causing cytotoxicity and leading to cell death [9].

2. Lipoprotein Lp(a)

It has been reported that high values of Lp(a) carry increased risk for IHD and CVD, however no correlation could be revealed between Lp(a) levels and other risk or antirisk factors for atherosclerosis. In our investigations the mean serum concentration of Lp(a) was significantly increased in atherosclerotic patients as compared to controls: 37.5, 39.0 and 27.6 mg/dl in IHD, CVD and control individuals, resp. ($p \leq 0.01$ vs. control). The elevation was more expressed in the case when atherosclerosis was associated with type II hyperlipidemia (52.3 and 47.6 mg/dl in type IIa and type IIb,resp.) or diabetes (47.6 mg/dl),however because of the wide range of distribution on the scatter diagram, the difference between the various groups of patients was statistically not significant,supporting the suggestion that Lp(a) is an independent risk factor for atherosclerosis.

It is accepted that Lp(a) is not only directly related to atherosclerosis, but is also genetically determined. The results of our screening studies, performed on children with familial risk for atherosclerosis, showed that the concentration of Lp(a) was very highly significantly increased ($p \leq 0.001$) in all but one (the diabetes) groups as compared to the controls (IHD 17.0, CVD 13.4, diabetes 7.2, multirisk 18.3, control 6.8 mg/dl). Elevated Lp(a) levels were measured in approx. 60% of the IHD group and of the multirisk group and in approx.40% of the CVD group.

Little is known concerning the atherogenicity of Lp(a). The data obtained in a series of in vitro studies might give a possible clue for the underlying molecular mechanisms [8]. It could be proved that Lp(a) is an even more favored substrate for the interaction with GAG and PG than LDL.It seems to be concievable that Lp(a) might react with soluble GAG of human plasma; this interaction not only may mask the uptake by the B/E receptor, but also may lead to the catabolism of the complexes by the scavenger pathway. Another explanation might be that Lp(a) that passed the endothelial layer and entered the intima might be complexed with arterial PG and retained to a much higher degree than LDL. There the complexes may be deposited extracellularly or, as rendered probable by our experiments performed on mouse peritoneal macrophages, might be taken up by monocytes/macrophages and be transformed into foam cells.

3. Natural inhibitory factors interfering with the lipoprotein - proteoglycan interaction

Studying the possibilities of the prevention or reversibility of LDL entrapment in the arterial wall the presence of natural inhibitory factor(s) in serum, interfering with the binding of LDL to PG has logically been assumed. This assumption was supported by our previous observation [10] that LDL, when added in the form of whole serum, had approx. 40% lower reactivity with PG than LDL of the same concentration. We also described that HDL had an approx. 25-30% inhibitory capacity when added to the mixture of GAG and LDL.
According to our recent investigations [11], a factor, isolated from the d>1.24 density fraction of human serum inhibits the GAG/PG - LDL interaction by approx. 50% at physiological concentration. Experiments [12], carried out with purified human plasma fibronectin suggest, that fibronectin may well be this (or one of these) inhibiting factors: the inhibitory capacity of fibronectin was 100% at approx. 50% of the physiological ratio in human serum. Furthermore, our results indicated that fibronectin can compete with GAG at the sites of GAG binding on LDL, and has a higher affinity for LDL than GAG/PG. Since fibronectin concentration is known to increase in the plaque area, it seems to be likely that fibronectin would not only dissociate GAG/PG - LDL complexes, but by replacing LDL - PG complexes by fibronectin - LDL complexes might accelerate the elimination of LDL particles from the arterial wall.

4. Factors interfering with the lipoprotein - elastin interaction

An important proccess leading to the development of the well-known appearance of atherosclerosis is the degradation of elastic fibres and the fragmentation of the elastic lamellae. The regulation of elastin metabolism both under physiological and pathological conditions is attributed to humoral and tissue elastases and their inhibitors. The mechanism of action of elastase consists of the selective degradation of lipid-bound elastin, by which elastase promotes the biosynthesis of newly formed elastin [13].
In our studies decreased elastase activity was measured in the serum of atherosclerotic patients (5.0, 7.9 and 9.3 ng/ml/24 h in IHD, CVD and control groups, resp., $p \leq 0.001$ vs. control). This phenomenon might reflect a causal relation.
The presence of elastase inhibitors in human serum has been identified. In healthy individuals we found a significant positive correlation ($p \leq 0.001$) between the elastase-type enzyme activity of the sera and their elastase inhibitory capacity [14]; this correlation could not be established in the sera of patients suffering from IVD, pointing to the possibility that in healthy individuals variation of elastase-type activity is counterbalanced by its inhibitors;

the lack of proportionality within the pathological population may well be related to the atherosclerotic proccess.

REFERENCES

1. Bihari-Varga,M.,Sztatisz,J.,Gal,S. (1981)'Changes in the physical structure of low-density lipoproteins in the presence of glycosaminoglycans and high-density lipoprotein' Atherosclerosis 39,19-23

2. Bihari-Varga,M.,Goldstein,S.,Lagrange,D.,Gruber,E. (1982)'Effect of limited tryptic treatment and sialic acid removal of low-density lipoproteins on the lipoprotein - glycosaminoglycan interaction'Internatl.J.Biol.Macromol. 4,438-442

3. Yamada,K.M.(1982)'Immunochemistry of the Extracellular Matrix'Furthmayr,H.(ed.),CRC Press,Boca Raton pp.111-123

4. Bihari-Varga,M.,Camejo,G.,Horn M.C.,Lopez,F.,Gruber E. (1983)'Structure of low-density lipoprotein comlexes formed with arterial matrix components'Int.J.Biol.Macromol.5,59-62

5. Lee,D.M. (1980)'Malondialdehyde formation in stored plasma'Biochem.Biophys.Res.Com.95,1663-1672

6. Krempler,F.,Kostner,G.M.,Bolzano,K.,Sandhofer,F. (1980) Turnover of lipoprotein Lp(a) in man'J.Clin.Invest. 65, 1483-1489

7. Bieth,J. (1978)'Elastases' in L.Robert (ed.),Frontiers of matrix biology,Karger,Basel,pp.1-8

8. Bihari-Varga,M.,Gruber,E.,Rotheneder,M.,Zechner,R., Kostner,G.M. (1988)'Interaction of Lipoprotein Lp(a) and Low Density Lipoprotein with Glycosaminoglycans from Human Aorta'Arteriosclerosis 8,851-857

9. Bihari-Varga,M.,Keller,L.,Csonka,E.,Landi,A.,Jellinek,H. (1988)'Oxidatively modified lipoproteins:humoral changes with age and atherosclerosis and interactions with endothelial cells'in G.Weber (ed.)Biology of the Arterial Wall, CIC Roma,pp.243-254

10. Bihari-Varga,M.(1978)'Influence of serum high-density lipoproteins on the low-density lipoprotein - aortic glycosaminoglycan interaction'Artery 4,504-511

11. Kempen,H.J.,Buytenhek,M.,GruberE.,Bihari-Varga,M.(1989) 'Factor present in plasma,inhibiting the interaction of low-density lipoprotein with arterial proteoglycan' Atherosclerosis 78,137-144

12. Labat-Robert,J.,Gruber,E.,Bihari-Varga,M.(1989)'Interaction between fibronectin,proteoglycans and lipoproteins' Int.J.Biol.Macromol. in the press

13. Katsunuma,H.,Shimizu,K.,Ebihara,T.,Iwamoto,T.(1983) 'Anti-atherosclerotic action of elastase'Age Ageing 12, 183-192

14. Bihari-Varga,M.,Keller,L.,Landi,A.,Robert,L.(1984) 'Elastase-type activity,elastase inhibitory capacity,lipids and lipoproteins in the sera of patients with ischaemic vascular disease'Atherosclerosis 50,273-281

ATHEROSCLEROSIS IN YOUTH

55

The WHO-ISFC study on pathobiological determinants of atherosclerosis in youth (PBDAY): a first morphometric approach to aortic lesions

G. WEBER, G. BIANCIARDI, L. CENTI, A. CICOGNANI*, G. FORTUNI*, M. SALVI, P. TANGANELLI and M. FALLANI*

*Istituto di Anatomia e Istologia Patologica, Centro di Ricerche Arteriosclerosi, via delle Scotte 6, 53100 Siena, Italy. *Istituto di Medicina Legale, Bologna, Italy*

INTRODUCTION

One of the aims of the PBDAY Study (WHO-ISFC) is to examine, both in children and young adults, the arterial structural changes which may determine the development of atherosclerosis, especially in its early stages and in relation to the social-cultural characteristics of different populations (1).
The Morphometric Reference Centre of the PBDAY Study in Siena, has been studying the extent, localization and composition of the aortic and coronary lesions, through the following approaches: 1) by using an automated image processing system in order to quantify the aortic intimal sudanophilia percentage and its spatial distribution; 2) using a manual input followed by image processing in order to evaluate the percentage of arterial raised lesions and their spatial distribution; 3) through a computerized manual assisted morphometry the histologic aspects of the lesions were examined.

Supported by NATO Grant 86/0446, CNR 88.00687.04, and M.P.I. 40%, 1988. We kindly acknowledge J.F. Cornhill and E.E. Herderick, The Ohio State University, Lab. of Experimental Atherosclerosis, Columbus, USA, for their help in the development of the morphometric techniques.

In this report we presented the preliminary data on aortic sudanophilia in order to study the spatial occurrence of fatty or fibro-fatty lesions in young Italian subjects.

MATERIALS AND METHODS

Twenty-five half left aortas, longitudinally cut from young Italian subjects (15-34 years of age) were stained with Sudan III, photographed on 35 mm color slides and sent to us from the Reference Centre of Malmö in Sweden (Prof. N.A. Sternby from the Patologiska Institutionen). In the Morphometric Reference Centre, the pictures of the aortas were digitized using a personal computer PC IBM AT-compatible (PC BIT, Rome), an Oculus-200 frame-grabber (Coreco, Canada; Pertel, Torino), a telecamera and our own software (C language). The digitized images (484 x 512 pixels, 256 gray levels) were filtered through linear stretch and a low-pass filter. Subsequently, a "follower" detected both the outline of the lipidic lesions and vessels. After the editing procedure (e.g. to erase shadows), the outlined images were stored on floppy disks. In order to remove anatomical variations among individual vessel specimens, the images collected from each vessel were subjected to linear transformation by subdividing each image into triangular sections which were successively transformed into corresponding triangles on a standard template (2). The standard templates were evaluated from the mean location of the anatomical landmarks of all the aortas studied. The anatomical landmarks, which corresponded to the apices of these triangles, were manually identified by using a graphic pen that was interfaced onto the computerized device. Finally, probability-of-occurrence maps were produced through subsequent algorhythms.

RESULTS

Our preliminary data show: 1) High variation of involvement among the individuals. 2) High (more than 50%) probabilities of sudanophilia in the thoracic dorsal surface (between the origin of the intercostal arteries), at the inflow of the celiac and mesenteric arteries, and in front of the 1st lumbar artery. 3) High (more than 50%) probabilities of sudanophilic lesions were also related to areas not associated with entrance regions or branching points (e.g. in the ventral surface of the abdominal aorta on the opposite side of the XII intercostal artery. 4) Low (less than 25%) probabilities of sudanophilia were present in the thoracic ventral surface and in the region close to the iliac bifurcation. Our preliminary results (3) agree with the results of the PDAY U.S. Study.

CONCLUSIONS

The probability-of-occurrence map represents an important advancement for the future exploration of the physical and metabolic differences between atherosclerotic lesion-prone and lesion-resistant areas. From our preliminary data on the study of aortic sudanophilia in the Italian specimens, though a major portion of sudanophilic lesions was associated with areas close to orifice regions (high shear stress regions), others were not linked to entrance regions or branching points and, viceversa, not all the areas associated with the entrance regions or branching points, appeared affected by sudanophilic lesions.

REFERENCES

(1) McGill HC Dr, ed. (1968). "The Geographic Pathology of Atherosclerosis". Baltimore, Waverly Press, pp. 126-133.

(2) Cornhill JF, Barrett WA, Herderick EE, Mahley RW, Fry D.L. (1985). Topographic study of sudanophilic lesions in cholesterol-fed mini pigs by image analysis. Arteriosclerosis, 5, 415-626.

(3) Cornhill JF, Herderick EE (1988). Localization of human atherosclerotic lesions with regard to hemodynamic forces. VIIIth International Symposium on Atherosclerosis, Roma. Poster sessions, abstract book, p. 157.

56
Atherosclerosis precursors in children. The Bologna study, an update

G. FALDELLA, S. ALATI, R. ALESSANDRONI, R. ROSSINI, M. LANARI, C. COLUCCI and G.P. SALVIOLI

Department of Preventive Pediatrics and Neonatology, University of Bologna, via Massarenti 11, 40138 Bologna, Italy

INTRODUCTION

In 1985, a prospective study was designed to obtain data on the risk factors of atherosclerosis and its determinants in Bologna school age children and to plan educational programmes in school that enable children to make informed choices concerning their health and lifestyle.
The study plan consisted of three successive stages. In the first stage, participants were enrolled and the cardiovascular risk factors prevalent among them were assessed. The second stage was an educational programme in which the results of initial blood tests and assessment of diet and lifestyle were discussed with the children, who were then informed about existing cultural and social trends and correct eating and lifestyle habits. In the third stage, at the end of the study the efficacy of the programme was evaluated by reassessing all the parameters considered at the outset.

SUBJECTS AND METHODS

The study was performed in three Bologna secondary schools. In January 1986, all first year students aged 12 +/- 0.5 years were invited to participate in the project and were informed about the study design. Then, data were collected on general health and development, lifestyle, nutritional habits and family health. Besides, the children underwent a medical examination for evaluation of height, weight, body mass index (BMI), ratio between real and ideal weight (RW:IW), triceps skinfold thickness (TST), blood pressure (BP) and a fasting venous blood sample was collected for evaluation of serum total cholesterol (TC), HDL-cholesterol (HDL-C), triglycerides (T), glucose and uric acid concentrations.

The educational program was carried out in schools. To make the intervention as feasible and as simple and possible and applicable to the general school population in the future, maximum teacher co-operation was sought. As adolescence is a critical period for adopting lifestyle habits which will be maintained throughout adulthood, the educational programme looked to develop children's awareness of primary health care and preventive medicine. Emphasis was placed on regular physical activity, maintenance of ideal body weight, discouraging smoking, and teaching the basic elements of a healthy diet. No individual dietary regimen was recommended.

Detailed methods on data collection procedures and laboratory analysis have been published elsewhere (1).

The data were processed using specific programmes developed for this study on an IBM computer linked to the Central University Computer (CINECA).

Statistical methods included Student's t test and correlation analysis.

RESULTS

At the beginning of the study (T1), the students present in the first middle school classes were 481 and 92.9% of the them agreed to enter. 33 of them were excluded as they were >13 years or <11 years old or had not had blood test. Thus the children eligible for longitudinal survey were 207 males, mean age = 11.80 years (SD=0.3), and 207 females, mean age = 11.74 years (SD=0.3).

Two years apart (T2), 385 students present in the third middle school classes were fully examined. 339 of them, 163 males and 176 females, were present both at T1 and T2 and thus the results of the study refer to them.

Cigarette smoking

At T1 3.5% males and 1% females admitted to having smoked. At T2 they were 16.3% and 15.3% respectively. Nobody was a regular smoker at T1 while 1.5% was at T2. Among the parents, prevalence of smokers slightly decreased from T1 (46% fathers and 36% mothers) to T2 (42% fathers and 34% mothers). 51% of the mothers of the children who had experienced cigarette smoking were regular smokers against 31% of the mothers of the children who had never smoked. No significant difference was found among fathers.Children with experience of smoking were clustered in school: in fact 69% of them were in 8 out of 23 classes.

Physical activity

Sedentary pattern of physical activity (i.e.: usually reads, watches television , goes to the cinema or spends leisure-time in sedentary activities) or moderately active pattern (i.e.: walks, rides a bicycle or spends at least four hours a week moving outdoors) concerned 48% males and 53% females at 12 years of age and 31% males and 45% females at 14 years of age. No correlation, either direct or indirect, was found between physical activity and experience of smoking. Thus, at this age, the attitute to smoking and to moving do not seem opposite behavioural models.
Among 14 year old males there was a good inverse correlation between physical activity and both triceps skinfold thickness and real weight:ideal weight ratio. Among females this correlation was found for RW:IW ratio but not for TST.

Height, weight, body mass index, skinfold

Mean and standard deviation of height, weight, BMI and triceps skinfold thickness, by sex, are summarized in table 1.

TABLE 1. Height, weight, body mass index and triceps skinfold in secondary school students at 12 and 14 years of age, 163 males and 176 females.

		12 years		14 years	
	Sex	Mean	SD	Mean	SD
H (cm)	M	149	7	163	8
	F	149	7	158	6
W (Kg)	M	45	10	57	11
	F	44	9	53	9
BMI (Kg/m2)	M	19.9	3.4	21.2	3.4
	F	19.6	3.1	21.5	2.9
TS (mm)	M	15.0	6.7	12.2	5.7
	F	15.8	5.6	15.8	5.1

Height and weight values of the subjects in study at both 12 and 14 years of age are above those referred in the tables of recommended dietary allowances for the Italian population (2). While they are equivalent in males and females at 12 years, they significantly differ at 14 years, related to the growth spurt of males. Thickness of triceps skinfold shows a significant reduction in boys ($p<.0005$) but not in girls.

Blood pressure

Mean systolic pressure was 125 mmHg (SD=13) in males and 126 mmHg (SD=15) in females at 12 years of age and 118 mmHg (SD=14) and 114 mmHg (SD=14) respectively at 14 years. Mean diastolic pressure was 77 mmHg (SD=10) in males and 77 mmHg (11) in females at 12 years and 66 mmHg (SD=13) and 67 mmHg (SD=12) at 14 years. The blood pressure levels significantly differ between 12 and 14 years of age. While blood pressure was measured with accurate instruments and procedures, environmental factors as anxiety should in part explain these differences. Blood pressure was correlated to body weight in males, both at 12 and 14 years, but not in females

Serum lipids

Mean and standard deviation of serum total cholesterol, high-density lipoproteins cholesterol and triglycerides, by sex, are summarized in table 2.

TABLE 2. Serum total cholesterol, HDL-cholesterol and triglycerídes in 339 secondary school students at 12 and 14 years of age, 163 males and 176 females.

		12 years		14 years	
	Sex	Mean	SD	Mean	SD
TC (mg/dl)	M	176	26	168	27
	F	179	27	177	26
HDL-C (mg/dl)	M	55	7	56	9
	F	54	8	60	9
TRI (mg/dl)	M	67	25	69	32
	F	71	27	68	26

Mean TC values were above the levels considered "at risk" for children by the NIH Consensus Conference, both in males and females and at 12 and 14 years of age (3). Mean T2 TC was significantly lower than T1 TC in males (P<0.005) but not in females. Conversely, mean HDL-C values were similar in males at T1 and T2, but significantly increased in females (P<0.005). No significant difference in triglycerides mean values was observed among males or females at either T1 or T2.
The overall correlation between the T1 TC determination and that at T2 was r=.73 (P<0.0001) both in males and in females. Individual TC levels at T1 and T2 showed a variation not greater than 10% in 57% males and 70% females; in most of the other children TC dropped by more

than 10%
Serum TC concentrations ranging from 180 to 199 mg/dl were found in 27% males and 28% females at T1 and in 18% and 22% respectively at T2. Values equal to or greater than 200 mg/dl of serum TC were found in 18% males and 19% females at T1 and 10% and 18% respectively at T2.

Nutrient intakes

The mean values and standard deviations of the intakes of energy-yielding nutrients, cholesterol and fibre (tab.3) were calculated from the dietary records of 213 children who participated in the dietary study both at 12 and 14 years of age.

TABLE 3. Mean daily intakes of energy and some nutrients in 213 children at 12 and 14 years of age.

	T1		T2		
	MEAN	S.D.	MEAN	S.D.	P
ENERGY (kcal)	2197	482	2203	596	N.S.
PROTEIN (% cal)	14.6	1.7	15.6	2.7	<.0005
ANIMAL PROTEIN (% cal)	9.8	1.9	10.3	2.9	<.025
FAT (% cal)	39.9	5.3	37.3	6.7	<.0005
ANIMAL FAT (% cal)	26.9	6.1	23.9	6.5	<.0005
CHOLESTEROL (mg%.cal)	191	46	199	77	N.S.
CARBOHYDRATE (% cal)	44.4	5.6	45.9	6.9	<.01
FIBRE (g)	14.9	5.0	17.2	7.2	<.0005

Correlations

A very good correlation ($p<0.0001$) between T1 and T2 values was found for BMI (r=.91 in M; r=.87 in F), TST (r=.75 in M; r=.73 in F), RW:IW (r=.87 in M; r=.84 in F), TC (r=.73 in M; r=.73 in F). A good correlation ($p<0.001$) was found for systolic BP (r=.44 both in M and F), HDL-C (r=.48 in M; r=.45 in F), TG (r=.52 in M; r=.42 in F). Diastolic BP correlated in M (r=.24) but not in F (r=.14).
Interrelationships between physical measurements and serum lipids are shown in tables 4 and 5 Systolic blood pressure values significantly correlated with anthropometric measurements at 12 and 14 years both in boys and in girls. This was less evident for diastolic blood pressure. Serum lipids were significantly correlated with each other. Total cholesterol was positively correlated with triceps skinfold thickness in males but not in females.
No correlation was found between serum cholesterol and fat and cholesterol intake, either at T1 and T2.

TABLE 4. Correlation coefficient (r) between studied variables in 163 boys at 12 and 14 years of age.

	T	RW:IW	BMI	TS	SBP	DBP	TC	HDL-C	TG
RW:IW	1		.94	.83	.52	.37	.17	-.10	.43
	2		.95	.76	.33	.25	.26	-.19	.13
BMI	1	.94		.83	.61	.42	.08	-.16	.40
	2	.95		.70	.37	.24	.19	-.25	.33
TS	1	.83	.83		.47	.33	.23	-.11	.41
	2	.76	.69		.23	.15	.31	-.02	.25
SBP	1	.52	.61	.47		.53	.05	-.09	.24
	2	.33	.37	.23		.46	.03	-.03	.06
DBP	1	.37	.42	.33	.53		.03	-.08	.12
	2	.25	.24	.15	.46		.02	-.01	-.02
TC	1	.17	.08	.23	.05	.03		.16	.31
	2	.26	.19	.31	.03	.02		.24	.26
HDL-C	1	-.10	-.16	-.11	-.09	-.08	.16		-.24
	2	-.19	-.25	-.02	-.03	-.01	.24		-.32
TG	1	.43	.40	.41	.24	.12	.31	-.24	
	2	.34	.33	.25	.06	-.02	.26	-.32	

if r> 0.25 P<0.001; if r>0.20 P<0.01; if r>0.15 P<0.05

TABLE 5. Correlation coefficient (r) between studied variables in girls at 12 and 14 years of age.

	T	RW:IW	BMI	TS	SBP	DBP	TC	HDL-C	TG
RW:IW	1		.95	.80	.41	.34	.07	-.06	.23
	2		.93	.68	.22	.00	.01	-.21	.08
BMI	1	.95		.80	.41	.34	.07	-.06	.23
	2	.93		.74	.24	.05	.01	-.20	.03
TS	1	.80	.82		.40	.33	.10	-.05	.14
	2	.68	.74		.17	-.03	-.04	-.14	-.03
SBP	1	.41	.50	.40		.67	-.11	-.13	.13
	2	.22	.24	.17		.53	.10	-.02	.05
DBP	1	.34	.39	.33	.67		-.08	-.08	.14
	2	.00	.05	-.03	.53		.04	-.00	-.06
TC	1	.07	.01	.10	-.11	-.08		.27	.21
	2	.01	.01	-.04	.10	.04		.38	.14
HDL-C	1	-.06	-.11	-.05	-.13	-.08	.27		-.23
	2	-.21	-.20	-.14	-.02	-.00	.38		-.25
TG	1	.23	.21	.14	.13	.14	.21	-.23	
	2	.08	.03	-.03	-.05	-.06	.14	-.25	

if r>0.25 P<0.001; if r>0.20 P<0.01; ifr>0.15 P<0.05

CONCLUSIONS

There is now general agreement that atherosclerosis prevention should begin in childhood. Adequate diet, regular physical activity, maintenance of ideal weight, avoidance of excess salt and cigarette smoking are the main steps of basic prevention. Identification and treatment of children at risk because of elevated blood cholesterol (TC) levels should be careful to avoid causing nutritional deficiencies or unjustified fear of illness. Moreover, during childhood TC varies and raised HDL-cholesterol (HDL-C) often accounts for elevated TC, so it would be better to evaluate non-HDL-C or LDL-C, using the formula of Friedewald et al.(4).
As in the USA and North Europe (5,6), serum cholesterol levels of Italian children are high, as appears from this and other studies. We found significant changes in nutritional habits, expecially in the fat intake, from T1 to T2. This apparently confirms the efficacy of the educational program. In fact, these changes did not occur among the children who had total cholesterol levels under 180 mg/dl at 12 years of age (fat intake = 39.5% cal at T1 and = 38.3% cal at T2), while they were consistent in those children with cholesterol levels above 200 mg/dl (fat intake = 41%cal at T1 and = 37.2% cal at T2). Moreover, it is difficult to ascertain the effect of diet on plasma cholesterol, at least at this age, as the above mentioned nutritional changes were evident both in children whose plasma cholesterol dropped under 200 mg/dl, with a very significant decrease in their previous level, and in those who maintained their elevated plasma cholesterol after our intervention in schools. Lastly, the tendency of plasma cholesterol to drop in males from 12 to 14 years of age and conversely the rise in HDL-cholesterol in females, during the same period, strongly suggest that hormonal and growth changes may have a notable effect on plasma cholesterol. Thus, according to the Nutrition Committee of the American Academy of Pediatrics (7) any widespread application of restrictive dietary patterns during childhood and adolescence should await demonstration of safety and efficacy of such restrictions in the population at risk.

Acknowledgements

We are grateful to Prof.G.C.Descovich for his helpful advice and suggestions and for analyzing the blood samples. This study was supported by the Emilia Romagna Region, Programma di ricerca sanitaria finalizzata per il triennio 1985-87.

REFERENCES

1. Salvioli G.P., Faldella G., Alessandroni R., Rossini R.,Lanari M., Alati S., De Marchis C. (1986) "Atherosclerosis precursors in children. The Bologna study. Preliminary data", in S. Lenzi and G.C. Descovich (eds.), Atherosclerosis and Cardiovascular Diseases, MTP Press Limited, Lancaster, pp. 205-213.

2. Turchetto E.(1986). LARN: i Livelli di Assunzione Raccomandati in Nutrienti per gli italiani. Pediatria, 1, 18-23.

3. Consensus Development Panel (1985). Lowering blood cholesterol to prevent heart disease. JAMA, 253, 2080-86.

4. Friedewald W.T., Levy R.I., Fredrickson D.S. (1972). Estimation of the concentration of low density lipoprotein cholesterol in plasma, without use the preparative ultracentrifuge. Clin.Chem. 18, 499-505.

5. Berenson, GS and Epstein, FH (1983). Conference on blood lipids in children: optimal levels for early prevention of coronary artery disease. Workshop Report: Epidemiological section. April 18 and 19, 1983. American Health Foundation. Prev Med, 12, 741

6. Viikari, J, Akerblom, HK and Uhari, M (1985). Atherosclerosis precursors in children. Acta Paediatr Scand, Suppl 318

7. American Academy of Pediatrics. Committee on Nutrition (1986). Prudent Life-style for Children: Dietary Fat and Cholesterol. Pediatrics, 78, 521-525.

57
Lipid and apolipoprotein in cord blood

M.R. AVERNA, C.M. BARBAGALLO, S. AMATO, G. DI PAOLA, G. MARINO, M. LABISI, U. DIMITA and A. NOTARBARTOLO

Internal Medicine and Geriatrics Institute, Department of Pathological Medicine, via del Vespro 143, 90127 Palermo, Italia

Abstract

In this study a series of Sicilian neonates was studied in order to investigate about the distribution of serum lipid and apolipoprotein at birth and the differences with adults. A series of 200 term, healthy newborns was studied. Total cholesterol (TC), triglyceride (TG), HDL-cholesterol (HDL-C), LDL-cholesterol (LDL-C), apo AI and apo B were assayed in all cord blood samples. TC mean value was 63.2 mg/dl and HDL-C represented about the 40 % of TC: no differences was found between male and female newborns. In neonates TC and LDL-C were about three-fold lower than adults, while HDL-C was about the 60 %; apo AI and apo B were respectively about 60 % and 30 % of adult levels. 3.5 % of newborns presented TC levels above the mean + 2 standard deviations. In conclusion lipid and apolipoprotein distributions in Sicilian newborns are not different from that of other population and there are no differences between males and females. It should be interesting the follow-up of "hypercholesterolemic" newborns in order to establish if it is possible to do a neonatal screening of familial hypercholesterolemia.

Introduction

Plasma lipids in cord blood have been studied by many authors in order to provide information on normal distribution of lipids in neonates and also to evaluate the feasibility of screening programs for early detection of hyperlipoproteinemia [1, 2]. At birth cholesterol, triglyceride and HDL-C levels in different population are very similar; in comparison to normal adult levels, LDL-C is about one third, triglyceride and VLDL are strongly reduced and the cholesterol of HDL is about 40 % of total serum cholesterol (3, 4, 5). Few studies, to our knowledge,have been carried out on apolipoprotein distribution in cord blood. Apo AI and apo B have been found present at 25% and 60% respectively of levels of adults [6, 7].In order to provide informations on cord serum lipid and apoliprotein AI and B distributions and to elucidate the differences between adult and neonatal lipid and apolipoprotein profiles, a series of 200 term neonates born in Sicily was studied.

Materials and methods

A series of 200 newborns, 100 males (M) and 100 females (F), born in a Department of Obstetrics and Neonatology in Palermo,between February 1989 and August 1989 was investigated. Cord blood was collected as soon as possible after birth from the umbilical vein. Clinical characterics (gestational weeks, Apgar score after 5', weight and lenght) are shown in table 1.

Tab. 1: Clinical characteristics of 200 Sicilian newborns.

	weeks	Apgar score	weight	lenght
All	39.4 ± 1.4	9.5 ± 1.1	3275.1 ± 469.2	49.4 ± 2.3
M	39.6 ± 1.2	9.5 ± 1.1	3404.4 ± 420.8	50.1 ± 1.9
F	39.1 ± 1.6	9.5 ± 1.1	3149.8 ± 479.5	48.8 ± 2.5

In cord blood samples total cholesterol (TC), triglyceride (TG) (enzimatic methods) and HDL-cholesterol (HDL-C) (PTA/Magnesium Chloride method) were assayed; LDL-cholesterol (LDL-C) was calculated by Friedewald formula. Apo AI and apo B were determined by nephelometric method (Behring nephelometer). Lipid and apolipoprotein quality controls were performed as previous described [8]. Newborns were compared with a group of 82 normolipidemic Sicilian healthy adults.

Results

In table 2 lipid and apolipoprotein levels in our series are shown. The cholesterol content of HDL-C represent about 40% of total cholesterol. TC, TG, HDL-C, LDL-C, Apo AI and B were not significantly different in male compared to female newborns.

Tab. 2: Lipid and apolipoprotein levels in 200 Sicilian newborns.

	TC	TG	HDL-C	LDL-C	AI	B
All	63.2 ± 23.9	42.2 ± 21.4	24.9 ± 7.1	35.2 ± 18.1	79.2 ± 13.8	27.9 ± 9.8
M	62.2 ± 26.5	43.2 ± 23.9	26.6 ± 7.1	33.5 ± 18.5	79.0 ± 13.2	27.0 ± 10.5
p	ns	ns	ns	ns	ns	ns
F	64.2 ± 21.0	41.3 ± 18.4	24.2 ± 6.9	36.9 ± 17.5	79.5 ± 14.5	28.6 ± 9.1

In table 3 newborns lipo-apoprotein profile has been compared to adult one. In newborns total cholesterol and LDL-C were about three-fold lower than adults, while HDL-C was about the 60% of adult level. Apo AI and apo B were respectively about 60% and 30% of adult values.

Tab. 3: Lipo-apoprotein profile: comparison of 200 Sicilian newborns (N) with 82 Sicilian adult controls (C).

	TC	TG	HDL-C	LDL-C	AI	B
N	63.2 ± 23.9	42.2 ± 21.4	24.9 ± 7.1	35.2 ± 18.1	79.2 ± 13.8	27.9 ± 9.8
%	38.2	49.8	56.2	33.9	60.5	29.1
C	165.1 ± 25.4	84.7 ± 33.3	44.1 ± 11.6	103.8 ± 23.6	130.8 ± 19.6	94.1 ± 16.4

In figure 1 the distribution curves of TC, LDL-C and apo B were depicted.

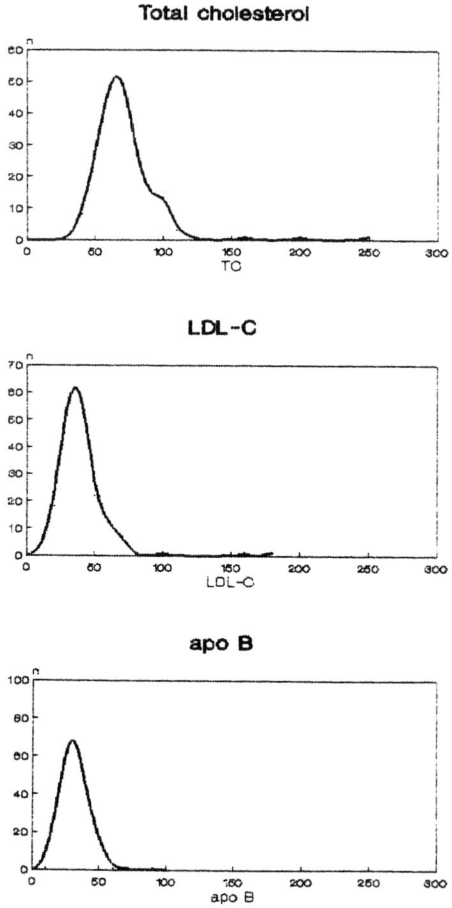

Fig. 1: Distribution of total cholesterol, LDL-cholesterol and apo B in 200 Sicilian newborns.

In order to establish the prevalence of abnormal cholesterol values, a mean + 2 standard deviations value was selected as cut-off. In table 4 the prevalence of "hypercholesterolemia" (evaluated as above) is shown. In our population 3.5 % of newborns showed cholesterol levels above the mean + 2 standard deviations. Lipo-apolipoprotein profile of "hypercholesterolemic" newborns was different from that of "normocholesterolemic" newborns: TC, TG, HDL-C, LDL-C and apo B were significanty higher.

Tab. 4: Lipids and apolipoproteins according to cholesterol levels.

	n	%	TC	TG	HDL-C	LDL-C	B
<2 SD	193		60.3 ± 14.7	40.6 ± 17.3	24.3 ± 6.2	32.9 ± 11.1	27.3 ± 8.6
p			*	*	*	*	*
>2 SD	7	3.5	149.1 ± 59.9	87.5 ± 51.9	38.4 ± 10.6	93.2 ± 46.8	49.0 ± 21.6

* $p < 0.0001$

Discussion

The results of this study confirm that cholesterol levels at born,in spite of geographical differences, are very similar in all population with values ranging from 60 to 82 mg /dl [1, 2, 3, 4, 5].In three previous studies in Italian newborns cholesterol levels were very similar to present data [9, 10, 11]. In perinatal period changes of cholesterol levels have been described: pre-term newborns show cholesterol levels higher than term ones. This finding has been explained by increased adrenal cholesterol uptake for steroidogenesis in the later gestational period;in fact LDL-receptor system reach complete maturity between 16 and 20 weeks of fetus development [12]. Cholesterol distribution between lipoprotein classes in cord blood differ from adult. VLDL are less represented than HDL and LDL. In this study plasma cholesterol was distributed for the 40 % in the HDL and for 60 % in the LDL and VLDL; in other studies HDL-C ranged between 40% and 50%. No differences sex-dependented was found. Apolipoprotein levels in cord blood have been studied by Dolphin [6] and McConathy [7]: apo AI and apo B levels have been found reduced, while apo CII, apo CIII and apo E presented values approaching adult's one. In this study apo B was about 30 %

of the adult levels and apo AI 61 %. Many authors have evaluated the feasibility of cord blood screening programs for early diagnosys of hypercholesterolemia. Kwiterovich concluded that LDL in cord blood is able to identify children with familiar hystory of hypercholesterolemia [13]. Glueck and co. have suggested the possibility of detection of hypercholesterolemia at birth by the evaluation of elevated cord, total and LDL, cholesterol [3]. On the contrary Darmady and co. stated that cholesterol assay can not be used as screening test for the existence of an high prevalence of false positive cases [14]. A prevalence of about 3 % of neonates with abnormal cholesterol levels have been found in this study (7/200). "Hypercholesterolemic" babies did not differ for gestational age, Apgar score after 5', weight and lenght from "normocholesterolemic" group. In conclusion the lipid and apolipoprotein distribution in Sicilian newborns population is very similar to that one of other population and no difference sex-dependented was been found. It is necessary a familial study and a follow-up of the newborns studied to establish if the abnormal cholesterol levels at born are predictive for an hypercholesterolemic condition in adult age.

References

1. Barnes, K., Nestel, P.J., Pryke, E.S., Whyte, H.M. (1972) "Neonatal plasma lipids", Med. J. Aust., 28, 1002-5.
2. Brody, S., Carlson, L.A., (1962) "Plasma lipid concentration in the newborn with special reference to the distribution of the different lipid fractions", Clin. Chim. Acta, 7, 694-99.
3. Glueck, C.J., Heckman, F., Schoenfeld, M., Steiner, P.M., Pearce, W., (1971) "Neonatal familial type II hyperlipoproteinemia: cord blood cholesterol in 1800 births", Metabolism, 20, 597-608.
4. Greten, H., Wengler, H., Wagner, H., (1973) " Early diagnosis of familial type II hyperlipoproteinemia" Nutr. Metab. 15, 1128-33.
5. Kaplan, A., Lee, V.F., (1965) "Serum lipid levels in infants and mothers at parturition", Clin. Chim. Acta 12, 258-63.
6. Dolphin, P.J., Breckenridge, W.C., Dolphin, M.A., Tan, M.H., (1984) "The lipoproteins of human: umbilical cord blood apolipoprotein and lipid levels", Atherosclerosis 51, 109-122.
7. McConathy, W.J., Lane, D.M., (1980) "Studies on the apolipoproteins and lipoproteins of cord serum", Pediatr. Res., 14, 757-61.
8. Averna, M.R., Barbagallo, C.M., Galione, A., Carroccio, A., Labisi, M., Marino, G., Montalto, G., Notarbartolo,

A., (1989) "Serum apolipoprotein profile of hypertriglyceridemic patients with chronic renal failure on hemodialytic therapy: a comparison with type IV hyperlipoproteinemic patients" Metabolism, 38, 601-2.

9. Magliano, E., Rusca, M., Samaja, U., Sirtori, C.R., (1978) "Diagnosi di ipercolesterolemia alla nascita: dosaggio del colesterolo nel sangue di funicolo ombellicale in 1000 gravidanze normali", Gaslini 10, 107-111.

10. Pagnan, A., Cerutti, A., Donadon, W., Ferrari, S., Tonolli, E., Bulian, I., Dal Palu', C., (1976) "Cord blood cholesterol, triglycerides and lipoprotein electrophoresis in 124 Italian infants", La Ricerca Clin. Lab., 6, 259-66.

11. Farinaro, E., Mancini, M., Trevisan, M.,Casullo, A., Di Mita, U., Rubino, A., Marotta, G., Mastranzo, P., (1979) "Plasma lipid and lipoprotein levels at birth in Naples, V International Symposium on Atherosclerosis, Houston, Texas, Abstract book, n. 399.

12. Parker, C.R.Jr., Carr, B.R., Simpson, E.R., McDonald, P.C., (1983) "Decline in the concentration of low-density lipoprotein-cholesterol in human fetal plasma near term", Metabolism 32, 919-23.

13. Kwiterovich, P.O.Jr., Levy, R.I., Frederickson, D.S., (1973), "Neonatal diagnosis of familial type-II hyperlipoproteinemia", Lancet, 1, 118-22.

14. Darmady, J.M., Fosbrooke, A.S., Lloyd, J.K., (1972) "Prospective study of serum cholesterol levels during first year of life", Br. Med. J. 2, 685-88.

NEW LIPID LOWERING AGENTS

58
Probucol revisited

J. DAVIGNON

Hyperlipidemia and Atherosclerosis Research Group, Clinical Research Institute of Montreal, 110 Pine Avenue West, Montreal, QC, Canada H2W 1R7

ABSTRACT. Probucol is a moderately potent cholesterol-lowering agent. It is a lipophilic substance with strong antioxidant properties and a long half-life. It lowers LDL-cholesterol, has no effect on triglycerides and is effective in familial hypercholesterolemia (FH). Its effect is additive to that of the diet and sustained. Its mode of action may involve a non LDL-receptor-mediated mechanism. Individual responses of LDL-cholesterol vary widely and appear to be influenced by apo E polymorphism, FH patients with the $\epsilon 4$ allele responding better. Probucol consistently lowers HDL-cholesterol, but this effect does not appear to be harmful and does not prevent xanthoma regression, even in homozygous FH subjects. There is indirect evidence that return of cholesterol to the liver is not impaired and may even be improved. An antiatherogenic effect in the LDL-receptor-deficient rabbit, attributed to its antioxidant properties, adds a new dimension to its use in the treatment of FH. In addition, preliminary results indicate a role in inhibiting the proliferative response to injury and a beneficial effect in experimental diabetes. Combination with drugs acting by different mechanisms to lower cholesterol may effectively control resistant cases. Compliance to resins is improved, as lower doses may be used, and the constipating effect is alleviated by probucol. Combination with lovastatin does not generally enhance the cholesterol-lowering effect but, in theory, may have a greater antiatherogenic potential. Combination with fibrates may lower plasma HDL-cholesterol without preventing xanthoma regression in FH patients, even when it induces a severe hypoalphalipoproteinemia.

Introduction

Probucol has a structural formula which bears little resemblance to any of the current lipid-lowering agents. Two tertiary butyl groups frame the hydroxyl radical of each of two phenol rings that are linked together by a dithiopropylidene bridge. The result is a highly lipophilic molecule with strong antioxidant properties which is poorly absorbed, circulates in plasma in association with lipoproteins, has a long half-life and tends to accumulate in adipose tissue [see ref. 1 for review]. Since its introduction in the early 1970's, this compound has been under close scrutiny because of undesirable side effects observed during pre-clinical studies and because of a propensity to lower plasma HDL-cholesterol in man. Attempts directed at explaining such side effects have yielded interesting results; a better understanding of its mode of action has accrued and new properties of the drug have emerged that are of potential benefit for the management and control of dyslipoproteinemias and atherosclerotic vascular disease. This brief review will examine the new face of a more than 10-year old drug that, in recent years, has been the focus of renewed interest [1-3].

Tolerance and safety

Probucol has been reported to sensitize the myocardium of the dog to epinephrine, an adverse effect which turned out to be species-specific. It also induced prolongation of the QT interval and sudden death in rhesus monkeys fed an atherogenic diet. These observations aroused concern for a cardiotoxic effect of potential clinical significance. In man, however, the drug has been remarkably well tolerated. In 252 men treated for over 5 years the rate of discontinuation because of adverse effects was 8% [2]. The side effects have been infrequent, mild, and mostly gastro-intestinal. Diarrhea, loose stools, flatulence, nausea and abdominal pain have been reported. Rarely, mention has been made of constipation, hyperhydrosis, fetid sweat, headache, dizziness, paresthesia, impotence, eosinophilia, skin rash, and palpitations. Probucol may lenghten the QTc interval in some individuals [1,2,4] and its combination with drugs known to have this effect, such as beta-blockers, should be avoided. Withdrawal of the drug has been advocated if QTc exceeds 470 msec. Palpitations are an infrequent side effect. Recently we have documented the onset of frequent ventricular premature contractions (VPCs) after more than one year of treatment with probucol in a patient with a mitral valve prolapse. They yielded rapidly to discontinuation of the drug. Prolongation of the QTc was not involved; it was 416 msec on therapy and 427 msec 27 days after stopping probucol. Prolongation of the QT interval does not appear to indicate a cardiotoxic effect of probucol [2]; in fact there is evidence that a modest QT prolongation *per se* would not indicate any harmful effect of a drug [5]. Indeed, QT prolongation appears to be a typical feature of many efficient anti-arrhythmic drugs of type Ic (such as quinidine) and type III (amiodarone, sotalol).

Browne et al. [6] measured 15,000 QT intervals and monitored the frequency of VPCs before and after 6 months of treatment with probucol or placebo in 16 patients with less than 600 VPCs per day. Although they could document a modest prolongation of the QTc interval in the probucol group (22 ±23 msec in the awake state and 20 ±18 during sleep), there was no increase in the number of VPCs in either group. There is one report of a lowered incidence of VPCs in patients receiving probucol [7].

Effect on low density lipoproteins (LDL)

Probucol lowers plasma cholesterol an average of 14% in heterozygous FH. [1,8]. This effect is sustained over years and is additive to the effect of the diet. It results from a decrease in both LDL- and HDL-cholesterol. Occasionally, the effect may persist for several weeks following discontinuation of the drug [9]. Triglycerides are virtually unchanged. LDL-cholesterol is lowered an average of 10% but the response is highly variable from subject to subject, tending to be more pronounced in milder cases of hypercholesterolemia [10]. This variability in response may be partly accounted for by apo E polymorphism. Patients with FH carrying the $\epsilon 4$ allele demonstrated the greatest reduction in cholesterol levels, but this effect did not appear to be shared by patients affected with other forms of hypercholesterolemia [11]. It was speculated that this greater response may represent enhanced catabolism of LDL in these individuals. There is evidence that the clearance of LDL is enhanced by probucol via the LDL-receptor pathway as well as through a new mechanism that is non-LDL-receptor mediated. Kesaniemi and Grundy [12] have shown that the fractional catabolic rate of apo-LDL is enhanced by probucol administration. The finding that probucol could lower plasma cholesterol and induce xanthoma regression in homozygous FH patients [13,14] led to the study of the effect of probucol in the Watanabe heritable hyperlipidemic rabbit (WHHL), deficient in LDL-receptors. Naruszewicz et al. [15] showed that native LDL are cleared from the plasma of WHHL rabbits at the same rate, whether the animal is treated with probucol or not. They were able to demonstrate, however, that LDL from probucol-treated animals (PB-LDL) were cleared about 50% more effectively than native LDL, whether injected in probucol-treated or untreated WHHL rabbits, or in normal New Zealand white (NZW) rabbits. Similarly, PB-LDL were degraded more effectively than native LDL by fibroblasts from WHHL or NZW rabbits. It was postulated that probucol, which gains access to the core of the LDL particles, somehow altered the conformation of its surface apolipoprotein B favoring enhanced clearance by a pathway independent of the LDL-receptor. These findings raised much speculation on the existence of an alternate receptor for cellular uptake and degradation of LDL. LDL composition is altered by probucol treatment [3], the particles are enriched in triglycerides and contain less cholesterol; the functional significance of these changes is not yet established.

Effect on high density lipoproteins (HDL)

Another source of concern for probucol was its HDL-lowering effect, since this fraction of plasma lipoproteins is involved in reverse cholesterol transport and ascribed an antiatherogenic role [1-3,10]. This is a very consistent effect of probucol, HDL-cholesterol being reduced on average 30%, mostly at the expense of the HDL_2 subfraction which correlates inversely with coronary artery disease (CAD) risk in epidemiological studies. The HDL_3 subfraction may be increased, especially in women. More specifically, the HDL_{2c} fraction is markedly reduced and the HDL_{3c} fraction increased [3]. Very early, a large number of arguments led us to believe that this effect was not harmful [16] and recent evidence indicates that reverse cholesterol transport is not impaired and may even be enhanced under the effect of probucol [3]. If the HDL-lowering effect of probucol, often resulting in a reduced LDL/HDL ratio, were deleterious, one would expect a markedly enhanced CAD mortality rate with long term exposure. Tedeschi et al. [17] showed that this was not the case; using the life table analysis method they calculated that the 5-year mortality rate for the probucol experience in 373 subjects was 1.0%, not any worse than the 1.8% 5-year rate observed in the control group of the WHO cooperative trial. In the Helsinki multifactorial primary prevention trial where CAD mortality was greater in the treated group than in the control groups, Miettinen et al. [18] observed that subjects treated with probucol had, in spite of a significant reduction in plasma HDL-cholesterol, a low CAD incidence rate and a very low CAD risk ratio (0.26) as compared to that of subjects treated with beta-blockers (5.27) or to that imparted by hypercholesterolemia alone (4.14). The fact that xanthomas regressed in both heterozygous and homozygous FH indicated that cholesterol was mobilized from the tissues and, paradoxically, reduction in tendon xanthoma thickness correlated with the reduction in HDL-cholesterol, but not with changes in LDL-cholesterol [14]. The concept emerged that probucol might enhance cholesterol mobilization and return to the liver. This view was supported by the work of Goldberg et al. [19] showing that probucol, in the presence of apo E-depleted HDL_3, enhanced cholesterol efflux from cultured human skin fibroblasts in a dose dependent fashion up to a 2 μM concentration. Cholesterol ester (CE) transfer from HDL to VLDL + LDL is reversed in a rare disease associated with very high levels of HDL_2, arcus corneae and CAD. Matsuzawa et al. [20] found that probucol could normalize CE transfer activity in these patients. More recently, Franceschini et al. [3] provided evidence that CE transfer activity is enhanced by probucol treatment in hypercholesterolemic patients. This finding, which indicates a beneficial effect of probucol on reverse cholesterol transport, has been confirmed by mass measurement of CE transfer protein (CETP) in preliminary experiments conducted by McPherson et al. [21].

Antioxidant and antiinflammatory properties

When LDL are oxidized they lose their affinity for the LDL-receptor and are taken up and degraded preferentially by the acetyl-LDL-receptor on macrophages [see ref. 22 for review]. This may result in the formation of foam cells. Oxidized LDL, in contrast to native LDL, are cytotoxic and may damage the vascular endothelium. Once they infiltrate the arterial wall, their chemotactic effect favors recruitment of blood monocytes that are eventually transformed into macrophages. They also have the ability to inhibit the motility of resident macrophages preventing their escape from the intima. These processes favor the development of atheromatous plaques and oxidized LDL have potent atherogenic properties. LDL oxidation and the resulting adverse effects, however, may be inhibited by antioxidants. The chemical formula of probucol is reminiscent of that of butylated hydroxy-toluene, a widely used antioxidant. In fact, probucol is, on a weight basis, 100 times more potent an antioxidant than vitamin E. LDL may be oxidized by exposure to endothelial cells (EC) in culture, an effect shared by smooth muscle cells and macrophages [23]. Exposure *in vitro* to Cu^{++} ions has the same effect. Parthasarathy et al. [24] showed that probucol, in a dose related effect, prevents the oxidative modification of LDL induced by exposure to EC or Cu^{++} as well as their uptake and degradation by macrophages. Moreover, LDL from the plasma of probucol-treated patients resist cell-induced and Cu^{++}-induced oxidative modification and enhanced macrophage degradation. These findings raised the possibility that probucol might have direct antiatherogenic effects because of its antioxidant properties. This was tested in the WHHL rabbit by Kita et al. [25]. They found that atherosclerosis progression could be prevented by feeding probucol 1% mixed with rabbit chow for 6 months. As compared to the control group, the percent surface area covered with plaques was inhibited by 87% in the thoracic aorta and 99.5% in the descending aorta for a mere 22% difference in plasma cholesterol between the two groups. In a similar experiment, Carew et al. [26] established that this was unrelated to the cholesterol-lowering effect of probucol alone, since lovastatin, given in a third group to achieve the same reduction in plasma cholesterol as that induced by probucol, failed to inhibit atheroma progression to the same extent. They also showed that probucol prevented the enhanced degradation of LDL by macrophages in the lesions of the probucol-treated animals while this process went on unabated in the control rabbits, thus linking the antiatherogenic effect to the antioxidant properties. Further work carried out by Finckh et al. [27] in the WHHL rabbit showed that atheroma formation was associated in this model with an increase in plasma oxidation products (measured as malondialdehyde equivalent) and a reduction in vitamin E concentrations. Probucol administration reversed these changes while preventing atheroma formation. They also obtained evidence that probucol may promote atheroma regression in this model and that its antiatherogenic effect is probably related to a combination of various effects. Stein et al. [28] have not observed a protective effect of probucol against atheroma formation in rabbits fed an atherogenic diet in contrast to other reports to the contrary [29,30]. So far the antiatherogenic potential of probucol has not been tested in man, but there is an ongoing study, the Probucol Quantitative Regression Swedish Trial (PQRST), which is contrasting the effect of cholestyramine alone with that of cholestyramine in combination with probucol on the progression of femoral atherosclerosis [31]. This combination effectively inhibits atheroma formation in the rhesus monkey [32].

Interleukin-1 (IL-1) is a cytokine that induces the synthesis of acute phase proteins [see ref. 33 for review]. Metallothionein is one such protein produced by the liver which binds zinc; its induction is associated with a reduction in plasma zinc levels. A reduction in zinc levels may therefore reflect IL-1 release and has been used as a bioassay for IL-1 release in the zymosan-primed mice challenged by lipopolysaccharides (LPS). IL-1 is a lymphocyte activating factor which potentiates the response of thymocytes to lectins such as phytohemagglutinin. A thymocyte proliferation assay has also been developed to measure IL-1 release. Since IL-1 is a proinflammatory mediator, it has been surmised that it might play a role in the atherogenic process as other cytokines, such as the platelet derived growth factor, do. In line with this hypothesis, Ku et al.[33] have presented evidence that modified LDL induce the release of IL-1 and that recombinant IL-1 causes aortic smooth muscle cell proliferation. They also demonstrated that large doses of probucol partly inhibit the fall in zinc induced by LPS in the zymosan-primed mouse, an indirect proof that IL-1 release is partly suppressed *in vivo*. They obtained direct evidence for inhibition of IL-1 release in an *ex vivo* system in which peritoneal macrophages from probucol-treated mice secreted 80 to 90% less IL-1 than controls, upon LPS stimulation, using the C3H/HeJ thymocyte proliferation assay. Probucol, however, has no direct influence *in vitro* on IL-1 release by macrophages. It is believed that probucol may have a beneficial effect in preventing *in vivo* IL-1 release with its mitogenic effect on arterial wall smooth muscle cells, release that may be mediated by oxidized LDL in the atherogenic process.

It has been shown that antioxidant therapy can prevent toxin-induced diabetes in animals. Probucol has no effect on plasma glucose or insulin levels in experimental diabetes. Drash et al. [34] however, showed that probucol may partially prevent or retard the onset of the spontaneous insulin-dependent diabetes mellitus which develops in the BB/W rat. Diabetes developed in 86.2% of the control rats (litter matched) at a mean age of 90.4 days. Probucol administration through 160 days of life was associated with a reduction to 62% and a delay in diabetes diagnosis to 99.6 days. This is a modest, albeit interesting, effect which was speculatively ascribed to a delay in beta cell destruction through an antiinflammatory effect of probucol.

Combination therapy with probucol

Combination drug therapy, added to a cholesterol-lowering diet, is often needed for the treatment of resistant cases of heterozygous FH. This allows for the potentiation of drug effects thereby reducing the amount of each drug used. Full advantage of complementary modes of action can then be derived. Furthermore, side effects of one medication may sometimes be compensated by those of another resulting in improved compliance. In the rhesus monkey, probucol acts in synergy with cholestyramine to induce a 35% reduction in aortic atherosclerosis, an effect at least 5 times greater than that achieved with either drug administered alone [32]. This combination is very effective at lowering plasma LDL-cholesterol and inducing xanthoma regression in FH. Adding probucol often alleviates the constipating effects of cholestyramine and may allow reduction of the amount of resin needed for optimal effect [35].

Combination of probucol with lovastatin does not generally result in a further decline in plasma cholesterol (although a marked additive effect has been observed in the occasional patient) [36,37]. In theory however, as suggested by the observations obtained in animals, it may potentiate the beneficial LDL-lowering effect of lovastatin, through an antiatherogenic effect associated with its antioxidant properties.

The association of probucol with a fibrate is logical for the treatment of hereditary forms of hypercholesterolemia with the IIb phenotype. Combination of probucol with clofibrate may indeed normalize the lipoprotein profile in some hypercholesterolemic patients. The HDL-reducing effect of probucol is enhanced in about 70% of patients receiving this association and a severe hypoalphalipoproteinemia may result [38]. This effect, paradoxically, does not appear to be deleterious; regression of xanthomas has been reported in one FH patient receiving this combination over 3.5 years with an average HDL-cholesterol of 11 mg/dL and a LDL/HDL ratio of 24.7.

Conclusions

Probucol has a diversity of effects which may act in synergy to oppose the atherogenic process: lowering LDL-cholesterol, preventing LDL oxidative modification and their damaging effects, improving return of cholesterol to the liver and, perhaps, curbing cell proliferation and inflammation in the arterial wall during this process. The ability of probucol to induce xanthoma regression was observed early. It should have been considered by the skeptics [39] as an indication of a potentially beneficial effect in spite of the HDL-lowering properties of the drug [16]. There was obviously more to probucol than met the eye. It retains, today, a place of choice among the lipid-lowering agents in being well tolerated, very efficient in combination, and uniquely effective in homozygous familial hypercholesterolemia.

References

1. Buckley, MM-T., Goa, K.L., Price, A.H. and Brogen, R.N. (1989) 'Probucol. A reappraisal of its pharmacological properties and therapeutic use in hypercholesterolaemia', Drugs 36, 761-800.
2. Strandberg, T.E., Vanhanen, H. and Miettinen, T.A. (1988) 'Probucol in long term treatment of hypercholesterolemia', Gen Pharmac 19, 317-320.
3. Franceschini, G., Sirtori, M., Vaccarino, V., Gianfranceschi, G., Rezzonico, L., Chiesa, G. and Sirtori, C.R. (1989) 'Mechanisms of HDL reduction after probucol', Arteriosclerosis 9, 462-469.
4. Dujovne, C.A., Atkins, F., Wong, B., Decoursey, S., Krehbiel, P. and Chernoff S. (1984) 'Electrocardiographic effects of probucol: a controlled prospective clinical trial', Eur J Clin Pharmacol 26, 735-739.
5. Roden, D.M. and Woosley, R.L. (1985) 'QT prolongation and arrhythmia suppression', Am Heart J 109, 411-415.
6. Browne, K.F., Prystowsky, E.N., Heger, J.J., Cerimele, B., Fineberg, N. and Zipes, D.P. (1984) 'Prolongation of the QT interval induced by probucol: demonstration of a method for determining QT interval change induced by a drug', Am Heart J 107, 680-684.
7. Weiss, R., Leitner, E.V. and Schwartzkopff, W. (1986) 'Probucol in the treatment of type IIA and type IIB hyperlipoproteinemia', IX International Symposium on Drug Affecting Lipid Metabolism. Florence, Italy, Abstract book p. 47.
8. LeLorier, J., Dubreuil-Quidoz, S., Lussier-Cacan, S., Huang ,Y.S. and Davignon, J. (1977) 'Diet and probucol in lowering cholesterol concentrations', Arch Intern Med 137, 1429-1434
9. Davignon, J., Lussier-Cacan, S., Dubreuil-Quidoz, S., LeLorier, J. (1982) 'Experience with probucol in the treatment of hypercholesterolemia', Artery 10, 48-55.

10. Davignon, J., Xhignesse, M., Mailloux, H., Nestruck, A.C., Lussier-Cacan, S., Roederer, G. and Pfister, P. (1988) 'Comparative study of lovastatin versus probucol in the treatment of hypercholesterolemia', Atheroscler Rev 18, 139-151.
11. Nestruck, A.C., Bouthillier, S., Sing, C.F. and Davignon, J. (1987) 'Apolipoprotein E polymorphism and plasma cholesterol response to probucol', Metabolism 36, 743-747.
12. Kesäniemi, Y.A. and Grundy, S.M. (1984) 'Influence of probucol on cholesterol and lipoprotein metabolism in man', J Lipid Res 25, 780-790.
13. Baker, S.G., Joffe, B.I., Mendelsohn, D. and Seftel, H.C. (1982) 'Treatment of homozygous familial hypercholesterolemia with probucol', S Afr Med J 62, 7-11.
14. Yamamoto, A., Matsuzawa, Y., Yokoyama, S., Funahashi, T., Yamamura, T. and Kishino B.I. (1986) 'Effects of probucol on xanthomata regression in familial hypercholesterolemia', Am J Cardiol 57, 29H-35H.
15. Naruszewicz, M., Carew, T.E., Pitman, R.C., Witztum, J.L. and Steinberg, D. (1984) 'A novel mechanism by which probucol lowers low density lipoprotein levels demonstrated in the LDL receptor-deficient rabbit', J Lipid Res 25, 1206-1213.
16. Davignon, J., Bouthillier, D. (1982) 'Probucol and familial hypercholesterolemia', Can Med Assoc J 126, 1024-1025 (Letter to the Editor).
17. Tedeschi, R.E., Martz, B.L., Taylor, H.A. and Cerimelle, B.J. (1980) 'Etude clinique à long terme (9 ans) de la tolérance et de l'efficacité du probucol', Nouv Presse Méd 9, 3021-3026.
18. Miettinen, T.A., Huttunen, J.K., Naukkarinen, V., Stranberg, T. and Vanhanen, H. (1986) 'Long-term use of probucol in the multifactorial primary prevention of vascular disease', Am J Cardiol 57, 49H-54H.
19. Goldberg, R.B. and Mendez, A. (1988) 'Probucol enhances cholesterol efflux from cultured human skin fibroblasts', Am J Cardiol 62, 57B-59B.
20. Matsuzawa, Y., Yamashita, S., Funahashi, T., Yamamoto, A. and Tarui, S. (1988) 'Selective reduction of cholesterol in HDL_2 fraction by probucol in familial hypercholesterolemia and hyperHDL_2 cholesterolemia with abnormal cholesteryl ester transfer', Am J Cardiol 62, 66B-72B.
21. McPherson, R., Marcel, Y.L., Milne, R. and Tall, A.R. (1989) 'Effects of probucol on plasma concentrations of cholesteryl ester transfer protein', *14th Canadian Lipoprotein Conference*, Oct.1-4, Thousand Islands, Ont. Canada

22. Steinberg, D., Parthasarathy, S., Carew, T.E., Khoo, J.C. and Witztum, J.L. (1989) 'Beyond cholesterol. Modification of low-density lipoprotein that increase its atherogenicity', New Engl J Med 320, 915-924.
23. Parthasarathy, S., Fong, L., Otero, D., Steinberg, D. (1987) 'Recognition of solubilized apoproteins from delipidated, oxidized low density lipoprotein (LDL) by the acetyl-LDL receptor', Proc Natl Acad Sci (USA) 84, 537-540.
24. Parthasarathy, S., Young, S.G., Witztum, J.L., Pittman, R.C. and Steinberg, D. (1986) 'Probucol inhibits oxidative modification of low density lipoprotein', J Clin Invest 77, 641-644.
25. Kita, T., Nagano, Y., Yokode, M., Ishii, K., Kume, N., Ooshima, ,A., Yoshida, H. and Kawai, C. (1987) 'Probucol prevents the progression of atherosclerosis in Watanabe heritable hyperlipidemic rabbit, an animal model for familial hypercholesterolemia', Proc Natl Acad Sci (USA) 84, 5928-5931.
26. Carew, T.E., Schwenke, D.C. and Steinberg, D.C. (1987) 'Antiatherogenic effect of probucol unrelated to its hypocholesterolemic effect: evidence that antioxidants *in vivo* can selectively inhibit low density lipoprotein degradation in macrophage-rich fatty streaks and slow the progression of atherosclerosis in the Watanabe heritable hyperlipidemic rabbit', Proc Natl Acad Sci (USA) 84, 7725-7729.
27. Finckh, B., Rath, M., Niendorf, A. and Beisiegel, U. (1989) 'Antiatherosclerotic effect of probucol in WHHL rabbit - Are there serum parameters to evaluate this effect?' *International Symposium on Lipid-Lowering Drugs: Mechanisms and Actions*. Ulm, F.R.G., Sept 21-22.
28. Stein, Y., Stein, O., Delplanque, B., Fesmire, J.D., Lee, D.M. and Alaupovic ,P. (1989) 'Lack of effect of probucol on atheroma formation in cholesterol-fed rabbits kept at comparable plasma cholesterol levels', Atherosclerosis 75, 145-155.
29. Kritchevsky, D., Kim, H.K. and Tepper, S.A. (1971) 'Influence of 4,4'-(isopropylidenedithio)bis(2,6-di-t-butylphenol) (DH-581) on experimental atherosclerosis in rabots', Proc Soc Exprl Biol & Med 136, 1216.
30. Tawara, K., Ishihara, M., Ogawa, H. and Tomikawa, M. (1986) 'Effect of probucol, pantethine and their combinations on serum lipoprotein metabolism and on the incidence of atheromatous lesions in the rabbit', Jap J Pharmacol 41, 211-222.

31. Walldius, G., Carlson, L.A., Erikson, U., Olsson, A.G., Johansson, J., Molgaard, J., Nilsson, S., Stenport, G., Kaijer, L., Lassvik, C. and Holme, I. (1988) 'Development of femoral atherosclerosis in hypercholesterolemic patients during treatment with Cholestyramine and Probucol/Placebo: Probucol Quantitative Regression Swedish Trial (PQRST): A status report', Am J Cardiol 62, 37B-43B.
32. Wissler, R.W. and Vesselinovitch, D. (1983) 'Combined effects of cholestyramine and probucol on regression of atherosclerosis in rhesus monkey aortas', Appl Pathol 1, 89-96.
33. Ku, G., Doherty, N.S., Wolos, J.A. and Jackson, R.L. (1988) 'Inhibition by probucol of interleukin 1 secretion and its implication in atherosclerosis', Am J Cardiol 62, 77B-81B.
34. Drash, A.L., Rudert, W.A., Borquaye, S., Wang, R. and Lieberman, I. (1988) 'Effect of probucol on development of diabetes mellitus in BB rats', Am J Cardiol 62, 27B-30B.
35. Dujovne, C.A., Krehbiel, P. and Chernoff, S.B. (1986) 'Controlled studies of the efficacy and safety of combined colestipol-probucol therapy', Am J Cardiol 57, 36H-42H.
36. Lees, A.M., Stein, S.W. and Lees, R.S. (1986) 'Therapy of hypercholesterolemia with mevinolin and other lipid-lowering drugs', Circulation 74(II), 200.
37. Witztum, J.L., Simmons, D., Steinberg, D., Beltz, W.F., Weinreb, R., Young, S.G., Lester, P., Kelly, N. and Juliano, J. (1989) 'Intensive combination drug therapy of familial hypercholesterolemia with lovastatin, probucol, and colestipol hydrochloride', Circulation 79, 16-28.
38. Davignon, J., Nestruck, A.C., Alaupovic, P.and Bouthillier, D. (1986) 'Severe hypoalphalipoproteinemia induced by a combination of probucol and clofibrate', in A. Angel and J. Frohlich (eds.), Lipoprotein Deficiency Syndromes, Plenum Press, New York, pp. 111-125.
39. Gagné, C., Lupien, P.J., Brun, D. and Moorjani, S. (1982) 'Probucol and familial hypercholesterolemia', Can Med Assoc J 126,1025 (Letter to the Editor)

59

Controlled US studies of fenofibrate in the treatment of dyslipidemias

G.F. BLANE

Laboratoires Fournier S.A., Centre de Recherche de Daix, 21121 Fontaine-les-Dijon, France

ABSTRACT. Data from mostly open, non-comparative European studies indicate that fenofibrate reduces total plasma cholesterol by approximately 20-25% in patients with various types of hyperlipoproteinemias, and reduces total plasma triglycerides by approximately 30-60% in patients with hyperlipoproteinemia. We review here two recent randomized, double-blinded, placebo-controlled clinical trials conducted in the United States which confirmed the European findings, firstly in patients with Type IIa or IIb hyperlipoproteinemia, secondly in patients with type IV or type V hyperlipoproteinemia.

1. First study : Double-Blind, Multicenter Trial in Patients With Type IIa or IIb Hyperlipidemia

Male and female hyperlipidemic patients aged 21 to 65 were considered eligible for the study if they had an average total plasma cholesterol concentration greater than 250 mg/dl at three successive visits and one of the three low-density lipoprotein cholesterol measurements exceeded 175 mg/dl. If, in addition, the plasma triglyceride concentrations averaged greater than 250 mg/dl at three initial visits, patients were classified as having combined hyperlipidemia or type IIB hyperlipidemia. Otherwise, they were considered to have pure type IIA hypercholesterolemia. All patients were instructed in a prudent American Heart Association Phase I diet at the first visit and three screening cholesterol measurements obtained over a six-week interval (see study outline in Figure 1).

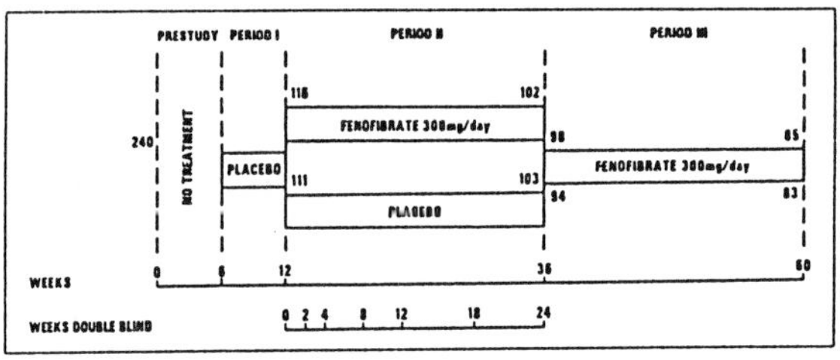

Figure 1. Outline of type IIA and IIB study protocol

227 subjects judged to be cooperative study candidates were randomly assigned to receive fenofibrate 100 mg three times daily or placebo, and then were followed for 24 weeks. During this double-blind phase, patients made six visits to the clinic at which blood samples were drawn for lipoproteins and clinical observations were made.

The 192 patients who elected to continue for another 24 weeks were all given active medication in an open-label design as shown in Figure 1 (Period III).

1.1. RESULTS

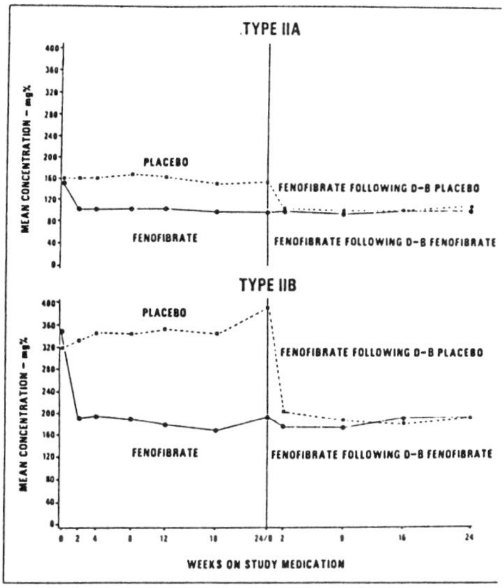

Figure 2. Mean total plasma triglyceride concentrations in patients randomly assigned to placebo or fenofibrate therapy for the 24-week double-blind (D-B) randomization phase and for a subsequent 24-week open-label phase

Effects of fenofibrate on total plasma triglyceride concentrations as compared with control concentrations are presented in Figure 2. In type IIA patients, comparing baseline with final results at the end of the double-blind phase, the triglyceride concentrations decreased 37.9% in the fenofibrate-treated group whereas they decreased 4.2% in the placebo group. In the type II B patients, triglyceride concentrations decreased 44.6% ; however, over the same time period triglyceride concentrations in the placebo-treated patients increased 22.3%. In both groups, during 24 weeks of open-label treatment, placebo group triglyceride concentrations became superimposable on those of the fenofibrate-treated group, which did not change from those of the previous double-blind treatment phase.

It is noteworthy that all of the triglyceride reduction achieved occurred in the first two weeks of therapy in both the double-blind, fenofibrate-treated patients as well as the fenofibrate-treated patients in the open-label phase.

Total plasma cholesterol concentrations in fenofibrate and placebo-taking patients are presented in Figure 3. Nearly all of the cholesterol-lowering effect was achieved within two weeks of fenofibrate administration. Total cholesterol concentrations declined 17.5% from the preceding baseline level in the type IIA group and 15.8% in the type IIB group. In the open-label phase, patients previously treated with placebo had a response to fenofibrate similar to those subjects treated with fenofibrate in the double-blind phase.

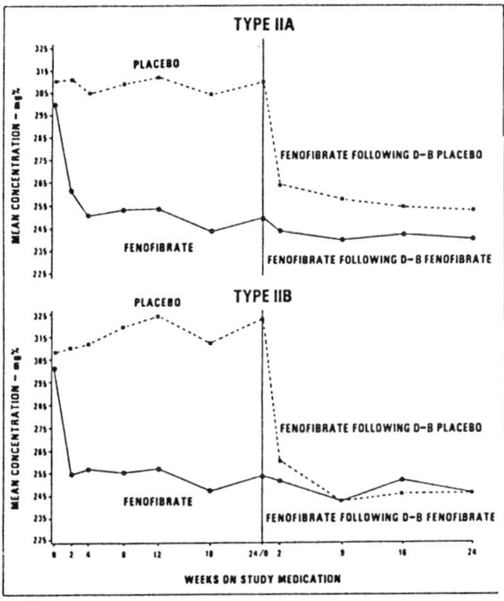

Figure 3. Mean total plasma cholesterol concentrations during the double-blind (D-B) randomization phase lasting 24 weeks and the subsequent 24-week open label phase.

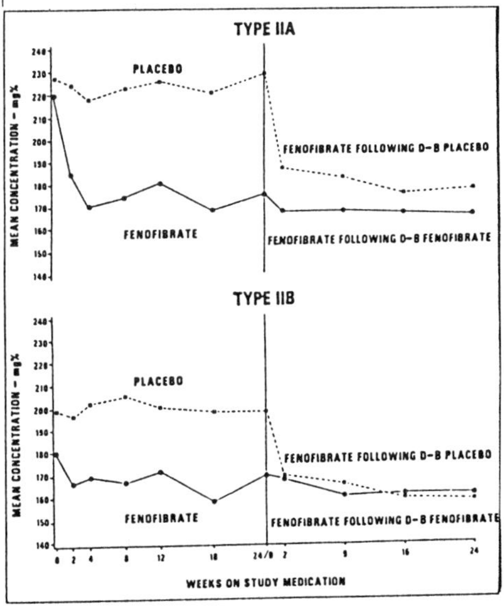

Figure 4. Comparison of mean low-density lipoprotein cholesterol concentrations in patients treated with placebo versus fenofibrate in a 24-week double-blind (D-B) randomization phase and the subsequent open-label treatment phase lasting 24 weeks.

Changes in plasma low-density lipoprotein cholesterol concentrations are presented in Figure 4. The pattern of results is similar to that seen for total cholesterol. In the case of low-density lipoprotein cholesterol in type IIA patients, a 22.3% reduction is observed compared with a 0.4% increase in the placebo group. In the type IIB group treated with fenofibrate, the low-density lipoprotein cholesterol concentrations decreased from 180 to approximately 168 mg/dl for a 6.1% reduction. However, when the placebo group was treated with fenofibrate in the open-label phase, the low-density lipoprotein cholesterol concentrations decreased substantially more, from 198 mg/dl to 158 mg/dl for a maximal 20.2% reduction at the end of the open-label phase.

Observations on changes in high-density lipoprotein cholesterol concentrations are presented in Figure 5. High density lipoprotein cholesterol concentrations increased 11.1% in the type IIA group and 15.3% in the type IIB group in the double-blind phase. Confirmatory changes were seen with the fenofibrate treatment in the open-label phase of previously placebo-treated patients. The time for the maximal increase in high-density lipoprotein cholesterol levels to be achieved is longer than in the other lipoprotein parameters described above.

In the case of the type IIA patients, high-density lipoprotein cholesterol concentrations reach an approximate maximum after four weeks of fenofibrate treatment and in type IIB patients after 12 weeks of fenofibrate treatment in the double-blind phase and 16 weeks in the open-label phase.

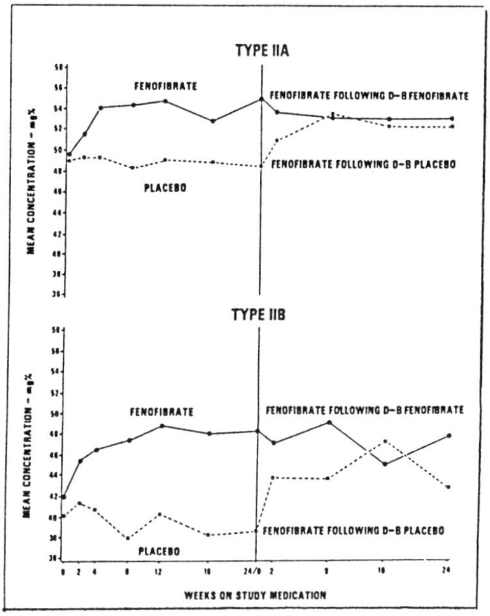

Figure 5. Mean plasma high-density lipoprotein (HDL) cholesterol concentrations comparing fenofibrate versus placebo-treated patients in a double-blind (D-B) randomization phase lasting 24 weeks and the subsequent 24 weeks of open-label treatment with fenofibrate.

1.2. CLINICAL ADVERSE EVENTS

Four patients experienced severe skin reactions while taking fenofibrate as compared with none taking placebo. Overall, 26% of patients had some kind of reported adverse reaction while taking fenofibrate as opposed to 20% taking placebo, giving a 6% excess attributable to fenofibrate. Of the side effects noted as severe, the most common was skin rash leading to the discontinuation of medication in three patients. A fourth patient, who stopped taking medication, reported fatigue and decreased libido. All patients experienced an uneventful recovery when treatment stopped. Results of blood pressure, pulse, and eye examinations showed no effect of fenofibrate administration.

1.3. LABORATORY VALUES

Three patients receiving fenofibrate and two taking placebo were withdrawn from the double-blind period of the study because of abnormal results from laboratory testing (increased liver enzymes). A further nine patients receiving fenofibrate and one receiving placebo were withdrawn due to adverse reactions. The relationship between these events and the study drug was assessed as "probable" in four of the total of 12 patients receiving fenofibrate and one of the three patients receiving placebo.

With respect to other laboratory studies, there was little difference in screening laboratory measurements between placebo and fenofibrate groups except for a reduction in uric acid concentrations and a slight increase in creatinine levels with 21 fenofibrate-

and 10 placebo-taking patients having levels above the normal range and 50% increased from baseline.

TYPE IIA
20% REDUCTION IN LDL-C
11% INCREASE IN HDL-C

TYPE IIB
6% REDUCTION IN LDL-C
15% INCREASE IN HDL-C
45% REDUCTION IN TG

Figure 6. Major Conclusions of First Study

2. Second study : Double-Blind Multicenter Trial in Patients With Type IV or V Hyperlipidemia

2.1. PATIENTS AND METHODS

An outline of the study is shown in Figure 7. The dietary stabilization period lasted 6-12 weeks and consisted of a National Institutes of Health or American Heart Association low-fat diet. Once maximal reduction of total plasma triglycerides had been achieved by means of this diet, patients whose 12-hour fasting total plasma triglycerides still ranged between 350-1500 mg/dl were enrolled in the treatment phase of the study. Written, informed consent was obtained from each patient and the use of diet was maintained throughout the remainder of the study.

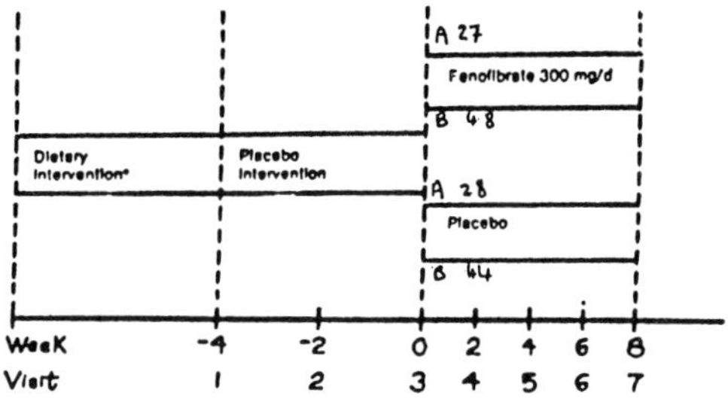

*Length varied from 6-12 weeks

Figure 7. Outline of type IV and V study protocol

The second portion of the protocol consisted of a single-blind placebo treatment of one placebo capsule given 3 times daily for four weeks (week -4 to 0). During this period, two separate fasting plasma lipid profiles were performed two weeks apart. Patients were entered into the next portion of the treatment phase if the mean of these determinations showed a total plasma triglyceride level between 350-1500 mg/dl.
The final portion of the treatment phase consisted of the double-blind treatment period for which patients were stratified into two treatment subgroups based on the mean fasting total plasma triglyceride level determined in the placebo treatment phase. Patients whose level ranged from 350-499 mg/dl were placed in treatment group A, while those with levels between 500-1500 mg/dl were placed in treatment group B.

2.2. RESULTS

One hundred and forty-seven patients were entered into the double-blind portion of this study. Fifty-five patients were stratified to group A and 92 to group B. 13 patients dropped out during the course of the study for various reasons, but were included in both the efficacy and safety evaluations.

Treatment results : Group A
For patients in group A (initial triglycerides 350-499 mg/dl) there was a statistically significant reduction in total triglyceride (- 46.2%), VLDL-triglyceride (- 44.1%), total cholesterol (-9.1%) and VLDL-cholesterol (-44.7%) in the fenofibrate-treated group. A statistically significant increase in HDL-cholesterol (+ 19.6%) was also observed in fenofibrate-treated patients. The LDL-cholesterol value was changed to a similar extent in both fenofibrate (+ 14.5%) and placebo (+ 12%) groups.

Most of the beneficial effect of fenofibrate on the plasma lipid profile was seen at the first visit following two weeks of therapy and was maintained for the remainder of the eight-week treatment period (Figure 8). One patient in each treatment group had chylomicrons present at one of the three placebo baseline visits. During the double-blind period, one patient in each treatment group had chylomicrons present at one of the four visits.

One patient in the fenofibrate group had a xanthoma present during the baseline period. This was no longer present at the end of fenofibrate therapy.

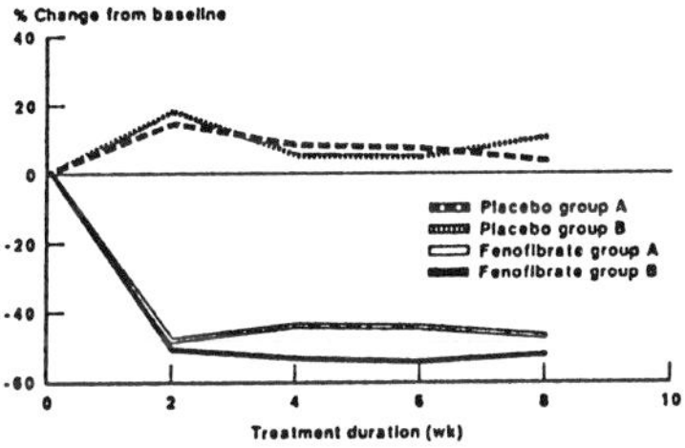

Figure 8. Change in triglycerides : Group A and Group B

Treatment results : Group B
In group B (initial triglycerides 500-1500 mg/dl) there was a statistically significant reduction in total triglyceride (-54.5%), VLDL-triglyceride (-50.6%), total cholesterol (-13.8%) and VLDL-cholesterol (-49.4%) in patients treated with fenofibrate. There was also a significant increase in HDL-cholesterol (+22.9%) in the fenofibrate group. However, patients in the fenofibrate group also experienced a significant increase in LDL-cholesterol + 45.0%) from a mean of 103.1 mg/dl ± 6.8 to a mean of 131.0 mg/dl ± 6.0.
Most of the effects of fenofibrate on the plasma lipid profile was again seen at the first visit following two weeks of therapy and was maintained for the remainder of the eight-week treatment period (Figure 8).
Xanthomas were initially present in two fenofibrate- and two placebo-treated patients during the baseline period. At the end of treatment, no fenofibrate-treated patient had a xanthoma, while two patients in the placebo group had xanthomas.

2.3. CLINICAL ADVERSE EVENTS

A combined total of 16/75 (21.3%) fenofibrate-treated and 11/72 (15.3%) placebo-treated patients from study groups A and B experienced at least one adverse event that was categorized as potentially drug related or of unknown relationship to therapy but the difference between fenofibrate and placebo was not significant.
Gastrointestinal tract abnormalities were the most commonly reported adverse events, and occurred 13 times in the fenofibrate- and 9 times in the placebo-treated groups. These events included dyspepsia, flatulence, dry mouth, nausea, vomiting, diarrhea, and constipation. One case of allergic hepatitis occurred in the fenofibrate group.

2.4. LABORATORY VALUES

Three patients who received fenofibrate and one who received placebo had elevations in one or more of their enzyme tests (i.e., SGOT, SGPT, alkaline phosphatase, CPK) to between two and three times the upper limit of normal. An additional five patients in the fenofibrate group and no patients in the placebo group had elevations of a single liver enzyme that were greater than three times the upper limit of normal.
For one or more hematologic values (Hb, Hct, and RBC), three fenofibrate-treated patients and no placebo recipients had a clinically significant change (< 10%) below the normal range.
Sixty-one of 66 fenofibrate patients in whom uric acid was measured before and after therapy had a decrease in this value compared with baseline as compared with 22/63 placebo recipients. The magnitude of this change was greater in those who received fenofibrate, being 1.4 mg/dl ± 0.2 in group A and 1.3 mg/dl ± 0.2 in group B, as compared with 0.1 mg/dl ± 0.2 and 0.3 mg/dl ± 0.2 in the two respective placebo groups.

3. Global Conclusions

A total of 374 patients were entered into the double-blind treatment phases of the two U.S. studies reviewed here. Of these 191 received fenofibrate under double-blind conditions and a further 76 were subsequently given the medication in an open fashion. The data confirm the lipid-modifying profile of fenofibrate, as previously established in short- to medium-term mostly open European trials.
The results of the study in Type II patients show striking improvement in total cholesterol levels in both sub-classes with reductions in low-density lipoprotein cholesterol in type IIA hyperlipidemia proportional to those seen in total cholesterol. In type IIB hyperlipidemic patients, low-density lipoprotein cholesterol concentrations decreased between 6 and 20 % in association with greater than 65% reductions in plasma triglyceride concentration. These observations are encouraging to the extent that they do not display any tendency for low-density lipoprotein cholesterol concentrations to rise during the treatment. HDL-cholesterol was increased significantly by of the order 12% in type IIA and 16% in type IIB patients, when allowing for changes in the placebo groups. Such HDL increases are similar to those seen in many European trials.
In the Type IV and V study, fenofibrate-treated patients in groups A and B had statistically significant reductions in total triglycerides (-46.2% vs. -54.5%), VLDL-triglycerides (-44.1% vs. -50.6%), total cholesterol (-9.1% vs.-13.8%), and VLDL-cholesterol (-44.7% vs. -49.4%), and had significant increases in HDL-cholesterol (+19.6% vs. +22.9%).

Patients with markedly elevated triglycerides often have a reduced LDL-cholesterol value due to a derangement in the normal composition of low-density lipoprotein. This produces a triglyceride rich and cholesterol depleted low-density lipoprotein. When triglycerides are reduced with therapy, the composition of low-density lipoprotein normalizes, which can produce an elevation in LDL-cholesterol.
The results of the present second study confirm this finding (Table 1) and are consistent with those reported for gemfibrozil. Taking into account the mean age of the study population (50-55 years), gender distribution (predominately male) and racial characteristics (predominately Caucasian) in both group A and B patients, the final mean LDL-cholesterol was well below the 50th percentile value of 144 mg/dl for healthy males in the 50-59 year age bracket. Some patients in group B, however, had LDL-cholesterol levels above 160 mg/dl.

	TREATMENT GROUP	
	A	B
Initial TG	432	726
Baseline LDL-C	128	103
After treatment LDL-C	137	131
Mean LDL-C normal U.S. males age 50-59	144	

Table 1. Effect of Fenofibrate on LDL-cholesterol in Type IV and Type V Patients

Fenofibrate therapy was generally well tolerated being associated, nevertheless, with a small excess of skin rash and occasional increases in liver enzymes. The percentage of patients experiencing an adverse event in the double-blind phase of the first trial (type IIA and IIB patients) was 26% for fenofibrate and 20% for placebo treatments. The corresponding figures for the second trial (type IV and V patients) were 21% and 15%.
Elevated blood cholesterol is a major cause of coronary artery disease, and it has been established in long-term studies with cholestyramine and gemfibrozil that lowering plasma cholesterol (and perhaps more specifically LDL-cholesterol) will reduce the risk of heart attacks. No epidemiological-scale study has been made with fenofibrate. However, the long-term total cholesterol and LDL-cholesterol reductions with this drug are considerably greater than those seen in the cholestyramine and gemfibrozil trials, and fenofibrate also increases HDL-cholesterol while cholestyramine has little effect. Thus, the prediction would be that if fenofibrate is considered to be free of long-term major adverse effects and if the lipid hypotheses of atherogenesis applies to the lipoprotein changes induced by fenofibrate as it does to cholestyramine and gemfibrozil, significant reductions in cardiovascular disease should result from fenofibrate treatment in type IIA and IIB hyperlipidemias.
Severe hypertriglyceridemia (plasma levels > 500 mg/dl) is a known health risk associated with eruptive xanthomata, abdominal pain, and/or pancreatitis which may be fatal. Dietary restriction and use of a fibrate such as clofibrate, fenofibrate or more recently gemfibrozil is indicated. However, the relationship between triglyceride, atherosclerosis and cardiovascular disease is more controversial. Persons with fasting plasma triglyceride levels in the intermediate range of 250-500 mg/dl have a two-fold excess risk of cardiovascular disease and should first diet and then be treated with appropriate drugs if still necessary. Fenofibrate is undoubtedly effective in this context.
Finally, although the association of elevated uric acid with coronary heart disease is unproven, the uric acid-lowering activity of fenofibrate may be of interest.

In global conclusion, the results of the two American studies confirm that fenofibrate therapy in both safe and effective for the treatment of primary types IIA, IIB, IV and V hyperlipoproteinemia in patients for whom dietary modifications have proved ineffective in reducing plasma cholesterol and/or triglycerides.

60

Effect of trapidil and its derivatives on the receptor-mediated low density lipoprotein metabolism by cultured human hepatic and extrahepatic cells

A. CORSINI, J. BEITZ*, S. BELLOSTA, F. BERNINI, R. FUMAGALLI, H.J. MEST* and R. PAOLETTI

Institute of Pharmacological Sciences, University of Milan, Italy;
**Department of Pharmacology and Toxicology, Martin Luther University, Halle-Wittenberg, G.D.R.*

ABSTRACT

The effect of trapidil (Rocornal^{R}) and some of its newly developed derivatives on the receptor-mediated low density lipoprotein (LDL) uptake and degradation was studied in human skin fibroblasts (HSF) and human hepatoma cell line Hep G2. One compound (AR 12456) influenced this pathway in a selective way: it enhanced the uptake and degradation of ^{125}I-LDL by Hep G2 cells in a dose-dependent manner, but inhibited it in HSF. When AR 12456 was preincubated with Hep G2 cells and then the incubation medium was transferred to HSF, a stimulation of specific LDL pathway occurred also in this cell line. The stimulation of the LDL pathway by AR 12456 in Hep G2 was modified by preincubation of Hep G2 cells with agents known to induce drug metabolism enzymes. These findings suggest that a metabolite(s) of AR 12456 might be responsible for the enhanced expression of LDL receptors in cultured human cells.

INTRODUCTION

Elevated plasma concentrations of low density lipoprotein cholesterol represent one of the major risk factors for development of atherosclerosis [1,2]. Epidemiological studies have clearly established a positive correlation between elevated plasma LDL-cholesterol and coronary heart disease (CHD) [1,2]. Since LDL transport over 60% of plasma cholesterol, they represent the key determinants of cholesterol homeostasis [3]. Plasma levels of LDL are largely controlled by expression and activity of LDL receptor in hepatic and extrahepatic tissues [3,4]. The goal of therapy in hypercholesterolemic patients is to lower plasma cholesterol by raising receptor-mediated LDL catabolism [5].

Trapidil, a coronary vasodilating drug, is capable of lowering serum levels of LDL cholesterol in hypercholesterolemic patients, while concurrently raising serum levels of high density lipoprotein (HDL) [6], a parameter inversely related to CHD. Recent studies have shown that trapidil and its newly developed derivatives (AR 12456, AR 12463, AR 12465, AR 12464) favourably affected events linked to atherogenesis, such as proliferation of smooth muscle cells of the arterial wall [7] phosphodiesterase activity [8], platelet aggregation and thromboxane formation [9]. Additionally, "in vitro" preliminary investigations [10,11] have shown that some of the trapidil derivatives, particularly AR 12456, were able to increase the expression of LDL receptors in cultured human cells and to enhance the consequent receptor-mediated uptake and degradation of LDL.

In the present study we have expanded our investigations on the stimulatory effect of these drugs on receptor-mediated LDL catabolism by cultured cells. For this purpose, studies were carried out in human skin fibroblasts (HSF) and in human hepatoma cell line Hep G2, as peripheral and central model of lipoprotein metabolism.

MATERIALS AND METHODS

Sodium ^{125}I-iodine (carrier free in 0.1N NaOH) was purchased from Amersham (Amersham, UK). Trapidil and trapidil derivatives, were synthesized by scientific laboratories of VEß DEUTSCHES HYDRIERWERK RODLEBEN (G.D.R.). For chemical nomenclature see references 7, 11. Reagents and disposable materials for cell cultures were obtained as previously described [12]. Low density lipoprotein (LDL) (d 1.019-1.063 g/ml) were isolated by sequential preparative ultracentrifugation from the plasma of clinically healthy volunteers [13].

Lipoproteins were iodinated with ^{125}I by the iodine monochloride method [14], exaustively dialyzed and sterilized by filtration. The final specific activity varied between 100 and 200 cpm/ng of LDL protein. Human lipoprotein-deficient serum (LPDS) was prepared by ultracentrifugation of plasma at d = 1.25 g/ml, 40000 rpm in 50.2 T, Beckman rotor for 72h [15].

Cell culture: Human skin fibroblasts (HSF) were grown from explants of skin biopsies obtained from normolipidemic clinically healthy volunteers, as previously reported [12]. The established human hepatoma cell line Hep G2 was obtained from American Type Culture Collection (Rockville, MD, USA) and was grown as previously described [12]. For all experiments cells were seeded in 35 mm plastic dishes ($1x10^5$ and $3\text{-}6x10^5$ cells for HSF and Hep G2, respectively) in 2 ml of medium containing 10% of fetal calf serum (FCS) and used six days after plating. Confluent monolayers of cells were preincubated, in the presence or absence of drugs, for the indicated times, as described in tables, at 37°C in the medium supplemented with 5% LPDS to up-regulate LDL receptors [16]. Drugs were dissolved in ethanol (1% final concentration); control cell dishes received the same volume of the solvent. After the preincubation period, ^{125}I-LDL was added to the cells which were incubated at 37°C for further 5h.

The uptake (binding + internalization) of ^{125}I-LDL was determined after digestion of cell monolayers in 0.1 N NaoH, following standard washing procedure [17]. The specific LDL uptake was computed by subtracting values observed in the presence of 100 fold excess of unlabelled LDL from those obtained in their absence. LDL degradation was measured from the accumulation of non-iodide trichloroacetic acid-soluble ^{125}I in the incubation medium in excess of that occurring in the absence of cells [17].

RESULTS AND DISCUSSION

Compound AR 12456, a trapidil derivative, selectively influenced the LDL-receptor pathway (Table 1). It enhanced the uptake and degradation of ^{125}I-LDL by Hep G2 cells, but inhibited this pathway in HSF. Compound AR 12465 displayed a minor effect in this respect. Neither trapidil nor the other derivatives affected the receptor-mediated LDL pathway in these "in vitro" models (data not shown). The central role of human hepatic LDL receptors in controlling the plasma level of cholesterol is now well established [18]. Human hepatoma cell line, although transformed, still retains several properties of normal human hepatocytes [19]. In particular, these cells have high affinity receptors for LDL with properties resembling those reported in extrahepatic and hepatc system [20-21]. Hep G2 cell line therefore was proposed as a suitable model for the study of lipoprotein metabolism in human liver cells [22]. Compound AR 12456 stimulated the uptake and degradation of ^{125}I-LDL by Hep G2 cells in a dose-dependent manner (EC_{50} were 14 μM and 11 μM for uptake and degradation, respectively). This action was time-dependent: a 24h preincubation was essential to observe the stimulatory activity.

An opposite picture (inhibition of LDL metabolism) occurred when compound AR 12456 was added to HSF. A possible explanation might be that the stimulating effect of the drug on LDL metabolism in Hep G2 cells occurred through biotransformation to active metabolite(s). To explore this hypothesis, the Hep G2 cells were preincubated for 48h with AR 12456 and then the incubation medium was transferred to HSF and the incubation carried out for further 24h. Under these experimental conditions a stimulation of specific LDL pathway occurred also in this

TABLE 1. Effect of AR 12456 on the specific uptake and degradation of ^{125}I-LDL by human skin fibroblasts and by human hepatoma cell line HEP G2

AR 12456 (mole/l)	HEP G2 uptake (% of control)	HEP G2 degradation (% of control)	HSF uptake (% of control)	HSF degradation (% of control)
1×10^{-5}	142.9	156.4	68.9	54.6
2×10^{-5}	177.4	211.9	64.1	35.0
3×10^{-5}	294.7	213.4	58.6	28.1

Cell monolayers were preincubated for 24h at 37°C in a medium supplemented with 5% LPDS and increasing concentrations of the drug. After addition of ^{125}I-LDL (20 μg protein/ml in Hep G2 and 7.5 μg LDL protein/ml in HSF), cells were incubated at 37°C for further 5h. Uptake and degradation of ^{125}I-LDL were then determined as described in Methods.
Control values for uptake and degradation were 150, 207.8, 27.8 and 36.6 ng ^{125}I-LDL protein/mg cell protein per Hep G2 and HSF, respectively.

cell line (Table 2). These findings suggest that a metabolite(s) of AR 12456 might be responsible for the enhanced expression of LDL receptors in cultured human cells.

To support this hypothesis, the influence of AR 12456 on Hep G2 cells preincubated with substances known to activate the hepatic drug metabolism, was investigated. It was recently reported that Hep G2 cells contain mixed function oxidases which respond to inducing agents [23-25]. The inducing agents activated distinct families of the P450 gene superfamily. Four out of the eight families primary code for catabolic microsomal enzymes are found in the liver [26]. We used inducing agents at the concentrations described to be active on the drug-metabolizing enzyme activities in this cell line [23-25]. The used inducing agents alone were inactive on the LDL-receptor-mediated uptake and degradation, excepted phenobarbital. This drug (0.5 and 1.0 mM) caused a dose-dependent increase of ^{125}I-LDL metabolism by Hep G2, and by HSF. This result required further studies, especially because Heller [27] has postulated an interrelation between hepatic microsomal enzyme induction and lipoproteins.

The influence of AR 12456 on the uptake and degradation of ^{125}I-LDL by Hep G2 cells, preincubated with or without inducers, is

TABLE 2. Effect of AR 12456 on the specific uptake and degradation of ^{125}I-LDL by human skin fibroblasts before and after preincubation of the drug with human hepatoma cell line HEP G2.

	AR 12456			
	1×10^{-5} M		2×10^{-5} M	
	uptake	degradation	uptake	degradation
	(% of control)		(% of control)	
Before pre-incubation	73 ± 7^{a}	50 ± 8^{b}	71 ± 9^{b}	34 ± 7^{c}
After pre-incubation with Hep G2 (48 h)	136 ± 1^{a}	137 ± 10^{a}	197 ± 6^{b}	219 ± 20^{c}

HEP G2 cells were preincubated in a medium containing 5% LPDS in the presence or absence of increasing concentrations of AR 12456 for 48 h. The preincubation medium was then transferred to HSF and the incubation carried out for further 24 h at 37°C. After addition of ^{125}I-LDL (7.5 μg LDL protein/ml) the incubation was continued for other 5h at 37°C. Uptake and degradation of ^{125}I-LDL were measured as described in Materials and Methods. Each point represents the mean of triplicate dishes ± SD. Drug vs control: $^{a}p < 0.05$; $^{b}p < 0.01$; $^{c}p < 0.001$ (Student's t test).

summarized in Tab. 3. The preincubation with phenobarbital (0.5 or 1 mM) completly abolished the ability of AR 12456 to enhance the LDL receptor pathway in Hep G2 cells. AR 12456 appears to inhibit such a pathway in Hep G2 cells pretreated with phenobarbital as it did in fibroblasts without enzyme inducers (see Table 1). Also a low concentration of 5,6-benzoflavone (1 μM), which caused a similar activation of P-450 species as 3-methylcholanthren [28], reduced the effect of AR 12456. 2 μM 5,6-benzoflavone was inactive. High concentrations of ethanol (0.5-1.0%) in the preincubation medium seemed to enhance the effect of AR 12456. More expended studies with a larger spectrum of inducers and/or inhibitors of distinct drug-metabolizing activities of the hepatoma cells are necessary to single out the most important P450-family for the metabolization of AR 12456.

Alternative mechanisms, however, cannot be ruled out at present:

TABLE 3. Influence of AR 12456 on the specific uptake and degradation of ^{125}I-LDL by HEP G2 cells, preincubated with or without inducers.

Inducers		% of control uptake	degradation
Without		152.5	149.9
5,6-benzo-	1 μM	106.7	111.1
flavone	2 μM	157.9	162.1
Ethanol	0.3%	135.6	132.0
	0.5%	152.4	166.9
	1.0%	182.3	196.2
Phenobar-	0.5mM	116.1	116.5
bital	1.0mM	68.2	77.8

HEP G2 cells were preincubated in a medium containing 5% LPDS in the presence or absence of the indicated concentrations of inducers. Three days after addition of inducing agents, the cells were washed twice with phosphate buffered saline. Thereafter the cells were incubated for 48 h in a medium supplemented with 5% LPDS in the presence of AR 12456 (10 μM), or absence of drug (controls). 20 μg of ^{125}I-LDL protein/ml were then added and the incubation was carried out at 37°C for further 5h. Uptake and degradation of ^{125}I-LDL were determined as described in Material and Methods. Each value in the average of triplicate determinations of 3 experiments.

for instance active metabolite(s) of compound AR 12456 could indirectly influence LDL metabolism in Hep G2 cells by decreasing endogenous biosynthesis of cholesterol thus evoking an up-regulation of LDL receptors by a feed-back mechanism [29]. In addition, since Hep G2 cells are able to synthesize and secrete insulin-like growth factors [30] which are possible candidates to up-regulate LDL receptors [30,31], the possibility exists that AR 12456 might act via this indirect mechanism.

The stimulating effect of compound AR 12456 on receptor-mediated LDL catabolism could be only a component of its hypocholesterolemic activity: in fact trapidil which shows the cholesterol lowering effect in human and animals [6] and AR 12463 which reduced elevated plasma cholesterol levels and the percentages of surface of aorta covered with fatty streaks in rabbits (Beitz et al., submitted for publication) do not interfere with LDL pathway, at least in "in vitro" systems.

The pharmacological significance of the observed "in vitro" effect of compound AR 12456 on LDL metabolism was investigated in cholesterol fed guinea pigs. The drug, when injected i.p. (5 mg/kg), decreased all ß-migrating lipoproteins and enhanced high density lipoprotein (unpublished results).

Altogether these findings suggest a hypocholesterolemic activity of compound AR 12456, which appears to be mediated, at least in part, by an increased receptor-mediated LDL catabolism.

ACKNOWLEDGEMENTS

This research was support in part by the Italiana M.P.I. (Italian Government).

The Authors are grateful to Miss Monica Zamati for typing the manuscript.

REFERENCES

1) Stamler J. (1979) 'Population studies', in R. Levy, B. Rifkind, B. Dennis, N. Ernst (eds.) Nutrition, Lipids, and coronary heart disease. Raven Press, New York, pp. 25-88.
2) Lowering blood cholesterol to prevent heart disease. Consensus conference. (1985) J. Am. Med. Assoc. 253:2080-2086.
3) Havel R.J., Goldstein J.L. and Brown M.S. (1980) 'Lipoproteins and lipid transport', in P.K. Bondy and L.E. Rosenberg (eds.), Metabolic control and disease. 8th ed. Saunders W.B., Philadelphia, PA, pp. 393- 494.
4) Goldstein J.L. and Brown M.S. (1983) 'Familial hypercholesterolemia. in J.B. Stanbury, J.B. Wyngaarden, D.S. Fredrickson, J.L Goldstein and Brown M.S. (eds.) The metabolic basis of inherited disease. 5th ed. McGraw-Hill, New York, pp. 672-712.
5) Brown M.S. and Goldstein J.L. (1981) 'Lowering plasma cholesterol by raising LDL receptors', N. Engl. J. Med. 305, 515-517.
6) Ohnishi H., Itoh C., Suzuki K., Nihot, Imaizumi Y., Yamazaki Y., Morishita S., Shmora M. and Ito R. (1980) 'Effect of 5-methyl-7-diethylamino-s-triazolo-(1.5-a) pyrimidine(trapidil) on various experimental hyperlipemias', Folia Pharmacol. J. AP. 76, 469-477.
7) Giessler C.H., Fahr A., Tertov V.V., Kudryashov S.A., Orekhov A.N., Smirnov V.N. and Mest H.J. (1987) 'Trapidil derivatives as potential antiatherosclerotic drugs', Arzneim-Forsch/Drug Res. 37, 538-541.
8) Krause E.G. and Karczewski P. (1976) Hemmung der zyklo-AMP spaltenden Nukleotid-Hydrolase des Herzens durch 5-Methyl-7-dial-

thylamino-s-triazolo(1,5-a)pyrimidin (Rocornal^{n})', Acta Biol. Med. Germ. 35, 167-172.

9) Ohnishi H., Kosuzume H., Yamaguchi K., Sato M., Umehara S., Funato H., Itoh C., Suzuki K., Kitamura Y., Suzuki Y. and Itoh R. (1980) 'Pharmacological properties of trapidil: comparison with other coronary vasodilators', Folia Pharmacol. Japon 76, 495-503.

10) Beitz J., Corsini A., Granata A., Fumagalli R., Mest H.J. and Paoletti R. (1988) 'Effect of derivatives of trapidil on the expression of LDL receptors', Biomed. Biochim. Acta 47, S153-S156.

11) Corsini A., Beitz J., Granata A., Fumagalli R., Mest H.J., Paoletti R. (in press) 'Trapidil derivatives and low density lipoprotein metabolism by human skin fibroblasts and by human hepatoma cell line Hep G2', Pharmacol. Res.

12) Corsini A., Granata A., Fumagalli R. and Paoletti R. (1986) 'Calcium antagonists and low density lipoproteins metabolism by human fibroblasts and by human hepatoma cell line HEP G2', Pharmacol. Res. Comm. 18, 1-16.

13) De Lalla O.F. and Gofman J.W. (1954) 'Ultracentrifugal analysis of serum lipoprotein', Methods Biochem. Anal. 1, 459-478.

14) McFarlane A.S. (1958) 'Efficient trace-labeling of proteins with iodine', Nature 182, 53.

15) Brown M.S., Dana S.E. and Goldstein J.L. (1974) 'Regulation of 3-hydroxy-3-methylglutaryl coenzyme A reductase activity in cultured human fibroblasts: comparison of cells from a normal subject and from a patient with homozygous familial hypercholesterolemia', J. Biol. Chem. 249, 789-796.

16) Goldstein J.L. and Brown M.S. (1977) 'The low-density lipoprotein pathway and its relation to atherosclerosis', A Rev. Biochem. 46, 897-930.

17) Goldstein J.L., Basu S.K. and Brown M.S. (1983) 'Receptor-mediated endocytosis of low-density lipoprotein in cultured cells', Methods Enzymol. 98, 241-260.

18) Bilheimer D.W., Goldstein J.L., Grundy S.M., Starzl T.E. and Brown M.S. (1984) 'Liver transplantation to provide low-density-lipoprotein receptors and lower plasma cholesterol in a child with homozygous familial hypercholesterolemia' N. Engl. J. Med. 311, 1658-1664.

19) Knowles B.B., Howe C.C. and Aden D.P. (1980) Human hepatocellular carcinoma cell lines secrete the major plasma proteins and hepatitis B surface antigen', Science 209, 497-499.

20) Hillingworht D.R., Lindsey S. and Hagemans F.C. (1984) 'Regulation of low-density lipoprotein receptors in the human hepatoma cell

line Hep G2', Exp. Cell. Res. 155, 518-526.

21) Havekes L., Ven Hinsbergh V., Kempen H.J. and Emeis J. (1983) 'The metabolism in vitro of human low-density lipoprotein by the human hepatoma cell line Hep G2', Biochem. J. 214, 951-958.

22) Cohen L.H., Griffion M., Havekes L., Schouten D., Ven Hinsbergh V., and Kempen H.J. (1984) 'Effect of compactin, mevalonate and low-density lipoprotein on 3-hydroxy-3-methylglutaryl-coenzyme A reductase activity and low-density-lipoproteins-receptor activity in the human hepatoma cell line Hep G2', Biochem. J. 222, 35-39.

23) Dawson J.R., Adams D.J. and Wolf C.R. (1985) 'Induction of drug metabolizing enzymes in human liver cell line Hep G2, FEBS letters 183, 219-222.

24) Sassa S., Sugita O., Galbraith R.A. and Kappas A. (1987) Drug metabolism by the human hepatoma cell, Hep G2' Biochem. Biophys. Res. Commun. 143, 52-57.

25) Grant M.H., Duthie S.J., Gray A.G. and Burke M.D. (1988) Mixed function oxidase and uDP-glucoronyltransferase activities in the human Hep G2 hepatoma cell line', Biochem. Pharmacol. 37, 4111-4116.

26) Gonzales F.J. (1989) 'The molecular biology of cytochrome P 450s', Pharmacol. Rev. 40, 243-288.

27) Heller R.F. (1981) 'Coronary heart disease, cancer, lipoproteins, and the effects of clofibrate in enzyme induction a common link and are lipoproteins red hettings?', Lancet II, 1258-1259.

28) Daimond L., McFall R., Miller J. and Gelboin H.V. (1972) 'The effects of two isomeric benzoflavones on aryl hydrocarbon hydroxylase and the toxicity and carcinogenicity of polycyclic hydrocarbons' Cancer Res. 32, 731-736.

29) Brown M.S. and Goldstein J.L. (1986) A receptor-mediated pathway for cholesterol homeostasis'. Science 232, 34-47.

30) Schwander J.C., Hauri C., Zapf J. and Froesch E.R. (1983) 'Synthesis and secretion of insulin-like growth factor and its binding protein by the perfused rat liver: dependence on growth hormone status', Endocrinology 113, 297-305.

31) Chait A., Bierman E.L. and Albers J.J. (1979) 'Low-density lipoprotein receptor activity in cultured human skin fibroblasts' J. Clin. Invest. 64, 1309-1319.

61
Bezafibrate: effects on serum lipoproteins and haemostatic factors

D. SOMMARIVA, A. BRANCHI*, A. ROVELLINI*, D. BONFIGLIOLI, L. SCANDIANI*, C. PINI*, M. TIRRITO and A. FASOLI*

*II Department of Medicine, L. Sacco Hospital and *Institute of Internal Medicine and Medical Physiopathology, University of Milan, via G.B. Grassi 74, 20157 Milan, Italy*

Abstract

After a period of dietary stabilization 68 patients with primary hyperlipoproteinemia have been treated with bezafibrate 200 mg t.i.d.. Cholesterol (C) and triglycerides (TG) were measured in lipoprotein fractions before and after 1 month of therapy. In type IIa patients, the main change was a 23% decrease of LDL-C. LDL-TG and VLDL lipids also underwent a reduction. In type IIb patients both VLDL and LDL lipids significantly decreased. In type IV patients VLDL lipids decreased and LDL-C rose. HDL-C significantly increased in all groups of patients owing to an increase of HDL3-C, while the C content of HDL2 subfraction significantly increased only in hypertriglyceridemic patients (type IIb and IV). The change in VLDL and LDL lipids resulted to be positively correlated with their pretreatment value. Apoprotein B decreased by 24% in type IIa and by 29% in type IIb patients. Apoprotein A-I increased by 19% in type IIb patients and underwent a small and non significant increase in type IIa patients. The change in serum lipoprotein lipid concentration was associated with a change in lipoprotein lipid composition. C:TG ratio decreased in LDL of type IIa, increased in LDL of type IV and in HDL of all groups of patients. Plasma fibrinogen resulted to be 10% lower after 1 month of bezafibrate than before. The diminution was greater in patients with plasma fibrinogen higher than average and was not related with the changes in serum lipoprotein lipid concentration.

Introduction

Bezafibrate, a clofibrate analogue, is a widely used hypolipidemic agent. The mechanism by which the drug reduces elevated lipid levels is not fully understood, though it has been shown that bezafibrate has multiple effects on lipid metabolism. The inhibition of peripheral lipolysis and of hepatic fatty acid synthesis and the increase of hepatic fatty acid beta-oxidation (Kohlmeier and Schlierf, 1982) may play a critical role in reducing hepatic triglyceride production and hence in decreasing the secretion of VLDL into the blood. Moreover, the catabolism of triglyceride-rich lipoproteins is enhanced through the activation of lipoprotein lipase (Klose et al., 1979) and this may account also for the increase in HDL cholesterol level. Studies in rat (Berndt et al., 1978) and in incubated (Blasi et al., 1989) and in fresh (Cosentini et al., 1989) human blood mononuclear cells demonstrated that bezafibrate suppresses the activity of 3-hydroxy-3-methylglutaryl Coenzyme A reductase. The inhibition of sterol biosynthesis may explain the hypocholesterolemic effect of the drug which seems to be due to the ensuing increased uptake and degradation of LDL owing to the increase of the expression of the high affinity receptors for LDL (Stewart et al., 1982). Besides having lipid lowering activity, bezafibrate has been reported to produce changes in haemostatic factors and in blood viscosity (Zimmermann et al., 1978; Arntz et al., 1981; Almer and Kjellstrom, 1986; Niort et al., 1988).

Aim of the present study was to evaluate the effects of the drug on serum lipoprotein concentration and composition and on plasma fibrinogen level in patients with primary hyperlipoproteinemia.

Materials and Methods

The study was carried out on 68 patients (39 males and 29 females) known to have primary hyperlipoproteinemia. According to WHO criteria (Beaumont et al., 1970), 33 patients were classified as type IIa, 25 as type IIb and 10 as type IV hyperlipoproteinemia. All the patients were on low cholesterol low fat diet since more than 2 months before entering the study and none of them was taking drugs known to affect lipoprotein

TABLE 1. Effects of bezafibrate on serum lipoprotein cholesterol and triglycerides in 33 type IIa patients

		basal	1 month	P
VLDL				
cholesterol	mg/dl	20.3± 3.20	12.7± 2.12	<0.05
triglycerides	mg/dl	55.4± 6.67	33.5± 4.76	<0.001
cholesterol:triglycerides		0.47± 0.07	0.55± 0.04	N.S
LDL				
cholesterol	mg/dl	237.8±13.70	183.0±12.58	<0.001
triglycerides	mg/dl	41.8± 2.02	37.2± 2.37	<0.05
cholesterol:triglycerides		6.05± 0.41	5.26± 0.33	<0.05
HDL				
cholesterol	mg/dl	58.9± 2.47	63.2± 2.74	<0.05
triglycerides	mg/dl	18.5± 0.98	16.6± 1.04	<0.05
cholesterol:triglycerides		3.39± 0.19	4.23± 0.32	<0.01

TABLE 2. Effects of bezafibrate on serum lipoprotein cholesterol and triglycerides in 25 type IIb patients

		basal	1 month	P
VLDL				
cholesterol	mg/dl	53.8± 4.40	15.3± 2.57	<0.001
triglycerides	mg/dl	170.1±10.93	67.7± 9.11	<0.001
cholesterol:triglycerides		0.33± 0.02	0.23± 0.04	<0.05
LDL				
cholesterol	mg/dl	199.6± 7.27	172.8± 8.54	<0.005
triglycerides	mg/dl	60.8± 5.82	43.2± 3.51	<0.05
cholesterol:triglycerides		4.50± 0.90	4.28± 0.24	N.S.
HDL				
cholesterol	mg/dl	48.8± 2.40	62.7± 3.30	<0.001
triglycerides	mg/dl	30.3± 2.26	22.2± 1.42	<0.005
cholesterol:triglycerides		1.69± 0.12	3.17± 0.26	<0.001

metabolism. The patients, after a run-in period, have been treated with bezafibrate 200 mg t.i.d. for 1-24 months.

Total and lipoprotein cholesterol (C) and triglycerides (TG) were determined by enzymatic methods (Miles Italiana S.p.A., Italy). Serum lipoproteins were fractionated by a mixed ultracentrifugation and precipitation procedure as described elsewhere (Sommariva et al., 1986). Apoprotein B and A-I were determined by an immunoturbidimetric method (Orion-Dasit, S.p.A., Italy). Plasma fibrinogen was determined by the method of Clauss (1957).

Results

During the run-in period no significant change in serum lipid level occurred. After 1 month of bezafibrate, in type IIa patients the main

TABLE 3. Apoprotein B and A-I before and after 1 month of therapy with bezafibrate in 18 hypercholesterolemic patients

	type IIa		type IIb	
	before	1 month	before	1 month
Apo B	168.1±18.02	127.2±17.42**	171.3±12.29	121.4±10.03*
Apo A-I	113.2± 7.98	122.5± 9.46	122.3±10.93	145.6± 8.13*

*P<0.05; **P<0.005 vs basal value

TABLE 4. Effects of bezafibrate on serum lipoprotein cholesterol and triglycerides in 10 type IV patients

		basal	1 month	P
VLDL				
cholesterol	mg/dl	86.8±11.00	36.3±11.28	<0.001
triglycerides	mg/dl	335.8±60.00	139.8±32.59	<0,05
cholesterol:triglycerides		0.28± 0.08	0.24± 0.05	N.S
LDL				
cholesterol	mg/dl	111.6±11.26	137.6± 8.89	<0.01
triglycerides	mg/dl	56.8± 7.04	46.5± 5.27	N.S
cholesterol:triglycerides		2.15± 0.28	3.22± 0.33	<0.05
HDL				
cholesterol	mg/dl	37.2± 2.17	46.3± 2.66	<0.05
triglycerides	mg/dl	43.2± 4.02	31.0± 3.54	<0.05
cholesterol:triglycerides		0.98± 0.14	1.71± 0.21	<0.05

change was the average 23% fall of LDL-C (54.8 mg/dl). VLDL-C decreased by 37% and HDL-C increased by 7%. TG significantly decreased in all the 3 main lipoprotein fractions. C to TG ratio decreased in LDL, increased in HDL and did not change in VLDL (table 1).

In type IIb patients, VLDL-C and TG decreased by 72% and 60% respectively, LDL-C by 13% and LDL-TG by 29%. HDL-C rose by 28% and HDL-TG fell by 27%. C to TG ratio significantly decreased in VLDL and increased in HDL (table 2). In a subgroup of hypercholesterolemic patients apoproteins B and A-I were measured before and after 1 month of bezafibrate. As it can be seen in table 3, Apo B decreased by 24% in type IIa and by 29% in type IIb patients. Apo A-I increased by 19% in type IIb and underwent a non significant increase in type IIa patients.

TABLE 5. Mean changes in cholesterol distribution between the 2 main HDL subfractions after 1 month of bezafibrate therapy

	HDL2-C		HDL3-C	
	before	1 month	before	1 month
type IIa	29.5±2.47	30.2±2.18	29.4±1.30	33.0±0.97**
type IIb	19.5±1.87	29.7±2.86**	29.3±1.29	33.1±1.24**
type IV	14.2±1.61	18.9±2.48*	24.1±1.61	27.4±1.82*

*P<0.05; **p<0.005 vs basal value

TABLE 6. Changes in plasma fibrinogen level during bezafibrate therapy

	N of subjects	mean+SEM mg/dl	P vs basal
basal	52	323.3±12.04	
1 month	52	294.0± 9.15	<0.005
4 months	36	296.2± 9.34	<0.001
8 months	18	285.4±16.23	<0.01

In type IV patients, VLDL-C and TG decreased by 58%, LDL-C and HDL-C increased by 23% and 24% respectively. C to TG ratio significantly increased in both LDL and HDL (table 4).

The C content of both HDL subfractions increased in all the 3 groups of patients. In type IIa patients, however, HDL2 C did not rise significantly (table 5).

Plasma fibrinogen was on the average 10% lower after 1 month of therapy than before (table 6). The changes of plasma fibrinogen, as well as the ones of lipoprotein lipids, resulted to be related to the pretreatment value (table 7).

In patients who continued the treatment for up to 2 years no further significant changes in plasma fibrinogen and in serum lipid level were recorded (table 6 and figure 1 and 2). Fasting blood sugar and alkaline phosphatase significantly decreased during the treatment.In no case safety laboratory parameters underwent pathological changes.

TABLE 7. Relationship between the diminution of lipoprotein lipids and of plasma fibrinogen and the respective pretreatment level

x		y	r	P
VLDL-C	vs	Δ VLDL-C	0.81	<0.001
VLDL-TG	vs	Δ VLDL-TG	0.87	<0.001
LDL-C	vs	Δ LDL-C	0.60	<0.001
LDL-TG	vs	Δ LDL-TG	0.78	<0.001
Fibrinogen	vs	Δ fibrinogen	0.67	<0.001

Discussion

Results of the present study confirm that bezafibrate lowers VLDL and LDL and increases HDL in the commonest types of hyperlipidemia (Olsson et al., 1977; Fellin et al., 1981; Lang et al., 1982; Olsson et al.,

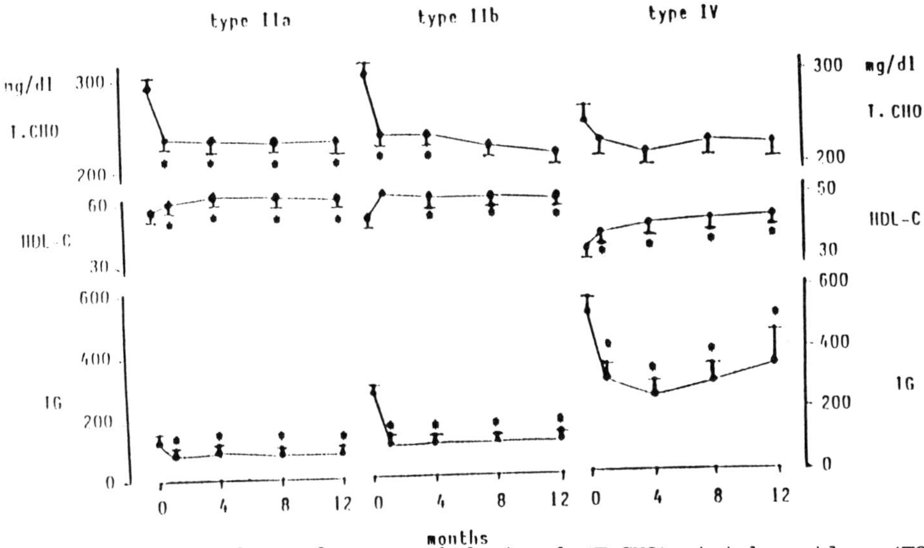

FIGURE 1: Mean values of serum cholesterol (T-CHO), triglycerides (TG) and HDL cholesterol (HDL-C) in 55 patients (25 type IIa, 18 type IIb and 12 type IV) treated for 1 year with bezafibrate 200 mg t.i.d.

1985). The changes produced by the drug are related to the type of the hyperlipoproteinemia and , possibly, to the basic metabolic defect. In fact, the decrease in serum lipid concentration was mainly due to a fall in LDL-C in type IIa patients and to a decrease of both VLDL and LDL lipids in type IIb. In type IV patients only VLDL lipids significantly decreased, while LDL-C rose. Parallel to the changes in C concentration of VLDL and LDL were the changes in apo B which strongly suggest that

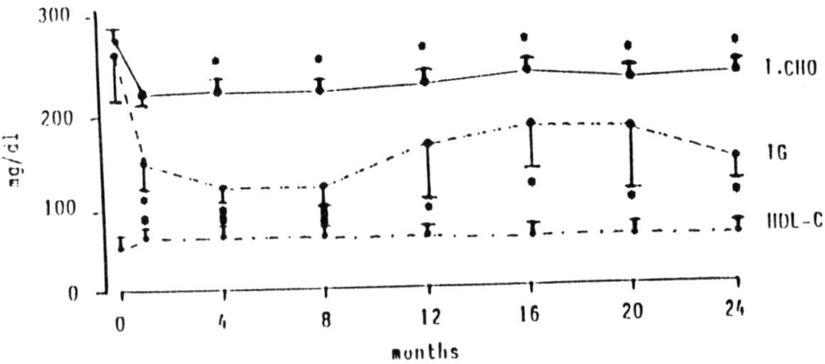

FIGURE 2: Mean values of serum cholesterol (T-CHO), triglycerides (TG) and HDL cholesterol (HDL-C) in 18 patients (9 type IIa, 5 type IIb and 4 type IV) treated for 2 years with bezafibrate 200 mg t.i.d.

bezafibrate decreases the number of circulating VLDL and LDL molecules. The drug seems to act also by modifying the lipid composition of the lipoprotein particles, in particular of LDL and HDL. C to TG ratio in LDL of hypertriglyceridemic patients and in HDL of all the 3 groups of patients increased, suggesting a partial deprivation in TG of these particles. These changes in lipid composition of lipoproteins in hypertriglyceridemia have been already observed after bezafibrate (Eisenberg et al., 1984) and may be accounted for by the activity of the lipid transfer proteins in front of a reduced VLDL mass.

Plasma fibrinogen was reduced by bezafibrate. Whether this is due to a reduction of hepatic synthesis of fibrinogen or to an increase of the fibrinolytic activity (Almer and Kjellstrom 1986) is at present unclear. At any rate, as in the case of serum lipoproteins, the lowering activity of bezafibrate appears to be related to the pretreatment plasma level of fibrinogen. A greater lowering effect in hyperfibrinogenemic than in normofibrinogenemic subjects may then be expected. Since plasma fibrinogen is believed to be an independent risk factor for atherosclerosis (Smith and Keen, 1986), its diminution by bezafibrate, toghether with the changes the drug produces on lipoprotein pattern might be of particular usefulness in prevention of coronary artery disease.

References

Almer, L.O. and Kjellstrom, T. (1986) 'The fibrinolytic system and coagulation during bezafibrate treatment of hypertriglyceridemia.' Atherosclerosis, 61, 81-85.

Arntz, H.R., Leonardt, H., Lang, P.D. and Vollmar, J. (1981) 'Effects of bezafibrate and clofibrate on blood rheology and lipoproteins in primary hyperlipoproteinemia.' Clin. Trial J., 18, 280-286.

Beaumont, J.L., Carlson, L.A., Cooper, G.R., Fejfar, Z., Fredrickson, D.S. and Stratter, T. (1970) 'Classification of hyperlipidemias and hyperlipoproteinemias.' WHO Bull., 43, 891-909.

Berndt, J., Gaumert, R. and Still, J. (1978) 'Mode of action of the lipid lowering agents clofibrate and BM 15075, on cholesterol biosynthesis in rat liver. Atherosclerosis, 30, 147-152.

Blasi, F., Sommariva, D., Cosentini R., Cavaiani, B. and Fasoli, A. (1989) 'Bezafibrate inhibits HMG-CoA reductase activity in incubated blood mononuclear cells from normal subjects and patients with heterozygous familial hypercholesterolemia.' Pharmacol. Res., 21, 247-254

Clauss, A. (1957) 'Rapid physiological coagulation method in determination of fibrinogen.' Acta Haemat., 17, 237

Cosentini, R., Blasi, F., Trinchera, M., Sommariva, D. and Fasoli A. (1989) 'Inhibition of cholesterol biosynthesis in freshly isolated blood mononuclear cells from normolipidemic subjects and hypercholesterolemic patients treated with bezafibrate.' Atherosclerosis, in press

Eisenberg, S., Gavish, D., Oschry, Y., Fainaru, M. and Deckelbaum R.J. (1984) 'Abnormalities in very low, low and high density lipoproteins in hypertriglyceridemia. Reversal toward normal with bezafibrate treatment.' J. Clin. Invest., 74, 470-475.

Fellin, R., Martini, S., Crepaldi, G., Senin, U., Mannarino, E., Avellone, G., Notarbartolo, A., Capurso, A., D'Agostino, C., Montaguti, U., Celin, D., Descovich, G.C. and Mantovani, E. (1981) 'Multicenter trial with bezafibrate in primary hyperlipidemias.' Curr. Ther. Res., 29, 657-666.

Klose, G., Behrendt, J., Vollmar, J and Greten H. (1981) 'Effect of bezafibrate on the activity of lipoprotein lipase and hepatic triglyceride hydrolase in healthy volunteers', in H. Greten, P.D. Lang and G. Schettler (eds), Lipoprotein and Coronary Heart Disease, G. Witzstrock Publ. House, New York, Baden-Baden, Cologne, pp. 182-184.

Kohlmeier,M. and Schlierf, G. (1982) 'Mode of action of bezafibrate', in G. Crepaldi, H. Schettler and G. Baggio (eds), Lipoprotein Metabolism and Therapy of Lipid Disorders, Excerpta Medica, Amsterdam, pp. 93-96.

Lang, P.D., Holler, H.D. and Vollmar, J. (1982) 'Tolerance of two years' treatment with bezafibrate in patients with hyperlipidemia', in G. Crepaldi, H. Schettler and G. Baggio (eds), Lipoprotein Metabolism and Therapy of Lipid Disorders, Excerpta Medica, Amsterdam, pp. 87-92.

Niort, G., Bulgarelli, M., Cassader, M. and Pagano, G. (1988) 'Effect of short-term treatment with bezafibrate on plasma fibrinogen, fibrinopeptide A, platelet activation and blood filterability in atherosclerotic hyperfibrinogenemic patients.' Atherosclerosis, 71, 113-119

Olsson, A.G., Lang, P.D. and Vollmar, J. (1985) 'Effect of bezafibrate during 4.5 years treatment of hyperlipoproteinemia.' Atherosclerosis, 55, 195-203.

Olsson, A.G., Rossner, S., Walldius, G., Carlson, L.A. and Lang, P.D. (1977) 'Effect of BM 15075 on lipoprotein concentrations in different types of hyperlipoproteinemia.' Atherosclerosis, 27, 279-287.

Smith, E.B. and Keen, G.A. (1987) 'Haemostatic factors and lipoproteins in atherogenesis', in S. Lenzi and G.C. Descovich (eds), Atherosclerosis and Cardiovascular Diseases, MTP Press, Lancaster, pp.319-325.

Sommariva, D., Tirrito, M., Bonfiglioli, D., Pogliaghi, I., Branchi, A. and Cabrini, E. (1986) 'Long-term effects of bezafibrate and of a bezafibrate and cholestyramine combination on lipids and lipoprotein lipids in type IIa hypercholesterolemic patients.' Int. J. Clin. Pharm. Res., 3, 249-253.

Stewart, J.M., Packard, C.J., Lorimer, A.R., Boag, D.E. and Shepherd, J. (1982) 'Effects of bezafibrate on receptor-mediated and receptor-independent low density lipoprotein catabolism in type II hyperlipoproteinemic subjects.' Atherosclerosis, 44, 355-365.

Zimmermann, R., Ehlers, W., Walter, E., Hoffrichter, A., Lang, P.D., Andrassy, K. and Schlierf G. (1978) 'The effect of bezafibrate on the fibrinolytic enzyme system and the drug interaction with racemic phenprocoumon.' Atherosclerosis, 29, 477-485

LDL APHERESIS

62
Efficiency and efficacy of LDL-apheresis performed at different intervals

G. FRANCESCHINI, L. CALABRESI, G. CHIESA and G. BUSNACH

Center E. Grossi Paoletti, Institute of Pharmacological Sciences, University of Milan and Department of Nephrology, Niguarda Cà Granda Hospital, Milan, Italy

ABSTRACT. Five heterozygous familial hypercholesterolemic patients have been treated with LDL-apheresis for a period of three months. The apheretic procedure was repeated four times at both biweekly and weekly intervals. A dextran-sulfate cellulose regenerating unit was used, processing one plasma volume at each time. The efficiency of the apheretic procedure was similar at both weekly and biweekly intervals, removing 60-70% of total cholesterol (TC), LDL cholesterol (LDL-C) and apo B. Weekly treatment was however more effective in lowering plasma lipid-lipoprotein levels: pre-apheresis TC, LDL-C and apo B levels were, in fact, 23-25% higher during the biweekly treatment.

1. Introduction

Non pharmacological treatments for the reduction of elevated plasma cholesterol levels, particularly those involving the extracorporeal removal of the atherogenic low density lipoproteins (LDL), have gained considerable interest in the last years. Since Thompson et al. (1) first used plasma exchange for the treatment of homozygous familial hypercholesterolemic (FH) patients, several more selective techniques, based on the use of affinity columns containing heparin (2), dextran sulfate cellulose (DSC) (3) or antibodies against apolipoprotein B (4) have been developed. In an effort to further improve the efficiency of the DSC apheretic procedure, a new device was designed, using two small DSC columns which can be regenerated automatically and used repeatedly during the procedure (5), thus overcoming saturation, a problem that can reduce the overall efficiency of LDL removal (6). In addition to these highly selective techniques, low cost, semi-selective systems, based on double membrane filtration, have been proposed (7, 8).

In spite of the wide diffusion of LDL apheresis, increasingly offered to patients with elevated cholesterol and/or coronary disease (9), a considerable confusion still exists on the criteria for the selection of patients amenable to the apheretic treatment and on the frequency of the apheretic procedures. In this study we evaluated the efficiency and the efficacy of a selective LDL apheretic procedure, performed at weekly and biweekly intervals, in a series of heterozygous FH patients.

2. Materials and methods

Five severe heterozygous FH patients, 3 females and 2 males (age: 54.2±3.4 y) were selected from those attending our Lipid Clinic. The diagnosis was based on the presence of tendon xanthomas and on a positive family history and checked by typing of lipoprotein receptor activity on skin fibroblasts. Lipid lowering treatments were stopped at least one month before the start of the study; the patients followed a standard low-lipid, low-cholesterol diet that was maintained throughout the study. LDL-apheresis was carried out using a double DSC column regenerating unit (5); one plasma volume was processed at each procedure. DSC-apheresis was repeated four times at biweekly intervals and then four more times at weekly intervals. Blood samples were collected before and after each apheretic procedure; total cholesterol (TC) and triglycerides were measured by enzyme methods. High density lipoprotein cholesterol (HDL-C) was evaluated after precipitation of apo B containing lipoproteins with dextran-sulfate $MgCl_2$ (10). Very low and low density lipoproteins (VLDL and LDL) were separated by sequential ultracentrifugation; apolipoprotein AI, AII and B levels were measured by immunoturbidimetry. Statistical analysis was carried out by the Student's t test; results are expressed as means±SD.

3. Results

The efficiency of the DSC apheretic procedure was nearly identical when performed at both weekly and biweekly intervals. Fifty-four percent of TC and 61% of LDL-C were removed on average by weekly DSC, compared to 60% ($p<0.05$) and 66%, respectively, by biweekly apheresis. Plasma apo B levels decreased by 67% and 69% after weekly and biweekly DSC; the selectivity of the procedure was maintained throughout the entire study, the plasma HDL-C, apo AI and apo AII levels decreasing by a maximum of 17%. By evaluating the absolute decrease of lipid/lipoprotein levels after the apheretic procedure, the biweekly treatment appeared to be more effective: TC decreased on average by 292 mg/dl (vs 220 mg/dl for weekly aphereses), LDL-C by 258 mg/dl (vs 189 mg/dl) and apo B by 212 mg/dl (vs 167 mg/dl; all $p<0.001$). A strong positive correlation ($r>0.95$) was found between the absolute post-apheresis decrease of TC, LDL-C and apo B and the starting, pre-apheresis level.

Weekly DSC treatment was significantly more effective in lowering plasma lipid/lipoprotein levels. In order to compare the general effect of the apheretic protocols, the pre- and post-apheresis mean levels during the biweekly and weekly treatments were calculated (Table). Considering the highest values, the hypocholesterolemic effect of weekly DSC was significantly better, compared to biweekly treatment, both for TC (-30% vs -14%) and LDL-C (-32% vs -15%). The HDL-C levels increased by 7% (weekly) and 9% (biweekly).

Plasma pre- and post-apheresis lipid and lipoprotein levels during biweekly and weekly treatment in 5 FH patients.

	Basal	Biweekly		Weekly	
		Pre	Post	Pre	Post
		mg/dl			
TC	555	480	195	388	166
VLDL-C	28	31	5	31	5
LDL-C	458	392	145	313	118
HDL-C	49	53	45	52	46
Triglycerides	151	163	49	156	53

4. Discussion

A comparison of the efficacy and efficiency of LDL apheresis performed at different intervals is justified by the growing diffusion of this type of procedures for the treatment of patients with elevated plasma cholesterol and/or coronary artery disease (2-9).

Despite the numerous studies, evaluating the efficacy of the various apheretic procedures in lowering plasma cholesterol levels, a considerable confusion exists on the protocols for apheretic treatment. The biweekly interval between two successive procedures is commonly used (7, 11), the hypocholesterolemic effect of treatment being generally unsatisfactory, especially in severe hypercholesterolemic patients (7). No data are available on the relative benefits of shorter vs longer intervals between procedures, particularly as pertains to the individual patient.

In the present study we evaluated the efficacy of one of the most selective and efficient apheretic procedures, the double DSC column regenerating unit (5), performed at weekly and biweekly intervals in five severe FH patients. To obviate possible confounding effects due to the variability in the amount of processed plasma, one plasma volume, calculated for each patient according to standardized formulas, was treated at each time. The efficiency of the apheretic procedure, ie the percentage removal of LDL, is clearly independent from the interval between two successive procedures. This indicates that the efficacy of the procedure critically depends from the amount of LDL amenable to apheretic removal, as confirmed by the strong positive correlation between the pre-apheresis LDL-C level and the post-apheresis decrease. Since this correlation is valid over a wide range of LDL-C levels, this imply that the hypocholesterolemic efficacy of the single procedure is much higher in severe hypercholesterolemic patients and make questionable the use of LDL-apheresis in subjects with moderately elevated cholesterol levels.

The present results clearly indicate that, in spite of a lower acute decrease of TC and LDL-C after weekly (vs biweekly) aphereses, the general hypocholesterolemic effect of weekly treatment is much more pronounced. This suggests that other factors, in particular the rate of lipid recovery after apheresis, can play a major role in determining the overall efficacy of the apheretic treatment. Thus, the combination therapy with LDL-apheresis and hypocholesterolemic drugs (12), possibly slowing-down the post-apheresis rebound of total and LDL-cholesterol, appears to be the most promising tool for the treatment of severe hypercholesterolemic patients.

5. References

1. Thompson, G.R., Lowenthal, R. and Myant, N.B. (1975) 'Plasma exchange in the management of homozygous familial hypercholesterolemia', Lancet i, 1208-1211.
2. Eisenhauer, T., Armstrong, V.W., Wieland, H., Fuchs, C., Scheler, F. and Seidel, D. (1987) 'Selective removal of low density lipoproteins (LDL) by precipitation at low pH: first clinical application of the HELP system', Klin. Wochenschr. 65, 161-168.
3. Yokoyama, S., Hayashi, R., Satani, M. and Yamamoto, A. (1985) 'Selective removal of low density lipoprotein by plasmapheresis in familial hypercholesterolemia', Arteriosclerosis 5, 613-622.
4. Stoffel, W. and Demant, T. (1981) 'Selective removal of apolipoprotein B-containing serum lipoproteins from blood plasma', Proc. Acad. Sci. USA 78, 611-615.
5. Mabuchi, H., Michishita, I., Takeda, M., Fujita, H., Koizumi, J., Takeda, R., Takada, S. and Oonishi, M. (1987) 'A new low density lipoprotein apheresis system using two dextran sulfate cellulose columns in an automated column regenerating unit (LDL continuous apheresis)', Atherosclerosis 68, 19-25.
6. Yokoyama, S., Hayashi, R., Kikkawa, T., Tani, N., Takada, S., Hatanaka, S. and Yamamoto, A. (1984) 'Specific sorbent of apolipopro-

tein B-containing lipoproteins for plasmapheresis', Arteriosclerosis 4, 276-282.

7. Franceschini, G., Busnach, G., Vaccarino, V., Calabresi, L., Gianfranceschi, G. and Sirtori, C.R. (1988) 'Apheretic treatment of severe familial hypercholesterolemia: comparison of dextran sulfate cellulose and double membrane filtration methods for low density lipoprotein removal', Atherosclerosis 73, 197-202.
8. Mabuchi, H., Michishita, I., Sakai, T., Sakai, Y., Watanabe, A., Wakasugi, T. and Takeda, R. (1986) 'Treatment of homozygous patients with familial hypercholesterolemia by double-filtration plasmapheresis', Atherosclerosis 61, 135-140.
9. Parker, T.S., Gordon, B.R., Saal, S.D., Rubin, A.L. and Ahrens, E.H.Jr. (1986) 'Plasma high density lipoprotein is increased in man when low density lipoprotein (LDL) is lowered by LDL-apheresis', Proc. Natl. Acad. Sci. USA 83, 777-781.
10. Warnick, G.R., Benderson, J. and Albers, J.J. (1982) 'Dextran sulfate precipitation procedure for quantitation of high-density lipoprotein', Clin. Chem. 28, 1379-1388.
11. Saito, Y., Shinomiya, M., Shirai, K. and Yoshida, S. (1988) 'Treatment of severe hypercholesterolemia by LDL-apheresis: cholesterol lowering effect and clinical evaluation', Contrib. Infus. Ther. 23, 160-171.
12. Mabuchi, H., Fujita, H., Michishita, I., Takeda, M., Kajinami, K., Koizumi, J., Takeda, R., Takegoshi, T., Wakasugi, T., Ueda, K., Miyamoto, S., Watanabe, A. and Oota, M. (1988) Effects of CS-514 (eptastatin), an inhibitor of 3-hydroxy-3-mehtylglutaryl coenzyme A (HMG-CoA) reductase, on serum lipid and apolipoprotein levels in heterozygous familial hypercholesterolemic patients treated by low density lipoprotein (LDL)-apheresis', Atherosclerosis 72, 183-188.

63

Ischemic heart disease and plasmapheresis for cholesterol

I. RICHICHI

Cardiovascular Prevention Center, Policlinico S. Matteo, P. le Golgi 2, 27100 Pavia, Italy

ABSTRACT. Risk factors influence growth factors of the atheromatous plaque. LDL hypercholesterolemia is a very important growth factor, and it has to be eliminated in order to arrest plaque evolution. Theoretically plaque regression can be achieved only with the reduction of total blood cholesterol below 150 mg/dl. To obtain such level plasmapheresis should be added to pharmacological treatment which alone would be insufficient. There are various methods of cholesterol plasmapheresis but the most commonly used ones remain: cascade filtration and plasmapheresis with dextran sulphate.

Introduction

Atherosclerosis is a chronic degenerative disease with multi-factorial etiology. The beginning of the pathological process in ischemic heart disease depends on the localisation of the atherosclerotic lesions. In Italy coronary atherosclerosis is the first cause of morbidity and mortality: about 150,000 myocardial infarcts annually, 30% of which die within a year. The high incidence has made it be considered a social disease. The pathological process starts right in the first decade of life, but it's not yet clear whether atheroma formation starts with the primitive lipid depositions or it follows arterial endothelial lesions. The evolution of the atherosclerotic plaque depends on multiple factors, the so called growth factors: endothelial, platelet, muscular and cholesterol. Recently plaque formation has been found to correlate well with mechanical, physical and chemical factors: raised arterial pressure causes mechanical stress on the endothelium, nicotine causes increased global arterial contractility resulting in endothelial microischemia. Catecholamines derived from stress activate both the above mechanisms. Low density lipoprotein (LDL) cholesterol enters endothelial cells by the process of internalisation; the transportation by lipoproteins in the blood stream makes possible the fixation of Apoprotein B to endothelial receptors thus initiating the process of cellular penetration and utilisation. This mechanism is regulated by the blood concentration of LDL and the quantity of cell receptors (these receptors are very limited in subjects with familial dyslipidemia). The excess in blood concentration of LDL determines the amount of penetration. When the endothelial surface is no longer intact or smooth, this activates other mechanism that induce the entrance of macrophages thus starting the process of atheroma formation. High density lipoprotein (HDL) has the very important role of transporting cholesterol from the cells into the blood stream and hence to the liver. Apoprotein B exerts an essential function of removal of excess cholesterol. Armstrong and Clarckson have demonstrated in a simple form the scheme of transport ► deposition ► reduction of atheroma. The experimental scheme is simple and comprehensible : putting a rabbit or a primate on a hypercaloric high lipid diet for 6 months results in the rapid formation of atheromas in arteries (carotid, femoral, coronary), and the thicknesses of these atheromas depend on the fatty excess or duration of the diet. Putting the same animals on a low lipid diet, and may be adding a hypocholesterolemic drug, results in regression of the atheromatous plaque.

In reality this mechanism or system is much more complex in man. Many of the contributing factors are not even recognised and cannot therefore be eliminated. However, it remains a valid system. In man the growth of the plaque remains silent, i.e. it doesn't produce symptoms, for some decades. As long as the arterial stenosis doesn't cause significant hypoxia of the area supplied, atherosclerosis remains silent. But when stenosis exceedes 75% then symptoms can appear, reflecting reduced blood flow. For this to occur it takes decades. In fact, the incidence of coronary atherosclerosis is highest after 30-40 years of age during which time the "experimental" growth mechanism has become very complicated as a result of spontaneous activation of other processes that modify the anatomical characteristics of the plaque. By this time the atheroma is no longer the soft fatty form but different and very complicated with a limited lipid content, after having undergone transformation processes. The characteristics of the atheroma depend on various elements: lipids, cells and fibres. A young atheroma is always rich in cholesterol, smootn and soft, and can therefore regress easily and rapidly. Whoreas an old atheroma contains little cholesterol but much fibrous or fibrocalcious tissue, and often becomes the site of ulceration, hemorrhage or thrombosis; and these complications accelerate the growth process.

Any attempts to achieve regression of the plaque must therefore take into account anatomical and pathological conditions and the prevalence or its histological and structural components. A serious therapeutic attempt must eliminate or reduce all factors that influence formation and growth of the atheromatous plaque. Any intervention should therefore include the following:

1) correction of all risk factors (cigarette smoking, stress, arterial

hypertension, diabetes, sedentary life style, obesity).
2) Low fat, low cholesterol diet.
3) Reduction of blood cholesterol levels.

Total blood cholesterol is certainly the foundamental factor in the formation and growth of atheroma.

Indications

It has not yet been well defined what levels of blood cholesterol can cmpleterly avoid the risk of coronary artery disease. In adult subjects (over 30 years) the safest mean value is 200 mg/dl. For an adult who is already affected by ischemic heart disease there's diffuse involvement of the coronary arteries, and the maintenance of a cholesterol level of 200 mg/dl is not enough to guarantee improvement of symtoms. This is maninly because at that level there's elimination of only the growth factor, while others factors remain active. Hence it's necessary to have the objective of achieving regression of the plaque.

Regression results from measures aimed at repairing and restructuring the plaque so as to increase the affected arterial lumen. The first objective of achieving is to eliminate cholesterol and lipids from the plaque. Theoretically this can be achieved by the reduction of cholesterolemia below 150 mg/dl. But a low cholesterol diet allows only 5-10% reduction in cholesterolemia, and even when intense cannot effect a reduction of over 20%; and the use of "statine" conses a reduction of 30-35%. The theoretical level of cholesterol compatibel, with regression can therefore not be reached by the above measures alon, hence the need for use of other methods of treatment.

LDL Cholesterol Plasmapheresis

The techniques of LDL plasmapheresis currently available are of the types:

a) Semiselective
b) Selective

a) The semiselective method, called also cascade filtration uses the principles of exclusion based on physical properties. LDL cholesterol a protein high molecular weight, is collected in the inside of a fibrous filtre of pores of 0.7 micron. Actually this method uses two filters: the first is a plasmaseparator with pores of 0.55 micron, which separates venous blood from the patient into corpuscular and plasma components. The plasma then undergoes cascade filtration during which proteins of high molecular weight remain inside the filter and are eliminated, while the rest is returned into the patient's circulation after remixing with the corpuscular part.

The advantages of this method are its flexibility, cost, easy reproducibility and diffuse use in centres for hemapheresis for the treatment of other pathologies.

The main disadvantage of semiselectivity is the loss of HDL cholesterol which amounts up to about 35%.

(b) The selective method utilises the biochemical property of LDL cholesterol to be fixed on a column-immobilised agent:

1) Plasmaperfusion on dextran sulphate (Kaneka method).

Dextran sulphate is capable of selectively binding LDL cholesterol, avoiding other plasma proteins principally HDL cholesterol. The system uses a plasma separator filter and two columns, each of 150 mls of dextran sulphate functionning alternately. The procedure goes through phases of saturation and regeneration of the two columns. The advantages of the Kaneka method are its selectivity, high efficiency and complete automation in the MA-01 system.

2) Plasmaperfusion on dextran sulphate (Cobe method).

plasma LDL cholesterol is absorbed by dextran sulphate particles which are then on their part removed by an appropriate filter. In the USA this system is in an advanced experimental stage. Its advantages would be the high degree of selectivity and easy execution.

3) The Heparin Extracorporeal LDL Precipitation System (Help-Braun)

Plasma separated by a filter is mixed with heparin solution at pH 5.12 capable of precipitation LDL cholesterol. The precipitate is then filtered of and excess heparin removed and concentration achieved using a hemofilter. High efficiency and selectivity are the advantages of the system, while the main disadvantages are high costs and difficulties with priming.

4) Immunoabsorbtion

This method, used at the University of Cologne (W. Germany), is based on the ability of monoclonal anti Apo B antibodies to bind LDL cholesterol in extracorporeal circulation. The system is analogous with the Kaneka method described above. Its advantages are high efficiency and selectivity. Disadvantages include high costs and the problem of reusing the columns for the same patient.

Objective and reports

Plasmapheresis is employed for the following end points:

a) Reduced blood cholesterol to desired levels.
b) Slow or arrest the progression of atheromatous plaques.
c) Induce regression of the plaque.

The criteria for patient selection is precise and a high degree of compliance is necessary in order to complete any protocol; therefore the the following are treated:

a) Patients with severe coronary artery disease and dyslipidemia.
b) Patients with coronary artery disease and severe dyslipidemia.
c) Patients with severe familial dyslipidemia.

In our Centre for the Prevention of Cardiovascular diseases 12 patients have been treated since October 1986. The protocol consists of history, clinical examination, antropometric examination, blood profile (total cholesterol, HDL cholesterol, Apo A1, Apo B100, tryglicerides, lipoprotein electrophoresis, electrolytes, fibrinogen), Ecg, exercise stress test every 3 months, dynamic Ecg every 3 months, and coronary arteriography at the beginning of treatment and 18 months afterwards.

Of the 12 patients (11 males, 1 female) who entered the treatment programme, 6 were excluded before the end because of poor compliance, 1 completed the cycle and 5 are still on treatment.

Seven patients had previous myocardial infarction, 4 had undergone aorto-coronary bypass surgery and 1 was affected by severe unstable angina.
The procedure of plasmapheresis consists of one session a week or two, a volume of plasma being processed each session.
In 5 patients the frequency of treatment was once every 15 days, while in the others it was weekly; 6 patients were treated with cascade filtration technique, while the other 6 with plasmaperfusion on dextran sulphate. The immediate effect of the procedure on the parametres measured are shown in the following table:

	F.C.I	F.C.II	C.S.D.
C.T.	-41.10%	-50.20%	-52.60
HDL	-31.10%	-32.40%	-13.10%
TG	-53.70%	-57.20%	-56.60%
Apo A1	-32.50%	-33.10%	-7.80%
Apo B	-41.90%	-45.90%	-46.2%
A1/B	+25	+29	+39

F.C.I = Standard Cascade Filtration
F.C.II = Modified Cascade Filtration
C.S.D. = Columns of dextran sulphate

The standard method of cascade filtration is characterised by semiselectivity (reduction of HDL cholesterol by 31.1% and Apo A1 by 32.5%) and low efficiency in reducing total cholesterol (by 41.1%).
The modified method brings some significant improvement in results with reduction of total cholesterol up to 50.1% without ulterior reduction of HDL cholesterol and Apo A1.
The Kaneka technique demonstrates high efficiency and selectivity. All patients tolerated the procedures well except on two occasions when side effects (vagal crises) were reported, both minor and during cascade filtration.
Extracorporeal removal of HDL cholesterol has proved to be extremely efficient in both methods employed, especially in modified cascade filtration and plasmaperfusion on dextran sulphate columns. The results of the trial will be reported after the completion of the experiment still underway. Subjective and clinical improvement has been achieved in 11 subjects, with the exception of one patient who after some session of plasmapheresis had bypass surgery; exercise stress testing showed stable or improved conditions.

References.

1) Glueck CJ. (1986) 'Role of risk factor management in progression and regression of coronary and femoral artery atherosclerosis. Am J Cardiol, 57: 35G-41G.

2) Friedman M. , Bayers SO. (1963) 'Observations concerning the evolution of atherosclerosis in the rabbit after cessation of cholesterol feeding. Am J Pathol, 43:349-59

3) Blankenhorn DH. (1982), 'Lipoproteins and the progression and regression of atherosclerosis. Cardiovasc Rev Rep, 3: 1063-71.

4) Thompson GR. (1980) 'Assessment of long-term plasma exchange for familial hypercolesterolemia'. Br Heart J. 43: 680-8.

5) Malinow MR. (1983) 'Regression of atherosclerosis in humans. A new frontier. Postgrad Med; 73: 232-5. 239-42.

6) Chait A. (1987) 'Progression of atherosclerosis: the cellular biology. Eur Heart J. 8 (suppl H): 15-22.

7) Anitschkow NN., Chacariw S. (1913) 'Uber experimentelle cholesterinstentose und ihr Bedeutung fur die Entstehung einiger pathologische Prozesse. Z. Allg Pathol Anat; 24: 1-9.

8) Armstrong ML., Megan MB (1972) 'Lipid depletion in atheromatous coronary arteries in rhesus monkeys after regression diets. Circ Res; 30: 675-80.

9) Clarkson TB., Lehner NDM. , Wagner WD. et al. (1980) 'A study of atherosclerosis regression in Macaca mulatta. 1 design of experiment and lesion induction. Am Pathol; 100: 633.

10) Malinow MR. (1981) 'Regression of atherosclerosis in humans. Fact or myth? Circulation 64: 1-3.

11) Blankenhorn DH, Nessim SA., Johnson RL et al. (1987) 'Beneficial effects of colestipolniacin therapy on coronary atherosclerosis and coronary venous bypass grafts. Jama 257: 3233-40.

64

Variables involved in the treatment of severe hyperlipoproteinemias by combined drug and LDL-apheresis treatment

C. STEFANUTTI, G.C. ISACCHI, B. MAZZARELLA, A. VIVENZIO, M. GOZZER[1], M. MASCI[1], A. BUCCI and G. RICCI

Istituto di Terapia Medica Sistematica & Cattedra di Ematologia, University of Rome "La Sapienza", Rome; [1]Policlinico Umberto I, viale del Policlinico (00161)

ABSTRACT. During clinical trials devoted to attaining the best possible control of severe hypercholesterolemia, a combination of adequate drug therapy and LDL-apheresis (LDL/A), should be put into practice. With relation to stopping the progression and/or obtaining the regression of preexisting coronary atherosclerotic lesions, this combination is a very promising one. Results depend on the intensity and frequency of this combination treatment. A long-term treatment with LDL/A can also be carried out without serious side effects, providing the patient's clinical status is satisfactory and his vascular accesses are well-represented.

INTRODUCTION. Overwhelming evidence demonstrated unequivocally that patients affected by high-risk plasma cholesterol levels (severe hypercholesterolemia), particularly those with hereditary hyperlipoproteinemia, will develop atherosclerosis even in the absence of additional coronary risk factors. As a matter of fact, the major complication of familial hypercholesterolemia (FH) is premature coronary heart disease (CHD). FH is highly resistant to medical treatment (diet and drugs). The advent of new powerful HMGCoA-reductase inhibitors, along with the possibility of making efficient drug combinations may allow for more satisfactory control of FH. However, different degrees of resistance and/or intolerance to an adequate drug treatment may be observed in at least 20-25% of patients with heterozygous FH. Obviously, homozygous patients are almost completely unresponsive to conventional medical treatment. In such cases, alternative treatment(s) must be considered. The most frequent metabolic disease for which plasma-exchange (PE) has been used is homozygous and heterozygous FH. This therapeutic approach was first described by De Gennes et al. (1967) [5] as a discontinuous plasma separation. Eight years later, Thompson et al. reported the use of continuous flow PE in the treatment of two homozygous patients affected by FH [6]. A more recent evolution of plasmapheresis technology, allowed the removal of LDL and VLDL by plasmaperfusion over filters or solid-phase affinity columns containing immobilized sorbents [7,8,9]. Plasma apoB-containing lipoproteins can also be precipitated or absorbed. Our current approach is devoted to develop a therapeutic schedule using LDL/A and combined drug treatment which would allow to keep as lowest as possible, LDL-cholesterol (LDL-chol) and apolipoprotein B (apoB) levels of patients whose response to diet and drugs was negligible and/or with clinically symptomatic CHD.

MATERIALS AND METHODS. We treated nine patients with FH unresponsive to an adequate, intensive LDL-chol lowering medical and dextransulfate cellulose LDL-affinity apheresis (DSC-LDL/A) treatment. Three patients affected by hypercholesterolemia and hypertriglyceridemia with/without CHD, were also treated. Patients were submitted to DSC-LDL/A with a frequency depending upon their clinical status. The most frequent treatment schedule was fourteen days. One-hundred and forty-one treatments have been performed without serious side effects. The longest continuous treatment was eighteen months. The clinical data of the patients are summarized in table 1. All patients have undergone to NIH "step two" diet, before starting and during the therapeutic cycle with LDL/A. Combined drug treatment before LDL/A was reported in table 2. LDL/A using dextransulfate cellulose column affinity apheresis (Liposorber, LA-15; Sulflux, FS-05; MA-01 System, Kanegafuchi Chemical Industries, Osaka, Japan) was performed as reported elsewhere [9]. Total cholesterol (T-chol) and triglyceride (Tg) levels, were evaluated in whole plasma and isolated lipoprotein fractions after ultracentrifugation (UC L5-65, Beckman) by enzymatic-colorimetric methods (CHOD-PAP for T-chol, GPO-PAP for Tg)[10]. HDL-cholesterol (HDL-chol) was evaluated after precipitation of apoB-containing lipoproteins with phosphotungstate $MgCl_2$[11].

Plasma apolipoprotein AI (apoAI) and apoB levels were evaluated by radial immunodiffusion using Nor-Partigen plates (Behring, Werke). Plasma lipoprotein and apolipoprotein levels were determined before and after each treatment with DSC-LDL/A.

RESULTS. Mean plasma lipoprotein, apolipoprotein and fibrinogen levels before starting and during the therapeutic cycle with LDL/A and combined drug treatment were shown in tables 3, 4, 5, 6. A combined intensive dietary and drug treatment which was begun before the therapeutic cycle with LDL/A, was not able to decrease mean plasma LDL-chol and apoB concentrations to lower levels than those reported in table 3 ("PRE" values). Mean apoB--containing lipoprotein and apolipoprotein concentrations after the beginning of therapeutic cycle with LDL/A were reduced to lower levels. However, an additive effect of combining drug treatment to LDL/A must be taken into account and evaluated on case-by-case basis. The effects of associating medical therapy to LDL/A in patients with familial and non familial hypercholesterolemia on mean plasma LDL-chol, VLDL-cholesterol (VLDL-chol), HDL--chol, HDL_2-, HDL_3-cholesterol (HDL_2-chol, HDL_3-chol), apoAI and apoB levels were reported in tables 3, 4, 5. The mean percent difference between pre- and post LDL/A values was remarkably significant. Mean plasma fibrinogen concentrations showed a statistically significant reduction after DSC-LDL/A ($p \leq 0.001$) (table 6).

DISCUSSION. An usual experience in the management of severe hyperlipoproteinemias, especially FH, is the individual variation in responsiveness to treatment with all lipid-lowering drugs. Even when medical therapy is appropriate and the patient's adherence is good, plasma cholesterol levels may still be far from desirability. Consequently, a partial treatment of hyperlipoproteinemia will obtain only a modest effect on the risk of CHD endpoints [2]. As a matter of fact, LRC-CPPT trial showed a "dose-response" relationship with regards of CHD endpoints. Furthermore, a large body of evidence suggests of lowering plasma cholesterol in hypercholesterolemic individuals with preexisting clinical CHD (secondary prevention) as well as in asymptomatic subjects (primary prevention). It has also been suggested that patients with coronary by-pass must be intensively treated to prevent vein grafts restenoses. The extracorporeal removal of apoB-containing lipoproteins with DSC-LDL/A, from plasma of patients with severe hyperlipoproteinemias without clinical control, showed to be highly efficient, safe and a substantially well-accepted approach for short- and long-term treatment cycles. Though combining drugs to LDL/A may be helpful to achieve a more pronounced lowering of plasma cholesterol level, the consequent possibility of getting advantage from prolonging or shortening the intervals between LDL/A procedures is still a matter of debate. Whether the treatment with LDL/A and drugs is aimed at stopping or regressing the development of coronary atherosclerosis, then, the therapeutic cycle must be intensive and continuous. The lesson from current knowledge teaches that the optimal therapeutic cycle cannot be shorter than 2-3 years [3]. However, a fraction of patients with severe hyperlipoproteinemia may get advantage from lowering of their atherogenic lipoproteins, within a short-time and within a relatively shorter therapeutic cycle. In our experience, patients with unstable angina (BD, DA, FG, PF) showed an appreciable short- and long-term clinical improvement after being treated by DSC-LDL/A. We can conclude that high risk individuals must be resolutely treated. Though the decision of using drugs and/or other kind of treatment must be made on case-by-case basis. Family history of CHD, preexisting clinical CHD, presence of other marked coronary risk factor/s, age and clinical state of the patient must be carefully considered. Clinical trials devoted to study a broader use of LDL/A in the treatment of CHD-related clinical complications (myocardial infarction, angina) and to secondary prevention of coronary surgery sequelae (restenoses), are to be performed. Finally, a better understanding of the mechanism of interaction between the treatment with LDL/A and hemostatic and rheologic functions, is also desirable and must be pursued.

TABLE 1. Patients general and clinical characteristics.
Familial hypercholesterolemia.

PATIENTS	SEX	AGE (yrs)	LIPOPROTEIN PHENOTYPE	CHD	DURATION of LDL-apheresis (months)	N. TREATMENT
FA	F	45	IIa	-	12	24
MJ	F	44	IIa	-	4	8
SM *	M	31	IIa	+	17	34
FG	M	40	IIa	+	12	24
PF	M	51	IIa	+	4	8
AD	M	30	IIa	-	3.5	7
CA	F	25	IIa	-	2	4
SV	M	30	IIa	-	0	1
DA	M	47	IIa	+	1	2
Nonfamilial hyperlipoproteinemia.						
BD	M	43	IV	+	30	15
FL	F	53	V	- §	1	2
CM	F	60	V	- §	0	1

*: receptor-defective homozygous FH

+: presence of exertional angina, and/or positive exercise stress test, and/or coronary artery by-pass grafting, and/or (previous) myocardial infarction

§: associated disease: amyloidosis diagnosed by liver and kidney biopsy.

TABLE 2. Medical treatment before starting DSC-LDL/A.

PATIENTS	DIET	DRUG	DOSE
SM	NIH Step 2	Cholestyramine	32 g/d
		Bezafibrate *	600 mg/d
		Simvastatin	40 mg/d
FG	"	Cholestyramine	24 g/d
		Simvastatin	40 mg/d
BD	"	Fenfibrate	300 mg/d
		Gemfibrozil	1200 mg/d
FA	"	Cholestyramine	24 g/d
		Gemfibrozil	1200 mg/d
MJ	"	Probucol	1500 mg/d
		Bezafibrate	600 mg/d
		Cholestyramine	24 g/d
		Gemfibrozil	1200 mg/d
CA	"	Cholestyramine	24 g/d
		Gemfibrozil	1200 mg/d
AD	"	Bezafibrate *	600 mg/d
		Lovastatin	20 mg/d
		Cholestyramine	30 g/d
PF	"	Cholestyramine	36 g/d
		Gemfibrozil	1200 mg/d
CM	"	Cholestyramine	24 g/d
		Bezafibrate	600 mg/d
SV	"	Fenfibrate *	300 mg/d
		Bezafibrate *	600 mg/d
		Gemfibrozil *	1200 mg/d
		Cholestyramine	12 g/d
		Lovastatin	40 mg/d
FL	"	Bezafibrate	600 mg/d
		Gemfibrozil	1200 mg/d
		Cholestyramine	24 g/d
DA	"	Simvastatin	40 mg/d

*: administered before of being submitted for medical care to the investigators.

TABLE 3. Acute effects of DSC-LDL/A on plasma lipoprotein and apolipoprotein levels. Familial hypercholesterolemia.

PATIENTS		LDL-chol*	Δ%	VLDL-chol	Δ%	apoB	Δ%	apoAI	Δ%
FA	PRE	280		19		220		160	
	POST	95	66	10	47	123	44	142	11
	$\overline{X}$	188		14		172		151	
MJ	"	274		21		231		142	
		131	52	6	71	129	44	128	10
		203		14		180		135	
SM	"	388		18		288		141	
		120	69	7	61	119	58	126	10
		254		12		204		134	
FG	"	276		23		234		131	
		109	60	8	65	109	53	113	14
		193		15		172		122	
PF	"	335		34		215		142	
		111	67	12	65	83	61	122	14
		223		23		149		132	
AD	"	243		18		177		120	
		101	58	5	72	90	49	115	4
		172		11		133		117	
CA	"	220		17		169		139	
		49	78	2	88	51	70	128	8
		134		9		110		133	
SV	"	287		16		236		134	
		100	65	6	63	105	55	125	7
		193		11		170		129	
DA	"	215		23		155		156	
		46	79	5	78	56	64	150	4

*: mg/dl; $\overline{X}$: (PRE + POST) / 2.

TABLE 4. Acute effects of DSC-LDL/A on plasma lipoprotein levels. Familial hypercholesterolemia.

PATIENTS		HDL-chol*	Δ%	HDL_2-chol	Δ%	HDL_3-chol	Δ%
FA	PRE	51		16		35	
	POST	44	14	12	25	32	8
	$\overline{X}$	47		14		33	
MJ	"	44		19		25	
		40	9	16	16	24	4
		42		17		24	
SM	"	48		16		32	
		44	14	12	25	30	6
		46		14		31	
FG	"	39		9		30	
		34	13	6	33	28	6
		36		7		29	
PF	"	60		26		34	
		55	8	22	15	32	6
		57		24		33	
AD	"	51		17		34	
		48	6	15	12	33	3
		49		16		33	
CA	"	48		12		36	
		43	10	10	16	33	8
		45		11		34	
SV	"	45		12		33	
		43	4	11	8	32	3
		44		11		32	
DA	"	52		22		30	
		51	2	21	4	30	-
		51		21		30	

*: mg/dl; $\overline{X}$: (PRE + POST) / 2.

TABLE 5. Acute effects of DSC-LDL/A on plasma lipoprotein and apolipoprotein levels. Nonfamilial hyperlipoproteinemia.

PATIENTS		LDL-chol*	Δ%	VLDL-chol	Δ%	apoB	Δ%	apoAI	Δ%
BD	PRE	140		82		177		138	
	POST	44	68	31	62	79	55	129	6
	$\overline{X}$	92		56		128		133	
FL	"	442		117		231		131	
		173	61	78	33	123	47	119	9
		307		97		177		125	
CM	"	515		69		291		135	
		126	75	20	68	109	62	128	5
		320		41		200		131	

PATIENTS		HDL-chol*	Δ%	HDL_2-chol	Δ%	HDL_3-chol	Δ%
BD	PRE	33		11		22	
	POST	31	6	10	9	21	4
	$\overline{X}$	32		10		21	
FL	"	37		9		28	
		31	16	7	22	24	14
		34		8		26	
CM	"	48		12		36	
		44	8	10	16	34	5
		46		11		35	

*: mg/dl; $\overline{X}$: (PRE + POST) / 2.

TABLE 6. Mean (± SD) plasma fibrinogen levels before and after DSC-LDL/A.

PATIENTS	SEX	FIBRINOGEN Before	FIBRINOGEN After	Δ%
SM	M	280*	195	30.3
FG	M	216	184	14.8
BD	M	230	182	20.8
FA	F	310	260	16.1
MJ	F	256	221	13.6
CA	F	220	160	27.2
AD	M	280	175	37.5
PF	M	270	192	28.8
SV	M	250	185	26.0
CM	F	280	176	37.1
FL	F	235	185	21.2
$\bar{X}$		**257**	**192** ◊	
SD		**28.4**	**25.6**	

*: mg/dl; ◊: $p \leq 0.001$ [t = 8.45].

REFERENCES.

1. Schaefer, E.J., Levy, R.I. (1985) 'Pathogenesis and management of lipoprotein disorders', New Engl. J. Med. 312, 1300.
2. Lipid Research Clinics Program: The Lipid Research Clinics Coronary Primary Prevention Trial Results: I and II (1984), JAMA 251, 351.
3. Blankenhorn, D.H. et al. (1987) 'Beneficial effects of combined colestipol-niacin therapy on coronary atherosclerosis and coronary venous bypass grafts', JAMA 257, 3233.
4. Brown, M.S., Goldstein, J.L. (1986) 'A receptor-mediated pathway for cholesterol homeostasis', Science 232, 34.
5. De Gennes, J.L. et al. (1967) 'Formes homozygotes cutanéo-tendineuses de xanthomatose hypercholestérolémique dans une observation familiale exemplaire - Essai de plasmaphérése à titre de traitement héroique', Bull. Mém. Soc. Méd. Hòp. Paris 118, 1377.
6. Thompson, G.R. et al. (1980) 'Assessment of long-term plasma exchange for familial hypercholesterolemia', Br. Heart J. 43, 680.
7. Homma, Y. et al. (1987) 'Comparison of selectivity of LDL removal by double filtration and dextran-sulfate cellulose column plasmapheresis, and changes of subfractionated plasma lipoproteins after plasmapheresis in heterozygous familial hypercholesterolemia', Metabolism 36, 419.
8. Mabuchi, H. et al. (1988) 'Effect of CS-514 (eptastatin), an inhibitor of HMGcoA-reductase on serum lipid and apolipoprotein levels in heterozygous familial hypercholesterolemic patients treated by low density lipoprotein (LDL)-apheresis', Atherosclerosis 72, 183.
9. Stefanutti, C. et al. (1988) 'Selective continuous removal of low density lipoproteins by dextran sulfate cellulose column adsorption apheresis in the therapy of familial hypercholesterolemia', Contrib. Infus. Ther. 23 172.
10 Havel, J. et al. (1955) 'The distribution and composition of ultracentrifugally separated lipoproteins in human serum', J. Clin. Invest. 34, 1345.
11 Burstein, M. et al. (1970) 'Rapid method for the isolation of lipoproteins from human serum by precipitation with polyanions', J. Lipid Res. 11, 583.

65

Multiple effects of LDL-apheresis against progression of atherosclerosis in patients with familial hypercholesterolemia

S. BERTOLINI, N. ELICIO, P. VIALE, F. NOBILI*, R. PIZZORNO, U. TORTOROLO, W. CAMPORA, C. ROTELLA, A. MARCENARO, G. RODRIGUEZ and R. BALESTRERI

*Atherosclerosis Prevention Centre, Department of Internal Medicine and *Institute of Neurophysiopathology, University of Genoa, Viale Benedetto XV, 6-16132 Genoa, Italy*

ABSTRACT. We studied some effects of two LDL-apheretic procedures, Cascade Filtration (CF) and Dextran-Sulfate Cellulose adsorption (DSC), in four patients with heterozygous Familial Hypercholesterolemia and severe coronary heart disease. We comfirmed the major efficacy and selectivity of DSC in comparison to CF and pointed out some changes which could contribute to the stabilization and regression of atherosclerosis in such patients; they include a reduction of LDL cholesterol to below the threshold levels of 150-100 mg/dl (combining LDL-apheresis with drug therapy), an improvement of the reverse cholesterol transport by HDL, a considerable reduction of the atherogenic and thrombogenic Lp(a), a decrease of fibrinogen and whole blood and plasma viscosity.

INTRODUCTION

Several different techniques have been developed for extracorporeal removal of Low Density Lipoproteins (LDL) from plasma in patients with Familial Hypercholesterolemia (FH), mainly homozygous patients or severe heterozygous low-responders to drug therapy. They include plasma exchange (Thompson 1987), affinity chromatography using heparin agarose gel (Lupien 1976), immunoadsorption by anti-LDL-antibody sepharose gel (Stoffel 1981), double membrane filtration (Homma 1986), heparin-induced LDL precipitation in low pH (HELP system) (Eisenhauer 1987) and Dextran-Sulfate Cellulose (DSC) adsorption (Homma 1986). Using these procedures alone or in combination with drugs a slowing of the progression or even a regression of atherosclerotic lesions have been documented (Thompson 1989, Oette 1989). The threshold levels of LDL cholesterol for stabilization and for regression of atherosclerosis seem to be below 150 and 100 mg/dl respectively (Oette 1989, Yamamoto 1989). The more recently developed techniques of LDL-apheresis, namely the adsorption on DCS columns and the HELP system, selectively remove LDL from plas ma and only sligtly affect High Density Lipoproteins (HDL). However, the beneficial effect of plasmapheresis does not seem limited to LDL removal.

In this paper we report our findings concerning two different methods of plasmapheresis used to treat four patients with heterozygous FH and severe coronary heart disease.

MATERIALS AND METHODS

Subjects and Procedures of LDL-apheresis. The clinical details of the four heterozygous FH patients are shown in Table 1.

TABLE 1. Clinical details of the four patients

Subject	age (years)	Plasma cholesterol (mg/dl) on diet	Medical history	LDL-apheresis
R.V.	41	500–600	MI,CABG,TIA	CF
A.E.	37	380–420	MI,CABG	CF,DSC
S.R.	44	420–480	MI,CABG,hemiparesis	CF,DSC
S.M.	62	420–470	MI,CABG	DSC

MI = myocardial infarction; CABG = coronary artery bypass graft; TIA = transitory ischemic attack.

Three patients were treated every 14 days for a year and a half with Cascade Filtration (CF) using Albusave filters BT 901 with an average pore size of 20nm (Dideco); two of the three and the fourth patient were more recently treated every 14 days with Liposorber system using Dextran-Sulfate Cellulose (DSC) adsorption columns LA-40 (Kaneka). During each procedure, lasting about 2h, 2-2.5 l of plasma were treated (flow rate: 18-20 ml/min).

Laboratory Methods. Plasma concentrations of total cholesterol (Tc), free cholesterol (Fc), HDL cholesterol (HDLc), triglycerides (Tg) were determined using enzymatic methods (Monotest Cholesterol High Performance, Test-Combination Free Cholesterol, Test-Combination Triglycerides Without Free Glycerol; Boehringer Mannheim GmbH); HDL cholesterol was determined using phosphotungstic acid and magnesium chloride as precipitating reagents, LDL cholesterol (LDLc) was calculated according to Friedewald (1972). Cholesteryl ester (cE) mass was calculated as (Tc - Fc) x 1.68. Plasma apolipoprotein AI and B levels were measured using immunoturbidimetric methods (Boehringer Mannheim GmbH) and Lp(a) lipoprotein by radioimmunoassay (Pharmacia). Serum lecithin:cholesterol acyltransferase (LCAT) activity was estimated according to Manabe et al (1987). The flotation rates of HDL subfractions were analyzed by rate-zonal density gradient ultracentrifugation in a Beckman SW41 Ti rotor (Franceschini 1985). Whole blood viscosity (WBV) was determined by the

rotational viscometer "Low-Shear 30" (Contraves, Zurich) at the shear rates of 0.471 sec^{-1} and 63.9 sec^{-1} in this order. Before each measurement, blood in the viscometer was sheared at 118.2 sec^{-1} for 30 sec. Plasma viscosity (PLV) was determined, after the blood sample had been centrifugated at 3000 rpm for 10 min at 37°C, at the shear rate of 18. 74 sec^{-1}. All the viscosity determinations were performed within 30 min of blood collection at 37°C by a thermostated water batch connected to the viscometer, according to ICSH guidelines (Report ICSH expert panel on blood rheology 1986). Plasma fibrinogen was measured by radial immunodiffusion (Nor Partigen, Behring Institute).
The statistical significance of differences between baseline and post-apheretic procedure for each parameter was evaluated using the t-test for paired data.

RESULTS AND COMMENTS
Table 2 reports the effect of CF in 2 patients (mean±SEM of 20 procedures) and the recovery of LDLc and apo B following the LDL-apheresis.

TABLE 2. Plasma concentration of LDL cholesterol and apoprotein B before and after CF (mean±SEM of 20 procedures; two patients)

	PRE-	POST-	after 24h	after 7d
LDLc (mg/dl)	336±19	199±14	214±14	315±17
(%)		- 41	- 36	- 6
apo B (mg/dl)	189±9	130±8		170±10
(%)		- 34		- 14

Seven days after LDLc recovered practically the pre-treatment level while apoprotein B remained significantly lower than its original level; this could mean that at this point LDL particles were enriched in cholesterol with respect to their protein content (LDLc/apo B ratio increased from 1.77 before CF to 1.85 after 7 days).
Comparing the effects of CF and DSC on plasma lipoprotein pattern (Table 3) it appears evident that DSC-apheresis removes atherogenic lipoproteins more effectively than CF and more selectively, because it affects the HDL system less (HDLc and apo AI decreased by 15% and 16% respectively after DSC and by 34% and 39% after CF).
During 14 different sessions of treatment (10 CF and 4 DSC) we measured HDLc and apo AI concentrations, free cholesterol content in plasma and in HDL and plasma LCAT avtivity. These measurements were performed before and at the end of LDL-apheresis, 24h after and 7 days after the procedure (Table 4). Moreover, we evaluated HDL subfraction distribution by rate-zonal ultracentrifugation (Fig. 1 and Table 5). After LDL-apheresis we observed an increase in the ratio between HDLc and apo AI

TABLE 3. Comparison between CF (22 procedures; three patients) and DSC (19 procedures; three patients); the values are mg/dl (mean±SD)

		PRE-	POST-	change (%)
LDLc	CF	373.7±60.1	225.5±44.4	- 39.6
	DSC	371.1±61.5	192.2±40.3	- 48.0
apo B	CF	219.4±33.7	140.7±28.8	- 35.7
	DSC	216.8±35.0	116.8±32.5	- 46.1
Tg	CF	100.0±28.8	58.4±20.8	- 41.6
	DSC	110.0±35.4	48.4±15.1	- 56.0
HDLc	CF	42.5±8.8	28.0±5.2	- 34.1
	DSC	40.6±6.7	34.5±5.5	- 15.0
apo AI	CF	135.2±23.7	82.8±17.4	- 38.7
	DSC	134.6+22.2	112.2+20.4	- 16.6

TABLE 4. HDL system before and after LDL-apheresis: mean±SEM of 14 treatments (10 CF and 4 DSC)

	PRE-	POST-	24h after	7d after
HDLc (mg/dl)	39.2±2.5	27.1±1.7§	32.4±1.3§	40.9±2.9
apo AI (mg/dl)	129.6±7.1	78.0±5.7§	86.8±4.7§	119.7±6.3*
HDLc/apo AI	0.300±0.01	0.360±0.01§	0.380±0.01§	0.340±0.01§
Fc/cE (plasma)	0.246±0.01	0.304±0.02*	0.319±0.02*	
Fc/cE (HDL)	0.211±0.01	0.254±0.01*	0.273±0.02*	
LCAT (nmol/ml/h)	538±46	300±38°	272±44*	559±23

°$P<0.05$, *$P<0.01$, §$P<0.001$

TABLE 5. Flotation rates of HDL subfractions before and after LDL-apheresis: mean±SEM of 14 treatments (10 CF and 4 DSC)

Elution volume	PRE-	POST-	24h after	7d after
Ve HDL3 (ml)	4.47±0.16	4.92±0.10°	5.42±0.13§	5.04±0.19°
Ve HDL2 (ml)	7.84±0.12	8.37±0.16°	8.67±0.22*	8.40±0.13*

°$P<0.05$, *$P<0.01$, §$P<0.001$

lasting at least seven days and an enrichment of free cholesterol in total plasma and in HDL. LCAT activity decreased after treatment but returned to baseline within 7 days. The elution profile of HDL subfractions in all patients changed at the end of apheresis and even more so 24h after because of the appearance of less dense, faster floating particles, as shown by the increase of the mean elution volume of both HDL3 and HDL2 subfractions. These changes were still evident (Table 5) after 7 days. All these findings taken together seem to suggest an im-

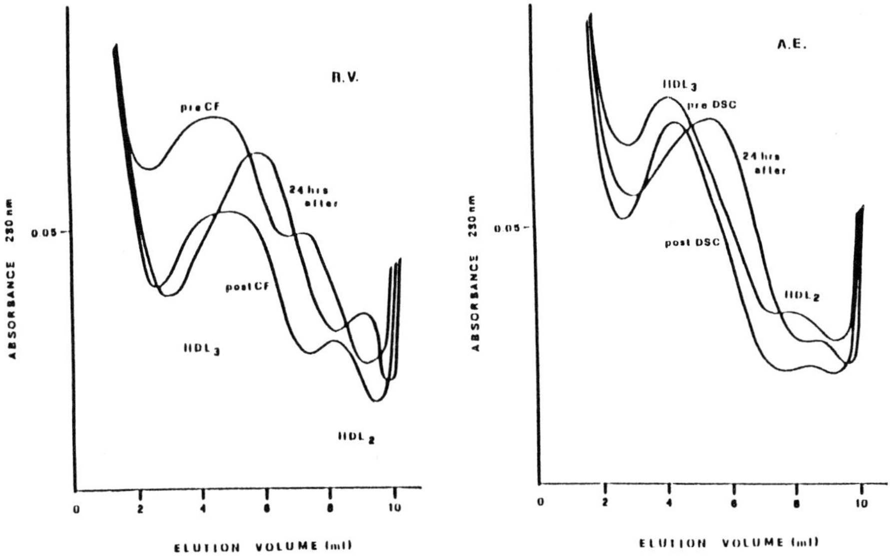

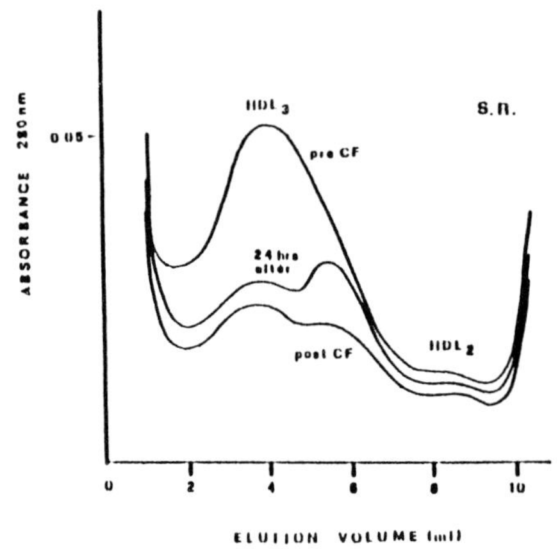

Figure 1. Elution profile of HDL subfractions before, at the end of LDL-apheresis and 24h after (patients R.V. and S.R.: CF; patient A.E.: DSC)

provement of reverse cholesterol transport by HDL following the removal of LDL.

Lp(a) has recently been found to be increased three-fold in patients with heterozygous FH (Utermann 1989); the mechanism which underlies this increase is still unclear. However, this lipoprotein, which contains apo B and apo (a) linked to each other by a disulphide-bridge, seems to be highly atherogenic because it interferes with the activation of plasminogen and so can lead to thrombogenesis (Scott 1989). Lp(a) is not affected by diet, and among the lipid-lowering drugs only combined nicotinic acid and neomycin treatment reduces its level (Scott 1989). Both CF and DSC-apheresis (Table 6) reduced to a large extent Lp(a) level in our FH subjects and this is another beneficial effect of these procedures against atherosclerosis progression in such patients.

TABLE 6. LDLc and Lp(a) concentrations before and after LDL-apheresis in the 4 patients treated with simvastatin 40 mg/day

Patient	LDL-apheresis	LDLc (mg/dl)	(%)	Lp(a) (mg/dl)	(%)
R.V.	n. 4 CF	315.0±18.0		28.3±3.6	
		188.0±11.0	- 40.3	15.4±3.8	- 45.6
S.N.	n. 2 DSC	322.5±14.8		8.1±0.6	
		162.5±14.8	- 49.6	3.6±0.3	- 55.5
S.R.	n. 2 DSC	214.0±8.5		94.5±3.0	
		101.5±2.1	- 52.6	38.8±1.5	- 58.9
A.E.	n. 3 DSC	238.0±16.7		64.5±4.4	
		99.5+2.7	- 58.2	31.8+5.9	- 50.7

Moreover, LDL-apheresis significantly lowered whole blood viscosity at the shear rate of 0.471 sec^{-1}, plasma viscosity and fibrinogen (Table 7) in our patients. The reduction of plasma viscosity may be the consequence of the decrease of both fibrinogen and cholesterol. While it is well known that fibrinogen is a major determinant of plasma viscosity, there is also increasing evidence that cholesterol itself (which is significantly reduced by LDL-apheresis) may be relevant in determining plasma viscosity (Schuff-Werner 1989).

TABLE 7. Change in fibrinogen, in whole blood viscosity and in plasma viscosity after DSC-apheresis

	PRE-	POST-	paired t-test
Hematocrit (%)	39.7±2.1	40.5±1.9	
Fibrinogen (mg/dl)	343±74	251±72	$P<0.05$
WBV (0.471 sec^{-1}; mPa/sec)	26.7±4.1	21.8±3.5	$P<0.01$
WBV (63.9 sec^{-1}; mPa/sec)	4.78±0.38	4.67±0.25	
PLV (18.74 sec^{-1}; mPa/sec)	1.52±0.07	1.36±0.11	$P<0.05$

The viscosity values are reported as the "peak" of the viscometric curve.

The reduction of low shear WBV is likely to depend mainly on fibrinogen decrease, through the reduction of erythrocyte aggregation which greatly influences low shear WBV; however, cholesterol level too seems to contribute in determining low shear WBV (Montefusco 1989). A decrease of high shear WBV had already been reported one and seven days after DSC (Montefusco 1989) and it was ascribed to the cholesterol reduction which improves erythrocyte deformability. In our study we did not find any change in high shear WBV; this was probably because the measurements were performed just after the end of the apheretic procedure. In conclusion several effects of LDL-apheresis may contribute to stabilization and regression of atherosclerotic lesions in FH patients. They include the reduction of LDLc and apo B to below the threshold levels required, the improvement of the reverse cholesterol transport by HDL, the reduction of the atherogenic and thrombogenic lipoprotein (a) and some hemorrheological changes which improve blood flow to the tissues.

REFERENCES

- Eisenhauer, T.; Armstrong, V.W.; Wieland, H.; Fuchs, C.; Scheler, F.; Seidel, D. (1987). 'Selective removal of low density lipoproteins (LDL) by precipitation at low pH: first clinical application of the HELP system',Klin Wochenschr 65, 161-168.
- Franceschini, G.; Tosi, C.; Moreno, Y.; Sirtori, C.R. (1985). 'Effects of storage on the distribution of high density lipoprotein subfraction in human sera', J Lipid Res 26, 1368-1373.
- Friedewald, W.T.; Levy, R.I.; Fredrickson, D.S. (1972). 'Estimation of the concentration of low density lipoprotein cholesterol in plasma without use of the preparative ultracentrifuge', Clin Chem 18, 499-502.
- Homma, Y.; Mikami, Y.; Tamachi, H.; Nakaya, N.; Nakamura, H.; Araki, G.; Goto, Y. (1986). 'Comparison of selectivity of LDL removal by Double Filtration and Dextran-Sulfate Cellulose column Plasmapheresis', Atherosclerosis 60, 23-27.
- Lupien, P.J.; Moorjani, S.; Awad, J. (1976). 'A new approach to the management of familial hypercholesterolemia: removal of plasma cholesterol based on the principle of affinity chromatography', Lancet i, 1261-1263.
- Manabe, M.; Abe, T.; Nozawa, M.; Maki, A.; Hirata, M.; Hakura, H. (1987). 'New substrate for determination of serum lecithin:cholesterol acyltransferase', J Lipid Res 28, 1206-1215.
- Montefusco, S.; Gnasso, A.; Scarpato, N.; Rubba, P.; Nappi, G.; Cortese, C.; Pandolfi, G.; Postiglione, A. (1989). 'Hemorheological effects of LDL-apheresis in familial hypercholesterolemia', Clin Hemorheol 9, 81-87.
- Oette, K.; Borberg, H. (1989). 'LDL apheresis by immunoadsorption' in G. Crepaldi et al (Eds.), Atherosclerosis VIII, Excerpta Medica, Amsterdam, pp. 819-822.
- Report ICSH expert panel on blood rheology (1986). 'Guidelines for measurement of blood viscosity and erythrocyte deformability', Clin Hemorheol 6, 439-453.
- Schuff-Werner, P.; Schutz, E.; Seidel, D. (1989). 'LDL-cholesterol, an understimated determinant of plasma viscosity?', Clin Hemorheol 9,

525.
- Scott, J. (1989). 'Lipoprotein(a). Thrombogenesis linked to atherogenesis at last?', Nature 341, 22-23.
- Stoffel, W.; Borberg, H.; Greve, V. (1981). 'Application of specific extracorporeal removal of low density lipoprotein in familial hypercholesterolemia', Lancet ii, 1005-1008.
- Thompson, G.R.; Lowenthal, R.; Myant, N.B. (1975). 'Plasma exchange in the management of familial hypercholesterolemia', Lancet i, 1208-1211.
- Thompson, G.R.; Barbir, M.; Michishita, I.; Larkin, S. (1989). 'Comparison of plasma exchange and LDL apheresis in the treatment of Hypercholesterolemia' in G. Crepaldi et al (Eds.), Atherosclerosis VIII, Excerpta Medica, Amsterdam, pp. 815-818.
- Utermann, G.; Hoppichler, F.; Dieplinger, H.; Seed, M.; Thompson, G.; Boerwinkle, E. (1989). 'Defects in the low density lipoprotein receptor gene affect lipoprotein(a) levels: multiplicative interaction of two gene loci associated with premature atherosclerosis', Proc Natl Acad Sci USA 86, 4171-4174.
- Yamamoto, A. (1989). 'LDL-apheresis: what we expect and what can be achieved' in G. Crepaldi et al (Eds.), Atherosclerosis VIII, Excerpta Medica, Amsterdam, pp. 843-844.

66
Long-term LDL apheresis in FH

A. MINARDI, P. ZUCCHELLI*, S. NUCCI*, G. SERMASI*, F.M. PICCHIO, M. BONVICINI**, G. BAROZZI, A. GADDI, Z. SANGIORGI and G.C. DESCOVICH**

*Department of Geriatrics, University of Bologna; *Immunohematology and Tranfusional Centre, S. Orsolo Hospital; **Department of Cardiology, University of Bologna, via Massarenti 9, 40138 Bologna, Italy*

The LDL-apheresis method permits a more adequate treatment of many cases of Familial Hypercholesterolemia (FH), previously resistant or poor responders to conventional hypolipemic diet and drug treatment.

With less selective methods [1-2] it is already possible to obtain a better control of plasma lipids, a reduction in lipid deposits and an improvement in cardiac symptoms [3-7].

Recent studies based on the LDL-apheresis technique confirm these encouraging results from a clinical and prognostic point of view [8-10].

There are therefore many ethical-scientific reasons in favour of this treatment for homozygous FH and severe forms of heterozygous FH with high LDL-cholesterol levels and/or the presence of advanced and rapidly progressing atheromatous lesions, requiring a more aggressive treatment to prevent further spreading of the vascular lesions.

One of the main problems with apheresis is the definition of a precise working protocol which can guarantee over time the effective stabilization (if not the regression) of atherosclerosis.

For this purpose many studies on LDL-apheresis have considered the value $\Delta/2$ ((post TC + pre TC)/2) as the mean cholesterolemia measurement between one treatment and the next. Even if this can be useful for simplifying treatment of the patient, to arrive at a non-empirical conclusion it is necessary to know: 1) the maximum threshold below which plasma LDL cholesterol should be kept to achieve stabilization or potential regression of atherosclerosis; 2) the mathematical parameter which best describes the mean cholesterolemia value and/or the (f)t function during apheretic treatment.

The aim of this study is to make a critical assessment of the variation in the value which may be attributed to the cholesterolemia trend during apheresis according to the parameter or function adopted.

Patients and Methods

An analysis is made of the results of two patients treated for two years, from our series of FH subjects submitted to LDL-apheresis (Tab.1).

Table 1: PATIENTS UNDER LDL-APHERESIS TREATMENT IN JULY 1989

PATIENT	AGE	SEX	DIAGNOSIS	ANGINA	A.M.I.	CHD*	BY-PASS	PERIOD OF TREAT.	METHOD
B.N.	59	M	HET.F.H.	+	+	+	+	2 YEARS	A
F.G	11	M	HOM.F.H.	-	-	+	-	~2 YEARS	B
P.F.	53	M	HET.F.H.	-	+	+	+	>6 MONTHS	A
P.I.	43	F	HOM.F.H.	+	±	+	+	<3 MONTHS	B
L.R.	39	M	HET.F.H.	-	-	-	-	>6 MONTHS	A
G.S.	54	F	HET.F.H.	+	+	+	+	<3 MONTHS	A
S.L.	47	M	HET.F.H.	-	+	+	+	<6 MONTHS	A

* diagnosed with treadmill exercise testing and/or myocardial scintigraphy and/or dynamic ECG according to Holter and/or coronary angiogram.

1) F.G. male, born on 3.23.1978, homozygous FH, was treated each month with selective removal of LDL (method B) starting in December 1987.

The family tree over the last six generations shows a clear vertical transmission of the gene (fig.1). Without treatment the father had cholesterolemia levels of between 320 and 380 mg/dl, the mother 400 and 480 mg/dl.

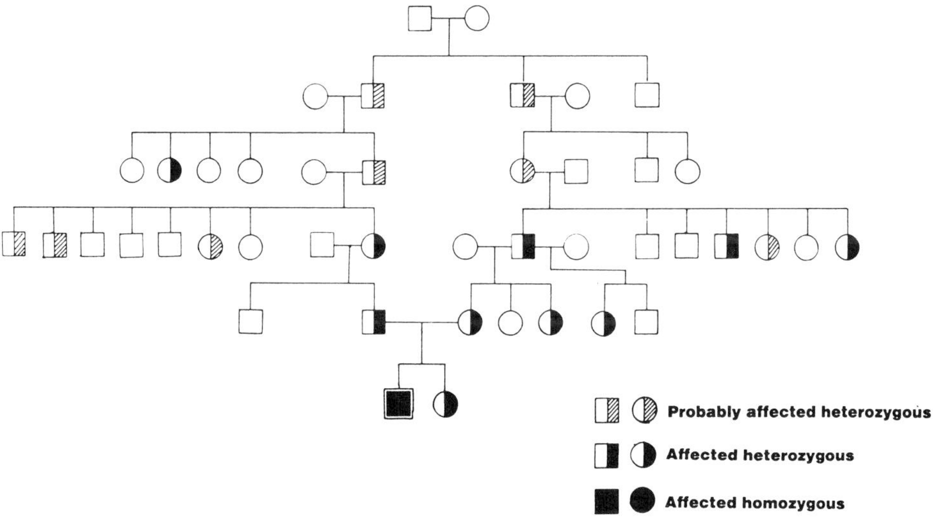

Fig.1: F.G. (male, 11 years old) homozygous F.H. Simplified pedigree of the family.

The LDL receptor activity measured on skin fibroblasts, was 5% in the propositus, 50% in the father and 25% in the mother.

Clinical examination revealed xanthelasmas, which appeared at an early age, corneal arch and cutaneous-tendon xanthomata at the phalangeal, elbow and knee joints, on the dorsal surface of the foot and in the gluteal region.

From a cardiovascular point of view the patient was asymptomatic and a myocardial scintigraphy at rest was negative. A first coronary arteriography, performed a few days before LDL-apheresis treatment began, showed: complete obstruction of the common trunk of the left coronary restored by a collateral vascular bed supported by the right coronary which revealed slight parietal ectases, as well as a stenosis at the beginning of the lower branch (fig.4).

Previous dietary and pharmacological treatment performed elsewhere between 1982 and 1987 had had little effect on the lipid pattern. During this period Total Plasma Cholesterol (TC) varied between 700 and 1100 mg/dl (LDL-C 650-1000 mg/dl, Apo B 350-500 mg/dl, HDL-C unmeasurable-15 mg/dl, Apo A1 20-50 mg/dl, VLDL-C 5-10 mg/dl, VLDL-TG 10-12 mg/dl) in the absence of other documented lipoprotein or apoprotein abnormalities.

In 1987, the association of a diet (replacing animal proteins with textured and delipidated soya proteins) with drugs (cholestyramine 20 mg/day; gemfibrozil 1.2 g/day) proved to be partially effective, lowering cholesterol to 647-520 mg/dl. This diet-drug treatment was maintained throughout the apheresis treatment.

2) B.N. male, born on 6.17.1930, heterozygous FH, was treated each month with LDL-apheresis (method A) starting in July 1987.

This patient (previous myocardial infarction, aorto-coronary and carotid by-pass) responded poorly to soya dietary protein plus cholestyramine and fenofibrate (TC between 400 and 450 mg/dl). Between all apheresis treatments the therapy used was: Simvastatine 40 mg/day.

Treatment of LDL-apheresis was carried out using dextran sulphate cellulose adsorption columns: Liposorber LA-40 (400 ml) and LA.15 (150 ml) (Kanegafuki).

Method A. The LA-40 column can be installed on an extracorporeal circulation machine using both plasma filtration and centrifugation for plasma separation.

In our study the LA-40 column was fitted on a blood-centrifuging continuous flow cell separator (DIDECO-VIVA). In this case the anticoagulant used was ACD-A (sodium citrate 2 H_2O 2.2 g; citric acid H_2O 0.80 g; anydrous glucose 2.25 g; distilled H_2O q.s. for 100 ml), which is mixed with the blood immediately after the sampling needle, before entering the cell separator, in a ratio varying from 1:8 to 1:16.

To prevent any reaction from the citrate, the patient is reinfused with slow drops during the procedure, for the entire apheresis period, with 5 vials of 10% Ca^{++} gluconate. The quantity of plasma to be treated depends on the initial TC level and the level to be obtained, considering that the column absorbs up to 7 g of cholesterol.

Method B. The LA-15 column is used with the MA-01 machine (Kanegafuki). Since it is automatically regenerable, this particular column permits the treatment of much larger quantities of plasma and is proposed for: 1) those patients of minute build or with a seriously damaged heart, to avoid hypovolemic reactions following an excessive volume of extracorporeal blood; 2) for those patients with cholesterol levels that are so high that they cannot be adequately treated with the LA-40 column. Polysulphone hollow fiber filter (Sulflux FS-05 Kanegafuki), with an average pore size of 0.2 m and an effective surface area of 0.2m^2, was used to separate plasma from the cellular components of the blood. Plasma and LDL separators, as well as all the tubes, were disposable.

Results

LDL-apheresis, using KANEKA MA-01 equipment proved to be highly effective and selective (absence of noticeable changes in other plasma lipid and protein fractions, except for some decrease in triglycerides due to partial VLDL removal) and was well tolerated. No significant changes in plasma albumine or blood cell counts were found.

After each treatment lipids were tested frequently to calculate cholesterol curves between one apheresis treatment and the next.

Fig.2 describes the cholesterolemia trend in the patient F.G. over the period 1985-1989.

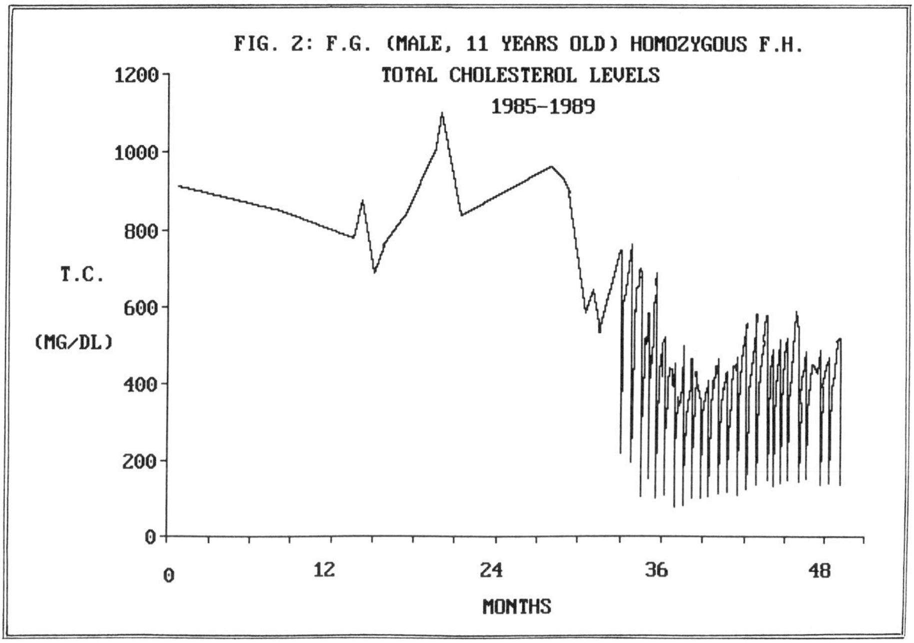

FIG. 2: F.G. (MALE, 11 YEARS OLD) HOMOZYGOUS F.H.
TOTAL CHOLESTEROL LEVELS
1985-1989

Fig.3 gives a more detailed analysis of the cholesterolemia trend in the same patient during the period in which he underwent LDL-apheresis treatment.

It can be observed that the first apheresis sessions were marked by a more rapid return of cholesterolemia to the starting levels; subsequently there was a certain slowing down (apheresis 5-12), reaching a plateau stage on the 7-10 day after apheresis; an alternating trend was then observed with negative stages (apheresis 14-16) followed by more favourable trends (apheresis 21-23).

After 14 months of apheresis treatment, a new coronary arteriography demonstrated that the atheromatous process had not progressed, with some signs which might indicate a reduction in the atheromatous plaque (fig.4).

FIG. 3: F.G. (MALE, 11 YEARS OLD) HOMOZYGOUS F.H.

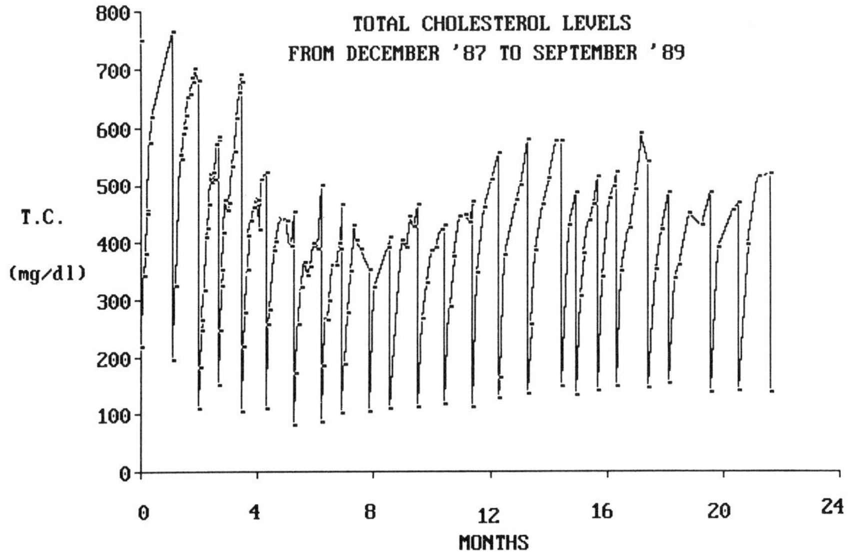

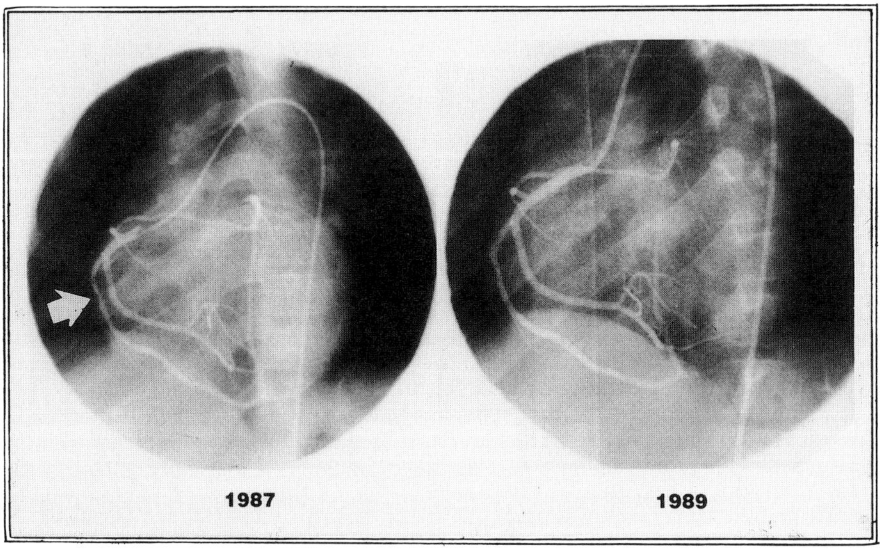

Fig.4: Coronary angiograms in F.G. (male, 11 years old) FH. Homozygous, before and after 14 months of LDL-apheresis treatment. Complete obstruction of the left common coronary trunk can be seen restored by a collateral vascular bed supported by the right coronary. The latter at the 1987 check-up showed slight parietal ectases, as well as stenosis (->) at the beginning of the lower branch which seemed to have disappeared in the 1989 angiogram.

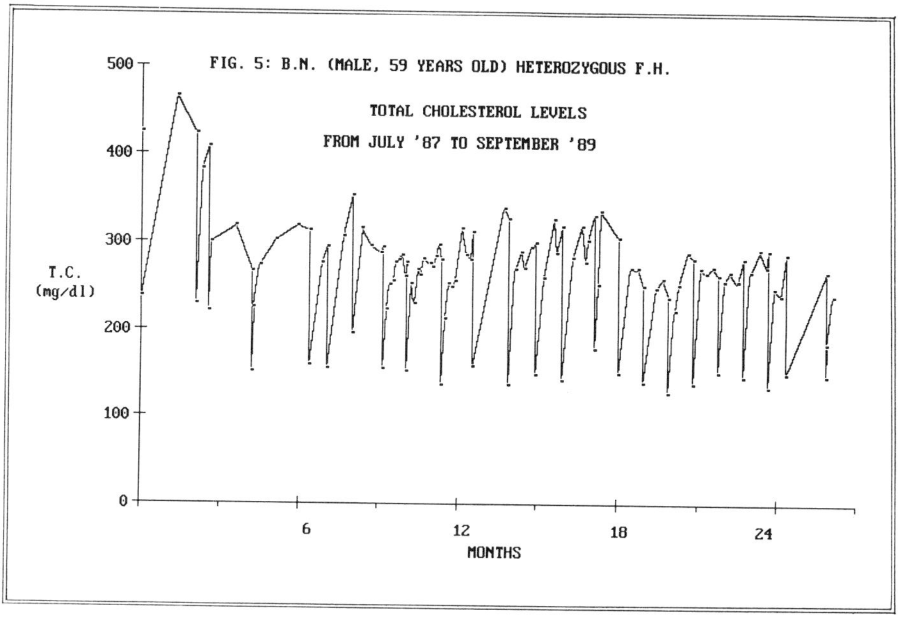

FIG. 5: B.N. (MALE, 59 YEARS OLD) HETEROZYGOUS F.H.
TOTAL CHOLESTEROL LEVELS
FROM JULY '87 TO SEPTEMBER '89

Fig.5 illustrates the cholesterolemia trend in the patient B.N. during LDL-apheresis treatment. Here again a negative trend in the first two treatments can be seen, with a fair homogeneity in subsequent sessions.

The patient in question clinically demonstrated a clear subjective improvement in the symptoms of stress angina after only 5-6 treatments.

The need to compare the rise in the post-apheresis curves in the individual patient and between the various patients derives from logical-ethical requirements. In fact the rhythm of apheresis treatment depends directly on the pattern of cholesterolemia increase obtained following dietary measures and different drug treatments; in particular the effect of the drugs in the steady-state must be studied and the effect of interactions as the result of the use of several drugs.

To this end, it is important to define which parameter or function is able to meet the mean cholesterolemia value during apheresis with the greatest precision.

Fig.6 gives an example of the mean cholesterolemia trend estimated according to two different parameters: a) the weighted average of several intermediate measurements multiplied by the time, b) the delta between post-apheresis cholesterol and the subsequent treatment pre-apheresis cholesterol.

A consistent divergence can be seen, with a tendency towards underestimation on the part of curve B.

On the other hand, it is clear that curve A, although empirically more expressive than the real mean (due to the larger number of points considered) cannot be considered other than a rough index.

FIG. 6: F.G. (MALE, 11 YEARS OLD) HOMOZYGOUS F.H.
MEAN PLASMA TOTAL CHOLESTEROL
WITH DIFFERENT INDEXES

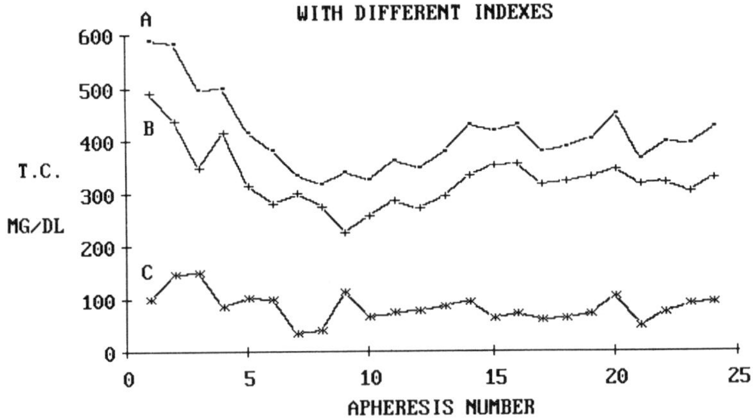

A) WEIGHTED MEAN OF SEVERAL INTERMEDIATE MEASUREMENTS MULTIPLIED BY THE TIME
B) DELTA OF PRE AND POST APHERESIS CHOLESTEROL
C) DIFFERENCE BETWEEN A AND B

Conclusions

It is known that LDL-apheresis is the only technique which can lower plasma cholesterol to the desired level, since the immediate lowering of LDL cholesterol depends merely on the volume of plasma passed through the LDL-apheresis device.

The rapid rebound of cholesterol after treatment does, however, represent a serious problem.

The efficacy of treatment will be guaranteed by maintaining cholesterolemia at a mean level which is able to inhibit the development of atherosclerosis.

It is therefore quite important to define the largest intervals possible between apheresis treatments within an effective margin, after establishing the dietary and drug therapy most suitable for slowing down the increase in cholesterolemia after treatment.

Here there is also the problem of treatment costs (so that the method can be made available to the high number of patients for whom it is indicated).

Thus it is necessary to study the rise in the cholesterol curve after apheresis with frequent intermediate samples, in an attempt to gauge the weight of the individual variables on which it is possible to intervene.

In our opinion this should be done even if it increases the difficulties and willingness of the patient to collaborate with the method.

In this way it will also be possible to assess with greater accuracy the importance of other variables, 1) interindividual (increase as compared to receptor activity) and 2) intraindividual (total cholesterol pool in the organism; variation in the speed of cholesterol synthesis).

At the same time it is necessary to study which parameter or mathematical function best describes the mean cholesterol value in the intervening period between one apheresis treatment and the next, also considering that the Δ/2 ((post-TC + pre-TC)/2) does not seem to been a sufficiently indicative value.

References

1. Thompson, G.R., Lowenthal, R. and Myant, M.B. (1975) 'Plasma exchange in the management of homozygous familial hypercholesterolemia', Lancet, *i*, 1208-1211.
2. Lupien, P.J., Moorjani, S. and Awad, J. (1976) 'A new approach to the management of familial hypercholesterolemia: removal of plasma cholesterol based on the principle of affinity chromatography', Lancet, *i*, 1261-1265.
3. Stoffel, W, Borberg, H. and Greve, V. (1981) 'Application of specific extracorporeal removal of low density lipoprotein in familial hypercholesterolemia', Lancet, *ii*, 1005-7.
4. Thompson, G.R., Miller, J.P. and Breslow, J.L. (1985) 'Improved survival of patients with homozygous familial hypercholesterolemia treated with plasma exchange', Br. Med. J., 291, 1671-1673.
5. Berger, G.M.B., Miller, J.L.,Bonnici, F. and Dubovsky, D.W. (1978) 'Continuous flow plasma exchange in the treatment of homozygous familial hypercholesterolemia', Am. J. Med., 65-243.
6. Saal, S.D., Parker, T.S., Gordon, B.R., Studebaker, J., Hudgins, L., Arthens, E.H. Jr and Rubin, A.L. (1986) 'Removal of low density lipoproteins in patients by extracorporeal immunoadsorption', Am. J. Med., 80-583.
7. Mabuchi, H., Michishita, I., Sakai, T., Sakai, Y., Watanabe, A., Wakasugi, T. and Takeda, R. (1986) 'Treatment of homozygous patients with familial hypercholesterolemia by double-filtration plasmapheresis', Atherosclerosis, 61, 135-140.
8 Saito, Y., Shinomiya, M., Shirai, K. and Yoshida, S. (1988) 'Treatment of severe hypercholesterolemia by LDL-apheresis: cholesterol-lowering effect and clinical evaluation', in Gotto, A.M. Jr., Mancini, M., and Scarpato, N. 'Treatment of severe hypercholesterolemia in the prevention of coronary heart disease', Karger, Basel, vol. 23, 160-171.
9. Shuff-Werner, P., Armstrong, V.W., Eisenhauer, Th., Thiery, J. and Seidel, D. (1988) 'Treatment of severe hypercholesterolemia by heparin-induced extracorporeal LDL precipitation (HELP)'in Gotto, A.M. Jr., Mancini, M., and Scarpato, N. 'Treatment of severe hypercholesterolemia in the prevention of coronary heart disease', Karger, Basel, vol. 23, 118-126.
10. Thompson, G., Barbir, M., Michishita, I. and Larkin, S. (1989) 'Comparison of plasma exchange and LDL apheresis in the treatment of hypercholesterolaemia' in Crepaldi, G. et al, 'Atherosclerosis VIII', Excerpta Medica, Amsterdam - New York - Oxford, 815-821.

67

Long-term double filtration LDL-apheresis in familial hypercholesterolemia

F. PINTUS, P. MASCIA, E. GANGA, A. BARRACCA*, V. SAU, P. ALTIERI* and S. MUNTONI

*Centro Regionale per le Malattie Dismetaboliche e l'Arteriosclerosi; *Divisione de Nefrologia e Dialisi, Ospedale Brotzu, via Peretti, 09134 Cagliari, Italy*

ABSTRACT.

Direct removal of LDL from plasma by plasmapheresis is an available method of treatment in FH homozygous patients and in the FH heterozygotes resistant to drug therapy.
Double filtration (DF) permits the removal of plasma components with molecular weight greater than about 300 kd.
We report the results of DF long-term therapy in 3 FH patients:one man (G.D.),aged 40 yr,and two women (C.S. and L.M.) aged 23 yr.All three had positive pedigree for FH,xanthomatosis since the age of 10,mean plasma total cholesterol levels ranging from 600 to 750 mg/dl.
DF was repeated every two weeks,and the total amount of plasma treated by each procedure was 3 litres.
DF causes a remarkable decrease in plasma total cholesterol (-53%),LDL-cholesterol (-55%),triglycerides (-54%) and HDL-cholesterol (-40%).
During the DF therapy a progressive reduction of Achilles tendon thickness and of tuberous xanthomata volume was recorded.
No significant side effects have been observed.

INTRODUCTION.

Liver transplantation (1) and direct removal of LDL from plasma by plasmapheresis (2) are the only available treatments in Familial Hypercholesterolemic (FH) homozygous patients,and in the FH heterozygotes resistant to drug therapy.
Different attempts have been made to remove cholesterol and LDL directly from the plasma of such patients.Among them there are plasma exchange (3),LDL immunoapheresis (4),double filtration LDL apheresis (DF) (5), heparin induced extracorporal LDL precipitation (6),dextran sulphate callulose column plasmapheresis (7).

SUBJECTS AND METHODS.

Here we report the results of long-term DF therapy in three FH patients: one man (G.D.), aged 40 yr, who has been suffering from angina since the age of 29, had a myocardial infarction in 1980 when he was 31 yr old; in 1989 he underwent coronary bypass operation. Two women (C.S. and L.M.) aged 23 yr, both free from overt symptoms of Coronary artery disease. All three had positive pedigree for FH, xanthomatosis since the age of 10, and mean total plasma cholesterol levels ranging from 600 and 750 mg/dl.

In the two women LDL-receptor activity, studied by the cultured skin fibroblast method, resulted less than 2% of normal; while in G.D. this has not been determined yet. The LDL-receptor activity was also virtually absent in a brother of C.S. and in a brother of L.M.

In all patients an arteriovenous shunt was constructed between the radial artery and the cephalic vein before the beginning of apheresis therapy.

DF was performed by two different filters. Hollow-fiber membrane filter, with an average pore size of 0.2μm and an effective surface area of 0.6 m^2, was used as plasma separator. The second filter for double-membrane filtration was hollow-fiber membrane filter of cellulose diacetate with an average pore size of 0.03μm and an effective surface area of 2.0 m^2. Blood was withdrawn at a rate of 100 ml/min by using a peristaltic pump from the arteriovenous fistula; plasma was separated through the filter at a rate of 30 ml/min by using a peristaltic pump and was then passed through the second filter. The filtrate was then infused into the patient with the cell-rich portion of the blood tha remained unfiltered by the first filter.

The DF procedure was repeated every two weeks, and the total amount of plasma treated by each procedure was about three litres. Each procedure lasted about 2½ hours.

G.D, C.S. and L.M. are being treated for 24, 14 and 12 months respectivily.

RESULTS.

The efficiency of the second membrane filter in trapping plasma components depends on its molecular weight. The decay of concentration of the component is also an exponential function of the plasma volume passing through the second filter (8).

As expected, DF causes a remarkable decrease in total cholesterol (TC), in LDL-cholesterol (LDL-C) and triglycerides (TG); it also causes a decrease in HDL-cholesterol (HDL-C), which, however, reaches pre apheresis levels in about 5 days (Table 1).

TABLE 1.Mean decrease (%) in serum lipid levels after double filtration

TC	LDL-C	HDL-C	TG
53	55	40	54

During long-term treatment,mean TC values range from about 550 mg/dl before,to 100 mg/dl after each apheresis.
The DF procedure also causes a reduction in immunoglobulins,C3,C4 and fibrinogen.IgA and IgG decreased by 28% to 44%,IgM and fibrinogen by 50% to 65%,C3 by 35% to 56% and C4 by 38% to 49%.We also found a decrease in albumin (-24%),and an increase in white blood cells (120-200%).
As the fibrinogen level plays an important part in the development of stroke and myocardial infarction,decreased fibrinogen levels may play an important role in preventing some complications of atherosclerosis (9).
Duting DF therapy a progressive reduction of tendon thickness and tuberous xanthomata volume was recorded.In particular we periodically measured the Achilles tendon thickness by ultrasonography,using the same landmarks,and,after one year of DF treatment,we found a reduction in the anteroposterior diameter of 27% in G.D. and of 38% in L.M. and C.S. (Table 2).

TABLE 2.Reduction in anteroposterior diameter of Achilles tendon after 1 year of double filtration therapy

	Men	Women
before	17 mm	16 mm
after	13 mm	9 mm
difference	27 %	38 %

No significant side effects have been observed.
In spite of the low selectivity in removing LDL-C,we conclude that DF is an effective and safe method of treatment for FH patients.

REFERENCES.

1) Starzl T.E.,Bilheimer D.W.,Bahnson H.T.,Shaw Jr B.W.,Hardesty R.L., Griffith B.P.,Iwatsuki S.,Zitelli B.J.,Gartner Jr J.C.,Halatack J.J.,

Urbach A.H. (1984) 'Heart-liver transplantation in a patient with familial hypercholesterolemia.'Lancet,i,1382-86.
2) Klinkmann H.,Behm E.,Ivanovich P. (1989) 'Removal of low density lipoproteins (LDL) from plasma:the state of the art.'The Int.J.of Artif. Org.,12,207-10.
3) Thompson G.R.,Miller J.P.,Breslow J.L. (1985) 'Improved survival of patients with homozygous familial hypercholesterolemia treated with plama exchange.'Brit.Med.J.,291,1671-3.
4) Stoffel W.,Bode C. (1984) 'Selective removal of low density lipoproteins.'In Pineda A.A. (ed.),Selective plasma component removal.Mount Kisko,New York,pp.1-22.
5) Agishi T. (1987) 'Double filtration plasmapheresis.'In Bambauer R., Malchesky P.S.,Folkenhagen D. (eds.),Therapeutic plasma exchange and selective plasma separation,Schattauer,Stuttgart,New York,pp.345-54.
6) Eisenhauer T.,Armstrong V.W.,Wieland H.,Fuchs C.,Scheler F.,Seidel P. (1987) 'Selective removal of low density lipoproteins (LDL) by precipitation at the low pH:first clinical application of the HELP system. Klin.Wschr.,65,161-8.
7) Odaka M.,Kobayashi H.,Soeda K. et al. (1987) 'Long term results of LDL selective plasma adsorption therapy on familial hypercholesterolemia.'Biomat.Art.Cells Art.Organs,15,113-24.
8) Yokoama S.,Hayashi R.,Satani M.,Yamamoto A. (1985) 'Selective removal of low density lipoproteins by plasmapheresis in familial hypercholesterolemia.'Arteriosclerosis,5,613-22.
9) Kannel W.B.,Wolf P.A.,Castelli W.P.,D'Agostino R.B. (1987) 'Fibrinogen and risk of cardiovascular death.'J.A.M.A.,258,1183-87.

STANDARDIZATION OF APOPROTEIN MEASUREMENT IN BLOOD

68
Apolipoprotein profile of a sample of Italian population. Correlations with coronary risk factors

A. CAPURSO, M. DI TOMMASO, A.M. MOGAVERO, F. RESTA, S. PALMISANO, D. CIANCIA, R. TAVERNITI and G. ANGELINI

Chair of Geriatrics, Institute of Clinical Medicine, University of Bari Medical School, Policlinico, 70124 Bari, Italy

ABSTRACT. Serum apolipoproteins (apo) A-I, A-II, B, C-II, C-III and E have been evaluated by R.I.D. in a population sample of nine italian cities, for a total of 490 males and 530 females, aged 20 to 60. The correlations among apolipoproteins and between apolipoproteins and some coronary risk factors (age, body mass index, blood pressure, glycemia, total cholesterol, HDL-cholesterol, triglycerides, smoke) have been calculated. In males, apo B was significantly correlated with age, blood mean pressure, total cholesterol, apo A-II and apo C-III. Apo A-I was significantly correlated only with apo A-II. Apo C-III was correlated also with apo E. In females, apo B was inversely correlated with body mass index and positively correlated with age and apo A-II. Moreover, apo C-II was correlated with apo C-III and apo E.

INTRODUCTION

Serum apolipoproteins (apo) have recently become matter of interest for diagnosis of coronary risk factors. Numerous studies have demonstrated that the measurement of serum apo A-I and apo B, in addition to the traditional serum lipid and lipoprotein parameters, may considerably improve the evaluation of coronary heart disease risk (Sniderman et al. (1980), De Backer et al. (1982), Noma et al. (1983), Kottke et al.(1986).

The present study was undertaken to know the mean values of serum apolipoproteins A-I, A-II, B, C-II, C-III and E in a sample of the italian population and to evaluate the correlation among apolipoproteins and between apolipoproteins and potential coronary risk factors i.e. age, sex, body mass index, blood mean pressure, blood glucose, serum cholesterol, HDL-cholesterol, serum triglycerides, cigarette smoking.

MATERIAL AND METHODS

The study population consisted of 1020 subjects (490 males and 530 females) who were randomly selected in the normal population. This study was part of a wider research programme promoted by the Italian "Consiglio Nazionale delle Ricerche - Progetto Finalizzato Medicina Preventiva - Aterosclerosi", to evaluate frequency and distribution of coronary risk factors in the italian population (The Nine Communities Study, Research Group ATS-OB43 (1987).

The population of nine italian cities (Padova, Pavia, Bologna, Siena, Roma, Napoli, Palermo, Cagliari and Venezia) was involved in this study. 1200 subjects of each city, for a total of 10.800 persons, were randomly selected from electoral lists and enrolled for the screening of the major coronary risk factors, i.e. systolic and diastolic blood pressure, fasting blood glucose, total cholesterol, HDL-cholesterol, triglycerides, heart rate, body mass index, physical activity at work, physical activity at leisure, stress at work, smoking (Research Group ATS-OB43 (1987). From each list of 1200 subjects a subset of 300 individuals was identified with random numbers and allocated in the present apoprotein study. Only 1020 subjects of the 2700 eligible individuals contacted for recruitment agreed to be enrolled.

Serum samples for apoprotein determinations were frozen at - 80 C until the day of processing. Serum apoproteins were assayed by radial immuno diffusion (R.I.D.) using polyclonal specific antibodies elsewhere described (Capurso et al., 1988). Anti apo E serum was prepared in our laboratory boostering rabbits with purified human apo E obtained by fractionation of apo-VLDL in preparative 21%-polyacrylamide gel electrophoresis with SDS, according to Neville (1971), modified. The specificity of antibodies was determined by electroimmunoblotting as elsewhere described (Capurso et al., 1988). The intra-assay coefficient of variation for all apoproteins was within 9%. The apoprotein reference standards for R.I.D. were those described elsewhere (Capurso et al., 1988).

The linear regression has been calculated between single variables, with each apoprotein serving in turns as dependent variable. The level of significance (p-value) has been calculated for single correlation coefficient.

RESULTS

The age standardized apoprotein mean values are reported in Table 1.

Univariate analysis of serum apoproteins are shown in Table 2. Single apoproteins are related to other apoproteins and to non-apoprotein variables described elsewhere (Research Group ATS-OB43 (1987).

TABLE 1. Age standardized mean values of serum apolipoproteins of the nine communities pool. The values are expressed in mg/dl

	Mean total	Males	Females	p (M/F)
Apo A-I	134 ± 16	132 ± 16	136 ± 17	< 0.001
Apo A-II	39.0 ± 7.6	37.8 ± 7.1	40.2 ± 7.7	< 0.001
Apo B	86.1 ± 14	88.9 ± 14	83.3 ± 13	< 0.001
Apo C-II	3.62 ± 0.7	3.75 ± 0.8	3.50 ± 0.7	< 0.001
Apo C-III	10.9 ± 2.2	11.1 ± 2.4	10.6 ± 2.0	< 0.001
Apo E	5.5 ± 1.2	5.5 ± 1.3	5.4 ± 1.6	N.S.
Apo B/Apo A-I	0.64	0.67	0.61	N.S.

DISCUSSION

Despite the number of epidemiological data on atherosclerosis and coronary risk factors, little data are still available on the discriminating power of serum apoproteins in the diagnosis of atherosclerosis risk.

The first aim of the present study was to state the mean values of serum apoproteins in a representative sample of the italian population. The values of serum apoproteins reported in this study are substantially similar to those published in the literature (Assmann (1982).

The apoprotein values have shown some significant differences between males and females. In particular, apo A-I and apo A-II were higher in females than in males while apo B, apo C-II and apo C-III, on the contrary, were higher in males than females. Apo E did not show significant differences between males and females.

By univariate analysis, significant correlations between serum apoproteins and some atherosclerosis risk factors were found.

In males, serum apo B was significantly correlated with age, apo A-II and apo C-III. The correlation coefficient between apo B and age was significantly high in the 20-40 age decades (p <0.001).
A significant correlation coefficient was also found between apo A-I and apo A-II, and between apo C-III and apo E. The smoke showed a significant correlation only with apo C-II.

In women, apo B was significantly correlated with age (particularly in the 40-60 age decades), with apo A-II (as in men) and with smoke. Moreover, apo A-I was highly correlated with apo A-II (as in men).

TABLE 2.1. (Males - 425 subjects). Linear correlation coefficients (r) between apoproteins and some coronary risk factors. (**) = p <0.01, for r >0.125. (***) = p <0.001, for r >0.178. BMI = body mass index. BMP = blood mean pressure = diastolic + 1/3(systolic - diastolic). TC = total cholesterol. HDLC = HDL cholesterol. TG = triglycerides.

	apo A-I	Apo A-II	Apo B	Apo C-II	Apo C-III	Apo E
AGE	0.072	0.078	0.242(***)	0.115	0.127	0.070
BMI	0.029	0.078	0.071	0.030	0.039	0.009
BMP	0.061	0.057	0.168(**)	0.043	0.087	0.046
GLUCOSE	0.012	0.020	0.005	0.045	0.069	0.031
TC	0.063	0.001	0.142(**)	0.100	0.136(**)	0.142(**)
HDLC	0.000	0.018	0.085	0.007	0.045	0.000
TG	0.010	0.059	0.107	0.053	0.105	0.010
SMOKE	0.071	0.017	0.007	0.159(**)	0.017	0.107
A-I		0.482(***)	0.093	0.038	0.115	0.037
A-II			0.202(***)	0.101	0.082	0.005
B				0.015	0.263(***)	0.163(**)
C-II					0.156(**)	0.157(**)
C-III						0.217(**)

TABLE 2.2. (Females - 481 subjects). (**) = p <0.01, for r >0.117. (***) = p <0.001, for r >0.167.

	apo A-I	Apo A-II	Apo B	Apo C-II	Apo C-III	Apo E
AGE	0.064	0.120(**)	0.320(***)	0.107	0.177(**)	0.131(**)
BMI	0.027	0.000	0.154(**)	0.029	0.047	0.026
BMP	0.020	0.017	0.137(**)	0.006	0.012	0.040
GLUCOSE	0.003	0.004	0.072	0.007	0.020	0.049
TC	0.015	0.024	0.042	0.012	0.121	0.043
HDLC	0.067	0.007	0.014	0.081	0.066	0.050
TG	0.055	0.097	0.069	0.032	0.030	0.047
SMOKE	0.014	-0.060	0.169(**)	0.048	0.000	0.101
A-I		0.352(***)	0.050	0.093	0.137(**)	0.034
A-II			0.266(***)	0.049	0.132(**)	0.098
B				0.076	0.111	0.130(*)
C-II					0.162(*)	0.154(*)
C-III						0.125

Surprisingly, HDL-cholesterol did not show a significant correlation with the major HDL apoproteins, i.e. apo A-I and apo A-II, in both sexes, indicating that cholesterol and apoproteins of HDL follow different metabolic pathways.

As far as the smoke is concerned, the significant correlation with apo B in women but not in men may indicate a greater increase of risk for atherosclerosis in smoking females than in smoking males.

REFERENCES

Sniderman, A., Shapiro, S., Marpole, D., Malcom, I., Skinner, B., Kwiterovich Jr.P.O. (1980) 'The association of coronary atherosclerosis and hyperapobetalipoproteinemia (increased protein but normal cholesterol content in human plasma low density lipoprotein)', Proc. Natl. Acad.Sci.(USA) 77, 604-608.

De Backer, G., Rosseneu, M., Deslypere J.P. (1982) 'Discriminative value of lipids and apoproteins in coronary heart disease', Atherosclerosis 42, 197-203.

Noma, A., Yokosuka, T., Kitamura K. (1983) 'Plasma lipids and apolipoproteins as discriminators for presence and severity of angiographically defined coronary artery disease', Atherosclerosis 49, 1-7.

Kottke, B.A., Zinmeister, A.R., Holmes, R.Jr., Kneller, R.W., Hallaway J., Mao, J.T. (1986) 'Apolipoproteins and coronary artery disease', Mayo Clin. Proc. 61, 313-319.

Research Group ATS-OB43 (1987) 'Cardiovascular risk factors in Italy. Up-date to the eithies of the Nine Communities Study', Card. Prev. Riab. 5, 73-140.

Capurso, A., Mogavero, A.M., Resta, F., Di Tommaso, M., Taverniti, R., Turturro, F., La Rosa, M., Marcovina, S. and Catapano, A.L. (1988) 'Apolipoprotein C-II deficiency detection of immunoreactive apolipoprotein C-II in the intestinal mucosa of two patients', J. Lipid Res. 29, 703-711.

Neville, D.M. (1971) 'Molecular weight determination of protein-dodecyl sulfate complexes by gel electrophoresis in a discontinuous buffer system', J. Biol. Chem. 246, 6328-6334.

Assmann, G., (1982) Lipid Metabolism and Atherosclerosis, F.K. Schattauer Verlag GmbH Publisher, Stuttgart, Germany.

69
A survey on apolipoprotein A-I and B: the CNR study

P. ROMA, S. FANTAPPIE, M.R. BAIOCCHI, R. FELLIN, P. AVOGARO, G. CAZZOLATO, S. MUNTONI, F. PINTUS, M. GIACCHI, M. SALVI, A. STRANO, G. AVELLONE, M. MANCINI, E. FARINARO, P. ORIENTE, L. POSTIGLIONE, G. URBINATI, R. ANTONINI, M.T. TENCONI, L. SOTTOCORNOLA and A.L. CATAPANO

Institute of Pharmacological Sciences, via Balzaretti 9, 20133 Milano, Italy

ABSTRACT. We report on a survey of apolipoprotein A-I and B measurements among 11 laboratories using a lyophilized serum to be evaluated for its possible use as "reference serum" in a large prospective study. Using a single method, radial immunodiffusion (RID), and a common antibody the partecipating laboratories evaluated the apo A-I and apo B concentrations in the proposed reference serum. Analyses were performed in quadruplicate in four consecutive days to estimate the day by day variation in a given laboratory. This value resulted to be 2% for apo A-I and 1.9% for apo B.

The grand mean values for apo B (92 mg/dl) and A-I (131 mg/dl) were very similar to those obtained with the same methods in the central laboratory. The serum was stable up to 1 year, thus it may be used as quality control serum in the determination of apo B and apo A-I concentrations for this study.

INTRODUCTION

The investigation on hyperlipoproteinemias has been focussed for many years on the determination of plasma lipids and lipids associated to lipoproteins. However, as the role of apoproteins has gained relevance, the need for their quantitative determination has been appreciated also in the clinical laboratory (1-4). Several retrospective studies have shown that apolipoprotein B (apo B) or apoprotein A-I (apo A-I) are better discriminators than plasma lipid or lipoprotein cholesterol levels for patients with a myocardial infarction (5-8). While these findings are encouraging, proof that apolipoproteins better predict myocardial infarction than plasma or lipoprotein cholesterol is still missing. One of the major problems hampering such a study in the lack of standardization among laboratories involved in a large prospective study.

In Italy the Progetto Finalizzato Malattie Degenerative obiettivo 43 has sponsored a trial to study the main risk factors for cardiovascular disease in nine demografically defined population samples across the country. Apoprotein A-I and B have been investigated among these factors.

In this paper we describe the production of a lyophilized serum, its characterization and labeling for apo A-I and apo B levels by the 11 laboratories partecipating in the study.

MATERIALS AND METHODS

The antisera were produced for this project in rabbits by Behring (Marburg, FGR) against purified human apoproteins. The monospecificity of the antisera was tested by immunodiffusion (9), immunoelectrophoresis (10) and immunoblotting (11). Apoprotein determinations were performed by RID. To avoid variability due to the use of different antisera or to the need of different pre-treatments of the samples. The plates were prepared by Behring using the common antiserum for all partecipants.

Two reference laboratories (Milan and Padua) developed a serum to be used as reference. This serum is a pool of fresh sera obtained from the local blood bank. Serum was lyophilized after addition of 0.14 M sucrose (12). The serum (0.5 ml) was dispensed with a calibrated pipette into Pierce hypovials (2 ml), lyophilized and then sealed with a silicone rubber plug with an aluminium ring. The sera were stored at -80°C until use except those vials used for the stability tests. The apoprotein content of the serum was determined by the two laboratories (Milan and Padua) using the same method to be used in the different laboratories against standards for apo B and apo A-I. For apo B determination, LDL freshly isolated by ultracentrifugation (d 1.025-1.050 g/ml) were used as standard; apo B was determined as tetramethylurea insoluble protein as described by Kane (13). Apo A-I was determined using purified HDL_3 (d 1.125-1.210 g/ml) whose apo A-I content was determined by SDS gel electrophoresis and scanning of the gel. The average apo A-I content of HDL_3 determined using this procedure was 66.5% (mean of 8 determinations) of the total protein in good agreement with data obtained with different methods (14,15). Using these standards, values of 130 mg/dl and 90 mg/dl were obtained for apo A-I and B respectively.

The stability of the reference sera was determined on sera stored up to 12 months at -80°, -20°, and 4°C and also on sera stored at the room temperature for up to 1 month.
The sera were then taken up with 0.5 $\pm$ 0.002 ml of distilled water and their apoprotein B and A-I content determined using appropriate standards. Six sera were reconstituted at every time point, and analyses were done in duplicate.

The RID method used required no sample dilution and no addition of detergent to the samples. Apo A-I values did not depend upon additions to the sample of detergent (Tween 20, Triton X-100 or tetramethylurea).

The sera were sent to the partecipating laboratories by registered mail and were received usually within 3 days from shipment. The lyophilized serum was brought to room temperature and 0.5 $\pm$ 0.002 ml of distilled water was added. The sample was mixed by gentle inversion every 5 min for a total of 20 min, avoiding bubble formation. Apo A-I and B determinations were repeated on 4 different vials in 4 consecutive days. Every partecipating laboratory used their standards.

A methodological stage was provided to all partecipating laboratories to explain the practical and theoretical implications of the method to be used. Reading of the plates was made after 48 h using a standard calibrated magnification lens.

RESULTS AND DISCUSSION

Apolipoproteins are a key component in the metabolic channeling of the different lipoprotein classes (16). Several authors have proposed that apolipoproteins are better discriminants than plasma lipids for subjects affected by coronary artery disease (CAD), however prospective studies demostrating that apolipoproteins are risk factors for CAD are still missing (5-8).

Methodological problems as well a lack of standardization among laboratories has been claimed to be responsible for the variation in apoprotein values found in different laboratories, therefore hampering large population studies in this field.

The first step in this study was to determine the monospecificity of the antisera. Immunoelectrophoresis and immunodiffusion showed that anti apo B serum did not cross react with apo A-I, apo A-II, C-I, C-II, C-III, and apo E; the antiserum to apo A-I did not cross react with LDL, apo A-II, C-I, C-II, C-III, and apo E. Immunoblotting analyses also demonstrated that the antisera reacted with the appropriate protein, in particular anti apo B reacted with apo B-100 and B-48 and anti apo A-I reacted with all major apo A-I isoforms (Data not shown).

The characteristics of the pooled sera used for preparing the "reference" material are reported in Tab.1; the serum had an averange cholesterol level of 185 mg/dl and of 79 mg/dl triglycerides.

The stability of the lyophilized serum was determined as described under methods and the results of the experiments are show in Tab.2. These data show that both apo A-I and apo B values were stable up to 1 year at -80°, -20° or 4°C. Furthermore storage at room temperature for up to 1 month did not affect the levels of immunodetectable apo A-I or apo B. The partecipating laboratories were therefore instructed to store the lyophilised sera for up to 6 months at 4°C. Furthermore sera were stable, after reconstitution with water, for up to 2 weeks at 4°C (data not shown). Further work is required to establish whether storage up to 1 year is also safe at this temperature. In a recent survey Cooper et al. (17) reported a reference lyophilized serum, however the serum stability for apo A-I and apo B measurements was not studied.

We also determined the serum stability up to 1 month at 20°C. No appreciable loss of immunodetectable apoproteins was found suggesting that shipment of these sera should not affect the levels of immunodetectble apo A-I or apo B. In our experience the apo B and, somewhat more, the apo A-I values of lyophilized sera not containing sucrose fell with time, similary to what reported for stored sera (18).

Much of the variability in determining apoproteins may depend upon the use of different antisera (19): for istance with some antisera apo A-I determinations require the structure of lipoproteins to be destroyed while other sera require no treatment of the semples (20,21). We therefore used a common antiserum and a commun method. The anti apo A-I serum we used did not require pre-treatment of the samples thus reducing the source of errors.

The values for apo A-I and B obtained by the 11 partecipating laboratories are reported in Tab.3. The grean mean values were 131 for A-I and 92 for apo B. The data reported from every laboratory did not differ significantly from each other with the exception of two laboratories for apo A-I and 1 laboratory for apo B (Duncan test). The among assay CV% was between 0.9 and 6.1 for apo A-I and from 0.3 to 4.6 for apo B. The CV% within assay for all laboratories was less than 3% (data not shown). Figure 1 depicts the within laboratory relation between apo A-I and apo B determinations. The lowest and highest values for vials 1 to 4 are reported and the two points are connected. The mean of the laboratories means is represented by the dotted lines. One laboratory had relatively low values for both apoproteins, one a relatively low value for apo A-I. Scattering of the data however was much less than that reported by Cooper et al. if data obtained using the RID method are compared (17). We suggest that the use of a common antiserum and the centrally prepared plates contribute to this finding.

In summary we have described the preparation of a lyophilized serum which meets the stability requirements necessary to be used for standardization in large prospective studies, furthermore calibration within each laboratory using this serum with the given values of apo A-I and B will allow comparison of the data obtained in different laboratories.

ACKNOWLEDGEMENTS

This work was supported, in part, by the CNR Progetto Finalizzato Malattie Degenerative ob.43. Miss Maddalena Marazzini typed the manuscript.

REFERENCES

1) Schonfeld, G., Lees R., George, P.K., Pfleger, B. (1974) 'Assay of total plasma apolipoprotein B concentration in human subjects', J Clin Invest 53, 1458-1467.
2) Avogaro, P., Bittolo-Bon, G., Cazzolato, G. (1978), 'Variations in apolipoproteins B and A during the course of myocardial infarction', Eur J Clin Invest 8, 121-129.
3) Onitri, A.C., and Lewis, B. (1977), 'Measurements of the

apoproteins of human serum lipoproteins by rocket immunoelectrophoresis', Clin Chim Acta 79, 39-45.
4) Fruchart, J.C., Kora, I., Cachera, C. (1982), 'Simultaneous measurement of plasma apolipoproteins A-I and B by electroimmunoassay', Clin Chem 28, 59-62.
5) Avogaro, P., Bittolo-Bon, G., Cazzolato, G., Quinci, G.B., Belussi, F. (1978) 'Plasma levels of apolipoprotein A-I and apolipoprotein B in human atherosclerosis', Artery 4, 385-394.
6) Riesen, W.F., Mordasini, R., Salzmann, G., Theler A., Gurtner, H.P. (1980) 'Apoproteins and lipids as discriminators of severity of coronary heart disease', Atherosclerosis 37, 157-162.
7) De Becker, G., Rosseneu, M., Deslypere, J.P. (1982) 'Discriminative value of lipids and apoproteins in coronary heart disease', Atherosclerosis 42, 197-203.
8) Maciejko, J.J., Holmes, D.R., Kottke, B.A., Zinsmelster, A.R., Dinh, D.M., Mao, S.J.T. (1983) 'Apolipoprotein A-I as a marker of angiographically assessed coronary artery disease', New Engl J Med 309, 385-389.
9) Ouchterlonly, O. (1953) 'Antigen-antibody reactions in gels. IV Types of reactions in coordinated system of diffusion', Acta Pathol Microbiol 32, 231-240.
10) Curry, M.D., Gustafson, A., Alaupovic, P., McConathy, W.J. (1978) 'Electroimmunoassay, radialimmunoassay, and radial immunodiffusion assay evaluation for quantification of human apolipoprotein B', Clin Chem 24, 280-288.
11) Burnette, W.N. (1981) 'Western blotting electrophoretic transfert of proteins from sodium dodecyl sulphate polyacrylamide gels to immunodified nitrocellulose and radiographic detection with antibody and radiodinated protein A', Biochemistry 112, 195-203.
12) Wieland, H., Seidel, D. (1982) 'Improved assessment of plasma lipoproteins patterns. IV simple preparation of a lyophilized control serum containing intact human plasma lipoproteins', Clin Chem 28, 1335-1337.
13) Kane, J.P., Sata, T., Hamilton, R.L., Havel, R.J. (1975) 'Apoprotein composition of very low density lipoprotenis in human serum', J Clin Invest 56, 1622-1634.
14) Alaupovic, P., Curry, M., McConathy, W., Fesmire, J. (1979) 'Electroimmunoassay of apolipoproteins accurring of high density lipoproteins of human plasma', in K. Lippel (ed.), Report of high density lipoproteins metabolism workshop. Bethesda, MD, USA, DHHS, NIH, NHLBI, 1661, 227-240.
15) Marcovina, S., Di Cola, G., Rapetto, C. et al. (1985) 'Development of a radial immunodiffusion technique employing monoclonal antibodies for apolipoprotein B determination of human plasma', Clin Chim Acta 147, 117-125.
16) Marcovina, S., France, D., Phillips, R.A., Mao, S.J.T. (1985) 'Monoclonal antibodies can precipitate low-density lipoprotein. I. Characterization and use in determining apolipoprotein B', Clin Chem 31, 1654-1658.

17) Cooper, G.R., Smith, S.J., Wiebe, D.A., Kuchmak, M., Hannon, W.M. (1985) 'International survey of apolipoproteins A-I and B measurements', Clin Chem 31, 223-228.

18) Albers, J.J., Cheung, M.C., Vahl, P.W. (1980) 'Effect of storage on the measurement of apolipoproteins A-I and A-II by radial immunodiffusion' J Lipid Res 21, 874-878.

19) Fesmire T.D., McConathy, W.J., Alaupovic, P. (1984) 'Use and significance of reference serum as secondary standard for electroimmunoassay of apolipoprotein A-I', Clin Chem 30, 712-716.

20) Fainaru, M., Glangeaud, M.G., Eisemberg, S. (1975) 'Radioimmunoassay of human high density lipoprotein apolipoprotein A-I', Biochim Biophys Acta 386, 432-443.

21) Curry, M.D., Alaupovic, P., Suenram C.A. (1976) 'Determination of apolipoprotein A and its constitutive A-I and A-II polypeptides by separate electroimmunoassay', Clin Chem 22, 315-322.

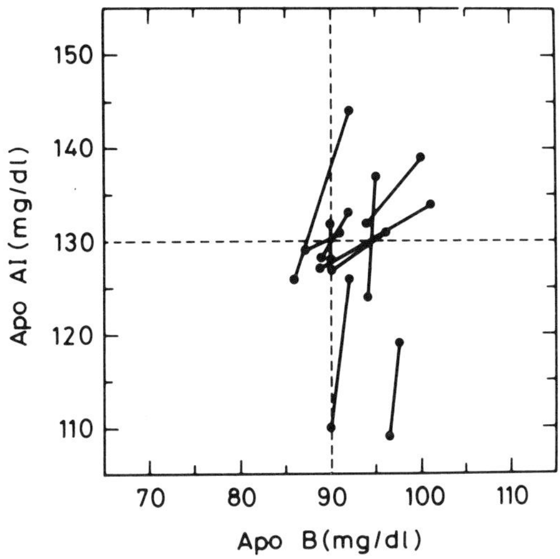

FIGURE 1. Within laboratory relation between apolipoprotein A-I and B determination. The lowest and highest values obtained for each laboratory are connected by a solid line. The dotted line represents the grand mean values.

TABLE 1. Characteristics of the serum pool (28 male donors) used as reference material.

	MEAN	RANGE
Total cholesterol mg/dl	185	120-240
Triglycerides mg/dl	79	51-190
HDL cholesterol mg/dl	48	34-65

TABLE 2. Stability of immunodetectable apo A-I and B in the serum pool. (Determinations were performed in a single laboratory).
mg/dl mean ± S.D.

		FRESH PREPARED	1 MONTH	6 MONTHS	1 YEAR
A-I	- 80°C	130±3.7	129±2.8	133±3.9	128±4.1
	- 20°C	130±3.7	128±4.3	127±4.1	132±3.1
	4°C	130±3.7	134±3.2	127±6.2	122±7.1
	20°C	130±3.7	127±4.8	N.D.	N.D.
B	- 80°C	89±2.7	90±1.9	88±3.2	90±3.1
	- 20°C	89±2.7	92±3.9	90±2.1	91±2.6
	4°C	89±2.7	91±1.7	90±2.1	89±3.7
	20°C	89±2.7	89±3.2	N.D.	N.D.

N.D. not determined.

TABLE 3. Apolipoprotein A-I and B determination by RID (mg/dl).

LAB.	Mean ± E.S.	
	Apo A-I	Apo B
1	136±2.38	87±1.41
2	114±4.64**,°°	97±0.50°
3	118±8.26°	91±1.15
4	129±1.50	93±3.37
5	129±5.45	94±0.59
6	131±2.06	91±2.87
7	132±2.50	95±5.51
8	135±9.60	88±2.64
9	135±3.09	95±2.71
10	130±1.70	90±0.39
11	129±1.92	90±0.50
GRAND MEAN	131±5.78	92±3.06

** $p < 0.01$ vs 1
°° $p < 0.05$ vs 4,6,7,8,9,10 and 11
° $p < 0.05$ vs 1

70
Reference standard for cholesterol evaluation in serum obtained by isotope dilution mass spectrometry

B. MALAVASI, D. COLOMBO and G. GALLI**

**Institute of Pharmacological Sciences, School of Pharmacy,*

***Department of Chemistry and Biochemistry, School of Medicine, University of Milan, Italy*

For the analysis by isotopic dilution, a sample containing the analyte to be measured is mixed with a known amount of the same analyte isotopically labelled. By gaschromatography-mass spectrometry (GC-MS), that allows to discriminate the labelled and the unlabelled compound on the basis of their molecular weight, it is possible to determine the intensity ratio of the two isotopes. The use as internal reference of the labelled analyte, that exhibits chemical-physical properties identical to the natural isotope, allows to not take into account the recoveries obtained from the different analytical steps, and the variability of the instrumental response, because the ratio between the two isotopic species remains unchanged during the overall analytical procedure. The analyte concentration is calculated on the basis of the volume of the specimen, the known amount of labelled analyte added, and the intensity ratio of specific ions of the two isotopes determined by GC-MS.

Through this procedure, described by Choen et al. (1) (National Bureau of Standard, Washington D.C.), utilizing deuterated cholesterol, we prepared two reference sera with different cholesterol concentration for the lipid clinics involved in the Italian National Program of Education for Cholesterol Control.

INTRODUCTION

In the last twenty years, necessity to monitor cholesterol concentration in biological specimens from large populations, turned this determination into a routine test for clinical chemistry.

A large number of different methodologies based on enzymatic or chemical reactions or gaschromatographic separations have been developed (2-5). For the assessment of precision and accuracy of these different analytical procedures, an absolute reference method based on isotope dilution GC-MS for the evaluation of BIAS of other techniques has been set up. This method meets all the necessary specifications to be considered the approach of choice for the assessement of absolute concentration (1,5-9).

For the analysis by means of isotope dilution, serum specimens containing unlabelled cholesterol to be measured are mixed with a known amount of a deuterated analogue, obtained by chemical synthesis. By means of mass spectrometry, that allows to discriminate between the labelled and unlabelled species of cholesterol on the basis of their different molecular weight, it is possible to determine the weight ratio between the two species.

This procedure was applied for the absolute cholesterol measurement in samples of two batches of lyophilized sera containing two different concentration of the sterol.

MATERIALS AND METHODS

Unlabelled and labelled cholesterol

To exclude the presence of cholest-7-en-3-beta-ol isomer, cholesterol (Merck) was submitted to bromuration-debromuration reaction (10). After recrystallization the compound was dried under vacuum. TLC analysis (Exane:Ethyl Ether: Acetic Acid 70:30:1) of the recrystallized product showed only one spot at the expected R_f. Selected ion monitoring analysis of the trimethylsilylated derivative (m/z 458) demonstrated the absence of signals at the expected retention times of others monounsaturated C_{27} sterols.

Deuterated cholesterol was synthetized according to BJoerkhem et al. (9). The labelled product was purified according to the procedure utilized for unlabelled cholesterol. Mass spectrum of the compound indicates that up to six deuterium atoms were introduced into the molecule.

Reagents

Solvents were purchased from Merck; Sylon HTP was obtained from Supelco.

Reference Serum

Two batches of 2000 vials each of lyophilized sera, A and B, with different cholesterol concetrations were supplied by Boehringer Biochemia Robin especially prepared for Italian National Program of Education for Cholesterol Control. Estimated cholesterol concentrations, evaluated by enzymatic method, were 170mg/dl for batch A and 238mg/dl for batch B respectively.

Preparation of the samples for SIM analysis

Three vials of lyophilized serum from batch A and B respectively have been reconstituted (2ml). From each vial three aliquots have been taken and diluted in order to achieve a final concentration of about 4µg of cholesterol in a volume of 100µl for batch A and 50µl for batch B respectively. 4µg of deuterated cholesterol were added to each specimen.

After hydrolysis of cholesterol esters and extraction performed according to the procedure described by Cohen et al. (1), the extracts were dried under nitrogen flow and added with 100µl Sylon HTP at 60°C for 20' to achieve the corresponding trimethilsilylethers derivatives. Aliquots (1µl) of the reaction mixture were injected into the gaschromatograph-mass spectrometer.

Preparation of calibration mixtures

Aliquots of purified deuterated and normal cholesterol were combined in order to obtain triplicate series of mixtures whose ratios by weight of unlabelled to labelled cholesterol were ranging between 0.61 and 1.01 in order to cover the range of the weight ratios of the isotopes in the two series of samples.

These mixtures were extracted and analyzed as described for serum specimens.

SIM analysis

Gaschromatography: a gaschromatograph HP 5988 equipped with a OV1 capillary column (20m; 0.2mm I.D.) was utilized. Instrumental conditions: column temperature varied between 150 and 290°C with an increment of 25°C/min; injector and transfer line temperature 280°C; Helium head pressure 7 PSI.

Mass-spectrometry: a VG 70SEQ instrument was used. Instrumental conditions: Temperature of electron impact ion source 250°C; electron energy 70 eV; accelerating voltage 8 KV; resolution 1000.

The two molecular ions 458 for unlabelled and 463 for deuterated cholesterol were monitored alternatively using voltage switched selected ion monitoring. Each mass was monitored with a dwell time of 80ms which, together with a settling time of 10ms between masses, gave a cycle of 180ms. Since the GC peak width at the base was about 12 seconds, about 66 measurements were made on each mass during the elution of the sample from the GC.

The intra and between-day instrumental accuracy, was estimated by repeated injections of a mixture containing the two cholesterol isotopes in a weight ratio of 0.703. The coefficient of variations were 0.33% and 0.42% respectively.

For each sample of calibration mixtures and lyophilized sera the ratio between normal and deuterated cholesterol have been calculated on the basis of three injections. Cholesterol concentrations of the two batches A and B represented the average of twenty-seven SIM analysis.

RESULTS

No signal in the ion trace 463 was found when purified unlabelled cholesterol was analyzed, whereas the chemically synthetized labelled cholesterol contains 6.9% of normal cholesterol, as demonstrated by the ratio between the ions 458/463. This isotopic contribution has been taken into account for the unlabelled sterol determination.

In table 1 are reported the concentrations found in samples of batch A and B respectively, and the corresponding CV.

This procedure allowed the achievement of the reference standard for the Italian National Program for Cholesterol Control.

TABLE 1

BATCH A			
sample	mg/dl	Means±d.s.	CV %
1	170		
2	172	171±1.25	0.73
3	173		

BATCH B			
sample	mg/dl	Means±d.s.	CV %
1	242		
2	239	240±1.25	0.52
3	240		

REFERENCES

(1) A. Cohen,H.S. Hertz, J. Mandel, R.C. Paule, R. Schaffer, L.T. Sniegoski, T. Sun, M.J. Welch, E. White V (1980) Clin. Chem. 26/7:860

(2) L.P. Cawley, B.O. Musser, S. Cambell, W. Faucette (1963) Am. J. Clin. Pathol. 39:450

(3) J.L. Driscoll, D. Aubuchon, M. Descoteaux, H.F. Martin (1971) Anal. Chem. 43:1196

(4) J.P. Blomhoff, (1973) Clin. Chim. Acta 43:257

(5) P. Roschlau,E. Berut, W. Gruber (1974) Z. Klin. Biochem. 12:403

(6) C.C. Sweeley, W.H. Holmsted, R. Ryhage, (1966) Anal. Chem. 38:1549

(7) C.G. Hammar, B. Holmsted, R. Ryhage, (1968) Anal. Biochem. 25:532

(8) J.P. Cali, Abstracts of the Xth International Congress of Clinical Chemistry, Mexico D.F., Avelar Hnos. Impresores, Mexico D.F., 1978, p.30.

(9) I. Bjoerkhem, R. Blomstrand, L. Svensson, (1974) Clin. Chim. Acta 54:185.

(10)L.F. Fieser (1953) JACS, 75:5421

CARDIOLOGISTS AND CHD AND ATHEROSCLEROSIS PREVENTION VERSUS THERAPY

71

Incidence and prognostic significance of silent myocardial ischemia in patients after acute myocardial infarction

D. BONADUCE, M. PETRETTA, T. LANZILLO, M.V. MONTEMURRO, V. BIANCHI, G. CONFORTI, G. MORGANO and P. ARRICHIELLO

Institute of Internal Medicine, Second School of Medicine, via S. Pansini 5, 80135 Naples, Italy

ABSTRACT. The incidence and prognostic significance of silent myocardial ischemia in 175 patients who survived a first acute myocardial infarction (AMI) were assessed by means of maximal exercise stress test and 24 hour continuous ECG monitoring performed before discharge. Thirteen patients showed silent ischemia with both techniques, 31 only with stress test, 5 only with ECG monitoring and 8 had a doubtful stress test but showed S-T segment depression during ECG monitoring, 118 were free from ischemia. Ten cardiac deaths and 31 coronary events including unstable angina, by-pass operation, and myocardial infarction occured during the one year follow-up period. S-T segment depression during ECG monitoring showed a lower sensitivity but a higher specificity and predictive accuracy for cardiac death and coronary events than did exercise stress test. When S-T segment depression is detected in the same patient with both techniques the sensitivity is lower and specificity higher. Whenever the presence of S-T segment depression is recorded, it shows a good sensitivity without significantly decreasing the specificity. Classifying patients according to the occurence of S-T segment depression on exercise test and/or ECG ambulatory monitoring, the Yates corrected chi-square test showed a significant pattern when cardiac deaths and coronary events are considered together ($p < 0.01$). However, the incidence of cardiac deaths and coronary events was comparable in patients with exercise S-T segment depression regardless of the occurence of S-T segment changes during continuous ECG monitoring. All 8 patients who stopped the exercise test before reaching target heart rate for dyspnea (5 patients), arrhythmias (2 patients), and hypertensive response (1 patient) had S-T segment depression during ECG monitoring: 2 of them died during follow-up and 3 suffered from unstable angina. Thus, ECG monitoring of these patients adds same helpful information but is less useful in patients who perform a maximal exercise stress test.

INTRODUCTION.

Spontaneous episodes of transient myocardial ischemia in absence of symptoms termed "silent ischemia" has been well documented in patients with known coronary artery disease and with previously undetected ischemic heart disease (1-6). The prevalence of these ischemic asymptomatic episodes, their hemodynamic correlates, and their therapeutic implications have been fully investigated (7-10). Many studies have also aimed to characterize the prognostic significance of asymptomatic episodes in patients with stable and unstable angina pectoris utilizing ECG monitoring (11-12). In patients who have survived an acute myocardial infarction, exercise stress test (13-15) and radionuclide techniques (16-18) are currently utilized to identify patients at high risk of subsequent cardiac events. At present few data are available about the prognostic significance in such patients of silent ischemic episodes recorded by continuous ECG monitoring. Furthermore, the relationships between continuous ECG monitoring and exercise stress test have not been fully clarified.

We have investigated the prevalence and short-term implications of silent ischemia at a maximal exercise stress test and during continuous ECG monitoring in 17 patients who survived a first myocardial infarction.

METHODS.

In all patients an exercise test was performed before discharge an average of 17 days after symptom onset, on a bycicle ergometer with stepwise increments of 25 watts every 2 minutes, after 2 initial minutes of zero load.

Twenty-four hours after exercise testing all patients underwent 24-hour ECG monitoring using a commercially available OXFORD MEDILOG II FM type two channel ECG.

RESULTS.

Exercise stress test. No complications resulted from the exercise stress test. Exercise test was stopped for the following reasons: maximal heart rate in 143 patients, angina in 17 patients, ST-segment depression ≥ 4 mm in 7, arrhythmias in 2, dyspnea in 5, and hypertensive response in 1. Twenty out of 143 patients who reached maximal heart rate and all 17 patients who stopped the test because of angina, showed ST-segment depression ≥ 1 mm. Therefore, 123 patients had no angina or occurence of ST-segment depression (70.3%), 44 had ST-segment depression (25.1%) (17 with angina, and 27 without), no patient suffered angina without ST-segment depression. In the 8 patients who stopped exercising for dyspnea, hypertensive response or arrhythmias, the test was considered doubtful for myocardial ischemia.

Mean heart rate at the onset of ST-segment depression was 123.2 b/min in the total study population, 122.5 in angina patients and 127.3 in asymptomatic ST-segment changes.

Continuous ECG monitoring. At least 1 episode of ST-segment depression was found in 26 of 175 patients (14.8%), while no patient presented episode of ST-segment elevation; 19 patients had only painless episodes (10.8%), 7 (4.0%) had both painless and painful episodes. Of a total of 65 identified episodes of ischemia, 53 (81.5%) were painless and the remaining 12 (18.5%) were associated with pain; of the 53 painless episodes, 12 were observed in patients who referred all painful episodes while 41 were observed in patients with exclusively painless episodes.

The total duration of episodes of ST-segment depression was 1166 minutes, 951 minutes without pain and 215 with pain. The mean duration of ischemic episodes was 17.9 minutes for painless and 17.9 for painful.

Mean heart rate at the onset of ST-segment depression was 97.6 b/min in the total study population, 94.8 b/min in painless episodes, and 99.2 b/min in painful.

Prognostic value of exercise stress test. The total one year mortality was 14 of 175 patients (8.0%) but only 10 of these were considered cardiac deaths (5.7%).

When ST-segment depression occurred during the exercise test it was highly predictive of mortality during follow-up (Table 1).

TABLE 1. Correlations between results of exercise stress test, coronary events, and mortality to one year follow-up after hospital discharge.

	No angina or S-T segment depression (123 patients)		S-T segment depression (27 patients)		Angina and S-T segment depression (17 patients)		Doubtful (8 patients)	
	No	%	No	%	No	%	No	%
CORONARY EVENTS								
None	103	83.7	18	66.7	6	35.3	3	37.5
Unstable angina	6	4.9	2	7.4	3	17.6	3	37.5
By-pass operation	6	4.9	0	0.0	4	23.5	0	0.0
Myocardial infarction	4	3.2	2	7.4	1	5.9	0	0.0
CARDIAC DEATHS	3	2.4	3	11.1	2	11.8	2	25.0
NON CARDIAC DEATHS	1	0.8	2	7.4	1	5.9	0	0.0

Five of 44 patients (11.4%) with ST-segment depression died as compared with only 3 of 123 (2.4%) without depression ($p < 0.01$). The occurrence of angina in the presence of ST-segment depression did not increase the prognostic importance of ST-segment depression. One-hundred and three of 123 patients without angina or S-T segment depression (83.7%) survived for one year without coronary events as compared to 24 of 44 (54.5%) with ST-segment depression associated or not with angina symptoms ($p < 0.01$). The occurrence of non fatal coronary events was higher in the subset of patients with angina than in those with only ST-segment depression without angina ($p < 0.05$) and those without angina or ST-segment depression ($p < 0.01$). In particular, unstable angina during the follow-up period was present in 8 patients (5.3%) who had no angina during exercise testing as compared with 3 patients (17.6%) who suffered angina symptoms.

Aorto-coronary by-pass grafting occured in 4 of 17 patients (23.5%) with angina and ST-segment depression and in 6 of 150 (4.0%) without angina ($p < 0.01$). No patient showing ST-segment depression without angina underwent aorto-coronary by-pass grafting. Recurrent myocardial infarction was seen in 1 of 17 patients (5.9%) with angina and in 6 of 150 (4.0%) without.

Prognostic value of continuous ECG monitoring. Five of 26 patients (19.2%) who showed ST-segment depression on ECG monitorinfg died of cardiac causes as compared to 5 of 149 (3.4%) without ST-segment depression (p< 0.01) (Table 2).

TABLE 2. Correlations between results of continuous ECG monitoring, coronary events, and mortality to one year follow-up after hospital discharge.

	No angina or S-T segment depression (149 patients)		S-T segment depression (19 patients)		Angina and S-T segment depression (7 patients)	
	No	%	No	%	No	%
CORONARY EVENTS						
None	117	78.5	11	57.9	2	28.6
Unstable angina	9	6.0	3	15.8	2	28.6
By-pass operation	9	6.0	1	5.3	0	0.0
Myocardial infarction	6	4.0	0	0.0	1	14.3
CARDIAC DEATHS	5	3.4	3	15.8	2	28.6
NON CARDIAC DEATHS	3	2.0	1	5.3	0	0.0

The occurrence of angina in the presence of ST-segment depression did not increase the risk of death. One hundred and seventeen out of 149 patients (78.5%) without angina or ST-segment depression survived one year follow-up without coronary events as compared to 13 out of 26 (50%) with ST-segment depression with or without angina symptoms (p< 0.01).

Unstable angina occurred in 9 out of 149 patients (6.0%) without angina or ST-segment depression, in 3 of 19 (15.8%) with painless ST-segment depression, and in 2 of 7 (28.6%) with painful ST-segment depression. There was a borderline difference (p<0.1) between patients without ischemic episodes and those with either painless or painful ST-segment depression while no significant difference was found in the incidence of by-pass operation or recurrence of non fatal myocardial infarction.

Relationship between determinants of prognosis on exercise stress test and continuous ECG monitoring. Patients were divided according to the occurrence of ST-segment depression at exercise stress test and/or continuous ECG monitoring and ordered on the basis of the incidence of cardiac death and coronary events (Fig. 1).

Thirteen patients showed ST-segment depression both at exercise test and ECG monitoring, and thirty one at exercise test alone; during follow-up cardiac deaths occurred in 2 (15.4%) and in 3 patients (9.7%) respectively. Coronary events occured in 3 of 13 (23.1%) and in 9 of 31 (29.0%) patients; the difference were not statistically significant. The exercise stress test showed no ST-segment changes in 123 patients and in only 5 of these ST-segment depressions were observed during ECG monitoring; cardiac death occurred during follow-up in 1 of these 5 patients (20.0%), while another patient (20.0%) referred unstable angina; of the remaining 118 patients 2 died during the follow-up (16.7%) and 15 presented non fatal coronary events (12.7%). The 8 patients who stopped the exercise stress test before reaching maximal heart rate showed all ST-segment depression on ECG monitoring; 2 of them (25.0%) died during the follow-up and 3 (37.5%) suffered a coronary event. The value of exercise testing soon after myocardial infarction in predicting mortality and cardiac events over the next year has already been well documented (19). Cardiac mortality over the one year after hospital discharge in our patients who underwent exercise stress test was 5.7%, and this rate is comparable to previous results. ST-segment depression was highly predictive of subsequent mortality. In fact cardiac death occurred in the following year in 5 of 44 patients (11.4%) who showed this abnormality and 3 of 123 (2.4%) without ST-segment depression. The presence or absence of angina adds no further prognostic information.

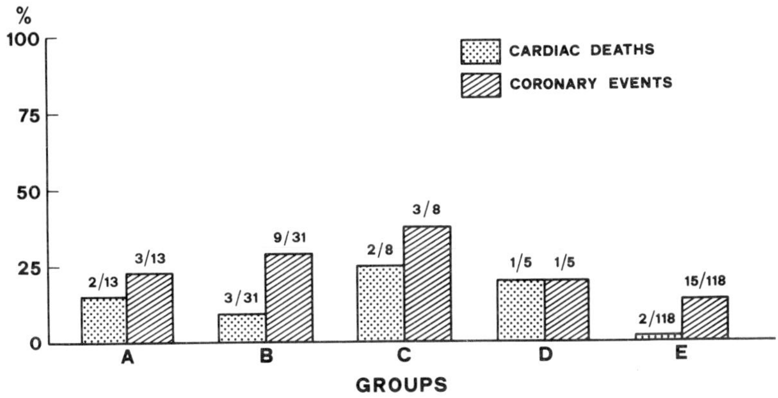

Figure 1. Patients distribution and incidence of cardiac deaths and coronary events according to S-T changes at ECG stress test and during continuous ECG monitoring. A = Patients with S-T segment depression both at exercise stress test and during continuous ECG monitoring. B = Patients with S-T segment depression at exercise stress test and without S-T segment depression during continuous ECG monitoring. C = Patients with doubtful exercise stress test and with S-T segment depression during continuous ECG monitoring. D = Patients without segment depression both at exercise stress test and during continuous ECG monitoring. E = Patients without S-T segment depression at exercise stress test and with S-T segment depression during continuous ECG monitoring.

DISCUSSION.

Continuous ECG monitoring has also been extensively applied in managing patients with coronary artery disease. It has been well documented, utilizing ECG monitoring, that the majority of ischemic episodes that occur in patients with angina syndromes are clinically silent. Silent ischemia has been shown to be closely correlated to the extent and severity of occlusive coronary artery disease and to be predictive of early clinical outcome in patients with unstable angina (12). Actually, the frequency and duration of myocardial ischemia revealed by continuous ECG recording may be useful in determining the risk profile and in evaluating therapy in patients with unstable angina (20). However, whether the magnitude of ischemia documented on ECG recording may constitute an index of prognosis in myocardial infarction patients has not yet been determined.

According to our results ECG monitoring also seems to be good predictor of cardiac death: cardiac death occurred during follow-up in 19.2% of our patients with ST-segment depression and in only 3.4% of those without. Angina symptoms observed via exercise stress test add little predictive value about cardiac mortality to ST-segment. Few data are available about the prognostic value of exercise stress test and ECG monitoring if the results of both techniques are considerd in the same patient.

Our data suggest that ECG monitoring adds little helpful information about cardiac death and coronary events in patients with exercise ST-segment depression. In fact, the incidence of cardiac deaths and coronary events was comparable in patients with exercise ST-segment depression regardless of the occurrence of ST-segment changes during ECG monitoring. According to these observations caution must be taken in the prognostic evaluation of patients with a negative ECG monitoring in the absence of an exercise stress test result. Only patients without ST-segment changes revealed by both techniques were at lower risk of subsequent fatal or non fatal cardiac events. ST-segment depression during ECG monitoring showed a higher specificity and predictive accuracy than exercise stress test for cardiac death and coronary events; the stress test seems more sensible but less specific. When ST-segment depression is detected in the same patient via both techniques the sensitivity is lower and specificity higher. On the contrary, whenever the presence of ST-segment depression, is recorded, it shows good sensitivity and not significantly decreased specificity.

The episodes of transient ischemia at ECG monitoring in patients with normal exercise response occurred during minimal physical activities or were related to different levels of mental activity. Previous studies performed in coronary artery disease patients, utilizing ECG monitoring, have clearly demonstrated that ischemic episodes are surprisingly prolonged, triggered by ordinary daily activities, and show a strong circadian rhythm (21-23). These newly recognized features suggest, even though they do not prove, that intermittent disturbances of coronary blood supply play an active role in triggering ischemia during everyday activities apart from increases in myocardial work and oxygen demand. Therefore the cardiac death of a patient with ST-segment depression during ECG monitoring but with normal exercise response might be explained by dynamic coronary obstruction.

Our study confirms the excellent predictive value of exercise stress test concerning 1 year prognosis after acute myocardial infarction. Also the detection of silent ischemia on continuous ECG monitoring offers helpful informations, however caution must be suggested in evaluating patients without ischemic episodes during ECG monitoring if the results of stress test is not available. In patients who stopped exercising before target heart rate without angina or ST-segment depression, ECG monitoring gives useful prognostic informations by means of ST-segment analysis.

REFERENCES.

1. Stern, S. and Tzivoni, D. (1974) "Early detection of silent ischemic heart disease by 24-hour electrocardiographic monitoring of active subjects", Br Heart J, 36, 481-490.
2. Langou, R.A., Huang, E.K., Kelly, M.J., Cohen, L.S. (1980) "Predictive accuracy of coronary artery calcification and abnormal exercise test for coronary artery disease in asymptomatic men", Circulation, 62, 1196-1203.
3. Deanfield, J.E., Selwyn, A.P., Chierchia, S., et al. (1983) "Myocardial ischemia during daily life in patients with stable angina: its relation to symptoms and heart rate changes", Lancet, 2, 753-758.
4. Deanfield, J.E., Shea, M., Ribeiro, P., de Landsheere, C.M., Horlock, P., Selwyn, P.A. (1984) "Transient ST-segment depression as a marker of myocardial ischemia during daily life", Am J Cardiol, 54, 1195-1200.
5. Cecci, A.C., Dovellini, E.V., Marchi, F., Pucci, P., Santoro, G.M., Fazzini, P.F. (1983) "Silent myocardial ischemia during ambulatory electrocardiophic monitoring in patients with effort angina", J Am Coll Cardiol, 1, 934-939.
6. Selwyin, A.P., Fox, K., Eves, M., Oakley, D., Dargie, H.J., Shillingford, J.P. (1978) "Myocardial ischaemia in patients with frequent angina pectoris", Br Med J, 2, 1594-1596.
7. Cohn, P.F. (1988) "Silent myocardial ischemia", Ann Intern Med, 109, 312-317.
8. Figueras, J., Singh, B.N., Ganz, W., Charuzi, Y., Swan, H.J.C. (1979) "Mechanism of rest and nocturnal angina: observations during continuous hemodynamic and electrocardiographic monitoring", Circulation, 59, 955-962.
9. Mulcahy, D., Keegan, J., Cunningham, D., et al. (1988) "Circadian variations of total ischaemic burden and its alteration with anti-anginal agents", Lancet, II, 755-759.
10. Singh, B.H., Nademanee, K., Figueras, J., Josephson, M.A. (1986) "Hemodynamic and electrocardiographic correlates of symptomatic and silent myocardial ischemia: pathophysiologic and therapeutic implications", Am J Cardiol, 58, 3B-10B.
11. Mody Vaghaiwalla, F., Nademanee, K., Intarachot, V., Josephson, M.A., Robertson, H.A., Singh, B.N. (1988) "Severity of silent myocardial ischemia on ambulatory electrocardiographic monitoring in patients with stable angina pectoris: relation to prognostic

determinants during exercise stress testing and coronary angiography", J Am Coll Cardiol, 12, 1169-1176.

12. Nademanee, K., Intarachot, V., Josephson, M.A., Rieders, D., Mody Vaghaiwalla, F., Singh, B.N. (1987) "Prognostic significance of silent myocardial ischemia in patients with unstable angina", J Am Coll Cardiol, 10, 1-9.
13. Fioretti, P., Brower, R.W., Simoons, M.L., et al. (1985) "Prediction of mortality during the first year after acute myocardial infarction from clinical variables and stress test at hospital discharge", Am J Cardiol, 55, 1313-1318.
14. De Busk, R.F., Kraemer, H.C., Nash, E., Berger, W.E., Lew, H. (1983) "Stepwise risk stratification soon after acute myocardial infarction", Am J Cardiol, 52, 1161-1166.
15. Starling, M.R., Crawford, M.H., Kennedy, G.T., O'Rourke, R.A. (1980) "Exercise testing early after myocardial infarction: predictive value for subsequent unstable angina and death", Am J Cardiol, 46, 909-914.
16. Leppo, J.A., O'Brien, J., Rothendler, J.A., Getchell, J.D., Lee, V.W. (1984) "Dipyridamole thallium-201 scintigraphy in the prediction of future cardiac events after acute myocardial infarction", N Engl J Med, 301, 1014-1018.
17. Corbett, J.R., Nicod, P., Lewis, S.E., Rude, R.E., Willerson, J.T. (1983) "Prognostic value of submaximal exercise radionuclide ventriculography after myocardial inafrction", Am J Cardiol, 52, 82A-91A.
18. Hakki, A.H., Nestico, P.F., Heo, J., Unwala, A.A., Iskandrian, A.S. (1987) "Relative prognostic value of rest thallium-201 imaging, radionuclide ventriculography and 24-hour ambulatory electrocardiographic monitoring after acute myocardial infarction", J Am Coll Cardiol, 10, 25-32.
19. Miller, D.H. and Borer, J.S. (1982) "Exercise testing early after myocardial infarction. Risks and benefits", Am J Med, 72, 427-438.
20. Gottlieb, S.O., Weisfeldt, M.L., Ouyang, P., Mellits, E.D., Gerstenblith, G. (1986) "Silent ischemia as a marker for early unfavorable outcomes in patients with unstable angina", N Engl J Med, 314, 1214-1219.
21. Rocco, M.B., Barry, J., Campbell, S., et al. (1987) "Circadian variation of transient myocardial ischemia in patients with coronary artery disease", Circulation, 75, 395-400.
22. Nademanee, K., Intarachot, V., Josephson, M.A., Singh, B.N. (1987) "Circadian variation occurrence of transient overt and silent myocardial ischemia in chronic stable angina and comparison with Prinzmetal angina in men", Am J Cardiol, 60, 494-499.
23. Deanfield, J.E., Shea, M., Kensett, M., et al. (1984) "Silent myocardial ischemia due to mental stress", Lancet, II, 1001-1005.

72
Chronic ischemic heart disease: prevention and therapy

P. PUDDU, G.M. PUDDU, C. BOZZOLI and A. MUSCARI

Istituto di Patologia Speciale Medica e Metodologia Clinica, University of Bologna, S. Orsola Hospital, via Massarenti 9, 40138 Bologna, Italy

In the term of "chronic ischemic heart disease" a series of different nosological, physiopathologic and etiological forms are included, which can differ even considerably in their therapy. Among these, stable, unstable, variant and microvascular angina are the most common, as well as the various forms in which chest pain is absent or is not the main symptom, such as "silent" ischemic heart disease and the arrhythmic or congestive forms. While at present the causes of microvascular angina are not well known, the forms affecting large epicardial vessels are mostly due to coronary atherosclerosis, although arterial diseases caused by different etiologies (infectious, dysreactive, malformative) may occasionally be involved. Therefore, from the point of view of both practical feasibility and interest due to incidence, the prevention of chronic ischemic heart disease actually coincides with atherosclerosis prevention.

1. Prevention

The prevention of atherosclerotic disease can start very soon, before the appearance of risk factors (Pre-primary prevention), or following risk factor appearance (Primary prevention), or after an acute cardiovascular event has occurred (Secondary prevention). Pre-primary prevention consists exclusively of hygienic-dietetic means, while other forms of prevention involve also the use of drugs (anti-hypertensive, lipid-lowering, anti-platelet and anti-anginal drugs). Obviously, the best results can be obtained with the earliest forms of prevention. However, this would require whole populations of young people complying to not easily acceptable dietetic habits and life-styles, especially taking into account that only a small percentage of those undergoing hygienic-dietetic restrictions would be destined to develop clinical symptoms. Conversely, finding subjects who do develop acute coronary events after having adequately controlled all risk factors, or having no risk factor at all, is not infrequent. New risk factors should come to light to allow the recognition of those subjects predisposed to atherosclerosis with more precision than is presently possible, so that they may actively and effectively be subjected to new or traditional means of prevention.

A few experimental studies have suggested that some factors of the immune system, especially of humoral immunity (antibodies, immune complexes, complement components), may be involved in atherogenesis [1,2]. On the other hand, apart from a considerable amount of evidence by Beaumont et al. concerning the existence of autoimmune forms of dyslipidemia [3], the clinical research on the immunological aspects of atherosclerosis has yielded only scanty or discordant results. This may be a consequence of the difficulty in performing adequately controlled studies, in consideration of the diffusion of atherosclerotic disease even in subjects without evident clinical symptoms. Taking into account these problems, we have recently studied [4] 2 groups of subjects highly selected for the presence or absence of significant atherosclerotic lesions (23 atherosclerotic subjects: 3 arterial stenoses greater than 75 % in different areas, documented by panangiography; 20 control subjects: absence of significant arterial stenoses in the arteriography of the aortic arch and normal response to exercise stress testing and Doppler ultrasonography of the lower limb arteries). In these subjects serum immunoglobulins (IgG, IgA, IgM) and 2 complement proteins (C3, C4) were assessed, as well as some traditional risk factors (serum total cholesterol, HDL-cholesterol, triglycerides, cigarette smoking, hypertension, diabetes, body mass index). The study showed that 2 immunological variables, serum IgA and C4, were higher in atherosclerotic subjects than in controls. This was demonstrated by both univariate analysis and multiple logistic regression. Serum IgA and C4 did not seem to be directly connected, since they were not correlated, IgA immune complexes do not bind complement factors and IgA aggregates can activate only the alternative pathway of complement, in which C4 is not involved. Therefore the subsequent attempts to obtain further explanations followed independent ways.

The production of IgA antibodies is normally stimulated in some body areas, including the intestinal area. Therefore we have considered the possibility that the antigens responsible for the production of specific IgA might be of alimentary origin. In 1967 Annand et al. proposed the theory, based on epidemiological data, that heat-denaturated milk proteins might be important risk

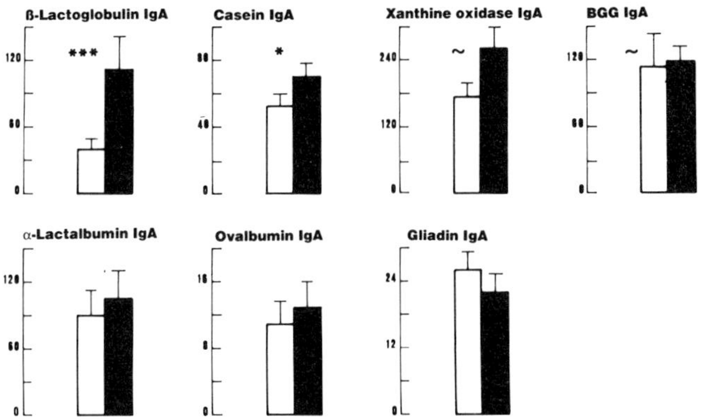

Figure 1. IgA antibodies against some food antigens in atherosclerotic subjects (solid bars) and controls (white bars). Values are mean ± 1 S.E.M. of absorbances at 405 nm X 1000. ~ P < 0.10, * P < 0.05, *** P < 0.005.

factors in the pathogenesis of coronary and cerebral thrombosis [5]. Subsequently Davis et al. [6] and Ross et al. [7] found that the titles of antibodies against milk proteins were higher in patients with myocardial infarction than in control subjects. After nearly a decade these researches were stopped since a few studies did not support the hypothesis of an association of anti-milk antibodies with coronary atherosclerosis [8, 9]. On the other hand, specific IgA antibodies against dietary antigens had never been investigated. For this reason we measured [10] by ELISA the IgA antibodies against ß-lactoglobulin, casein, α-lactalbumin, xanthine oxidase and bovine IgG (BGG) present in bovine milk, as well as the IgA antibodies against ovalbumin and gliadin, in the sera of the subjects selected in our previous study. Results (Fig. 1) showed that IgA antibodies against ß-lactoglobulin and casein were higher in atherosclerotic than in control subjects. No significant differences were found for IgG and IgM antibodies against the same antigens. We have considered some possible explanations according to which these findings might be caused by atherosclerosis, but none of them was convincing. Instead, the formation of circulating IgA immune complexes might be damaging to the arterial wall. This would agree with the fact that in some diseases in which generalized vascular injury occurs, such as Shönlein-Henoch purpura and diabetic microangiopathy, high concentrations of circulating IgA immune complexes have been found [11, 12]. Since we found no difference in the consumption of milk and milk products between atherosclerotic and control subjects, it is possible that atherosclerotic subjects have an abnormal tendency, perhaps genetically established, to produce IgA antibodies in excess in response to a normal absorption of undigested milk (and possibly of other origin) proteins.

A recent study by Beaumont et al. [13] showed the presence of LDL- or HDL-containing IgA immune complexes, mostly of the IgA class, in the sera of coronary artery disease subjects. Therefore we were prompted to measure, again by ELISA, the IgA antibodies against the 3 main lipoproteins (LDL, HDL, VLDL) and the apoproteins B and AI in the same sera previously studied, to ascertain possible correlations with IgA antibodies to milk proteins. This study (to be published) showed that: 1) All the IgA antibodies to apoproteins and lipoproteins, except anti-apo AI, were significantly higher in the sera of atherosclerotic subjects than in controls. The most significant difference concerned anti-apo B IgA; 2) These autoantibodies were present in at least 50 % of atherosclerotic subjects; 3) Most of the possible correlations of anti-apoprotein and anti-lipoprotein IgA with IgA antibodies to milk proteins were significant. The correlation of anti-ß-lactoglobulin with anti-apo B IgA ($P < 0.0005$) and all the correlations involving anti-BGG IgA were the most significant; 4) All the IgA antibodies associated with atherosclerosis (especially anti-lipoprotein IgA) correlated strongly with total IgA. According to all these data, the hypothesis that modified apoproteins may cause the formation of antibodies cross-reactive with milk proteins seems worth consideration. However, the inverse cannot be excluded, that is to say antibodies originally produced against some milk proteins might subsequently interact with apoproteins due to some structural similarity of the molecules. The interaction of lipoproteins with antibodies seems to increase their atherogenicity significantly and in fact the transformation of macrophages into foam cells is induced or considerably accelerated, in vitro, by the presence of antibody-lipoprotein immune complexes [14]. On the other hand, macrophages incubated with even large amounts of non-complexed or non-modified lipoproteins do not become foam cells [15].

As far as the association between C4 and atherosclerosis is concerned, another study by our group (unpublished data) showed the existence of a highly significant correlation between serum C4 and total cholesterol ($P < 0.0001$ in univariate analysis, Fig. 2; $P = 0.005$ in multiple linear regression, only in men). Crystalline cholesterol present in atherosclerotic plaques is a highly immunogenic structure which causes the production of complement-fixing

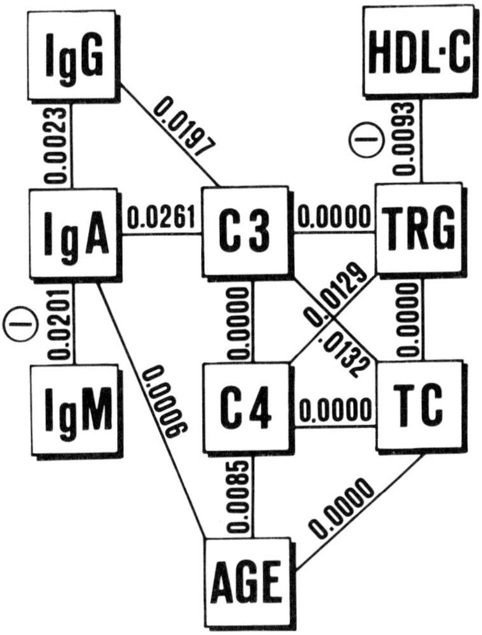

Figure 2. Simple correlations (P values) among immunological and lipid variables in 87 control subjects aged 20-75. Minus signs indicate inverse correlations.

antibodies [16]. Indeed, cholesterol has been shown to activate complement through the classic pathway [17], where C4 is involved. Serum C4 might therefore increase secondarily to the presence of atherosclerotic lesions, due to accelerated synthesis stimulated by chronic activation. On the other hand, the damaging properties to cell structures of complement activation products might contribute to the progression and aggravation of atherosclerotic lesions.

In conclusion, at present some humoral immunological variables can be considered as markers of atherosclerosis. Prospective studies are needed to ascertain whether they can also be used as new independent risk factors and whether this may provide some additional advantage, with respect to traditional risk factors, in the prevention of coronary events.

2. Therapy

Most of the therapeutic means commonly employed in chronic ischemic heart disease are actually preventive means of coronary atherosclerosis, coronary thrombosis or acute ischemic events. The main classes of drugs used, as everybody knows, are beta-blockers, calcium antagonists and nitrates, with non-substantial differences among the single components of each class. Their mechanisms of action, even at the molecular level, have been almost entirely elucidated and are reported in every textbook, as well as the benefits of anti-platelet, anti-thrombotic, anti-arrhythmic, inotropic and vasodilator drugs. What appears worth emphasizing, in a certainly non-exhaustive critical review, is the therapeutic approach to some particular clinical forms that have been recently included in the vast field of chronic ischemic heart disease, namely microvascular angina, silent ischemia and ischemic cardiomyopathy.

Microvascular angina (syndrome X) is a clinical syndrome characterized by episodes of effort and sometimes also rest angina, positive exercise stress testing, episodes of silent ischemia and angiographically normal coronaries with no signs of coronary spasm. This type of angina had been previously related to an impaired vasodilator capacity of the coronary micro-circulation, perhaps due to calcium imbalance. Actually, microvascular angina seems to be a consequence of a general disorder affecting the smooth muscle, involving both coronary and peripheral vessels, caused by hypersensitivity to neurogenic or humoral vaso-constrictor stimuli or by diffuse alteration of the myogenic tone. The therapy of these forms of angina has not yet been established. Although some beneficial but variable effects heve been obtained with calcium antagonists [18], recent studies have shown the effectiveness of propranolol [19], which abolished or sharply reduced the frequency and duration of ischemic episodes in some patients with syndrome X. This seems to suggest that ischemia and the decrease in coronary reserve are almost exclusively induced by an increase in oxygen demand, probably caused by sympathetic hyperactivity, similarly to what is thought to occur in silent ischemia.

Silent ischemia is defined as an objective evidence of myocardial ischemia in the absence of anginal pain or other symptoms. It occurs in coronary patients during exercise, rest or even sleep, has short duration and sometimes is induced by mental stress or cigarette smoking. Silent ischemia may not be associated with an increase in heart rate, due to primary reduction of myocardial blood flow. This may be referred to a functional abnormality of the endothelium in the atherosclerotic coronary arteries or to vasoconstriction caused by pulsatile hyperincretion of epinephrine. The drugs commonly used for the treatment of symptomatic ischemia are usually effective in decreasing the incidence of silent ischemic episodes, but higher doses are often needed. The administration of metoprolol in the forms with epinephrine increase [20] has been shown to reduce the duration of myocardial ischemia.

In ischemic cardiomyopathy the coronary disease is associated with a severe myocardial dysfunction often undistinguishable from primary congestive cardiomyopathy. Heart failure symptoms are pre-eminent and progressively overwhelm the initial angina or silent ischemia. Although Q waves may be present in the electrocardiogram, chronic ischemia may cause loss of contractility with maintainance of myocardial viability ("hibernating myocardium") [21]. If inotropic drugs are effective, indicating that a significant contractile reserve is still present, coronary by-pass or angioplasty, if practicable, may prolong survival. Very little can be done with medical treatment alone, although an appropriate medical therapy may be of benefit in the forms with prevalent arrhythmic disturbances, which nevertheless sometimes require subsequent electric or surgical therapy.

3. References

1 Howard, A.N., Patelski, J., Bowyer, D.E. and Gresham, G.A. (1971) 'Atherosclerosis induced in hypocholesterolaemic baboons by immunological injury and the effects of i/v polyunsaturated phosphatidyl choline', Atherosclerosis, 14, 17.

2 Muir, C., Taylor, T.G. and Munday K.A. (1977) 'An investigation in rabbits of the immunological theory of atherogenesis', Proc. Nutr.Soc., 36, 95A.

3 Beaumont, J.L. and Beaumont, V. (1977) 'Autoimmune hyperlipidemia', Atherosclerosis, 26, 405.

4 Muscari, A., Bozzoli, C., Gerratana, C., Zaca', F., Rovinetti, C., Zauli, D., La Placa, M., and Puddu, P. (1988) 'Association of serum IgA and C4 with severe atherosclerosis', Atherosclerosis, 74, 179.

5 Annand, J.C. (1967) 'Hypothesis: heated milk protein and thrombosis', J. Atheroscler. Res., 7, 797.

6 Davies, D.F., Davies, J.R. and Richards, M.A. (1969) 'Antibodies to reconstituted dried cow's milk protein in coronary heart disease', J. Atheroscler. Res., 9, 103.

7 Ross., J. and Oster, K.A. (1975) 'Milk-protein antibodies and myocardial infarction', Lancet, ii, 1037.

8 Toivanen, A., Viljanen, M.K. and Savilhati, E. (1975) 'IgM and IgG anti-milk antibodies measured by radioimmunoassay in myocardial infarction', Lancet, ii, 205.

9 Gibney, M.J., Gallagher, P.J., Sharratt, G.P., Benning, H.S. Taylor, G. and Pitts, J.M. (1980) 'Antibodies to heated milk protein in coronary heart disease', Atherosclerosis, 53, 119.

10 Muscari, A., Volta, U., Bonazzi, C., Puddu, G.M.,

Bozzoli, C., Gerratana, C., Bianchi, F.B. and Puddu, P. (1989) 'Association of serum IgA antibodies to milk antigens with severe atherosclerosis', Atherosclerosis, 77, 251.

11 Levinsky, R.J. and Barratt,T.M. (1979) 'IgA immune complexes in Henoch-Schönlein purpura', Lancet, ii, 1100.

12 Triolo, G., Giardina, E., Rinaldi, A. and Bompiani, G.D. (1984) 'IgA- and insulin-containing (C3-fixing) circulating immune complexes in diabetes mellitus', Clin. Immunol. Immunopathol., 30, 169.

13 Beaumont, J.L., Doucet, F., Vivier, P. and Antonucci, M. (1989) 'Immunoglobulin-bound lipoproteins (Ig-Lp) as markers of familial hypercholesterolemia, xanthomatosis and atherosclerosis', Atherosclerosis, 74, 191.

14 Klimov, A.N., Denisenko, A.D., Vinogradov, A.G., Nagornev, V.A., Pivovarova, Y.D., Sitnikova, O.D. and Pleskov, V.M. (1988) 'Accumulation of cholesteryl esters in macrophages incubated with human lipoprotein-antibody autoimmune complex', Atherosclerosis, 74, 41.

15 Brown, M.S. and Goldstein, J.L. (1983) 'Lipoprotein metabolism in the macrophage: implications for cholesterol deposition in atherosclerosis', Annu. Rev. Biochem., 52, 223.

16 Swartz, G.M.Jr., Gentry, M.K., Amende, L.M., Blanchette-Mackie, E.J. and Alving, C.R. (1988) 'Antibodies to cholesterol', Proc. Natl. Acad. Sci. USA, 85, 1902.

17 Hammerschmidt, D.E., Greenberg, C.S., Yamada, O., Craddock, P.R. and Jacob, H.S. (1981) 'Cholesterol and atheroma lipids activate complement and stimulate granulocytes. A possible mechanism for amplification of ischemic injury in atherosclerotic states', J. Lab. Clin. Med., 98, 68.

18 Ferrini, D., Bugiardini, R., Galvani, M., Gridelli, C., Tollemeto, D. and Puddu P. (1986) 'Opposing effects of propranolol and diltiazem on the angina threshold during an exercise test in patients with syndrome X', G. Ital. Cardiol., 16, 1224.

19 Bugiardini, R., Borghi, A., Biagetti, L. and Puddu, P. (1989) 'Comparison of verapamil versus propranolol therapy in syndrome X', Am. J. Cardiol., 63, 286.

20 Lee, D.D-P., Kimura, S., De Quattro, V. (1989) 'Noradrenergic activity and silent ischemia in hypertensive patients with stable angina: effect of metoprolol', Lancet, i, 403.

21 Braunwald, E. and Rutherford, J.D. (1986) 'Reversible ischemic left ventricular dysfunction: evidence for the "hibernating myocardium"', J. Am. Coll. Cardiol., 8, 1467.

73
Cholesterol and coronary heart disease - the pros and cons for action

M.F. OLIVER

Wynn Institute for Metabolic Research, London NW8 9SQ

UNWISE OPINIONS

The voice of the moderate regarding policies for lowering cholesterol levels is not often heard. By their nature, the propagandists for lowering everyones cholesterol shout louder and the voices of the more cautious are in danger of being silenced. The vociferous entry of self-appointed health educationalists into the cholesterol-coronary heart disease (CHD) field has led to unwise claims and excesses. These include, for example, the unqualified statement of the National Heart Lung Blood Institute Consensus[1] "Reduction of blood cholesterol levels will reduce the rate of coronary heart disease" and "all patients after myocardial infarction should have their cholesterol brought down to 160 mg/dl" (Rifkind, this conference). There have been equally unwise statements from the ultraconservative such as "the ideology behind the current health promotion rhetoric is an unhealthy mix of Utopian and totalitarian thinking".[2]

This sort of polarisation is not only irresponsible but, more important, it has introduced an unnecessary emotional element into a complicated subject. More scientific rigour and intellectual honesty and discipline are needed in order to give real perspective and also to identify the problems which require further research and new initiatives. I shall endeavour to provide some perspective regarding these issues: I will summarise this briefly and refer the reader to a fuller analysis recently published.[3]

ACTION FOR THOSE AT HIGH RISK

The data provided through the follow-up of the control group of the Multiple Risk Factor Intervention Trial[4] has clearly indicated the nature of the relationship between serum cholesterol and total mortality, on the one hand, and between serum cholesterol and CHD mortality, on the other hand (Fig 1). The relationship between serum cholesterol and CHD mortality is a continuum. It is curvilinear and not linear. It follows from this that a proportionately greater yield can be expected through successful intervention to lower serum cholesterol

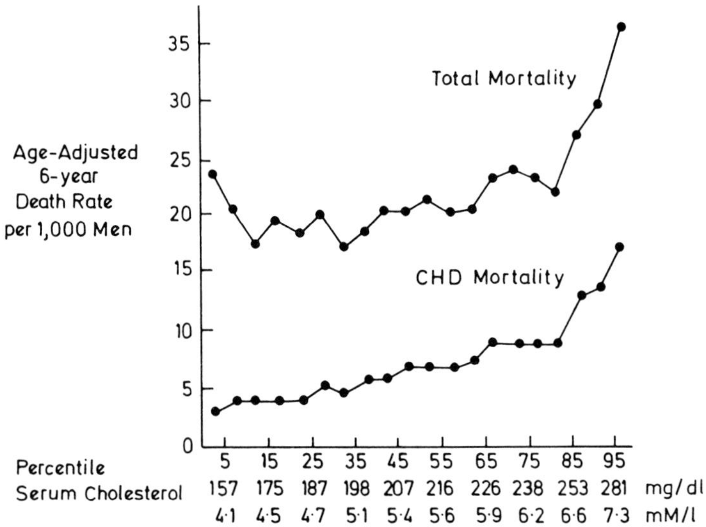

Age-adjusted CHD and total 6-year death rate per 1000 men screened for MRFIT according to serum cholesterol percentiles.

Figure 1

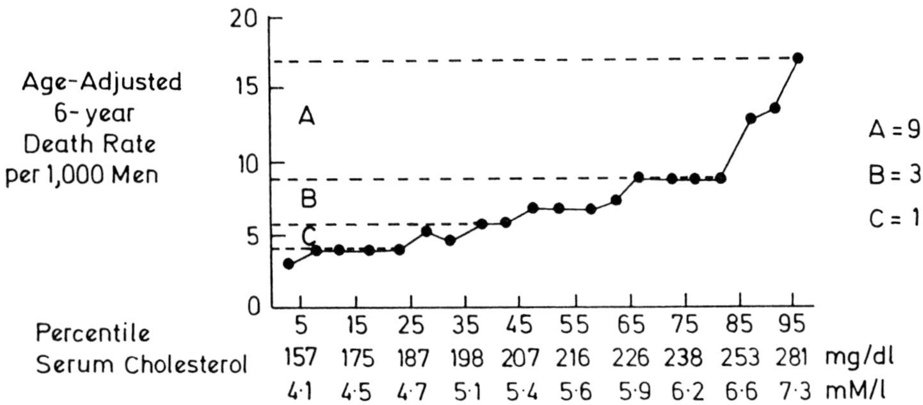

Age-adjusted CHD and total 6-year death rate per 1000 men screened for MRFIT according to serum cholesterol percentiles.

Figure 2

when initially high in comparison with intervention at lower levels (Fig 2); even although there are fewer people with high levels. From Fig 2 it can be seen that completely successful reduction of serum cholesterol from a level of approximately 7.3 mmol/L to 6.6 mmol/L might be associated with 9/1000 fewer deaths over a six year period. Similarly, reduction of serum cholesterol from a level of about 5.9 mmol/L to 5.1 mmol/L might be associated with three fewer deaths per thousand over a six year period. Whereas reduction below about 5 mmol/L produces very little theoretical benefit and none has yet been shown in practice.

It is interesting to translate this information into a population and for the United Kingdom, where there are 9 million men between the ages of 30 and 65, the best that would be expected is 3,600 fewer deaths per year in those with serum cholesterol concentrations above 6.5 mmol/L and the total reduction is in the region of 6,000 fewer deaths per year. Thus, most of the protection has been derived from intervention in the group with the highest serum cholesterol concentrations. (Table 1).

Supporting the high risk strategy are the results of the three major cholesterol lowering intervention trials.[5-7] All of these were conducted in middle-aged men with initial serum cholesterol levels above the 66th percentile and, in the case of the LRC-CPPT[6] and Helsinki Heart Study[7], the initial serum cholesterol was above the 90th percentile. These studies are consistent in showing an impressive and significant reduction in the incidence of non-fatal myocardial infarction. They did not show a significant reduction in cardiac mortality. It must be emphasised that the intervention trials were

TABLE I

ESTIMATE OF BENEFIT FOR CHOLESTEROL REDUCTION

Men 30 – 65 in UK

Cholesterol (mmol/l)	Nos	Reduction in CHD Deaths Over 6 years*	Best estimate/year
< 5.2	3000000	1/1000	500
5.2 – 6.5	3600000	3/1000	1800
> 6.5	2400000	9/1000	3600
All	9000000		6000

Derived from MRFIT (361000 men) estimates

all conducted in men between the ages of 30 and 64 and that initially they had marked elevation of serum cholesterol. The trials all involved drugs not diets. None were conducted in women.

Postponement of myocardial infarction is an important contribution to the quality of life and it is reasonable to assume that this would be associated in time with some reduction of cardial mortality, even although this was not possible to demonstrate during the 5-7 year period of the trials.

If any further argument is needed to support the high risk stragegy, it can be derived from the fact that 30%-35% of myocardial infarction "attributable" to serum cholesterol concentrations occurs above the 85th percentile.[8] There has been remarkable consistency in epidemiological surveys to indicate that the graded risk, demonstrated in the MRFIT data, applies in almost all Western populations. Additionally, the motivation from persons with a family history of premature CHD and from those with known high cholesterol levels is great. Similarly, the enthusiasm for doctors to lower serum cholesterol in such individuals is high.

ACTION IN THOSE WITH MILD ELEVATION OF SERUM CHOLESTEROL

There is a considerable temptation, not resisted enough by some of the professional trial investigators, to extrapolate the successful results of the cholesterol intervention trials in those with hypercholesterolaemia to otherwise healthy people with mild elevation of serum cholesterol. This is understandable but not, in my opinion, justified until formal clinical trials proving efficacy have been conducted. It is even less justifiable to recommend lowering of serum cholesterol below 5 mmol/L. Such advice is based on opinions and not facts.

From Fig 2 it will be seen that the number likely to benefit - assuming that it really is possible to lower mild elevation of serum cholesterol safely and consistently over many years - will be only in the region of 3/1000 fewer deaths from CHD over 6 years. But it can also be calculated that there will be in the region of 20-25 fewer non-fatal myocardial infarcts over a 6 year period and this is a worthwile contribution to public health.

The costs of drugs maybe punitive, both to the individuals and to governments. The annual cost of gemfibrozil may be calculated as £200 per year, of most HMGCoA reductase inhibitors as being in the region of £500 per year and of the anion-exchange resins in the region of £800 per year. If one assumes an average cost of £500 per man per year, then for the UK, - where there are three million men with serum cholesterol levels of 5.2 - 6.5 mmol/L, - the cost will be £1.5 billion per year. Additionally, the adverse effects of these drugs will have to be taken into account. It is not possible at this particular time to assess the safety of the HMGCoA reductase inhibitors, although few serious adverse effects have been reported.

The alternative is a strict diet but experience, outside control diet conditions, indicates that compliance to a strict diet is extremely poor. Even within the conditions of clinical trials, such as the MRFIT, compliance to a diet sufficient to reduce serum cholesterol significantly was bad. No large scale dietary trial has been conducted and it is not possible to conclude with certainty that reduction of serum cholesterol through dietary means reduces non-fatal myocardial infarction or even cardiac death. Nevertheless, epidemiological data is strong enough to advocate a reduction in total fat calories, particularly from saturated fats. The wisest policy, therefore, for individuals with mild elevation of serum cholesterol is to give them specific attention to every risk factor and include advice regarding a prudent diet. This is consistent with the recommendations of the European Atherosclerosis Society.[9]

UNRESOLVED PROBLEMS

RELATIONSHIP OF CHOLESTEROL TO CANCER

There is little doubt that there is a relationship between serum cholesterol and disease, as illustrated in Fig 3. There have been sufficient reports to indicate an increased incidence of cancer, particularly colon cancer, in individuals with low serum cholesterol concentrations for the issue to be taken seriously. The relationship between low serum cholesterol and cancer remains at least six years after baseline serum cholesterol estimations were made and longer in

POSSIBLE RELATION BETWEEN PLASMA CHOLESTEROL AND DISEASE

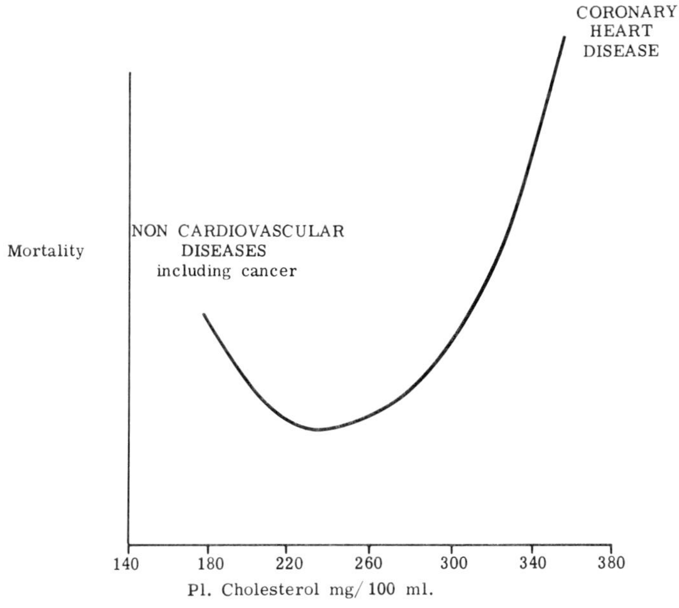

some studies and cannot be explained away by the presence of undetected cancer. While Epstein[10] has provided a review indicating no study has been large enough to confirm the association, none has - by the same token - been large enough to refute the relationship. Therefore, more data requires to be collected. The matter becomes more relevant as a result of the fact that two of the three major intervention trials to lower very high serum cholesterol were associated with an increased incidence of cancer. This was significant in the case of the WHO Clofibrate Trial. It was not significant in the case of the LRC-CPPT trial, even although there was an excess of colon cancer in the cholestyramine group compared with the control (21 compared with 11). I have raised the question on a preceding occasion[11] about the extent of reduction of body cholesterol or of membrane cholesterol which occurs with a 10% reduction in plasma cholesterol over 10-20 years and the extent that reduction of membrane cholesterol can occur without impaired biological function of membranes. These questions remain unanswered. An answer is certainly needed before reduction of mild hypercholesterolaemia below levels in the region of 5.0 mmol/L becomes a universal policy. The answer should be derived from the ongoing primary prevention trials using HMGCoA reductase inhibitors, since these drugs lower serum cholesterol profoundly, but will not be available for at least 5 years. It is encumbent on investigators concerned with these trials to ensure accurate and complete monitoring of non-cardiovascular deaths, particularly cancer.

LOW CHOLESTEROL AND VASCULAR DISEASE

Low cholesterol appears also to be associated with an increased incidence of haemorrhagic, as distinct from thrombotic, stroke.[12] The explanation of this is not clear but it has been recorded sufficiently frequently to require attention in a brief review such as this.

Those who promote the view that cholesterol-lowering is the answer to CHD do not seem to realise that the commonest cause of death in persons with low serum cholesterol is coronary heart disease. They argue that most people's cholesterol is not low enough and that were it to be lowered to levels in the region of 4 or 3.5 mmol/L then CHD would not be the principal cause of death. This is an entirely theoretical argument because such levels of cholesterol have not been achieved in a large population for long periods. An alternative approach is to conclude that there are potent, and as yet ill-defined, factors determining the development of CHD other than serum cholesterol and that more research into and control of these should be the priority.

SIGNIFICANCE OF HYPERCHOLESTEROLAEMIA IN WOMEN

There are important differences regarding the relationship of serum cholesterol and CHD between women and men. This needs to be emphasised, since more than half of the adult population comprises women and neither screening nor aggressive intervention is supported by the facts.

There are three main points to make regarding serum cholesterol concentrations in women. The first is that there is no statistical relationship internationally between serum cholesterol and coronary mortality: for the 19 countries with accepted good death certification for CHD, there was a correlation coefficient of 0.67 for serum cholesterol in men and a non-significant correlation of 0.24 for women[12]. Second, there is no significant relationship between serum cholesterol and CHD prognosis in women, in contrast to the well-known and clearly identified graded difference between serum cholesterol and prognosis in men[13]. Third, no clinical trials of the effect of reducing hypercholesterolaemia have ever been conducted in women. It should not be assumed, therefore, that women will benefit by reducing hypercholesterolaemia as men. Clinical observations have provided many, although anecdotal, reports that hypercholesterolaemia is well tolerated in women into their seventies. It has been argued that elevation, postmenopausely, of serum LDL in women is likely to have the same deleterious effect on coronary arteries as in men but the exposure will, of course, be very much shorter and any related excess of CHD is not likely to be seen until the seventies.

SECONDARY PREVENTION

There are advocates of lowering the serum cholesterol of every patient following a myocardial infarct. This is a complex area which appears to be overshadowed recently by two reports suggesting that the use of nicotinic acid has reduced cardiac mortality after myocardial infarction. One of these, the Coronary Drug Project, was a nine year follow-up of patients who received niacin for 5 years at the end of which time there was a marginally significant reduction in non-fatal myocardial infarction. At the end of the follow-up, there was a reduction in cardiac mortality[14]. The other study was an unblinded and relatively small uncontrolled clinical trial in which compliance to niacin was very variable[15]. Even if it is true that the administration of nicotinic acid reduced cardiac mortality, it should not be concluded that this is a result of lowering serum cholesterol since the principal effect of nicotinic acid is on triglyceride rich VLDL. Additionally, nicotinic acid has well-established and prolonged vasodilator activity. The most important determinant of prognosis after myocardial infarction is reduction of left ventricular ejection fraction or reduction of systolic volume. In other words, myocardial damage sustained at the time of the infarct determines long-term outcome. Additionally, there is almost certainly a thrombotic tendency in some patients following myocardial infarction and it is unlikely that this will be influenced by lowering serum cholesterol. Nevertheless, it is certainly wise to attempt to reduce very high levels of serum cholesterol particularly in patients with angina and those who have had coronary by-pass surgery in order to maintain graft patency. But to use expensive drugs for those with mild elevation of cholesterol levels will add an unnecessary additional economic burden to patients with myocardial infarction, who are probably already taking some combination of drugs for reduction of symptoms and improvement of effort tolerance.

CONCLUSION

Every effort should be made to lower marked hypercholesterolaemia and raised LDL - those in the top quartile of cholesterol distribution - in young and middle aged men and probably also in patients with angina. The aim of this is to postpone non-fatal myocardial infarction. Action at lower levels will be of limited benefit.

The extension of the above recommendation to young and old men and to women is not founded on fact. The relationship between serum cholesterol and CHD in women is different from that in men and is not significant. Nor is there a relationship between serum cholesterol concentrations and prognosis in women.

At present, it does not appear that reduction of hypercholesterolaemia reduces cardiac mortality significantly. Clinical trials of successful reduction of hypercholesterolaemia have been associated with an increase in non-cardiovascular mortality. Total mortality has remained unchanged.

The relationship of low serum cholesterol concentrations to cancer remains unresolved. It is a sufficiently important question for an increased research effort to be made.

The most well documented indication for cholesterol-lowering after the development of symptoms of CHD is post-coronary artery by-pass grafting.

1. Consensus Conference. Lowering blood cholesterol to prevent heart disease. JAMA 1985; 253: 2080-2086.

2. McCormick J, Skrabanck P. Coronary heart disease is not preventable by population interventions. Lancet 1988; 2: 839-841.

3. Oliver MF. Should hypercholesterolaemia be treated aggressively. Debates in Medicine 1990; Vol.3 (In press).

4. Martin MJ, Hulley SB, Browner WS, Kuller LH, Wentworth D. Serum cholesterol, blood pressure and mortality: implications from a cohort of 361,662 men. Lancet 1986; 2: 933-936.

5. Committee of Principal Investigators. WHO co-operative trial in the primary prevention of ischaemic heart disease using clofibrate. Brit Heart J 1978; 40: 1069-1118.

6. The Lipid Research Clinic Coronary Primary Prevention Trial Results. 1. Reduction in incidence of coronary heart disease. JAMA 1984; 251, No. 3: 351-374.

7. Frick MH, Elo O, Haapa K, Heinonen OP, Heinsalmi P, Helo P, Huttunen JK, Kaitaniemi P, Koskinen P, Manninen V, Maenpaa H, Malkonen M, Manttari M, Norola S, Pasternack A, Pikkarainen J, Romo M, Sjoblom T, Nikkila EA. Helsinki Heart Study: Primary Prevention Trial with Gemfibrozil in middle-aged men with dyslipidaemia. NEJM 1987; 317: 1237-1245.

8. Heller RF, Chinn S, Tunstall-Pedoe HD, Rose G. How well can we predict coronary heart disease? Findings in the United Kingdom heart disease prevention project. Br Med J 1984; 288: 1409-11.

9. Study Group, European Atherosclerosis Society. Strategies for the prevention of coronary heart disease: A policy statement of the European Atherosclerosis Society. Euro Heart J 1987; 8: 77-88.

10. Epstein FH. This meeting - Editor please complete.

11. Oliver MF. Serum cholesterol - the knave of hearts and the joker. Lancet 1981; ii: 1090-5.

12. Simons LA. Interrelations of lipids and lipoproteins with coronary artery disease mortality in 19 countries. Am J Cardiol 1986; 57: 5G-10G.

13. Anderson KM, Castelli WP, Levy D. Cholesterol and mortality: 30 years of follow-up from the Framingham Study. JAMA 1987; 257: 2176-2180.

14. Canner PL, Berge KG, Wenger NK, Stamler J, Friedman L, Prineas RK, Friedewald W. Fifteen year mortality in Coronary Drug Project patients: Long-term benefit with Niacin. JACC (1986) 8 No. 6: 1245-1255.

15. Carlson LA and Rosenhamer G. Reduction in mortality in the Stockholm Ischaemic Heart Disease Secondary Prevention Study by combined treatment with Clofibrate and Nicotinic Acid. Acta Med Scand 1988; 223: 405-418.

74
Diagnosis and evaluation of ischemic heart disease

M. SANGIORGI and D. DE NARDO
Department of Internal Medicine, Institute of "Clinica Medica", II University of Rome "Tor Vegata", Italy

Methodology for clinical procedure

Diagnostic approach to coronary artery disease patients primarily involves the internist. Anamnesis, physical examination and evaluation of risk factors enable the internist to assess a priori the pretest probability of coronary artery disease (CAD). Therefore a diagnostic iter will be started employing a sequence of independent tests. The goal of the sequence is to obtain a growing acquisition of knowledge in order to place the patient into a sufficiently low or high disease probability category.This approach is based on the sequential bayesian analysis, the statistical law of conditional probability, which states that the posttest probability can not be directly assessed only by the test result but it is influenced by the prevalence of disease, namely pretest probability. This clinical procedure is effective in the vast majority of patients, and yet some limiting factors to a strict bayesian approach have to be considered. Sometimes the tests employed are not independent, the test results are not absolutely negative or positive and prominently we have not an adequate gold standard representing an ideal marker of myocardial ischemia.

Provocative tests for inducing ischemia

CAD remains the dominant cause of myocardial ischemia, and yet their relationship is not straightforward when considering that,on one hand, coronary atherosclerosis is not necessarily associated with myocardial ischemia and,on the other hand,functional variations as coronary spasm, vasomotor tone and platelet aggregation may primarily provoke a transient hypoperfusion. Functional abnormalities associated to development of myocardial ischemia may be revealed by clinical or laboratory markers. Regional myocardial perfusion impairment is reflected by transient defect of Thallium-201 myocardial uptake, metabolic impairment by abnormalities of radiolabeled fatty acids turnover, regional and global ventricular dysfunction by Echocardiography and radionuclide angiocardiography changes, ST segment changes by conventional ECG or Holter monitoring, and finally angina pectoris in the anamnesis.
Sometimes it is possible to identify some markers of myocardial ischemia using ECG Holter monitoring and ambulatory radionuclide monitoring of left ventricular function or in patients with numerous daily anginal episodes using radionuclide studies during a spontaneous episode. In the vast majority of patients, however, a physiologic or pharmacologic provocative test of inducible ischemia will be needed both to evaluate the presence of CAD and to determine its functional and prognostic significance, so contributing to assess the need for and efficacy of therapeutic options. A variety of procedures has been

proposed.Schematically some tests reveal ischemia induced by increased demand in front of a reduced flow reserve (isotonic stress test,atrial pacing, dipyridamole test); ergonovine and hyperventilation test may reproduce a primary blood flow reduction due to a dynamic vascular obstruction; additionally other tests may provoke in susceptible patients ischemia both increasing metabolic demand and producing a corresponding inadequate response in myocardial blood flow (isometric exercise, cold pressor test, mental stress, Beta-adrenergic stimulants administration).

Angina pectoris: the key symptom

Anginal pain is, indeed, the prominent symptom in CAD patients but it must be considered in the context of a careful history and clinical examination, evaluating the possible association with other symptoms and the characteristics of the pain. Approximately three-fourths of patients of our study population complained as a first pain syndrome a chest dysconfort related to exertion (just during physical stress 53.9 % of cases,both during physical activity and spontaneously 22.7 %) and only 13.7 % of patients suffered as first clinical manifestation from angor at rest and 9.7 % of patients had as first symptom of CAD a myocardial infarction.In a patient population (17) of 1465 males and 580 females studied with coronary angiography, CAD was detected in 89 % of males and 62 % of females with typical angina, in 70 % of males and 40 % of females with a probable history, whereas only in 22 % of males and 5 % of females with non anginal pain. In our study(9) of 121 males and 56 females suspected of CAD with combined use of ECG and Tl-201 stress tests, we had a statistically significant difference between patients with typical angina and patients with atypical chest pain when considering that in the first group combined test was positive in 82.4% and negative in 4.6 %,whereas 20.3 % had a positive test and 50 % had a negative combined test in the second group ; of significance in this regard,the patient group with typical angina had a higher mean age. The prevalence of CAD decreases substantially as chest pain becomes less typical.

ECG findings in myocardial ischemia

In patients with an intermediate probability (range of 10 % to 90 %)of CAD, the ECG stress test is generally the first test performed, unless ECG will be nondiagnostic a priori. On the other hand ECG has limited diagnostic value in women with atypical pain when considering that prevalence of CAD in patients with atypical angina is 2.5 times greater in men than in women while the incidence of false positive exercise ST segment responses is 4.5 times greater in women than in men. On the other hand, in male patients with atypical chest pain a positive exercise ST response provides a significant increase of the probability of CAD especially if ST segment depression is marked, appears early at low workloads, is associated to chest pain, has a long postexercise duration > 6' , and is associated to an abnormal systolic blood pressure response. Most commonly the ischemic exercise response consists of a horizontal or downsloping ST segment depression greater than 1 mm 0.08" after the end of QRS complex. Less frequently a ST segment elevation is exercise induced and it reflects, in the absence of previous infarction and a history of variant angina, a fixed coronary stenosis of marked hemodynamic severity. Additionally an exercise induced U wave inversion in the absence of electrolyte abnormalities, suggests a high grade stenosis in left anterior descending or in left main coronaries. Beyond the above mentioned criteria, other parameters associated with increased severity of CAD and poor prognosis are represented by onset of signs and symptoms of ischemia at heart rate < 120/min, appearance of ST segment depression in multiple leads and the occurrence of exercise induced ventricular tachicardia. Cumulative experience has demonstrated that sensitivity of ECG stress test for CAD detection (2, 13) is about 60% among the symptomatic patients and specificity 82 %. An important determinant of sensitivity seems to be the number of leads used. However, false negative rate is most likely due also to the level of exercise achieved. In patients who are unable to perform a treadmill or bicycle testing because of an impairment of lower extremities, arm ergometry represents an useful but less sensitive procedure. Other alternatives are represented by atrial pacing, an invasive procedure, which has a reported sensitivity ranging between 21 and 100 % and dipyridamole test with a reported sensitivity ranging between 8 and 53 %. Intravenous administration of Beta-adrenergic agonists appears promising. One important question is whether Holter monitoring for detection of myocardial ischemia improves diagnostic efficacy of ECG exercise test. Data of Tzivoni (16) show that only 74 of 118 patients who had a positive ST segment exercise response also had ischemic abnormalities detected by Holter monitoring during daily activity, so demonstrating a 37 % lower sensitivity for Holter monitoring in comparison with stress test for the detection of ischemic changes. On the other hand in subjects yet diagnosed as CAD patients, Holter monitoring may represent a valuable contribute to identify different mechanisms of ischemic cardiac pain also in the same patient, to detect silent myocardial ischemia and to characterize the incidence of the episodes, their duration and daily occurrence.

Nuclear medicine studies
Myocardial perfusion imaging

The sensitivity of ST segment depression on the ECG stress test is strictly influenced by the level of exercise achieved. On the contrary this is not the case with Tl-201 stress scan. In a study of Esquivel et al (7) the overall prevalence of Tl-201 initial defects is higher than ST segment depression on ECG and remains the same for all levels of effort except for patients with 1-vessel disease; additionally the prevalence of redistribution on delayed scan is higher than ST segment depression, except at higher levels of effort when they are similar. In this context it should be stressed that an impairment of regional relative myocardial blood flow and the subsequent regional ventricular metabolic and motion abnormalities develop earlier than ECG changes during an exercise test. That may well explain the clinical and experimental evidence that exercise radionuclide studies are both more sensitive and more specific than exercise ECG in CAD diagnosis. The overall sensitivity and specificity of Tl-201 stress scan by a visual analysis came to 83 % and 90 % respectively in a recent review of 22 published series (2) encompassing 2048 patients. Our experience with Tl-201 stress scan in 13 years regards more than 2000 patients. In this period we have observed an overall sensitivity of 86 % of Tl-201 and a sensitivity of combined stress test ECG and Tl-201 of 95 % with a specificity of Tl-201 ranging between 95 and 78 % as a function of patient population studied. It has been reported (2) that sensitivity and specificity of Tl-201 scan are both around 90 % when computer processing is used to obtain quantitative assessment. Sensitivity of CAD detection in patients with 1-, 2-, 3-vessel disease is respectively 80, 83, 96 %. However the location of stenosis and the extension of ischemic myocardium influence its detection. When, togheter with visual analysis, which has never to be omitted in our opinion, quantitative approach and analysis of segmental wash out is performed the sensitivity for detection of stenosis of left descending artery increases from 74 to 82 %, for circumflex artery from 40 to 61 % and for right coronary artery from 78 to 90 % without reduction of specificity. Computer quantitation of Tl-201 uptake and wash out provides incremental information for the detection of left main or multivessel coronary disease. In fact, 72 % of patients demonstrating a diffuse slow wash out has either 3-vessel or left main disease. Other parameters predictive of the proportion of myocardium at ischemic risk corresponding to the extent of CAD are represented by the number and location of defects in more than one vascular region and furthermore by an increased pulmonary Tl-201 uptake on stress scan reflecting an exercise-induced left ventricular failure (13). Additionally a cardiac dilatation on the first stress scan due to diffuse subendocardial ischemia and global left ventricular dysfunction is considered a high risk indicator (13) . Instead, only a minority of patients with left main disease shows the typical pattern of septal and posterolateral defects whereas more frequently the other indices of high risk are detected. In this context it should be stressed as index of hemodynamically severe disease a markedly severe defect which demonstrates slow reversibility (13). Of significance in this regard, some defects reverse after 4 hours,some defects reverse after 24 hours postexercise, some defects do not reverse and some defects are observed at rest Tl-201 scan, and yet viable myocardium is present. In these last istances a repeated injection of Tl-201, in our experience during acute administration of amyl nitrite (3), may aid in detecting severely underperfused but viable myocardium when a homogeneous Tl-201 uptake is gained by the drug.Thus Tl-201 stress study represents a valuable technique both for detecting CAD and for establishing patients management decisions, such as the need for coronary angiography and revascularization procedure (13). In view of an adequate interpretation of Tl-201 findings it is noteworthy that Tl-201 defects,sometimes reversible, may be observed in the absence of CAD in patients with idiopathic dilated or hypertrophic cardiomyopathies,or myocardial diseases due to sarcoidosis,scleroderma or in some patients with mitral valve prolapse. An intriguing problem arises in patients with LBBB. In such patients diagnosis of presence or absence of CAD remains frequently undetermined using noninvasive tests.This was the case in 45 % of patients in our study. In fact LBBB per se causes ECG is nondiagnostic a priori, Tl-201 shows an anteroseptal defect and radionuclide angiocardiography shows impaired global left ventricular function and septal wall motion abnormalities also in the absence of CAD. For these reasons in LBBB patients CAD may be diagnosed only under the condition that a transient Tl-201 defect is observed in areas other than anteroseptal. It is evident that the above mentioned defects in the absence of CAD have to be considered false positive findings of CAD, but they suggest the role of perfusion impairment due to microvascular abnormalities in some idiopathic or secondaries cardiomyopathies. In this context it should be stressed that also in CAD patients coronary angiography is only an imperfect descripter of coronary anatomy and it provides scarce information concerning regional myocardial blood flow, functional significance of a stenosis and of the visualized collateral vessels and regarding the proportion of myocardium at ischemic risk (13). Basing on this assumption, discordant findings between Tl-201 scan results and coronary angiography do not constantly mean that radionuclide test is wrong, when considering the possible inadequacy of the gold standard. In fact, Tl-201 false positive results are more frequently observed in patients with 25 to 50 % narrowing of coronary arteries than in patients with stenosis less than 25 % . A note of caution, however, is needed when considering that Tl-201 scan is prone to artifacts of the attenuation type caused, for istance, by breast tissue or a high diaphragm overlying the heart. Probably for this reason Tl-201 scan results have a reduced specificity in the female patients. In our study population of 79 females (1), suspected of CAD because of a chest pain with typical characteristics in 45 patients,just 18 % of combined stress test ECG and Tl-201 did not provide findings adequate to a diagnosis whereas a CAD was detected in 57 % of patients and excluded in 25 % . Of significance in this regard, the frequency of positive tests was significantly higher in patients with typical angina than in patients with atypical chest pain ($p<0.001$), whereas no significant differences were observed between the subgroup of patients with a rest ECG normal and the subgroup of patients with an abnormal baseline pattern of ST-T at rest. By contrast false negative results should be caused by superimposition of normoperfused myocardium, reduced size of hypoperfused area, an early redistribution in the presence of a long imaging time. However a normal stress Tl-201 study is associated with an excellent prognosis when considering that in these patients a cardiac death rate of 0.5% /year and a myocardial infarction incidence of 0.6% /year have been reported.

In our opinion, patients having an intermediate probability of CAD who need a Tl-201 scintigraphy are: asymptomatic patients with a positive exercise ECG, patients with nonanginal chest pain and a positive or nondiagnostic exercise ECG, patients with atypical angina, patients with typical angina and a negative exercise ECG.

An useful alternative to exercise in perfusion imaging is Dipyridamole test(administration of 0.75 mg/Kg in 4' i.v.)(4).The drug provokes arteriolar vasodilatation secondary to accumulation of adenosine, thus causing a maldistribution of blood flow in the subendocardial areas supplied by stenotic arteries whereas an increase of regional blood flow in areas perfused by normal coronary vessels occurs. The resultant dyshomogeneity of myocardial perfusion can be imaged by Tl- 201 scan. Some authors suggested also a mechanism of passive collapse of the stenosis operating during dipyridamole administration. In one study of ours in CAD patients (4), no changes of coronary angiography findings were observed during pharmacologic effect of dipyridamole; additionally dipyridamole caused angor and ischemic ECG changes in 50 % of patients and Tl-201 scan during dipyridamole demonstrated a sensitivity for CAD detection of 90 % comparable to exercise scintigraphy in the same patients. Similar high values of sensitivity have been reported by numerous studies. Thus this approach is adequate for patients who are unable to perform a satisfactory exercise test.

Radionuclide angiocardiography

Following Tl-201 stress test or dipyridamole test, a small percentage of patients will still have an intermediate probability of CAD.

In these patients a second radionuclide test should be employed in an attempt to define diagnosis: radionuclide angiocardiography (RNA).

Using RNA a positive test result may be represented by an abnormal ejection fraction (EF) response during exercise and the development of regional wall motion abnormalities (RWMA). Initially RNA had gained respect as diagnostic tool. Now, however, it is evident that an abnormal EF response to exercise can occur in the presence of cardiomyopaties, valvular diseases, hypertensive cardiopathy, and also in normal female subjects. Additionally, RWMA are detected, in the absence of CAD, in patients with LBBB, cardiomyopathies and mitral valve prolapse. A marked decline in the apparent specificity (14) of exercise RNA has been reported, whereas cumulative experience at many centers (2,10, 13) has demonstrated a sensitivity around 89 %. For these reasons RNA does not play a key role in the diagnosis of CAD; in fact a positive response represents a poorly specific result. Thus RNA should be employed, as diagnostic tool, only as second radionuclide test in patients with inconclusive Tl-201 stress scan. By contrast, in patients with known CAD,RNA provides useful parameters for the functional evaluation, risk stratification,thus aiding in patients management decision and in assessment of the efficacy of therapy. In this regard,absolute value of left ventricular EF, the degree of fall in EF at the peak of exercise, the number and location of exercise induced RWMA, transient left ventricle dilatation and the response of right ventricle EF are valuable indices of extent of CAD (13). Additionally, cumulative experience has reported as predictor of severe stenosis the magnitude of exercise induced RWMA and the low level of exercise to onset of RWMA. The combined use of myocardial perfusion imaging and RNA may be needed to assess functional significance of a stenosis or establish myocardial viability, thus contributing to decide the need for and the choice of the more adequate revascularization procedure (13). Furthermore, following revascularization surgery or in postangioplasty patient RNA and Tl-201 have a key role in assessing the effectiveness of the procedure in abolishing ischemia, the patency of grafts or restenosis occurrence.

The recent proposal of a new Tc-99m labeled isonitrile compound (MIBI- Tc99m) has been suggested to ameliorate the study of myocardial perfusion, when considering the better physical characteristics of Tc-99m than Tl-201. Because of high count rates it is now possible, with this radiopharmaceutical, to obtain during the same procedure of stress test(5) a ventricular function study by first transit angiocardiography, a myocardial perfusion imaging, and an ECG study, that could represent a valuable grid for the identification of CAD patients. Unfortunately, despite favourable promises, MIBI-Tc99m did not provide,at least using planar imaging,findings comparable to Tl-201 scan; these results seem to be unsatisfactory in the detection of periinfarction ischemia and ischemia induced by high levels of exercise. Better results were achieved with MIBI-Tc99m using single photon emission computed tomography. More accurate, indeed, seem the reults obtained using MIBI-Tc99m with SPECT acquisition during dipyridamole test. This is the case,probably,because a longer period of dyshomogeneous myocardial blood flow during dipyridamole test allows the myocardial uptake of MIBI-Tc99m to be different in ischemic and normoperfused areas.

Echocardiographic studies

Mechanical consequences of ischemia may well be detected by 2D- Echocardiography. Cumulative experience of several exercise studies has demonstrated (10) that the overall sensitivity of exercise 2D-Echocardiography is around 70 % while the specificty is around 90%.Technique limitations concerning image acquisition procedure should be overcome when considering that,accordingto some authors,images acquired immediately in the postexercise period in the decubitus position provide diagnostic information which is similar to that during peak exercise. It should be stressed that, using a new regional dysfunction or the worsening of preexisting dyssinergy as the marker of ischemia,most likely the level of exercise achieved influences test result. More recently some Authors have proposed Dipyridamole Echocardiography in the diagnosis of CAD. With the use of ECHO-Dipyridamole, a sensitivity around 56 % has been reported in patients with effort angina and 62 % in patients with angina at rest. In one study of ours in CAD patients with effort angina with the use of Dipyridamole test (4), echocardiographic study was positive in 40 % of patients , while an ischemic ST depression and angor were observed in 50 % of patients.

Coronary angiography: appropriate uses

Noninvasive methods we have above mentioned are able to provide an adequate diagnostic and functional evaluation in the vast majority of patients. Neverthless, coronary angiography remains the only technique available at present time for evaluating the anatomy of coronary arteries, so representing the unavoidable reference standard of the other methods and the basis of preoperative evaluation whenever a revascularization procedure is required. The use of coronary angiography is in expansion at present time because of the increasing development of various forms of therapeutic approach. However, in this regard it should be stressed that numerous variables other than anatomy have a key role in clinical decision making and in determining prognosis.According to this point of view and considering that coronary angiography is an invasive procedure associated to a low but finite morbidity, it should be recognized that its use is not justified just for improving diagnostic accuracy in patients who can not be considered a priori candidates for definitive treatment of angioplasty or surgery and in patients who have not been adequately studied by noninvasive methods. In our opinion, the use of coronary angiography is not justified also in patients with mild, stable angina in the absence of an impaired left ventricular function and of high risk criteria. Coronary angiography is, indeed.mandatory: in patients with evidence of high risk on noninvasive tests , when myocardial ischemia is detected in presence of prior myocardial infarction, in patients unresponsive to the treatment with an angina limiting the usual activities, in patients with unstable angina, in patients with Prinzmetal's angina. It is justified the use of coronary angiography: in male patients with typical angina aged less than 40 years, in female patients with typical angina aged less than 40 years when an objective evidence of ischemia has been obtained by Tl-201 scan.

Myocardial ischemia despite normal coronary angiograms

In a certain percentage (ranging between 10 and 30 %) of patients who had undergone coronary angiography because of typical effort angina and ischemic pattern at radionuclide and ECG studies coronary arteries are normal. In these subjects coronary spasm is inducible by ergonovine only in a small percentage of cases ranging between 2.2 and 6.8 % . A certain percentage of false negative ergonovine test results has to be considered. furthermore a certain percentage of false positive radionuclide and ECG studies really is obtained. Neverthless myocardial perfusion abnormalities, wall motion impairment,ECG changes and angor in the presence of normal coronary angiograms frequently suggest a substantial number of problems, unsolved at present time.

In our group of 9 patients with effort angina and normal coronaries, stress Tl-201 showed transient defects in 6; in these 6 patients Dipyridamole test caused in 2 cases angor, in 1 ECG ischemic changes, in 1 wall motion changes at Echocardiography,and transient defects of Tl-201 uptake in 6. Hypertension,diabetes, valvular and myocardial diseases,collagen diseases were not present in these 6 subjects having myocardial ischemia despite normal coronaries. Thus, a reduced dilatory reserve of the small coronary arteries could be hypothized(4) on the basis of the same ischemic pattern observed both at exercise and Dipyridamole scintigrams. An abnormal coronary vasomotion involving both epicardial and intramural vessels has been demonstrated(12) in similar patients by some authors. On the other hand,on the basis of histologic studies and contractility findings,other authors suggest that an early stage cardiomyopathy should be present in some cases (15), while microvascular abnormalities should be the explanation in other cases because of typical angina. The last two hypotheses, however, are not entirely conflicting. On one hand,in these patients frequently a LBBB is found and may represent the sole manifestation of an arrythmogeneous cardiomyopathy.Moreover it has been demonstrated that LBBB per se is able to provoke septal perfusion impairment, increase of lactate concentrations in coronary sinus during exercise test (11) and global and regional left ventricular dysfunction (6) trough the inefficiency of the abnormal sequence of ventricular contraction. On the other hand, on the basis of experimental studies (8) Factor and Sonnenblick have suggested that also human dilated cardiomyopathies could be caused by inhomogeneous blood flow to the myocardium due to microvascular spasm. At present time, a relationhip between idiopathic cardiomyopathies and "X syndrome" represents only a hypothesis when considering that their clinical presentation and course and prognosis appear very different.

In clinical practice, decision making must rely just on well defined and accepted criteria. However, diagnosis and functional evaluation of patients suspected of ischemic heart disease deserve a broad minded nonconformist approach. Myocardial ischemia occurs as a result of numerous,complex,dynamic and variable phenomena among which metabolic, neurogen,myogen, umoral factors and extravascular compressive forces play a role, at present time not well recognized, in the regulation of myocardial perfusion. The application with criticism of knowledge derived from research and technological resources use may result in a better comprehension of the various clinical entities.

References

1) Autore, C., Fragola, P., Pitucco, G. et al (1983) "La cardiopatia ischemica nella donna. Validita' diagnostica dell'uso combinato della prova da sforzo e della scintigrafia miocardica con Tallio-201", Clin Ter Cardiovasc 2,5, 247-258.

2) Beller, George A. and Gibson, Robert S.(1987) "Sensibilita', specificita' e significato prognostico delle metodiche di valutazione non invasiva per la coronaropatia occulta o manifesta", Prog in Pat Cardiovasc 30, 3, 187-221.

3) Caputo, V., De Nardo, D., De Angelis, A. et al (1983) "Possibilities of Thallium-201 myocardial scintigraphy in effort angina diagnosis", in M. Salvatore and E.Porta (eds.) Radioisotopes in Cardiology, Plenum Publishing Corporation, pp. 295-300.

4) Caputo, V., De Nardo, D., Antolini M., et al (1987) "Il test al Dipiridamolo e la scintigrafia miocardica con Tl-201 nella diagnosi della patologia ischemica miocardica", Radiol Med 73, 390-393.

5)Ciavolella, M., Giannitti, C., Scali, D. et al (1989) "Incremento di accuratezza nella diagnosi di cardiopatia ischemica mediante valutazione radioisotopica simultanea della funzione ventricolare regionale e della perfusione miocardica ed unico test ergometrico", Atti L Congresso Soc It Cardiol.

6) De Nardo,D., Antolini,M., Pitucco,G. et al (1988) "Effects of left bundle branch block on left ventricular function in apparently normal subjects.Study by equilibrium radionuclide angiocardiography at rest", Cardiology 75, 5, 365-371.

7) Esquivel, L., Pollock, Stewart G., Beller, George A. et al (1989) "Effect of the degree of effort on the sensitivity of the exercise Thallium-201 stress test in symptomatic coronary artery disease", Am J Cardiol 63, 160-165.

8)Factor, S. and Sonnenblick, E.(1982) "Hypothesis: Is congestive cardiomyopathy caused by a hyper-reactive myocardial microcirculation (microvascular spasm) ?", Am J Cardiol 50, 1149-1152.

9) Fragola, P., Autore, C., Pierangeli, L. et al (1984) "L'uso combinato dell'elettrocardiogramma da sforzo e della scintigrafia miocardica con Tallio-201 in soggetti con sospetta cardiopatia ischemica", Clin Ter Cardiovasc 3-4, 105-113.

10) Kaul, S. (1989) "Cardiac imaging in conjunction with exercise stress testing in patients with suspected coronary artery disease: a comparison of the techniques", Cardiovasc Imag 1, 20-28.

11) Mora, B., Douard, H., Barat, J.P. et al (1987) "Apparition simultanee d'un bloc de branche gauche et d'une douleur thoracique a' l'effort", Arch Mal Coeur 80,12, 1807-1811.

12) Pozzati, A., Morgagni, GL., Ottani, F. et al (1989) "Abnorme risposta coronarica a stimoli vasomotori: analogie tra angina variante e sindrome X", Cardiologia 34,5, 411-418.

13) Rozanski, A. and Berman, Daniel. S. (1987) "The efficacy of cardiovascular nuclear medicine exercise studies", Seminars in Nuclear Medicine 17,2, 104-120.

14)Rozanski, A., Diamond G., Forrester, J. et al (1983) " The declining specificity of exercise radionuclide ventriculography", N Engl J Med 309, 518-522.

15)Tartagni, F., Melandri, G., Tomassini, F. et al (1986) "Significato della positivita' della scintigrafia miocardica da sforzo nei pazienti a coronarie indenni: correlazioni clinico-strumentali", Cardiologia 31,1, 23-27.

16)Tzivoni, D., Gavish, A., Gottlieb, S. et al (1988) "Prognostic significance of ischemic episodes in patients with previous myocardial infarction", Am J Cardiol 62, 661-664.

17)Weiner, D., Ryan, T., McCabe, C. et al (1979) "Exercise stress testing. Correlation among history of angina, ST segment response and prevalence of coronary artery disease in the Coronary Artery Surgery Study (CASS)", N Engl J Med 301, 230-235.

ADDRESS: Prof. M. Sangiorgi, Director of Clinica Medica
II University of Rome, Ospedale S. Eugenio
p.le dell'Umanesimo. 00144 Rome Italy

75

Antioxidant metabolic mechanisms in hypertensive and atherosclerotic arterial wall

F. CUCCURULLO[1], D. LAPENNA[1], E. PORRECA[1], A. PENNELLI[2], G. RICCI[2] and G. DEL BOCCIO[2]

Istituto di Patologia Speciale Medica[1] and Istituto di Scienze Biochimiche[2], Università G. D'Annuzio, via dei Vestini, 66013 Chieti, Italy

ABSTRACT. In 7 rabbits subjected to suprarenal aortic coarctation (SAC: mean pressure gradient 37.6±4 mmHg, after 16 days), the aortic wall antioxidant system and lipid peroxidation of the hypertensive segment were tested. Aortic wall antioxidant system and lipid peroxidation were also studied in 24 rabbits fed a 0.5% cholesterol-enriched diet for 10, 30 and 60 days (groups A1, B1 and C1: 8 rabbits each), as compared to controls receiving a standard diet for the same periods (groups A, B and C).

After 16 days of SAC, a significant rise in Total thiol content (Tot-SH), Selenium-dependent Glutathione peroxidase (GSH-Px), Glutathione reductase (GS-SG Red) and Thiobarbituric acid reactive substances (TBARS) was observed. There was also evidence of Selenium-independent Glutathione peroxidase activity (GST-Px), whereas Glutathione transferase (GT) increased not significantly.

In cholesterol-fed rabbits, the percentage of intimal sudanophilia was negligible in group A, but progressively rose in group B (22±6%) and C (57±9%). Significant rise in Tot-SH and GSH-Px was observed in groups A1, B1 and C1. Total Superoxide dismutase activity underwent a significant rise only in groups B1 and C1. On the contrary, the activities of Catalase, GS-SG Red and GT underwent a persistent decrease in the experimental groups. GST-Px activity was not detectable. Finally, aortic TBARS levels reached the peak at 10 days and persisted unmodified at 30 and 60 days of atherogenic diet.

In conclusion, antioxidant metabolic mechanisms and lipid peroxidation are significantly modified in the hypertensive and atherosclerotic rabbit aortic wall, thus suggesting the involvment of free radical-mediated oxidative stress in the pathophysiology of these disease entities.

Introduction.

The problem of free radical-vascular wall interaction has recently emerged in the literature.Particularly, free radicals have been implicated in the pathophysiology of acute hypertension-induced vascular damage and atherosclerosis. Kontos et al. demonstrated that free radicals are produced in the brain microvasculature during experimental acute hypertension, inducing functional, biochemical and morphological changes (1).Furthermore, there is growing evidence that free radical-mediated oxidative injury plays a focal role in the pathophysiology of atherosclerosis, resulting in crucial events, such as endothelial damage and LDL oxidation (2, 3).

Moreover, any susceptibility of the vascular wall to the oxidative stress is critically influenced by the adequacy of the cellular antioxidant system. The present study investigates antioxidant metabolic mechanisms and lipid peroxidation in: a) the hypertensive aorta of rabbits subjected to suprarenal aortic coarctation ; b) the aortic tissue of rabbits fed on hyperlipidic diet.

Matherials and Methods.

Experimental hypertension. Male New Zealand white rabbits (2.5-2.8 kg.) were anesthetized with i.m.ketamine hydrochloride (75 mg/kg) and a midline laparotomy was performed. A silk ligature was passed around the abdominal aorta between mesenteric and renal arteries. In 7 rabbits (group B),the ligature was tightened until distal blood pressure was less than 30 mmHg (4). Seven sham-operated rabbits (group A) were treated in an identical manner, except for the ligature, which was not tightened. The blood pressure above the coarctaction was recorded by direct puncture of the central ear artery at the time of surgery and before sacrifice (16 days later). The blood pressure below the coarctaction was determined from the femoral artery. After sacrifice, the aorta from the aortic valve to the ligature was quickly removed and placed in ice-cold 0.1 M potassium phosphate buffer with 1 mM EDTA, ph 7.4 (buffer A).The vascular wall was carefully cleaned from the fat and connective tissue.
Experimental atherosclerosis. Male New Zeland white rabbits (age 2 months and weight 1.7-2 Kg) were divided at random in six groups, with 16 rabbits in each group.Eight animals were used for biochemical study and 8 for morphological study. The experimental groups received an atherogenic diet composed by 89.5% rabbits pellets, 5% lard, 5% peanut oil and 0.5 % cholesterol (5) for 10,30, and 60 days (groups A1, B1 and C1). The control groups were given a standard rabbit diet for the same period (groups A, B,and C). Another control group (8 rabbits) was studied right after an initial adaptation period of 2 weeks (group 0). The daily amount of pellets was 100 g for all rabbits, and water was given ad libitum.After sacrifice,the aortas were removed from the aortic valve to the iliac bifurcation for morphological or biochemical studies.
Sudan red staining. The aortas were fixed with 10% formalin for 24 h, rinsed in 70% ethanol and immersed in Sudan IV for 15 min (6).The percentage of aortic intimal involvement by lipid infiltration was determined by planimetry distribution of sudanophilia in the photographs.
Biochemical analysis. The vessels were weighed and homogenized (1:5 w/v) in buffer A. Thiobarbituric acid reactive substances (TBARS), an index of lipid peroxidation, were determined on this homogenate, according to the method of Ohkawa et al. (7) and expressed as nmoles of TBARS/g wet tissue. Total thiol compounds (Tot-SH: of which GSH represents the main biochemical pool) were assayed in the supernatant obtained after centrifugation at 1,000 rpm for 5 min. at 4°C, according to Ellman's method (8) and expressed as nmoles of R-SH/g wet tissue. Catalase (Cat) and Superoxide dismutase (SOD) activities were measured after centrifugation of the initial homogenate at 3,000 x g for 10 min. at 4°C. The Cat activity was assayed on the appropriate supernatant (made 1% by adding Triton X-100) by spectrophotometric method, following the decrease in absorbance at 240 nm and 25°C, due to the hydrogen peroxide decomposition by catalase (9). Specific activity was expressed as U/mg of supernatant protein; one unit (U) is the amount of enzyme which decomposes 1 µmole of H_2O_2. The total SOD activity was determined by using the xanthine oxidase-nitroblue tetrazolium system (10), after sonication of the centrifugate at 50 watt for 2 min. in ice-bath and further centrifugation at 20,000 x g for 30 min. SOD specific activity was expressed as U/mg protein. One unit (U) was defined as the amount of enzyme that inhibits 50% of the rate of nitroblue tetrazolium reduction in the assay condition. Selenium-dependent (GSH-Px) and selenium-independent glutathione peroxidase (GST-Px) activities were measured on the cytosol harvested after further centrifugation at 105,000 x g for 60 min. GSH-Px activity was

measured by the Paglia and Valentine's method (11), using 0.25 mM hydrogen peroxide as substrate and expressed in units (U), each representing the oxidation of one µmole of NADPH/min. GST-Px activity was measured by Lawrence and Burk's method (12), using 1.2 mM cumene hydroperoxide as substrate and expressed as U/mg protein. GS-SG Red activity was determined as previously reported (13). Enzyme activity was performed at 37°C by measuring the disappearance of NADPH at 340 nm and expressed as U/mg protein. One unit (U) is 1 µmole of NADPH oxidized/min. GST activity was determined according to the method of Habig et al. (14). One unit (U) is defined as the amount of enzyme required to catalyze the formation of 1 µmole of CDNB-GSH conjugate/min. Protein concentrations were determined by Bradford's method (15).

Statistical analysis. The results were calculated as mean±SD. Comparisons between hemodynamic and biochemical values in rabbits subjected to aortic coarctation hypertension and controls were computed by the Student's t-test. In cholesterol-fed rabbits, biochemical and morphological data were analyzed by analysis of variance for repeated measures in each group. Where an overall difference was detected, Bonferroni's test was used to determine which means differed significantly. When comparisons involved control and cholesterol-fed rabbits, significance was determined by the t-test for independent means. $p<0.05$ was considered as significant.

Results.

The biochemical results obtained in the hypertensive and cholesterol-fed rabbits, as compared to control animals, are summarized in Table 1 and 2. In cholesterol-fed rabbits, the percentage of aortic surface area covered by sudanophilia was 22±6 and 57±9% in groups B1 and C1, but negligible in Control and A1 groups.

Tables

TABLE 1. Thiobarbituric acid reactive substances and antioxidant defence mechanisms in the hypertensive aorta of rabbits subjected to suprarenal aortic coarctation hypertension (group B) as compared to sham-operated animals (group A)

	Group A	Group B	Significance
Tot-SH (nmoles R-SH/g wet tissue)	129.4±13.8	295.3±20	p<0.0005
GS-SG Red (U/mg protein)	0.093±0.013	0.112±0.015	p<0.05
GSH-Px (U/mg protein)	0.064±0.012	0.207±0.023	p<0.0005
GST-Px (U/mg protein)	0	0.014±0.007	
GST (U/mg protein)	0.480±0.037	0.507±0.085	NS
TBARS (nmoles TBARS/g wet tissue)	12.71±3.73	27.56±2.4	p<0.001

TABLE 2. Changes in the aortic antioxidant defence system and thiobarbituric acid reactive substrances in 24 rabbits fed on a 0.5% cholesterol - enriched diet for 10, 30 and 60 days (Gr. A1,B1 and C1,respectively). Gr. 0,A,B and C : control rabbits.
All enzymatic activities are expressed as U/mg protein; Tot-SH and TBARS levels are expressed as nmoles R-SH or TBARS/g wet tissue.
*, p<0.05 vs values that precede; °, p<0.01 and °°, p<0.001 vs control rabbits

	GR. O	GR. A	GR. B	GR. C
SOD	52.75 ±4.1	54.9 ±4.6	53.5 ±3.8	59.1 ±5.6
Cat	18.51 ±2.3	17.65 ±2	19.25 ±2.6	20.4 ±3.5
Tot-SH	145.4 ±12.6	148.05 ±12.9	151.2 ±11.7	144.4 ±9
GSH-Px	0.057 ±0.04	0.056 ±0.014	0.052 ±0.012	0.063 ±0.01
GS-SG Red	0.092 ±0.011	0.086 ±0.013	0.098 ±0.08	0.094 ±0.01
GST	0.462 ±0.042	0.455 ±0.049	0.446 ±0.037	0.457 ±0.04
TBARS	12.6 ±2.45	13.26 ±2.9	11.75 ±3.1	14.7 ±2.6

	GR. O	GR. A1	GR. B1	GR.C1
SOD	52.75 ±4.1	58.8 ±3.5	72.7* ±6.9°°	92.1* ±8.2°°
Cat	18.51 ±2.3	8.3* ±2.6°°	7.95 ±1.9°°	8.5 ±3°°
Tot-SH	145.4 ±12.6	186* ±18.7°	243.9* ±56°°	238.4 ±32°°
GSH-Px	0.057 ±0.04	0.087* ±0.05°	0.132* ±0.01°°	0.147 ±0.02°°
GS-SG Red	0.092 ±0.011	0.065* ±0.011°	0.077 ±0.014°	0.074 ±0.008°
GST	0.462 ±0.042	0.301* ±0.002°°	0.307 ±0.045°°	0.323 ±0.012°°
TBARS	12.6 ±2.45	31.07* ±5.87°°	35.67 ±5.93°°	33.42 ±9.15°°

Discussion.

The present study demonstrates that aortic lipid peroxidation and antioxidant defence system of the aortic wall are significantly modified in rabbits subjected to aortic coarctation hypertension and in cholesterol-fed animals. Higher values of total thiol compounds with respect to the controls were observed in the hypertensive animals.This phenomenon could be partly explained by increased glutatione reductase activity.It is well known that two forms of glutatione peroxidase exist in mammalian cells (16). The first is a selenium-dependent enzyme, that reduces hydrogen peroxide and organic hydroperoxides.The other is a selenium independent enzyme , that reduces only the organic hydroperoxides and seems to be associated with glutatione trasferases belonging to class Alpha (17). The marked activation of selenium-dependent glutatione peroxidase in the hypertensive aorta emphasizes the primary role of this enzyme in modulating the vascular susceptibility to the hypertension-induced oxidative stress. When glutathione peroxidase activity was assayed with cumene hydroperoxide, higher values with respect to those assayed with hydrogen peroxide were observed only in the hypertensive animals, whereas these values were identical in control rabbits. This phenomenon seems to suggest the appearance of a "new" enzymatic activity associated with glutathione transferase in the hypertensive aorta, which could contribute to the vascular scavenging of cytotoxic byproducts of lipid peroxidation. In this context, a slight activation of glutathione trasferase in the hypertensive aorta was observed. Finally, the increased levels of TBARS, a well known index of lipid peroxidation, emphasize the occurence of vascular oxidative stress in the hypertensive rabbits.

In cholesterol-fed rabbits, significant changes in the aortic antioxidant defence mechanisms and lipid peroxidation were observed. Aortic superoxide dismutase and glutathione peroxidase activities were significantly increased at 30 and 60 days; however, only the second underwent a significant rise at 10 days, thus stressing the primary role of this enzyme in the arterial wall protection. On the contrary, catalase activity was significantly depressed throughout the study. Since superoxide radical (18) and hydrogen peroxide (19) may inactivate catalase, this mechanism could be involved in our model. Concomitant with the increased activity of glutathione peroxidase, a significant and progressive rise in total thiol compounds was also observed in cholesterol-fed rabbits. It is intringuing to explain this phenomenon in front of a persistently decreased glutathione reductase activity, even though the inhibition of glutathione reductase has been recently shown to increase the tissue GSH levels, probably via feedback activation of GSH synthesis (20, 21). Aortic glutathione transferase activity underwent a persistent depression in all experimental groups. It is well known that this enzyme detoxifies the cells from cytotoxic byproducts of lipid peroxidation, such as hydroxyalkenals (17). There is experimental evidence that 4-hydroxynonenal appears during LDL oxidation and may be responsible for part of the cytotoxicity of oxidized LDL (22). Although our study does not clarify the mechanisms of the decreased activity of glutathione transferase in atherosclerotic aorta, a role may be hypothesized for this enzyme in the pathophysiology of oxidized LDL-induced vascular injury. TBARS levels significantly increased in cholesterol-fed rabbits, reaching the peak at 10 days and persisting unmodified at 30 and 60 days. Finally, aortic lipid infiltration was extensive and progressive from 30 to 60 days, but negligible at 10 days.

In conclusion, our study suggests that: 1) suprarenal aortic coarctation hypertension is associated with a free radical-mediated oxidative stress of the hypertensive aortic wall; 2) hyperlipidic diet involves remarkable modifications in the antioxidant defence mechanisms of the rabbit aorta, some of which are stressed (superoxide dismutase, selenium-dependent glutathione peroxidase, total thiol compounds), whereas others (catalase, glutathione reductase, glutathione transferase) are significantly depressed, thus potentially modulating the vascular susceptibility to the oxidative injury.

References.

1) Kontos, H.A. (1985) 'Oxygen radicals in cerebral vascular injury', Circ. Res, 57, 508 516.

2) Henning, B. and Chow, C.K., (1988)' Lipid peroxidation and endothelial cell injury: Implications in atherosclerosis', Free Radic. Biol. Med. 4, 99-106.

3) Ross, R. (1986)' The pathogenesis of atherosclerosis. An update' New Engl. J. Med. 314, 488-500.

4) Miller, H.J.S., Pinto, A. and Mullane, K.M. (1987)' Impaired endothelium-dependent relaxation in rabbit subjected to aortic coarctation hypertension' Hypertension 10, 164-170.

5) Peterson, D.W., Griffith, D.W. and Napolitano, C.A. (1979)' Decreased myocardial contractility in papillary muscles from atherosclerotic rabbits' Circ. Res. 45, 338-346.

6) Holman, R.L., McGill, H.C., Strong, J.P. and Geer, J.C. (1958)' Technics for studyind atherosclerotic lesions' Lab. Invest. 7, 42-47.

7) Ellman, G.L. (1959)' The sulphydril groups' Arch. Biochem.Biophys. 82, 70-77.

8) Ohkawa, H., Ohishi, N. and Yagy, K. (1979)' Assay for lipid peroxides in animal tissues by thiobarbituric acid reaction' Anal. Biochem. 95, 351-358.

9) AEBI, H. (1974)' Catalase', in H. U. Bergmeyer (ed.), Methods in Enzymatic Analysis, Academic Pres, New York, pp. 673-684.

10) Beauchamp, C. and Fridovich, I. (1971)' Superoxide dismutase: Improced assay and an assay applicable to acrylamede gels' Anal. Biochem. 44, 276-287.

11) Paglia, D. E. and Valentine, W. N. (1967)' Studies on the quantitative and qualitative characterization of erythocities glutathione peroxidase' J. Lab. Clin. Med. 29, 143-148.

12) Del Boccio, G., Casaccia R., Aceto A., Casalone E., De Remigis P. and Di Ilio, C. (1987)' Glutathione metabolizing enzyme activities in human thyroid' Gen. Pharmacol. 18, 315-320.

13) Lawrence, R. A. and Burk, R. F. (1976)' Glutathione peroxidase activity in selenium deficient rat liver' Biochem. Biophys. Res. Comm. 71, 951-958.

14) Habig, W. H., Pabst, M. J. and Jakoby, W. B. (1974)' The first enzymatic step in mercapturic acid formation' J. Biol. Chem. 249, 7130-7139.

15) Bradford, M. M. (1976)' A rapid and sensitive method for the quantitation of microgram quantities of protein using the principle of protein-dye binding' Anal. Biochem. 72, 248-254.

16) Flohe', L., Gunzler, W. A. and Loschen, G. (1979) 'The glutathione peroxidase

reaction: A key to understand the selenium requirement of mammals', in N. Kharasch (ed.), Trace Metals in Health and Desease, Raven Press, New York, pp. 262-286.

17) Mannervik, B. (1985)' The isoenzymes of glutathion transferase' in A. Meister (ed.), Advances in Enzymology and Related Area of Molecular Biology, John Wiley & Sons, New York, pp 357-417.

18) Kono, Y. and Fridovich, I., (1982)' Superoxide radical inhibits catalase ' J. Biol. Chem.257, 575 -5757

19) Schonbaum, G. R. and Chance B., (1976) 'Catalase' in P. D. Boyer (ed.), The Enzymes, Academic Press, New York pp. 363-387.

20) Smith, A. C. and Boyd, M.R., (1984) 'Preferential effects of 1,3-bis- (2-Chloroethyl) - 1-Nitrosourea (BCNU) on pulmunary glutathione reductase and glutathione/glutathione disulfide ratios: Possible implications for lung toxicity' J. Pharmacol. Exp. Ther. 229, 658-663.

21) Jenkinson, S.G. Jordan J. M. and Lawrence, R.A., (1988) 'BCNU-induced protection from hyperbaric hyperoxia: Role of glutathione metabolism' J. Appl. Physiol. 65 2531-2536.

22) Morel, D. W., Vargo E., Jurgens G., Esterbauer H., Hoff H.F. and Chisolm G. M. (1988) '4-hydroxynonenal is a cytotoxic component of oxidized LDL' FASEB J. 2, A809 (Abstr.).

76
Magnetic resonance of the heart

C. GAUDIO

II Department of Cardiology, University "La Sapienza" Rome, Istituto Neurotraumatologico Italiano (I.N.I.), Rome, Italy

ABSTRACT. The use of spectroscopic and tomographic NMR techniques in cardiology is still in its early stage. However, the results obtained so far in some sectors of cardiovascular pathology indicate that this noninvasive technique can play a major role, providing structural information along with in vivo determination of cardiac metabolism in a well defined range of diseases. Further inquiry is however needed to define the role and diagnostic effectiveness of NMR in cardiology and to standardize its findings with reference to the advantages and disadvantages of its clinical application.

Introduction.

An excellent resolution of cardiac morphology has been made possible on the sagittal, axial and coronal planes by synchronization of the ECG R-wave with NMR pulse sequence. Low or non-existent signal strength produced by blood flow is a natural radiopaque agent between the cardiac chambers and the cardiac walls, which can be easily distinguished from both the endocardial and epicardial surface, thus making it possible to measure wall and septum thickness as well as chamber size. Angulated transverse tomographies have permitted the simultaneous visualization of the "four cardiac chambers" view, in which cardiac anatomy is thus well outlined: atria, ventricles, interatrial and interventricular septa, mitral valve and tricuspidal plane, papillary muscles, the moderator band of the right ventricle, aortic and pulmonary cusps, the proximal tracts of the right and left coronaries are all structures clearly shown by NMR. The pericardium appears as a thin curvilinear structure sending out a weak NMR signal between 2 more powerful signals sent out by the myocardium and pericardium fat.

Methods.

Early tomographies of a beating heart were made difficult by cardiac wall motion. This problem, however, has been solved by synchronizing NMR images with such a physiological parameter as the ECG R-wave. In other words, images are always obtained at the same point of successive cardiac cycles. The application of this method has improved the quality of cardiac images and provided more detailed description of internal cardiac anatomy. Furthermore, when NMR imaging is used, the blood is like a natural radiopaque agent inside the heart chambers and blood vessels so that no injection of a radiopaque agent is required. In this paper we shall deal with current clinical applications of NMR and report the results which we achieved with the use of a Philips Gyroscan 15 Superconducting System, operating at 1.5 Tesla. In our study we examined 82 patients (50 men, 32 women; average age: 45 years) and, in order to standardize our technique, 30 normal volunteers (19 men, 11 women: average age: 42 years). The Spin Echo sequence was always used (TE=20 ms; TE=80% R-R). 1 cm thick images were obtained with a multislice technique on all conventional planes: transverse, sagittal, coronal) with or without angulation.

Congenital malformations.

Several congenital malformations have been studied by means of NMR, thus obtaining accurate images. NMR has proved extremely effective in detecting: interatrial septal defects; interventricular septal defects; Ebstein's anomaly; transposition of the great vessels; persistent truncus arteriosus; cor triatriatum; congenital mitral stenosis. The anomalies of the pulmonary valve have also proved easy to visualize (Fig.1).

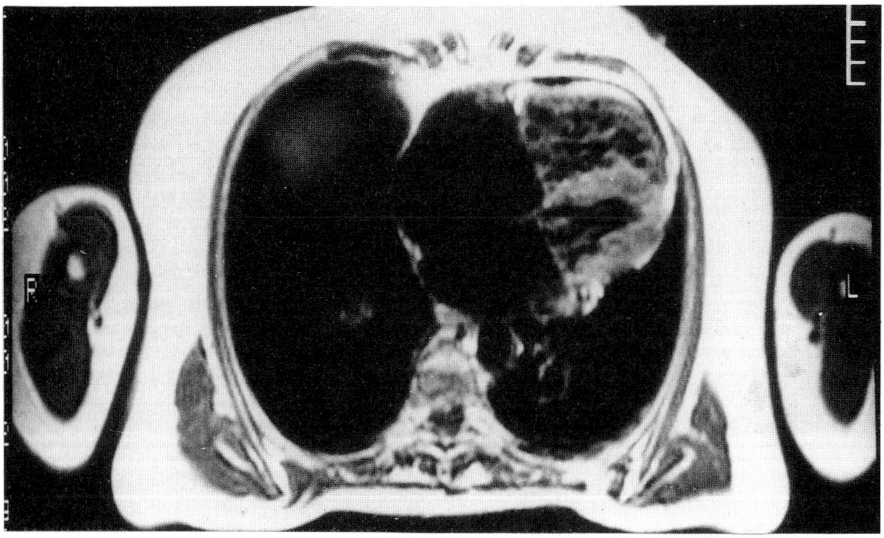

Figure 1. Interatrial septal defect.

Cardiomyopathies.

NMR has proved useful in the assessment of restrictive, congestive and hypertrophic cardiomyopathies. NMR makes it possible to distinguish hypertrophic forms affecting the basal septum alone, from those affecting the anteroapical segment, the whole interventricular septum or the apical wall and the left ventricular lateral wall. In such cases both transverse and sagittal tomographies provide clear images of the longitudinal extent of hypertrophy. Wall thickness can be easily measured both in diastole and in systole by means of the images obtained through ECG synchronization. Comparison of the images obtained by means of 2 dimensional echocardiography confirms the reliability of MRI in detecting the presence and extent of hypertrophy (Figg. 2,3).

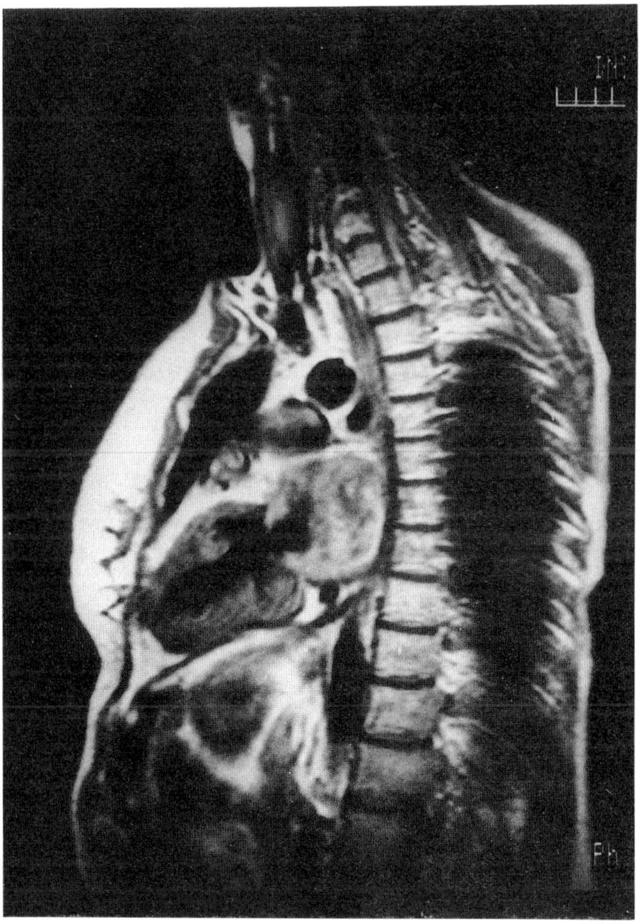

Figure 2. Restrictive cardiomyopathy.

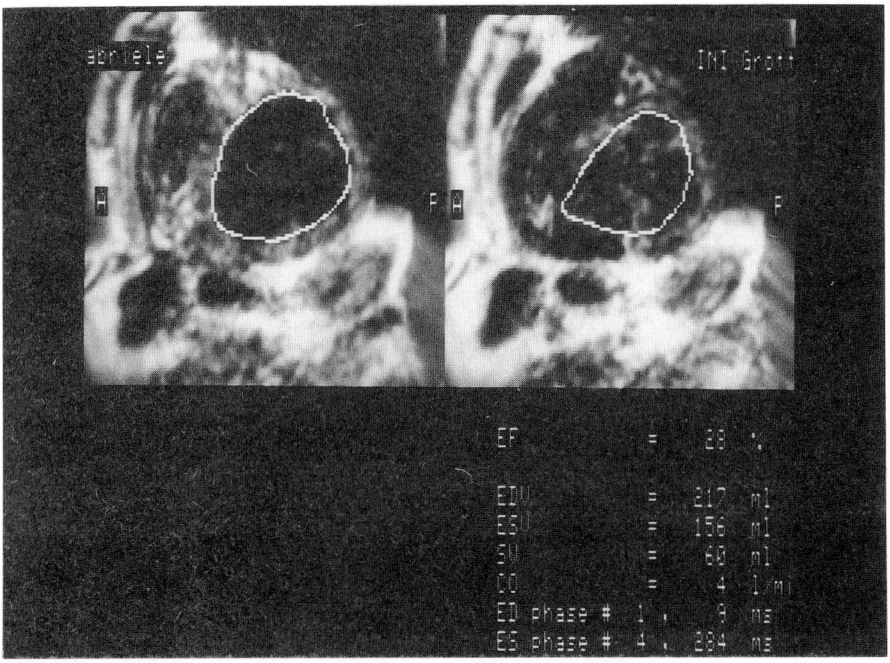

Figure 3. Congestive cardiomyopathy: volume ejection fraction.

Coronary diseases.

NMR makes it possible to study both ventricular walls and interventricular septum and to detect previous myocardial infarctions (MI). The localization of a previous MI is clearly shown by myocardial thinning of the relative ventricular free wall or septum, and its extent is measured by examining multiple adjacent axial planes. Comparison with angiographic and echocardiographic data has confirmed the validity of NMR. In addition to structural information NMR provides information on tissue characterization making use of T1 and T2 relaxation times andon proton density.
Changes in T2 have been detected in acute MI of dogs. The values of T2 in such cases do not overlap the ones detectable in a normal myocardium. If there has been a previous MI, NMR can show not only the portion of myocardium affected, but also the presence of an aneurysm, indicated by thinning and bulging of the wall both at the level of the ventricular wall and of the interventricular septum. Comparison of end-diastolic with end-systolic images allows the detection of dyskinetical or akinetical regions with a slow-down or stasis of blood flow; in fact the relative images show a more powerful signal in the ventricular portion affected(Fig. 4).

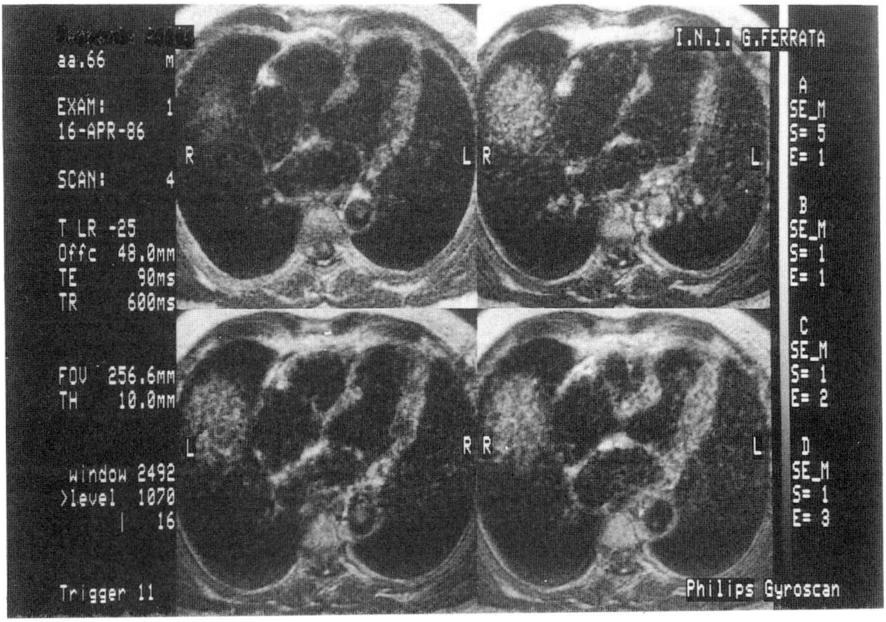

Figure 4. Myocardial bulging in antero-septal MI.

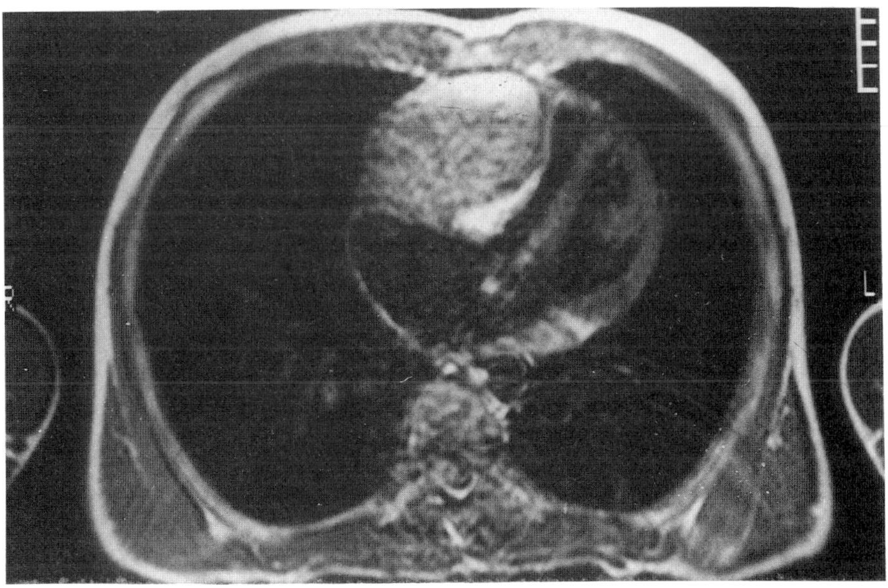

Figure 5. Haemorrhagic saccate pericarditis.

Pericardites.

NMR has proved extremely useful in the study of pericardites. It shows the pericardium as a 1-2 mm thick structure which sends out a weak signal on account of the fibrous composition of the tissue. When subject to NMR examination, exudative pericardites show, between the parietal and visceral pericardia, the presence of exudate. Constrictive, saccate, chronic and haemorragic forms are also recognizable(Fig. 5).

Conclusion.

The application of NMR in cardiovascular clinical medicine has turned over a new leaf in diagnosis and research. Heart performance results from several cellular biochemical reactions as well as from related electrophysiological phenomena. The heart's functional integrity depends on the integrity of its anatomical structure and, at the cellular level, on metabolic integrity. Over the last 30 years the main techniques of inquiry into the heart's structure and function have made use of ionizing radiations. Little more than 15 years ago echocardiography was added to more traditional techniques, hushering in the era of non invasive instrumental diagnosis, providing a quicker and cheaper clinical examination than more traditional ones. Echocardiography can provide detailed structural images and, with the help of the Doppler technique, information on the global and regional functioning of the heart, the cardiac valves and great vessels.
However, neither ultrasonic nor radiographic techniques can provide information on the metabolic state of the myocardial fibres. NMR is widely used in research and diagnosis owing to its ability to provide the structural and metabolical information required.

References.

Lanzer P. Botvinick EH. Schiller N.B. Crookes L.E. Arakawa M. Kaufman L. Davis P.L. and Herfkens R. (1984) Cardiac imaging using gated magnetic resonance. Radiology, 150: 121-127.

Phost G.M. Canby R.C. (1987) Nuclear magnetic resonance imaging: current applications and future prospects. Circulation, 75: 88-94.

Stark D.D. Higgins C.B. Lanzer P. Lipton M.J. Schiller N. Crooks L.E. Botvinick E.B. and Ksugmsn L. (1984) Magnetic resonance imaging of the pericardium: normal and pathological findings. Radiology, 150: 469-474.

Sechtem U. Higgins C.B. Sommerhoff B.A. Lipton M.J. Huyche E.C. (1987) Magnetic resonance imaging of restrictive cardiomyopathy. Am J Cardiol, 59: 480-482.

White R.D. Caputo G.R. Mark A.S. Modin G.W. and Higgins CB. (1987) Coronary artery bypass graft patency: noninvasive evaluation with MR imaging. Radiology, 164: 681-686.

RATIONALE FOR THE PREVENTION IN HIGH RISK SUBJECTS

77
The role of HDL-subfractions in reverse cholesterol transport and its disburbances in Tangier disease and HDL-deficiency with xanthomas

G. SCHMITZ, T. BRÜNING and E. WILLIAMSON

Institut für Klinische Chemie und Laboratoriumsmedizin and Institut für Arterioskleroseforschung, Westfälische Wilhelms-Universität, Albert-Schweitzer-Str. 33, D-4400 Münster, Federal Republic of Germany

High density lipoproteins (HDL) represent one of four major classes of lipoproteins that circulate in human plasma. They are involved in different metabolic processes such as lipid transport, bile acid formation, steroidogenesis, cell proliferation and interfere with plasma proteinase systems. HDL are perfect acceptors of free cholesterol and in concert with cholesteryl ester transfer protein (CETP), hepatic lipase (HL) and lecithin:cholesteryl acyl-transferase (LCAT), they play a major role in reverse cholesterol transport and bile acid formation. HDL do not only transport lipids from peripheral cells to the liver but also deliver cholesterol to steroid producing cells, and thereby are important for steroidogenesis, too.
The precursors of HDL are secreted from the intestine (1,2) and liver (3) from which the circulating spherical HDL particles are formed (4). The intestinal "nascent HDL" contain apo A-I and apo A-IV and the hepatic "nascent HDL" contain apo A-II, apo E and apo A-I as major apolipoproteins. The lipid part of both particles consists of phospholipids and small amounts of free cholesterol and triglycerides (Fig. 1). These precursor particles appear in the plasma compartment as discoidal HDL or spherical HDL as larger triglyceride-rich particles and small phospholipid-rich HDL. In addition, HDL precursors are produced within the plasma compartment during lipolytic processing of chylomicrons by lipoprotein lipase which leads to the formation of phospholipid, apo A-I, apo C disks arising from the surface of the lipolyzed chylomicrons (5). Besides these "surface remnants", "core remnants" are formed from chylomicrons as residual particles, which are taken up by the liver via the remnant receptor (6). The HDL precursors are transformed to large cholesterol enriched HDL particles after interaction with peripheral cells and involvement of several enzymes and proteins such as LCAT, HL and CETP. The HDL-cholesterol metabolism of the mature HDL in the plasma compartment is summarized in Fig. 2.

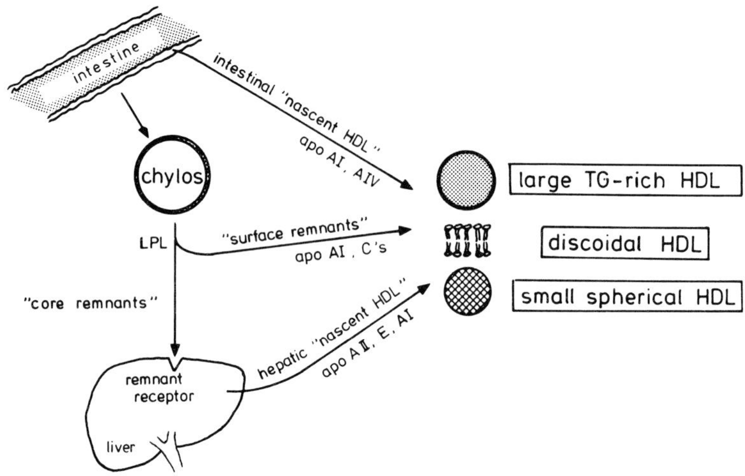

Figure 1: Origin of HDL precursors.

It has been demonstrated from various laboratories, that specific HDL-subclasses play a central role in the transport of cholesterol to peripheral tissues from the liver for removal in the bile. Excess unesterified cholesterol from cholesterol-rich peripheral cells is taken up by HDL and undergoes esterification through the action of LCAT. The transfer of most of this newly generated cholesteryl esters to triacylglycerol-rich lipoproteins such as VLDL is mediated by serum cholesteryl ester transfer proteins (8). VLDL-remnants, or the ultimate product LDL can then be removed from the plasma by receptor-mediated uptake in the liver. This process provides an indirect mechanism for the reverse cholesterol transport and plays a major role in species with high cholesteryl ester transfer activity. Apart from this mechanism, there is evidence of an alternative direct pathway of reverse cholesterol transport. The core expansion of HDL by the accumulation of cholesteryl esters is associated with enrichment of the particles with apo E (9). It has been proposed that apo E serves as a ligand which then promotes the internalization of the lipoprotein by apo E receptors on the liver. The apo E mediated, direct reverse cholesterol transport to the liver in humans is approximately 11% of the HDL cholesterol (10).

Additionally, HDL-with apo-E seem to be able to deliver cholesterol to cholesterol-poor peripheral cells. This delivery of peripherally derived cholesterol to nonhepatic cells would represent a pure redistribution of cholesterol among cells. It has been hypothesized that hepatic lipase, by mediating an increase in the concentration of cholesterol within HDL, may promote the partitioning of cholesterol into hepatocytes. Although there is support for this hypothesis this stili remains to be proven (for review see 11).

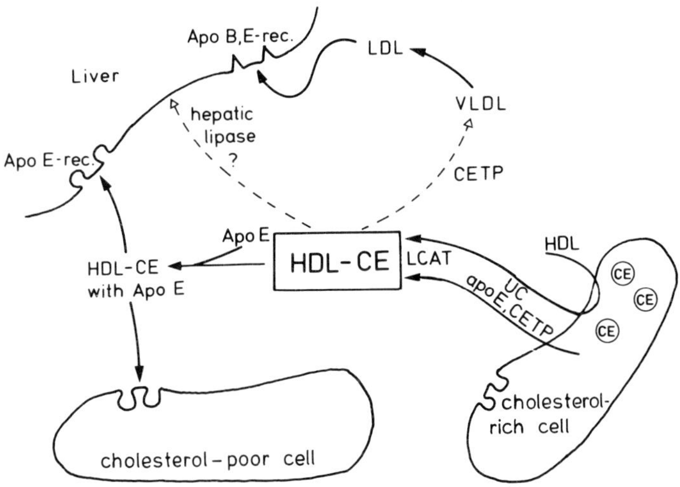

Figure 2: HDL-cholesterol metabolism in the plasma compartment modified according to Weisgraber et al. (7).

The importance of HDL in reverse cholesterol transport is confirmed by the well known observation that HDL levels are negativly correlated with coronary artery disease. Since macrophages participate in the formation of atherosclerotic plaques, cholesterol metabolism in macrophages has been intensively investigated in recent years. It has been demonstrated that atherogenic lipoproteins are ingested by macrophages and degraded in lysosomes. The cholesterol component is released from the lysosomes and either reesterified in the cytoplasmic compartment or resecreted from the cells, promoted by cholesterol acceptors such as HDL (12,13). Macrophages, in contrast to B,E-receptor cells such as fibroblasts, are critically dependent on mechanisms of reverse cholesterol transport to maintain their cholesterol homeostasis. Here we propose a mechanism by which different HDL subfractions are involved in the coordinate regulation of cholesterol and phospholipid metabolism.

The cellular interaction of HDL-subclasses with macrophages was studied in great detail in our laboratory and we have isolated HDL-subpopulations by preparative free flow isotachophoresis (14). With this technique three HDL-subpopulations with fast, intermediate and slow electrophoretic mobility could be separated. The fast migrating HDL are rich in apo A-I and phosphatidylcholine (PC) and bind with high affinity to HDL-receptors on macrophages. The subpopulation with intermediate mobility is rich in apo A-II, apo E, apo C-apolipoproteins, cholesteryl esters and sphingomyelin. The slow migrating HDL subpopulation consists of particles rich in apo A-I and apo A-IV, is associated with high LCAT activity and exhibits high nonspecific binding besides a small portion of specific interaction. Since both, the fast and the slow migrating HDL-subpopulations are good promoters for cholesterol efflux, it is concluded that the HDL-subpopulations rich in apo A-I seem to promote cholesterol efflux via the interaction with HDL receptors, while apo A-IV rich HDL can receive their driving force for cholesterol efflux from the concomitant action of LCAT via a predominantly nonspecific interaction of these particles with the cell surface and thereby extract cholesterol from the cell membrane. Further experiments were performed by monitoring the distribution of HDL-subpopulations by analytical capillary isotachophoresis after incubation of freshly drawn human serum for up to 8 h at 37°C with and without inhibition of LCAT (15). Serum incubation at 37°C leads to a time dependent increase in the concentration of the fast migrating high affinity type apo A-I/PC HDL particles, with a concomitant decrease in the slow migrating LCAT-rich HDL particles. When Ellman's reagent is added as an LCAT inhibitor during in vitro incubation, no significant interconversion of these HDL-subpopulations is visible. The results indicate that LCAT plays a major role in the formation of high affinity binding apo A-I/PC-rich HDL particles by converting apo A-I/A-IV-rich HDL particles into apo A-I/PC rich HDL particles. These results are underlined by the isotachophoretic analysis of the HDL pattern in patients with LCAT-deficiency and Fish eye disease. In both disorders the fast migrating apo A-I/PC-rich HDL particles are absent while the slow migrating apo A-I/A-IV particles are present in non-incubated sera and no interconversion of the HDL subpopulations is observed upon serum incubation in these patients. From these results and our recent studies (16-19) on the regulation of cellular cholesterol and phospholipid metabolism in macrophages we propose the model shown in Fig. 3.

Two major routes exist by which macrophages, in addition to physicochemical exchange, can release excess cholesterol:

1. Upon cholesterol loading macrophages form cholesterol- and phospholipid containing "lamellar bodies" which originate from lysosomes. These lamellar bodies move towards the cell periphery, attach to the cell membrane and

release their lipid components into the extracellular medium or into the cell membrane. This mechanism of cholesterol release is promoted by apo AI/AIV-LCAT rich HDL particles which preferentially bind nonspecifically to the cell membrane.

2. An HDL receptor-mediated cholesterol efflux where apo A-I-rich HDL bind specifically to a 110 KDa HDL binding protein on macrophages. These apo A-I-rich HDL particles are internalized into a nonlysosomal compartment and take up cholesterol from "lamellar bodies" which are formed from cytoplasmic lipid droplets upon attachment of endoplasmic reticulum. The latter mechanism is promoted by ACAT-inhibitors such as Octimibate which increase cellular free cholesterol. It may not be ruled out that also apo A-IV/PC particles which are formed during the LCAT reaction may interact specifically with the cell membrane as suggested by Dvorin et al. (20).

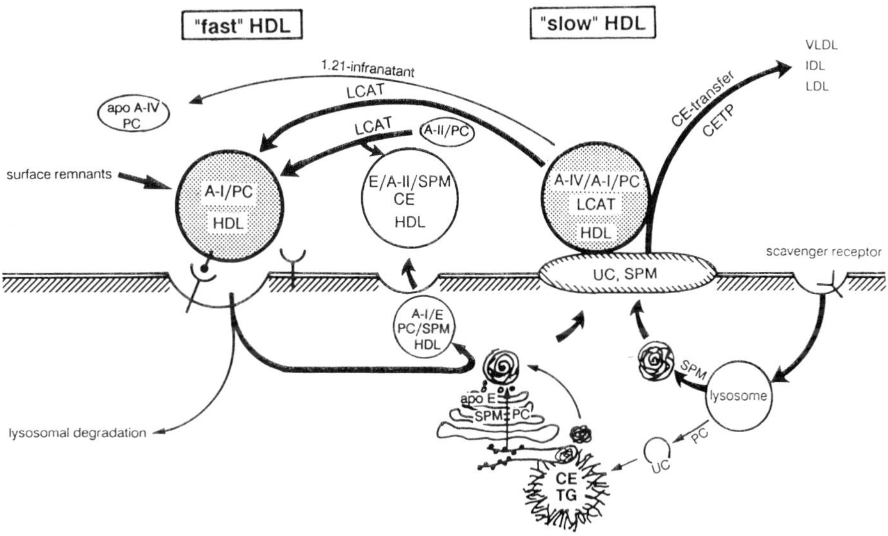

Figure 3: Interaction of HDL-subclasses with macrophages

However the apo AI/PC particles seem to be the major ligands for the HDL-receptor. Since both mechanisms involve the formation of "lamellar bodies", we have studied phospholipid metabolism in macrophages in great detail (21) and found that upon cholesterol loading of macrophages with acetyl-LDL, after an initial increase in phospholipid synthesis, the rate of synthesis continuously declined upon further cholesterol loading. The turnover rate of cellular phospholipids was not affected under the same conditions. The lysosomal inhibitor chloroquine abolished the inhibition of the phospholipid synthesis rate during acetyl-LDL incubation, revealing a strong correlation between cholesterol influx and the rate of phospholipid synthesis.

The reduction in phospholipid synthesis induced by cholesterol loading is reversible by the addition of HDL to the tissue culture medium. When HDL_3 was added to cholesterol loaded macrophages a 2 - 3 fold increase in PC-synthesis and a 2-fold increase in sphingomyelin (SPM) formation was observed after 3 h.

The dihydropyridine Ca^{++}-antagonist Nifedipine which promotes the formation of "lamellar bodies" from the lysosomal route and downregulates HDL-binding, enhanced SPM-synthesis, while PC-synthesis remained constant. However, ACAT inhibitors which promote HDL receptor-mediated cholesterol efflux and the formation of "lamellar bodies" from cytoplasmic lipid droplets induce the synthesis of both phospholipid classes.

The internalized apo AI/PC-rich HDL may also take up cholesterol from apo E containing "lamellar bodies" which appear in the trans-Golgi region and the newly formed products obviously represent the precursors of apo E/AII-rich HDL with intermediate mobility.

Various HDL-deficiency syndromes have been described (22) including Tangier disease (23) and HDL-deficiency with plane xanthomas (24-26). They represent genotypically heterogenous syndromes and we have recently shown that the gene defect in HDL-deficiency with plane xanthomas is a base insertion in the codon for amino acid 5 of apo A-I leading to a frame shift with a subsequent nonsense peptide premature termination (25,26). The defect in Tangier disease is related to a cellular defect in the translocation of cellular cholesterol where HDL-precursors are erroneously degraded in lysosomes (23). However, in Tangier disease the underlying defect could not yet be precisely defined.

We compared the lipid metabolism in monocyte-derived macrophages (MNP) from normals with MNP from patients with Tangier disease or HDL-deficiency with plane xanthomas (Fig. 4).

In Fig. 4, uppermost panel, the binding of HDL_3 at 4°C to MNP (27) under fasting and 3 h postprandial conditions are shown. No significant differences in the affinity of the HDL_3 particles to the cells could be observed between the fasting and 3 h postprandial state and between the patient-MNP and normal MNP. The K_D ranged between 7.5 - 7.9 x 10^{-8} M. However, the maximum HDL_3-binding capacity on Tangier-MNP in the fasting, as well as in the postprandial state is increased by about 20 % (fasting state) and 25 % (postprandial state). The B_{max}-values are indicated in Fig. 4. MNP from patients with HDL-deficiency with plane xanthomas reveal also a higher B_{max}-value in the fasting state as compared to normal cells, but in the postprandial state no reduction in the maximum binding capacity could be observed as found in normal- and Tangier MNP.

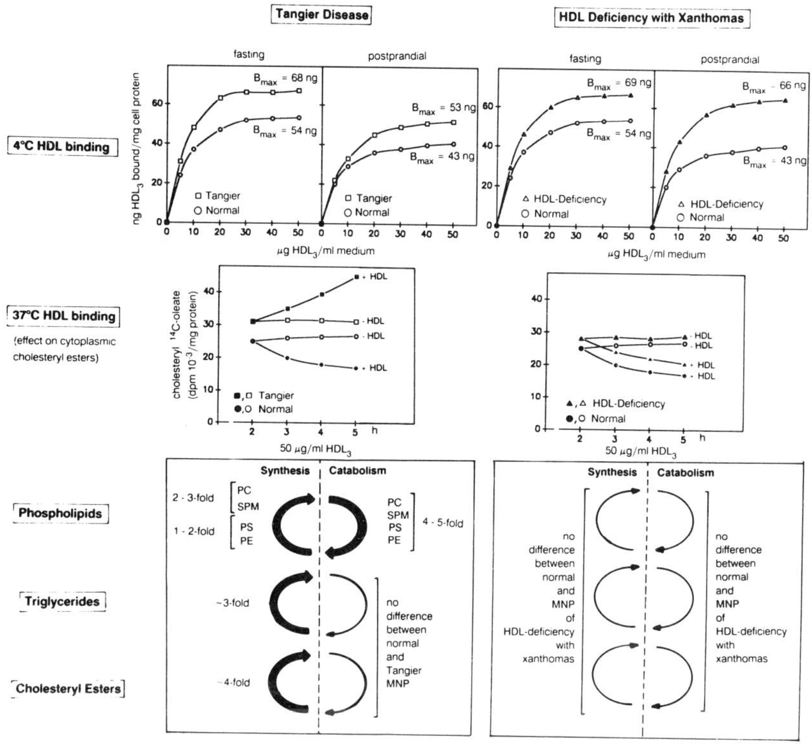

Figure 4: Lipid metabolism in normal-MNP and MNP from Tangier-disease and HDL-deficiency with plane xanthomas.

The influence of HDL_3-incubation at 37°C on the metabolism of cytoplasmic cholesteryl esters of cholesterol loaded MNP was monitored at various time intervals and the results are shown in Fig. 4, middle panel.

In normal MNP and in cells from the patient with HDL-deficiency with plane xanthomas HDL_3 induces cholesterol efflux which leads to a reduction in the cholesterol reesterification by ACAT. In contrast, Tangier-MNP exhibited already an increased starting activity of cholesterol esterification due to a higher total cholesterol content in the cell and in addition HDL_3 incubation induced the formation of cytoplasmic cholesteryl esters, which is due to the lysosomal degradation of HDL_3 in Tangier-MNP (28).

The regulation of phospholipid-, triglyceride- and cholesteryl ester synthesis and catabolism was also analyzed and the results are shown in Fig. 4, lower panel. When normal MNP were compared with cells from patients with HDL-deficiency with plane xanthomas, no dysregulation of the synthesis and catabolism of phospholipids, triglycerides and cholesteryl esters could be observed.

Binding of normal HDL_3 to Tangier MNP is increased due to a higher expression of HDL binding sites. The bulk of the internalized HDL_3 was found in lysosomes and only minor amounts of the internalized HDL_3 were resecreted from the Tangier monocytes and most of it was degraded (28). Furthermore, in Tangier disease the cellular defect is associated with a dysregulation of cellular lipid metabolism, leading to an overproduction of triglycerides and esterified cholesterol and to an enhanced synthesis and intracellular catabolism of phospholipids.However, in Tangier-MNP the cellular defect is associated with significant abnormalities in cellular phospholipid-, triglyceride- and cholesteryl ester metabolism. Tangier-MNP have about 2-fold increased rates of synthesis for phospholipids, about 5-fold for triglycerides and about 3-fold for cholesteryl esters as compared to normal MNP. The turnover rate of cellular phospholipids is also enhanced while the turnover rates for triglycerides and cholesteryl esters are normal (29).The interaction of HDL-subclasses with normal MNP and MNP of patients with Tangier disease or HDL-deficiency with plane xanthomas is summarized in Fig. 5.

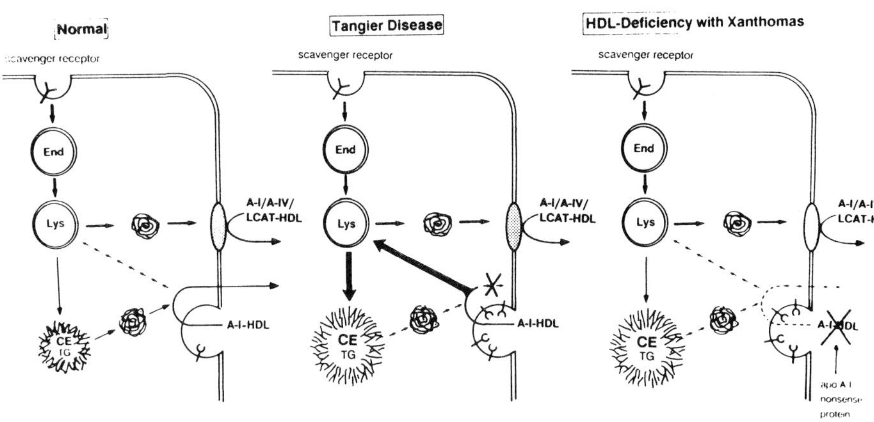

Figure 5: Interaction of HDL subclasses with normal MNP and MNP from patients with Tangier disease or HDL-deficiency with plane xanthomas.

Tangier MNP fail to respond to the HDL-interaction with a coordinated regulation of phospholipid-, triglyceride- and cholesteryl ester metabolism and thus finally accumulate cholesteryl esters in the affected cells (29). Therefore, we have defined Tangier disease as "a disorder of intracellular traffic" where HDL precursors which bind to the receptor are erroneously degraded in lysosomes of the affected cells. In contrast, monocyte/macrophages of patients with HDL-deficiency with plane xanthomas exhibit normal intracellular traffic and lipid metabolism, but the number of HDL binding sites is elevated to the same extent as in Tangier-MNP. The identified HDL-deficiency with Xanthomas is of an asynthetic type, due to a defect in apo A-I synthesis and release from the intestinal mucosa cell (25, 26) which is different from the hypercatabolic type found in Tangier disease where the apo A-I gene is unaffected (23). The lack of apo A-I containing HDL as a cholesterol acceptor for reverse cholesterol transport leads to the accumulation of cholesteryl ester containing lipid droplets in cutaneous macrophages.

The comparison of HDL-metabolism of cells as well as plasma in HDL-deficiency with xanthomas, Tangier disease and other genetic defects of HDL metabolism will give new insights into abnormalities of the HDL-receptor mechanism and the reverse cholesterol transport.

1. Green, P.H.R.; Glickman, R.M.: Instestinal lipoprotein metabolism. J.Lipid Res. 22: 1153-1173 (1981).
2. Bisgaier, C.L.; Glickman, R.M.: Intestinal synthesis, secretion and transport of lipoproteins. Annu. Ref. Physiol. 45: 625-636 (1983).
3. Marsh, J.B.: Apoproteins of the lipoproteins in a none recirculating perfusate of rat liver. J. Lipid Res. 17: 85-90 (1976).
4. Mahley, R.W.; Innerarity, T.L.; Rall, S.C. Jr.; Weisgraber, K.H.: Plasma lipoproteins: Apolipoportein structure and function. J. Lipid Res. 25: 1277-1294 (1984).
5. Tall, A.R.; Small, D.M.: Plasma high-density lipoproteins. N.Engl. J.Med. 299: 1232-1236 (1978).
6. Hui, D.Y.; Innerarity, T.L.; Milne, R.W.; Marcel, Y.L.; Mahley, R.W.: Binding of chylomikrone remnants and ß-very low density lipoproteins to hepatic and extrahepatic liporotein receptors: A process independent of apolipoprotein B-48. J.Biol.Chem. 259:15060-15068 (1984).
7. Weisgraber, K.H.; Rall, S.C. Jr.; Innerarity, T.L.; Mahley, R.W.: HDL - with apolipoprotein E: important considerations and metabolic significance of this high density lipoprotein subclass; in Lippel, proceedings of the workshop on lipoprotein heterogeneity; national institut of health publication no. 87-2646, pp. 111-121 (1987).
8. Tall, A.R.: Plasma lipid transfer proteins. J. Lipid Res. 27: 361-367 (1986).
9. Koo, C.; Innerarity, T.L.; Mahley, R.W.: Obligatory role of cholersterol and apolipoprotein E in the formation of large cholesterol-enriched and receptor-active high density lipoproteins. J. Biol. Chem. 260: 11934-11943 (1985).
10. Weisgraber, K.H.; Mahley, R.W.: Subfractionation of human high density lipoproteins by heparin-sepharose affinity chromatography. J. Lipid Res. 21:316-325 (1980).
11. Phillips, M.C.; Johnson, W.J.; Rothblat, G.H.: . Mechanisms and consequences of cellular cholesterol exchange and transfer. Biochim. Biophys. Acta 906: 223-276 (1987).

12. Brown M.S.; Goldstein, J.L.: Lipoprotein metabolism in the macropahge : implications for cholesterol deposition in atherosclerosis. Ann. Rev. Biochem 52: 223-261 (1983).
13. Ho Y.K.; Brown M.S.; Goldstein, J.L.: Hydrolysis and excretion of cytoplasmic cholesterol esters by macrophages: stimulation by high density lipoproteins and other agents. J. Lipid Res. 21: 391-398 (1980).
14. Nowicka, G.; Brüning, T.; Böttcher; A; Kahl, G.; Schmitz, G.: The macrophage interaction of HDL subclasses separated by free flow isotachophoresis. J Lipid Res (submitted 1989).
15. Nowicka, G.; Dieplinger, H.; Williamson, E.; Böttcher, A.; Stender, S.; Schmitz, G.: Lecithin: cholesteryl acyltransferase converts apo A-I/A-IV rich HDL particles into high affinity apo A-I/phosphatidylcholine rich HDL particels. (In preparation).
16. Schmitz, G.; Robenek, H.; Lohmann, U.; Assmann, G.: Interaction of high density lipoproteins with cholesteryl ester-laden macrophages: biochemical and morphological characterization of cell surface receptor binding, endocytosis and resecretion of high density lipoproteins by macrophages. EMBO J. 4: 613-622 (1985).
17. Schmitz, G.; Niemann, R.; Brennhausen, B.; Krause, R.; Assmann, G.: Regulation of high density lipoprotein receptors in cultured macrophages: role of acyl CoA: cholesterol acyltransferase. EMBO J. 4: 2773-2779 (1985).
18. Schmitz, G.; Robenek, H.; Beuck, M.; Krause, R.; Schurek, A.; Niemann, R.: Ca^{++} antagonists and ACAT inhibitors promote cholesterol efflux from macrophages by different mechanisms: I. Characterization of intracellular lipid metabolism. Arteriosclerosis 8: 46-56 (1988).
19. Robenek, H.; Schmitz, G.: Ca^{++} antagonists and ACAT inhibitors promote cholesterol efflux from macrophages by different mechanisms: II. Characterization of intracellular morphological changes. Arteriosclerosis 8: 57-67 (1988).
20. Dvorin, E.; Gorder, N.L.; Benson, D.M.; Gotto, A.M. Jr.: Apolipoprotein A-IV. A determinant for binding and uptake of high density lipoproteins by rat hepatocytes. J. Biol. Chem. 261: 15714-15718 (1986).
21. Schmitz, G.; Beuck, M.; Fischer, H.; Robenek, H.: Regulation of phospholipid biosynthesis during cholesterol influx and high density lipoprotein-mediated cholesterol efflux in macrophages. J. Lipid Res. (submitted 1989).
22. Schaefer, E.J,: Clinical, biochemical and genetic features in familial disorders of high density lipoprotein deficiency. Arteriosclerosis 4: 303-322 (1984).
23. Assmann, G.; Schmitz, G.; Brewer, H.B. Jr.: Familial high density lipoprotein deficiency: Tangier disease; in Scriver, Beaudet, Sly, Valle, The metabolic basis of inherited disease. 6 th ed. chapt. 50, pp. 1267-1282 (Mc-Graw-Hill, New York 1989).
24. Gustavson, A.; Mc Conathy, W.J.; Alaupovic, P.; Curry, M.D.; Persson, B.: Identification of apoprotein familiesin a variant of human plasma apolipoprotein A deficiency. Scand. J. Clin. Lab. Invest. 39: 377-388 (1979).
25. Schmitz, G.; Lackner, K.: High density lipoprotein deficiency with xanthomas : a defect in apo A-I synthesis. J. Clin,. Invest. (submitted 1989).
26. Lackner, K.; Schmitz, G.: High density lipoprotein deficiency is caused by a point mutation in the apo A-I gene. J. Clin. Invest. (submitted 1989).
27. Schmitz, G.; Wulf, G.; Brüning, T.: Flow-cytometric determination of HDL_3 binding sites on human leukocytes. Clin. Chem. 33: 2195-2203 (1987).
28. Schmitz, G.; Assmann, G.; Robenek, H.; Brennhausen, B.: Tangier disease: a disorder of intracellular membrane traffic. Proc. Natl. Acad. Sci. USA 82: 6305-6309 (1985).
29. Schmitz, G.; Fischer, H.; Beuck, M.; Hoecker, K.-P.; Robenek, H.: Dysregulation of phospholipid synthesis in Tangier-monocyte derived macrophages. Arteriosclerosis (in press 1990).

78
HDL cholesterol and triglycerides as risk factors for CHD

P.W.F. WILSON and K.M. ANDERSON
Framingham Heart Study, Framingham, MA 02167, USA

ABSTRACT. Lipoprotein cholesterol data from the Framingham Study show that triglycerides, total cholesterol, LDL cholesterol (LDL-C) and HDL cholesterol (HDL-C) levels are both important in determining risk for coronary heart disease (CHD) occurring among individuals 45-84 years. In general, a 10 mg/dl difference in LDL-C is associated with a 5-7 per cent difference in coronary disease over 14 years, and a 10 mg/dl difference in HDL-C is associated with a 18-22 per cent difference in the opposite direction in CHD over 14 years. Such effects are seen over and above the usual coronary risk factors such as cigarette use and hypertension. The association of CHD with HDL-C levels are uniformly stronger than with triglyceride levels in Framingham cohort where the tests were performed simultaneously. The lipid fraction HDL-C is associated with the occurrence of subsequent myocardial infarction even at cholesterol levels below 200 mg/dl in both men and women. About 20 per cent of myocardial infarctions occur among men and women with cholesterol levels in the bottom quartile, and about half of these individuals, or 10% of the total number of infarction victims have simultaneously low HDL-C levels.

Introduction

While blood cholesterol and LDL-C receive most of the attention as markers for future CHD (1,2), there is considerable evidence that HDL-C and triglycerides play an important role (3,4,5). Early data from Framingham was largely confined to total cholesterol and total triglycerides measurements, but more recent data collections allow assessment of the role of various lipid fractions and their effect on CHD outcomes. In particular, recent analyses from clinical trials show that favorable changes in HDL-C during the course of cholesterol lowering therapy may help to identify individuals who achieve greater benefit and protection from CHD (6,7). On the horizon is the impact of apolipoprotein A1 and apolipoprotein B levels and their importance in determing coronary risk, but there are no large prospective studies with data to assess the lipoproteins at this time.

Materials and Methods

Data are based upon the experience of the Framingham cohort, a sample of 5209 men and women 30-62 years of age in 1948 when the study was begun. Triglycerides were measured on participants attending biennial exam eight (non-fasting) and eleven (fasting) in 1966-68 and 1972-74 respectively, using the Kessler technique (8). The cholesterol in HDL was determined first at the eleventh examination in 1972-74 following precipitation of non-HDL particles with heparin-manganese, according to a modification of the Lipid Research Clinics program method (9). Other variables used in the analyses include total cholesterol measured by the Abell-Kendall method (10), sitting blood pressure, number of cigarettes smoked daily during the past year, presence of glucose intolerance if casual glucose levels exceed 120 mg/dl, and presence of left ventricular hypertrophy on the electrocardiogram (LVH-ECG) (11).

Coronary heart disease incidence was determined from information obtained at regular clinic visits and review of outside hospitalizations. Persons with coronary heart disease at baseline examinations (angina pectoris, history of myocardial infarction (MI), or coronary insufficiency) were excluded from the incidence analyses. Statistical methods include both logistic and proportional hazards regression. The effect of various factors on coronary heart disease outcome was determined by exponentiating the specific beta coefficients from logistic regression analysis.

Results

After 20 years of follow-up from the initial measurement of triglycerides (non-fasting) in Framingham, there was a significant association with later CHD in both men and women after age adjustment (Table 1). The triglyceride to CHD association was weaker ($p=0.06$ in both sexes) after multivariate adjustment for age, systolic blood pressure, cigarettes smoked per day, glucose intolerance, and LVH-ECG. In age group analyses, which are not shown, the strongest associations between triglycerides and 20 year incidence of CHD among men occurred in those 45-54 years ($p=0.016$) and 65-74 years ($p=0.031$). Similarly, among women the strongest associations between triglycerides and CHD were seen for individuals 35-44 years ($p=0.028$) and 45-54 years ($p=0.065$) at baseline.

Weaker relationships with fasting triglycerides were seen for 14 year CHD incidence subsequent to the 1972-74 baseline examination (Table 2). In the overall analysis, after age adjustment the triglyceride levels were not associated with later CHD in men, but were in women. The triglyceride relationship for women was not significant in multivariate analysis undertaken as in Table 1 ($p=0.84$). On the other hand, age-group specific analyses of the relationship between triglyceride levels and CHD in women remained statistically significant for women 55-64 years ($p=0.04$) and 65-74 years ($p=0.04$).

TABLE 1. 20 Year Incidence of CHD according to non-fasting triglycerides. Framingham Cohort Age 35-84, Follow-up 1966-86.

Men: Triglycerides (mg/dl)	Men: Rate (per 1000 per 10 yr)	Women: Triglycerides (mg/dl)	Women: Rate (per 1000 per 10 yr)
<50	154	<50	76
50-64	159	50-64	78
65-79	238	65-79	110
80-94	228	80-94	116
>94	217	>94	152
At risk	867		1215
Cases	288		234
Age adjusted test for trend	p=0.0019		p=0.0024

The HDL-C to CHD relationships after the 1972-74 baseline are stronger than for triglycerides (Table 3). Age-group specific analyses of interest showed at least borderline significance levels for HDL-C and 14 year incidence of CHD in men 55-64 years (p=0.015) and women 45-54 (p=0.094), 55-64 (p=0.003), 65-74 (p=0.039), and 75-84 years (p=0.068).

TABLE 2. 14 Year CHD Incidence and fasting triglycerides. Framingham Cohort Age 45-84, Follow-up 1972-1986

Men: Triglycerides (mg/dl)	Men: Rate (per 1000 per 10 yr)	Women: Triglycerides (mg/dl)	Women: Rate (per 1000 per 10 yr)
<80	190	<70	74
80-109	169	70-99	107
110-139	257	100-129	115
140-159	273	130-159	160
>159	345	>159	170
At risk	935		1317
Cases	232		203
Age adjusted test for trend	p=0.410		p=0.005

TABLE 3. 14 Year Incidence of CHD according to HDL-C. Framingham Cohort Age 45-84, Follow-up 1972-1986

Men: Triglycerides (mg/dl)	Men: Rate (per 1000 per 10 yr)	Women: Triglycerides (mg/dl)	Women: Rate (per 1000 per 10 yr)
<35	230	<40	205
35-39	244	40-49	146
40-44	185	50-59	150
45-49	175	60-69	72
>49	193	>69	66
At risk	935		1317
Cases	232		203
Age adjusted test for trend	p=0.0012		p<0.0001

The relative impact of various fasting lipid measures on the 14 year incidence of coronary heart disease is shown in table 4. These relationships are obtained from the beta coefficient for each lipid measure in the multivariate logistic regression analysis. For example, a 10 mg/dl positive difference in HDL-C in men is associated with an 18% negative effect on CHD incidence.

TABLE 4. Impact of Lipids on 14 year CHD incidence. Framingham Cohort 1972-86

Type of Lipid	Per Cent Risk Difference Per 10 mg/dl lipid difference: MEN	WOMEN
Cholesterol	4 *	5 *
HDL-C	-18 *	-22 **
LDL-C	5 *	7 **
Number at risk	935	1317
Number of cases	324	291

Key: * $0.001 \leq p < 0.01$, ** $p < 0.001$

Total cholesterol and HDL-C are commonly measured simultaneously and some men and women with low cholesterol levels develop coronary disease. Such a tabulation is shown for the endpoint MI for Framingham cohort men and women in tables 5 and 6 (12). A total of 136 men developed MI over 12 years; 18% had cholesterol levels less than 192 mg/dl (bottom quartile of cholesterol for men), and about half of that group (9% of the cases) had HDL-C levels under 36 mg/dl (bottom quartile of HDL-C for men).

TABLE 5. Lipids and 12 year incidence of myocardial infarction. Framingham cohort 1972-84. Men--136 cases.

		HDL-C (mg/dl)	
		≤36	>36
Cholesterol (mg/dl)	>192	18%	65%
	≤192	9%	9%

Twenty-three per cent of the women developing MI had cholesterol levels under 212 mg/dl (bottom quartile of cholesterol for women), and about half of that group (11% of the total) had cholesterol levels under 45 mg/dl (bottom quartile of HDL-C for women).

TABLE 6. Lipids and 12 year incidence of myocardial infarction. Framingham cohort 1972-84. Women--92 cases.

		HDL-C (mg/dl)	
		≤45	>45
Cholesterol (mg/dl)	>212	41%	33%
	≤212	11%	12%

Discussion

This article summarizes some of the recently updated information on CHD incidence in the Framingham cohort (13,14). The triglyceride data show associations with CHD, but the analyses are not uniformly statistically significant. Large biological variation in triglyceride levels is partly responsible for the weaker relationships, and a small number of cases in some of the subgroups also plays a role. It is possible that triglyceride acts similarly to blood cholesterol as a risk factor for CHD, and the strength of its association is weaker at greater ages. Additionally, when multivariate CHD prediction equations include HDL-C, LDL-C, triglycerides and other risk factors, the impact of triglycerides is blunted considerably because of the highly significant negative correlation between HDL-C and triglycerides. Independent of HDL-C levels, there is a residual effect of triglyceride level on CHD in women in such analyses, but not in men (4).

The HDL-C and CHD data have now been extended to 14 years and show relationships which are less strong than reported earlier (4). For instance, after adjustment for multiple variables, a 10 mg/dl difference in HDL-C is associated with a 20% difference in CHD over the course of 14 years. This estimate is highly significant, emphasizing the salutary role of higher HDL-C levels. A recent review has highlighted this favorable impact of HDL-C on CHD, and found remarkably consistent effects of HDL-C on CHD incidence in men from Framingham, the Lipid Research Clinics Program, the Multiple Risk Factor Intervention Trial, and the British Regional Heart Study (15).

About 20 per cent of myocardial infarctions past age 50 in the Framingham cohort occur in individuals with relatively low HDL-C (tables 5 and 6). The relative importance of such a finding is still not fully understood and needs replication in other studies.

References

1. Stamler J, Wentworth D, Neaton J (1986) 'Is the relationship between serum cholesterol and risk of death from coronary heart disease continuous and graded?' JAMA 256, 2823-2828

2. Grundy SM (1986) 'Cholesterol and coronary heart disease: A new era' JAMA 256, 2849-2858

3. Hulley SB, Rosenman RH, Bawol RD, and Brand RJ (1980) Epidemiology as a guide to clinical decisions' N Engl J Med 302, 1383-1389

4. Gordon T, Castelli WP, Hjortland MC, Kannel WB, Dawber TR, (1977) 'High density lipoprotein as a protective factor against coronary heart disease: The Framingham Study' Am J Med 62, 707-714

5. Castelli WP (1988) 'Cholesterol and lipids in the risk of coronary artery disease--The Framingham Heart Study' Can J Cardiol 4(A), 5-10

6. Lipid Research Clinics Program (1984) 'The Lipid Research Clinics Coronary Primary Prevention Trial Results II. The relationship of reduction in incidence of coronary heart disease to cholesterol lowering' JAMA 251, 365-374

7. Manninen V, Elo MO, Frick H. et al. (1988) 'Lipid alterations and decline in the incidence of coronary heart disease in the Helsinki Heart Study' JAMA 260, 641-651

8. Kessler G and Lederer H (1965) 'Fluorometric measurements of triglycerides' in Technicon Symposia Automation in Analytical Chemistry, Skeggs LT (ed) New York, pp. 341-344

9. Lipid Research Clinics Program. Manual of Laboratory Operations (1974) vol 1: Lipid and Lipoprotein Analysis. DHEW publ. no (NIH) 75-628. Bethesda MD, NIH, 1974

10. Abell LL, Levy BB, Brodie BB, and Kendall (1952) 'Method of cholesterol measurement' J Biol Chem 195, 357-366

11. Shurtleff D (1974) Some characteristics related to the incidence of cardiovascular disease and death. Framingham Study, 18 year follow-up. DHEW publ. No. (NIH) 74-599

12. Abbott RD, Wilson PWF, Kannel WB, Castelli WP, (1988) 'High density lipoprotein cholesterol, total cholesterol screening and myocardial infarction: The Framingham Study' Arteriosclerosis 8: 207-211

13. Castelli WP, Garrison RJ, Wilson PWF, Abbott RD, Kalousdian S, Kannel WB (1986) 'Coronary heart disease incidence and lipoprotein cholesterol levels: The Framingham Study' JAMA 256, 2835-2838

14. Kannel WB, Wolf PA, Garrison RJ (1988) The relationship between sporadically measured variables and the risk of cardiovascular disease and death: Framingham Heart Study, 30-34 year follow-up Section 38. NIH Publication

15. Gordon DJ, Probstfield JL, Garrison RJ, et al, (1989) 'High-density lipoprotein cholesterol and cardiovascular disease: Four prospective American Studies' Circulation 79, 8-15

79

The ATS-Sardegna prevention campaign. Background and features

S. MUNTONI

Centre for Metabolic Diseases and Atherosclerosis, Ospedale "G. Brotzu" (San Michele), via Peretti, I-09134 Cagliari, Italy

ABSTRACT. The ATS-Sardegna Campaign is a community-oriented undertaking of prevention of cardiovascular diseases, and of health promotion. The campaign has been planned by the Centre for Metabolic Diseases and Atherosclerosis, Cagliari, and funded by the Sardinian Department of Public Health. Both population and individual (high risk) strategies are features of the campaign. The population strategy is accomplished through both the mass media and special media. The individual strategy relies upon the general practitioners. The campaign spreads throughout the whole island of Sardinia.

Cardiovascular diseases and, in particular, coronary heart disease account for almost half of the deaths and for a great deal of morbidity in Western European Countries, included Italy. This holds true, although at somewhat lower absolute incidence rates, also for Sardinia (11), where, however, in late years we recorded an unfavourable trend of some major risk factors for atherosclerosis.

In fact, two surveys of the major risk factors for atherosclerosis were carried out by us in Sardinia with identical procedures: in 1976-78 the Italian National Research Council (CNR) special project ATS-RF2 (15), and in 1982-84 the Sardinian special programme of epidemiology of risk factors for atherosclerosis: the ATS-Sardegna project (9). Therefore, we found ourselves in a position to survey the changes in the mean levels of risk factors during a six-year period in Sardinian demographic samples of both sexes, aged 20-59 years at entry.

Considering serum total cholesterol, the age-standardized mean levels had risen, in the six-year period (in a random sample of the same age as the previous one), from 189 to 203 mg/dl in men, and from 184 to 197 mg/dl in women: an average increase of about 2 mg/dl per year in both sexes. This was paralleled by the doubling of the score of consumption of foodstuff rich in saturated fats, as obtained from a semiquantitative food-frequency questionnaire: from 6 to 15 in men, and from 6 to 13 in women (13).

As for smoking habit, while the age-standardized prevalence of smokers in the same period decreased slightly in males (from 58% to 49%), it rose in females from 13% to 21%, and particularly in young females (20-29 years) up to 41% (9).

Such a trend of the two risk factors (serum cholesterol in both sexes, and smoking in women) doubtlessly heralded a surge of cardiovascular disease morbidity in our island in the next years.

On the other hand, during the last 20 years a number of preventive trials demonstrated the feasibility and effectiveness of a population strategy for prevention of cardiovascular diseases (1).

Therefore, a strong and urgent need of a preventive intervention in Sardinia was clearly evident.

Although our Institution (the Regional Centre for Metabolic Diseases and Atherosclerosis, Cagliari) was already engaged in the Italian CNR community-based special programme "Preventive and Rehabilitative Medicine" (16) , and, furthermore, also in the implementation of a multicenter trial on epidemiology and prevention of atherosclerosis in Sardinia (the ATS-Sardegna Project) (9), we felt that at that moment (late 1986) Sardinian population needed more a community-oriented prevention campaign, rather than further preventive trials in limited, though multiple, intervention areas versus reference areas. Moreover, the budget of the Sardinian Department of Health allotted larger funds to preventive campaigns than to clinical trials.

As a matter of facts, the unfavourable trend of cardiovascular disease risk factors we had recorded in Sardinia had also been detected at the same time in other Northern (5) and Southern (6) Italian areas. Therefore, a nation-wide action would have been the most appropriate response to such a threat to the public health.

However, the feasibility of a national population strategy implies that whole communities, their leadership and national institutions should participate in preventive programs (1). But all this requires such complex and co-ordinate legislative measures, that a national programme very seldom develops, unless "initiative, experience and example at the local level" (18) acts as an initiation process.

With all the above considerations in mind, in late 1986 we planned a community-oriented campaign of multifactorial prevention of cardiovascular diseases in Sardinia: the ATS-Sardegna Campaign.

On the other hand, Sardinia is not new to campaigns of health education, which in recent years have been addressed to some health issues peculiar to the Sardinian population.

Some years ago, a campaign against favism (the G-6-PD-deficient condition is highly prevalent among Sardinians) through illustrated messages on mass media caused a sharp drop in hospital admissions for acute hemolytic anemia from fava bean ingestion.

Likewise, a campaign of health education on thalassemia (the beta-thalassemia trait is very frequent in Sardinia) caused a decline in the births of babies affected with thalassemia major.

Other examples could be mentioned.

Consequently, the question was to consider that, if the above campaigns proved to be fruitful, not less could have been one addressed to an epidemic which, though different in kind from the typical Sardinian pathology, causes higher morbidity and mortality than do all other "traditional" diseases taken together.

Therefore, we proposed the implementation of the ATS-Sardegna Campaign to the Sardinian Department of Public Health, which in 1988 officially announced its launch (2).

We were fully aware that a population strategy for prevention raises far more principle issues than does a community-based scientific trial. In fact, while a preventive clinical trial has only to count on its own scientific and ethical design, a public health action must reconcile and harmonize at least four components (1, 12):

1. scientific and ethical base;
2. political involvement;
3. financial support;
4. educational and advertising means.

Therefore, our great effort has been devoted to build a model of campaign based on the above four components, so as to fulfil what we consider the basic requirements for its validity as an ethical and effective undertaking, with, in addition, the features of a first stage in the development of a national programme (18).

1. As for its ethical-scientific content (feasibility, effectiveness, safety, favourable cost/benefit ratio) such a campaign has received the guide-lines from recognized scientific communities, such as the Italian Rimini Report 84 (8), the WHO Reports (17, 18), the USA (4), Italian (3) and European (14) Consensus Conferences, the Italian CNR Guide-lines (10), the Italian National Institute for Nutrition Guide-lines (7).

2. Action aimed at influencing and helping a population change in knowledge, attitude and behaviour, i.e. a public health undertaking (1), should be carried out, on principle, under the responsibility of the political authorities and institutions (18), though with scientific advice from a capable, devoted and well trained expert acting as an initiator and co-ordinator, and with the involvement of a local research institute (18). This is the case for the ATS-Sardegna Campaign.

Obviously, voluntary organizations and, above all, health profession organizations may play a role in the prevention programme, making it possible also to identify individuals at particular risk of cardiovascular disease, and to support the population strategy with the individual (high risk) strategy, so leading to a proper balance between the two (10). This is also a feature of the ATS-Sardegna Campaign.

3. The involvement of political institutions is also necessary in order to appropriate adequate funds for the implementation of the programme, through legislative measures which are more likely to be taken if the cost/benefit relations are correctly appraised, and the funds needed are regarded as investment for future benefit (18). The ATS-Sardegna Campaign has been financed by the Sardinian Department of Public Health.

4. The involvement of the mass media has been considered as indispensable (18), though not sufficient, so that other means of capillary health education have also been envisaged. Furthermore, collaboration from the beginning between mass communication experts and the medical team of the campaign has been particularly tight.

Owing to the necessary complexity of the main four components of the campaign, some unforeseen snags have been met with, particularly as far as politica, financial and bureaucratic aspects are concerned. I think that a short list of the major difficulties we met with might come useful to future planners of such a kind of undertakings:

(a) some disappointment came from the political component, whose sensibility towards this issue must however be fairly acknowledged. In fact, just after the official announcement of the appropriation for the ATS--Sardegna Campaign by the Sardinian Department of Public Health at the Joint-Meeting CNR-Sardinian political dignities, Rome, June 28th, 1988 (2), the funds allotted were cut down without notice;

(b) a subsequent recovery of the missing amount was prevented, so far, by necessity to divert financial resources towards the country afflicted with an exceptional drought;

(c) some other rubs came from the front of bureaucracy, inasmuch as the Health Administration of the Cagliari District was entrusted by the Department of Health with the task of managing the financial operations of the campaign. As a consequence, the preparatory phase of the campaign got stuck for half a year into the sluggish bureaucratic machinery, with ensuing delay of the start of the campaign.

Anyhow, almost everything is now (September 1989) at the starting point. The campaign is aimed at the major risk factors for atherosclerosis; however, it is above all a campaign of health promotion.

The target of the ATS-Sardegna Campaign is the general population. Special action has been planned towards three target groups: the family, the school, the medical profession.

The communication is accomplished through both the mass media and special media.

In Sardinia, two local newspapers have a wide circulation, and some local television networks enjoy a widespread audience. Spaces for reiterative messages have been made available on these media.

The special media consist of:

(a) a vade-mecum of prevention entitled "La Macchina-uomo" (The Human Machine) and featured as a maintenance hand-book. It is an illustrated means of health education for the family and the school;

(b) the volume "Guide-lines for the community-based prevention of coronary heart disease", edited in 1987 by the Italian CNR (10). This volume has been reprinted under licence from the Editor, as a means of involvement of the general practitioners in the accomplishment of the individual (high risk) strategy of the campaign.

What we expect of the ATS-Sardegna Campaign is, above all, a general improvement in the health of the Sardinian population. Moreover, as it is the first regional programme in Italy, we also expect it to catalyse the spread of cardiovascular prevention in the whole Country.

References

1. Blackburn, H. (1988) 'Development of public policy', in S. Muntoni, F.H. Epstein and G. Lamm (eds.), Epidemiology of Atherosclerosis (Satellite Meeting to 8th International Symposium on Atherosclerosis, Porto Cervo, October 14-15, 1988), CIC Edizioni Internazionali, Roma, pp. 97-104.

2. 'Collaborazione CNR-Sardegna sulle Malattie Cardiovascolari' (1988) Il Medico d'Italia 47, 3.

3. Consensus Conference Italiana (1986) 'Abbassare la colesterolemia per ridurre la cardiopatia coronarica', Giorn. Arterioscl. 11, 163-170.

4. Consensus Conference (1985) 'Lowering cholesterol to prevent heart disease', J.A.M.A. 253, 2080-2086.

5. Descovich, G.C. (1988) 'From the Brisighella Study to the Brisighella Project, in S. Muntoni, F.H. Epstein and G. Lamm (eds.), Epidemiology of Atherosclerosis (Satellite Meeting to 8th International Symposium on Atherosclerosis, Porto Cervo, October 14-15, 1988), CIC Edizioni Internazionali, Roma, pp. 71-76.

6. Farinaro, E., Trevisan, M., Giumetti, D., Panico, S., Krogh, V., Jossa, F., Fusco, G., Celentano, E., Coraggio, S., Ferrara, A.L. (1984) 'Time trends

of risk factors for CHD in a population sample of Southern Italy: the Olivetti Survey' in S. Lenzi and G.C. Descovich (eds.), Atherosclerosis and Cardiovascular Diseases, Editrice Compositori, Bologna, pp. 301-305.

7. Gruppo di Esperti dell'Istituto Nazionale della Nutrizione (1986) Linee guida per una sana alimentazione italiana, Roma.

8. Gruppo di Lavoro del G.I.E.P. e del CNR-ATS-Ob43 (1984) 'Prevenzione della cardiopatia coronarica in Italia. Rapporto Rimini 84, Giorn. Arterioscl. 9, 249-256.

9. Gruppo di Ricerca ATS-Sardegna (1987) 'I fattori di rischio dell'arteriosclerosi in Sardegna. La Fase A del Progetto Finalizzato Regionale ATS-Sardegna', Giorn Arterioscl. 12, 115-191.

10. Gruppo di Ricerca CNR-ATS-Ob43 (1987) Linee guida per la prevenzione comunitaria della cardiopatia coronarica, Direzione del Progetto Finalizzato Medicina Preventiva e Riabilitativa, Roma.

11. ISTAT (1987) Annuario Statistico Italiano, ISTAT, Roma, p. 106.

12. Menotti, A. (1989) La Prevenzione della Cardiopatia Coronarica. Seconda Edizione, Il Pensiero Scientifico Editore, Roma.

13. Muntoni, S. on behalf of the ATS-Sardegna Research Group (1986) 'Parallel increase in saturated fat intake and mean plasma cholesterol levels in Sardinia, during a six-year period', X World Congress of Cardiology, Washington, D.C., Abstr. No. 2593.

14. Study Group, European Atherosclerosis Society (1987) 'Strategies for prevention of coronary heart disease: a policy statement of the European Atherosclerosis Society, Eur. Heart J. 8, 77-88.

15. The Research Group of the Italian National research Council (1981) 'Distribution of some risk factors for atherosclerosis in nine Italian population samples', Am. J. Epidemiol. 113, 338-346.

16. The Research Group for Atherosclerosis Risk Factors (ATS-RF2), Rome, Italy (1986) 'Three year intervention on risk factors for atherosclerosis in the Italian Nine Communities Study', Clin. Ter. Cardiovasc. 3, 151-158.

17. World Health Organization (1982) Prevention of Coronary Heart Disease, Technical Report Series 687, WHO, Geneva.

18. World Health Organization (1985) Primary Prevention of Coronary Heart Disease, WHO-Euro reports and Studies 98, WHO, Copenhagen.

80
The Brisighella heart study report from 1984 to 1989

G.C. DESCOVICH, S. D'ADDATO, A. DORMI, G.L. MAGRI, A. MINARDI, Z. SANGIORGI, C. TURCHI[1], G. MANNINO[2] and M. SANTARELLA[3]

Department of Geriatrics, University of Bologna; [1]Department of Agriculture and Nutrition, Emilia-Romagna Region; [2]Head of Numerical Analysis Department, University of Modena; [3]Head of Brisighella Hospital, Italy

Epidemiological research in the cardiovascular field, with particular reference to coronary heart disease (CHD) and other pathologies linked to atherosclerosis, has in recent years revealed the need for an exact assessment of the individual risk factors (RF) together with an evaluation of the preventive results which can be obtained with their correction.

Total plasma cholesterol has been confirmed as a strong predictive RF for CHD and, furthermore, its reduction in entire populations appears to be largely responsible for a simultaneous drop in CHD mortality rates in the same countries (U.S.A., Canada and Australia in the first place) [1-3].

In fact, clinical trials of primary and secondary prevention have demonstrated that relatively small reductions in plasma cholesterol lead to a substantial drop in the number of new fatal and non-fatal cardiac events [4-7].

The Brisighella Heart Study proposed to apply these conclusions, by setting up a prevention programme for a whole population, not only on the basis of the entry data, but also considering the figures obtained subsequently, since this population was followed during a longitudinal study, started in 1972, and completely re-examined every 4 years until 1984.

The need for preventive measures was in fact prompted by the results of the longitudinal study [8-11], which are reported in another chapter in this book. In particular, in the males, a solution with five MLF parameters, applied taking account of the entry values of some of the main FRs, gave the coefficients listed in Table 1.

Tab.1: Brisighella Study Longitudinal Survey (1972-1988)
Males (age 35-75 years old at entry)
Cardiovascular death: 5 MLF parameters

Parameter	Coefficient	SD	t	p
Constant	-8.0463	0.5860	-	-
Age (yr)	0.0476	0.0068	7.0	<0.001
Physical Act. (code)	-0.1297	0.0277	4.7	<0.001
Smoking (cig/day)	0.0963	0.0367	2.6	<0.005
SBP (mmHg)	0.0167	0.0024	7.0	<0.001
TC (mg/dl)	0.0042	0.0013	3.2	<0.005

THE BRISIGHELLA HEART STUDY

The fourth observation in the longitudinal study (in 1984) [9] revealed that preventive intervention had become necessary and urgent for the Brisighella population as regards ischemic heart disease, given the high mortality rates for this cause (markedly higher than the national Italian rates) [12], and the rising cholesterol levels (2 mg/dl/year in men and 3 mg/dl/year in women) in relation to the deterioration in nutritional habits.

As regards the type of intervention, the hypothesis adopted was that of using the already existing health structures as much as possible, so as to limit the costs to a minimum and establish an example which could be extended to larger areas of the country.

At first an ad hoc committee was set up, with the aim of planning the intervention; a number of public bodies were invited to take part in the committee, including the Emilia-Romagna Department of Agriculture and Nutrition, which also helped to finance the project, the Emilia-Romagna Health Department and the University of Bologna.

During the first stage a feasibility study was carried out, involving intervention on the behavioural and nutritional habits of the entire adult population (approximately 9000 persons).

In 1985 a "Centre of Information on Nutrition" was set up in the local hospital; four dieticians began work on a nutrition programme.

To inform the population of the new service available, 3012 letters were sent out to the head of each family in the town; informative brochures were subsequently also prepared and distributed. The material made available to the citizens consisted of official documents from Institutes and Italian scientific structures [13-15].

The guide lines followed by the dieticians of the Nutrition Information Centre consisted mainly of suggesting a reduction in the quantity of saturated fats and cholesterol in the everyday diet, in encouraging an increase in the consumption of complex carbohydrates and vegetable oil, in particular corn oil, olive oil and soft polyunsaturated margarine, attempting as far as possible to integrate this advice with the traditional diet of the population. A reduction in salt consumption was also advised.

During this first year of the intervention the practice of rapid cholesterolemia measurement was also adopted using the Reflotron technique (dry-chemistry rapid method) on a capillary blood sample taken from a finger.

The reliability of this method was assessed as compared with the traditional enzymatic technique (Eppendorf), guaranteed by means of quality control carried out together with the WHO laboratory in Prague [11].

During the first year of activity, 1147 subjects were observed by the Nutritional Information Centre; total plasma cholesterol was measured in these subjects every four months.

During the first eight months there was a reduction of 15% in total plasma cholesterol in females and 19% in males, whereas after twelve months there was a change in the trend, due partly to the seasonal modifications and partly to the fact that less attention was given to nutritional habits (fig.1).

For this reason a permanent educational activity is very important: a decrease in compliance was observed immediately after the summer holidays, when other interests are more relevant for people.

Once the feasibility of the study had been assessed, a detailed programme was drawn up which aimed at reinforcing the intervention on the entire population by means of action directed towards two particular sub-groups: the high-risk subjects (HR) and the school population (fig.2).

Fig 1: **BRISIGHELLA HEART STUDY**

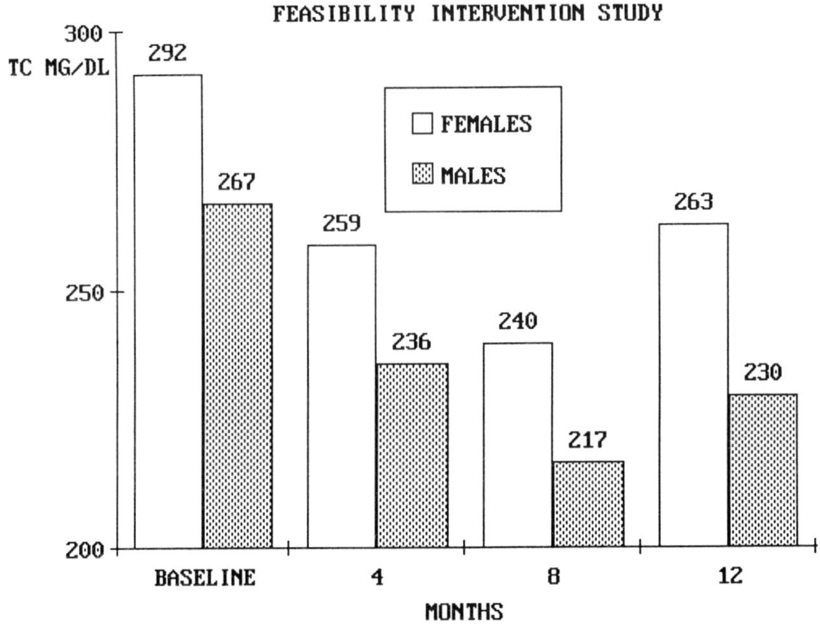

Fig. 2

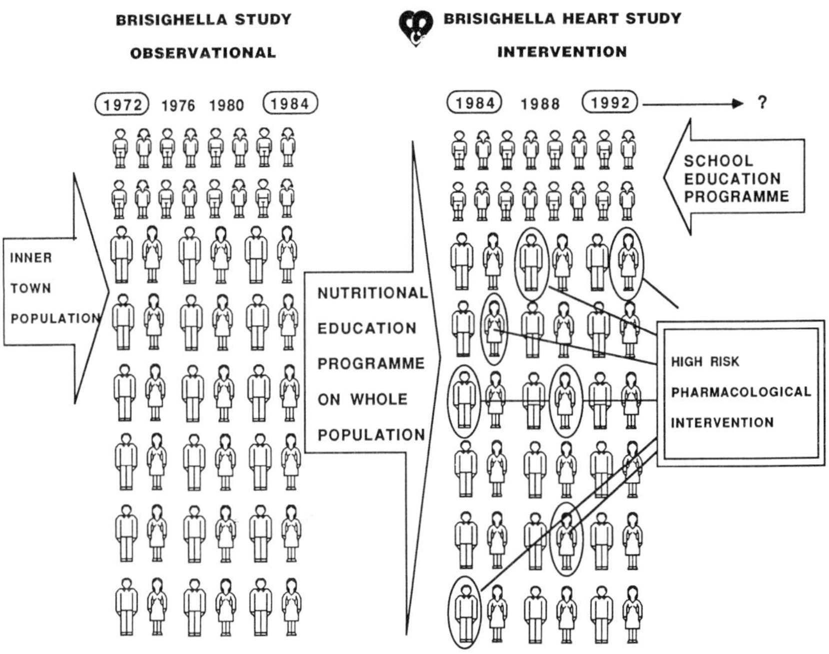

The need to intervene in the high-risk subjects with more severe dietetic measures, and even drugs, derived from the fact that most subjects had such high cholesterol values that they could not be corrected with mere nutritional intervention.

The TC cut-off point adopted to define the boundary between medium and high-risk was 240 mg/dl, in accordance with the American Consensus Conference and the Panel of the National Cholesterol Education Program [16-17].

The protocol envisaged that subjects who, after at least six weeks of nutritional treatment, did not drop below the critical threshold, would be started on a drug treatment based on Gemfibrozil (600 mg b.i.d.).

Subsequently these patients were followed up for an overall period of five years with six-monthly check-ups.

A special Service for outpatients, similar to the Bologna Lipid Clinic, was opened at the Brisighella Hospital.

In October 1988, the 5th mass screening was started on the Brisighella "historical" citizen, i.e. those subjects who had taken part in the 1972 Brisighella Study.

At the same time other Brisighella citizens were studied, who had not taken part in the initial study (1972) and who had come to the Centre as a result of the publicity aimed at the entire population.

At the end of the first screening period, 2640 citizens had been examined, 1854 "historical" and 786 new subjects; 1180 of all citizens examined had TC >239 mg/dl.

The HR percentage was very high (44.6%), but was much lower than the 1984 check-up (61%).

Fig. 3

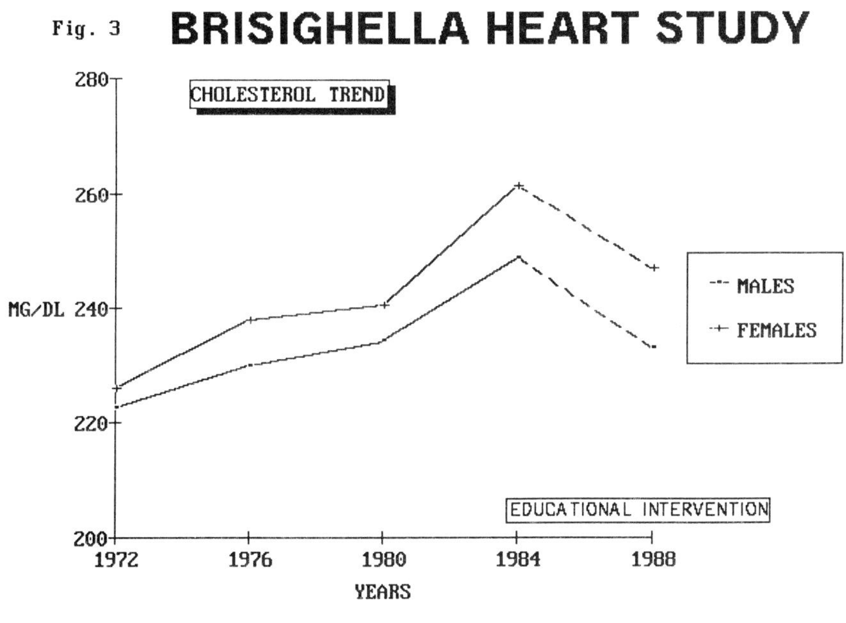

Figure 3 shows in more detail how, considering the average total cholesterol values in the "historical" subjects in 1988 and comparing these values with the average values of the same subjects at previous check-ups, there had been an inversion of the constantly rising trend recorded earlier, both in males and in females.

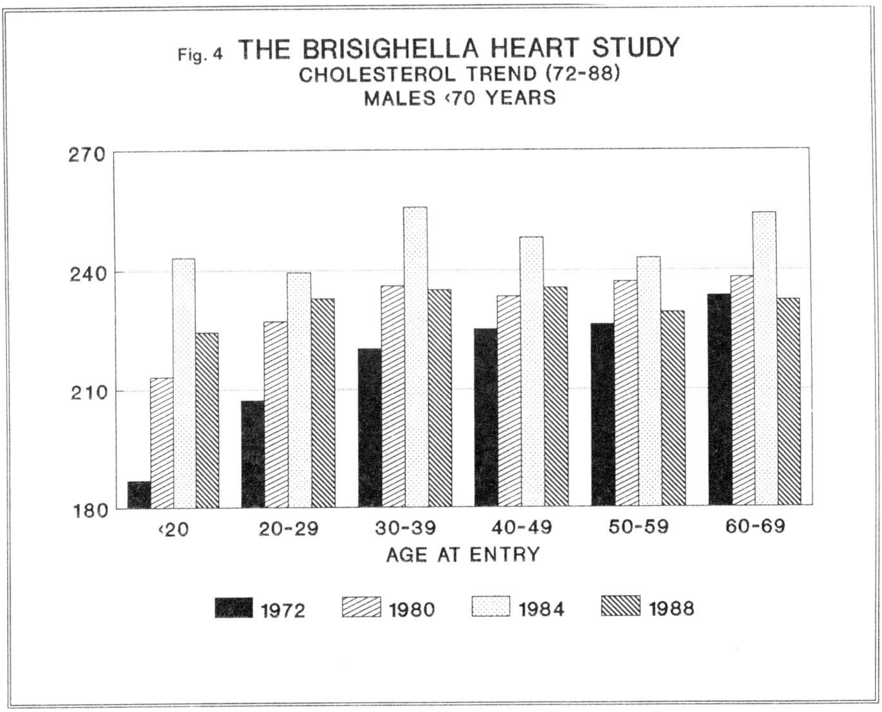

Figure 4 also shows how this inversion of the trend had occurred in all the age classes considered.

This, in our opinion, is due to the Nutritional Education Programme operating in Brisighella.

A clear marker for this interpretation is the very impressive rise in the consumption of soft margarine in Brisighella (900% vs 14% in the whole of Italy).

All the HR subjects underwent a more intense nutritional approach; 593 of these completed 6 weeks of correct dietary habits and TC fell to the "medium risk" level (200-239 mg/dl) in 213 (35.9%). The citizens who, at the checkup following 6 weeks of dietary education, had TC values >239 mg/dl were treated with Gemfibrozil (600 mg b.i.d.). Approximately 450 HR citizens continued this drug treatment for at least six months and approximately 200 for at least a year. During this period no adverse side effects were reported and approximately 650 Brisighella citizens are still under treatment with Gemfibrozil.

The second population group for which specific intervention was decided was the school population (nursery school, primary and secondary school), the aim being not only to carry out pre-primary prevention but also to create children who were active propagandists in their own families of the messages received at school.

During the school year 1987-88, the "ad hoc Committee", with the help of a mass media expert and a pedagogist, prepared a great deal of material for teachers and for school children.

The methods employed were aimed at developing in the children a critical attitude towards the reading of publicity messages (in particular those referring to food) and attempted to trigger the educational message from real experiences, so that personal experience interacted with information received.

The results obtained were generally encouraging, since the children demonstrated a good and correct understanding of the nutritional messages which were given to them (Tab.2) and a readiness to put them into practice.

Tab.2: Brisighella Heart Study School Education Programme Correct replies given by students after one year of intervention

Which foods contain most cholesterol?	96%
Which diseases provoke cholesterol?	98%
Which foods should you eat least?	97%
Which foods should you eat most?	100%
Have you talked about cholesterol in the family?	81%
Has your family changed its eating habits?	51%

Figure 5 compares the cholesterolemia distribution in a school class before the intervention and the following year: a change in the median from 160-180 mg/dl level to 140-160 mg/dl level can be seen and a shift to the left of TC values which also leads to the disappearance of the 220-240 mg/dl TC plasma concentrations.

Fig. 5 **BRISIGHELLA HEART STUDY**

SCHOOL EDUCATION PROGRAMME

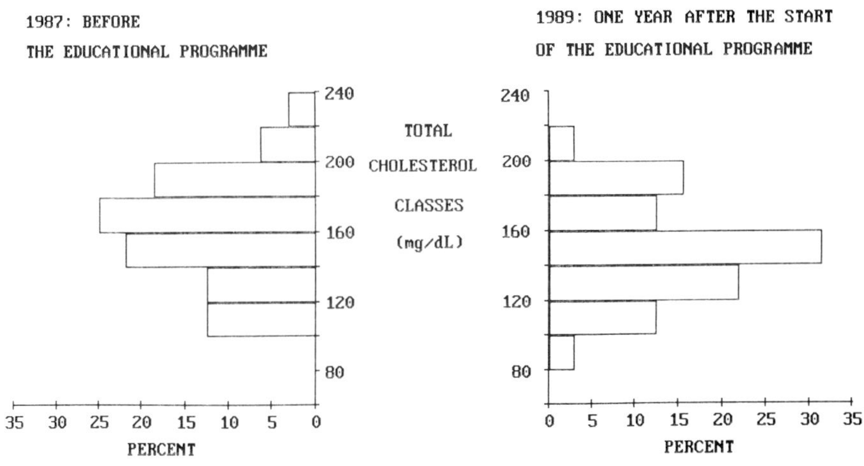

Conclusions

Both studies, first the feasibility study and subsequently the long-term intervention study, appear to confirm the validity of the initial idea. It was possible to enroll a large number of free-living subjects into the intervention programme without special care units. Moreover, the initial inversion of the rising TC trend may testify a substantial change in the nutritional habits of the entire population. With the continuation of the nutritional programme and pharmacological treatment it is reasonable to expect a marked drop in new fatal and non-fatal cardiac events at the end of the five-year intervention programme.

References

1. World Health Statistics Annual (1987) 'Mortality from ischaemic heart disease in industrialized countries'. Geneva, 25.
2. Stamler, J. (1985) 'The Marked Decline in Coronary Heart Disease Mortality Rates in the United States, 1968-1981; Summary of Findings and Possible Explanations', Cardiology, 72, 11-22.
3. Hardes, G.R., Dobson, A.J., Lloyd, D.M. and Leeder, S.R. (1985) 'Coronary Heart Disease Mortality Trends and Related Factors in Australia', Cardiology, 72, 23-28.
4. Lipid Research Clinic Program (1984) 'The Lipid Research Clinic Coronary Prevention Trials Results: I. Reduction in the incidence of coronary heart disease', JAMA, 251, 351-364.
5. Lipid Research Clinic Program (1984) 'The Lipid Research Clinics Coronary Prevention Trials Results: II. The relationship of reduction in incidence of coronary heart disease to cholesterol lowering', JAMA, 251, 365-374.
6. Frick, M.H., Elo, O., Haapa, K., Heinonen, O.P., Heinsalmi, P., Helo, P., Huttunen, J.K., Kaitanjemi, P., Koskinen, P., Manninen, V., Maenpaa, H., Malkonen, M., Manttari, M., Norola, S., Pasternack, A., Pikkarainen, J., Romo, M., Sjoblom, T. and Nikkila, E.A. (1987) 'Helsinki Heart Study: Primary prevention trial with gemfibrozil in middle-aged men with dyslipidemia', N. Engl. J. Med. 317, 1237-1245.
7. Blankenhorn, D.H., Nessim, S.A., Johnson, R.L., Sanmarco, M.E., Azen, S.P. and Cashin-Hemphill (1987) 'Beneficial effects of combined colestipol-niacine therapy on coronary artery atherosclerosis and coronary venous bypass grafts', JAMA 257, 3233.
8. Descovich, G.C., Dalmonte, G., Dormi, A., Braiato, A., Mannino, G., Benassi, M.S., Gaddi, A., Magri, G.L., Perini, P., Sangiorgi, Z., Trivelli, N. and Lenzi, S. (1984) 'The Brisighella Study: a community survey' in S. Lenzi and G.C. Descovich (eds.), Atherosclerosis and Cardiovascular Diseases, MTP Press, Lancaster, Boston, The Hague, Dordrecht pp 467-477.
9. Descovich, G.C., Dormi, A., Gaddi, A., Magri, G.L., Mannino, G., Rimondi, S., Sangiorgi, Z. and Lenzi S. (1987) 'From observational to intervention programmes. The Brisighella study' in S. Lenzi and G.C. Descovich (eds.), Atherosclerosis and Cardiovascular Diseases, MTP Press, Lancaster, Boston, The Hague, Dordrecht pp 215-221.
10. Descovich G.C. (1988) 'From the Brisighella Study to the Brisighella Project' in S. Muntoni, F.H. Epstein and G. Lamm (eds.), 'Epidemiology of Atherosclerosis' (Proceedings of 8th International Symposium on Atherosclerosis, Satellite Meeting), CIC Edizioni Internazionali, Roma pp 71-76.
11. Descovich, G.C., Gaddi A., Minardi A., Magri G.L., Dormi A., D'Addato S., Vigna M., Sangiorgi Z. (1989) 'The Brisighella Heart Project' in 'Biotechnology of Dyslipoproteinemias: Clinical Applications in Diagnosis and Control', Raven Press New York (in press).
12. Menotti, A., Capocaccia, R., Farchi, G., Pasquali, M. (1985) 'Recent trends in coronary heart disease and other cardiovascular diseases in Italy', Cardiology, 72, 88-96.
13. G.I.E.P. (1986) 'Rapporto Rimini 84: Prevenzione Primaria della Cardiopatia Coronarica', Giornale della Arteriosclerosi, 3, 249.
14. Consensus Conference Italiana (1986) 'Abbassare la colesterolemia per ridurre la cardiopatia coronarica. CNR Direzione del Progetto Finalizzato di Medicina Preventiva e Riabilitativa', Roma.
15. Istituto Nazionale della Nutrizione (1986) 'Linee guida per una sana alimentazione', Roma.
16. Consensus Conference (1985) 'Lowering blood cholesterol to prevent heart disease', JAMA 253, 2080-2086.

17. The Expert Panel (1988) 'Report of the National Cholesterol Education Program Expert Panel on Detection, Evaluation, and Treatment of High Blood Cholesterol in Adults', Arch. Intern. Med. 148, 36-69.

Acknowledgements

We would like to thank the Quaker-Chiari & Forti company for supplying the Cuore corn oil and Parke Davis for the Gemfibrozil drug and for the advice and cooperation generously provided on the basis of their experience gained in the Helsinki Heart Study.

Appendix

BRISIGHELLA HEART STUDY MEMBERS (All Researchers listed here must be considered "Authors" of the present papers)

Coordinator:	G.C. Descovich - Bologna
Cholelitiasis Staff:	Chairman E. Roda
Bologna Medical Staff:	G.C. Descovich, G. Barozzi, A. Cavina, C. Ceredi, M. Colletta, A. Ciarrocchi, G. De Simone, A. Gaddi, A. Minardi, C. Naldoni, S. Paci, A. Romagnoli, M. Vigna
Bologna Biochemical Laboratory Staff:	Dir. Z. Sangiorgi, G. Copparoni, I. Faenza, G. Gamberi, G. La Regina, C. Meotti
Bologna Nutritional Laboratory Staff:	M.L. Borlotti, F. Brini, E. Faggioli, G. Negro, E. Tabanelli, G. Tarrini
Bologna Biometrics Laboratory Staff:	Dir. G. Mannino, A. Dormi, A. Braiato
Bologna ECG Reading and Coding Staff:	Dir. S. Rimondi, L. Finazzo
Bologna Echographic Reading and Coding Staff:	S. D'Addato, D. Festi, G.L. Magri, G. Manganaro, A. Matteucci
Bologna Rheumatic Staff:	S. Ferri
Medical Students Field Operators:	M. Ceccardi, G. Sisca, B. Descovich, C. Descovich
General Secretariat:	C. Maurizzi, M. Nanni
Brisighella Gen. Practitional Staff:	J. Drei, I. Gamberi, A. Naldi, F. Onofri, C. Samore' L. Savorani, G. Trere', F.M. Valpondi, P. Viozzi
Brisighella Hospital Staff:	Dir. M. Santarella, A. Callea, D. Casadei-Giunchi, C. Colombi, M. Gualdrini, S. Milletti, F.M. Montanari G. Pagano, O. Quercia, R. Ramponi, A. Sarti F. Tavoni, A. Zambon, A. Zamboni, R. Zucchini
Brisighella Biochemical Laboratory Staff:	E. Folco-Zambelli
Brisighella Coordination Staff:	E. Pelliconi, R. Bandini, B. Alboreti, F. Silvestrini
Brisighella Anagraphic Staff:	L. Sbarzaglia

Emilia-Romagna Region:	
Assessorato all'Agricoltura e all' Alimentazione:	G. Ceredi, M.C. Turchi
Press Office:	F. Gencarelli, I. Cattania
U.S.L. 37 Faenza:	F. Laghi, R. Bertoni, P. Fabbri

Mass media Staff:	E. Marino	Pedagocic Staff:	R. Bianco Finocchiaro

International Board:	G. Lamm	(Heidelberg)	Epidemiology
	A. Menotti	(Roma)	Epidemiology
	G. Grafnetter	(Praga)	Laboratory
	G. Sprovieri	(Bologna)	Laboratory
	A.M. Gotto Jr.	(Houston)	Lipids
	J. Iacono	(Washington)	Nutrition
	A. Mariani Costantini	(Roma)	Nutrition

HYPERLIPOPROTEINAEMIA THERAPY: WHEN TO OPT FOR DRUG COMBINATIONS

81
Drug combination therapy for selected hyperlipidemic patients

C.A. DUJOVNE, M.I. SZTERN and W.S. HARRIS

The Lipid and Arteriosclerosis Prevention Clinic, Division of Clinical Pharmacology, University of Kansas Medical Center, 1348 Bell 39th and Rainbow, Kansas City, KS 66103, USA

ABSTRACT. We performed individual patient clinical trials with hypolipidemic drug combinations in thirty-one patients who failed to either tolerate or normalize their lipid profile with single drug treatment. Type IIA, IIB or IV hyperlipoproteinemics were randomly assigned to sequential treatment with resins, lovastatin, fish oil, niacin or gemfibrozil alone or in combination. In successful cases, lovastatin plus resin exerted greater hypolipidemic effect than either one alone or than twice the lovastatin dose. Lovastatin suppressed the hypertriglyceridemic effect of resins. Fish oil plus resin prevented the undesirable effects of resin on triglycerides and of fish oil on LDL-C levels. Fish oil plus niacin resulted in better control of LDL-C and triglycerides than either alone. Fish oil and gemfibrozil had additive hypotriglyceridemic effects. In selected patients, hypolipidemic drug combinations may result in more effective control of serum lipid levels than monotherapy.

Introduction

The practicing physician is often confronted with the need to perform single-patient clinical trials to evaluate the potential therapeutic benefit of combined hypolipidemic drug therapy. The different reasons for combined drug therapy are depicted in Table I. The most common reason in our trial was the failure to attain normalization of serum lipoprotein levels using a single agent at its usual dose. We report here the efficacy of a variety of drug combinations in 31 patients with various types of serum lipoprotein abnormalities.

Methods

Patients with the following lipoprotein disorders were considered candidates for combined drug therapy: type IIA (isolated hypercholesterolemia) defined by serum triglycerides levels <250mg/dl with an LDL cholesterol level >170mg/dl, type IIB (mixed hyperlipidemia) defined by a serum triglyceride level >250mg/dl with an LDL cholesterol level >170mg/dl, and type IV (isolated hypertriglyceridemia) defined by a serum triglyceride level >250mg/dl and LDL cholesterol level <170mg/dl.

All patients were between 18 and 65 years of age and of either sex. They were non-diabetic/non-obese, euthyroid and without clinical or laboratory evidence of renal, hepatic or pancreatic diseases. They were not taking any other drugs known or suspected to affect blood lipoprotein levels.

TABLE 1. Reasons for drug combination for hypolipidemic therapy

1. Partial failure to correct single or multiple serum lipoprotein level abnormalities with a single drug.
2. A single drug causing desirable effects on one lipoprotein parameter, but undesirable effects on another. (see Table 4)
3. Intolerance to fully effective dose of a single drug.
4. Increased cost of larger doses of a single agent.
5. Dose related toxicity by larger doses of a single drug.

Lipoprotein Measurements

These were performed by methods described previously from our laboratory (1), which is at Phase III of the Lipid Standardization program of the United States Centers for Disease Control.

Choice of Drugs and Dosages

The drug combination to be tested in a given patient was chosen based on the lipoprotein abnormality as follows: For type IIA: cholestyramine (Questran™) or colestipol (Colestid™) plus lovastatin (Mevacor™). For type IIB: cholestyramine or colestipol plus lovastatin (Mevacor™); fish oil (FO) capsules rich in eicosapentaenoic acid (MaxEPA™ or Promega™) plus cholestyramine, or FO plus niacin in slow release preparations (Nicobid™ or Nicolar™ or generic equivalents). For type IV: FO plus gemfibrozil (Lopid™) or FO plus niacin.

The doses employed were titrated up from and to arbitrarily predetermined limits as follows: cholestyramine, 8 - 16gm/day; colestipol, 10 - 20 gm/day; niacin, 250mg to 1.5gm/day; gemfibrozil, 600 to 1,200mg/day; lovastatin, 20 - 80mg/day; fish oil capsules (containing 30 to 37% of n-3 fatty acids), 10 - 18 capsules/day providing 4 - 6gm of n-3 fatty acids/day.

Treatment Protocol

Upon initiation of the drug trial, every patient had been on supervised low fat, low cholesterol diet at Phase I or II of the AHA guidelines for at least 2 months. Most of them were monitored for diet compliance by a method of dietary records developed at our Clinic (2). Baseline serum lipoproteins were obtained on 2 to 3 occasions; the patient was then assigned to a treatment sequence which always started with a single drug and was followed randomly by 2 - 3 months of the alternate single drug or the drug combination treatments (Table 2). Serum lipoproteins were measured and clinical laboratory safety assessments were performed every 4 - 6 weeks throughout the trial.

TABLE 2.

BASELINE	>	SINGLE DRUG	>	ALTERNATE SINGLE OR COMBINATION	>	REMAINING ALTERNATE TREATMENT	>	INCREASED DOSE OF SINGLE DRUG

Patients

We studied a total of 7 type IIA patients with the lovastatin - resin combination; 10 type IIB patients with the FO - niacin combination; 2 type IIA and 5 type IIB patients with the FO - resin combination; and 7 type IV patients with the FO - gemfibrozil combination. In this trial we did not test combinations which have been proven efficacious in previously published studies, such as niacin plus resins, probucol plus resins, gemfibrozil plus resins, and gemfibrozil plus niacin.

Results

Because of the wide variety of responses and the relatively small number of patients in each group, we have chosen to present selected examples of responses in individual patients. For each of the drug combination trials, we arbitrarily divided responses in three categories: positive, equivocal and negative. In comparing combination treatment to each single drug treatment, a response to combination therapy was considered to be positive when it led to changes in all serum lipoprotein parameters that were more beneficial than either drug alone. A response to a combination treatment was considered to be equivocal when the combination produced better effects in some of the lipoprotein parameters, but not in others; and a response was considered to be negative when combination therapy was not better than either drug alone for most lipoprotein parameters. The minimum goal of therapy was to reduce triglyceride serum levels to ≤250mg/dl and LDL cholesterol to ≤150mg/dl. Based on these criteria, our patients responded as shown in Table 3. Individual examples of response to some of the combinations are presented in Figures 1 - 4. The legends in each figure describe the results and interpretation of drug combination advantages in each patient. The order of treatment was random, but is presented always in the same sequence in the figures. The bars represent means of three determinations done at 4-6 weeks intervals.

TABLE 3.

Combination	Total Patients	Negative	Responses Equivocal	Positive
Lovastatin-Resin	7	0	3	4
Fish Oil (FO)-Resin	7	1	5	1
FO-Niacin	10	2	5	3
FO-Gemfibrozil	7	3	3	1

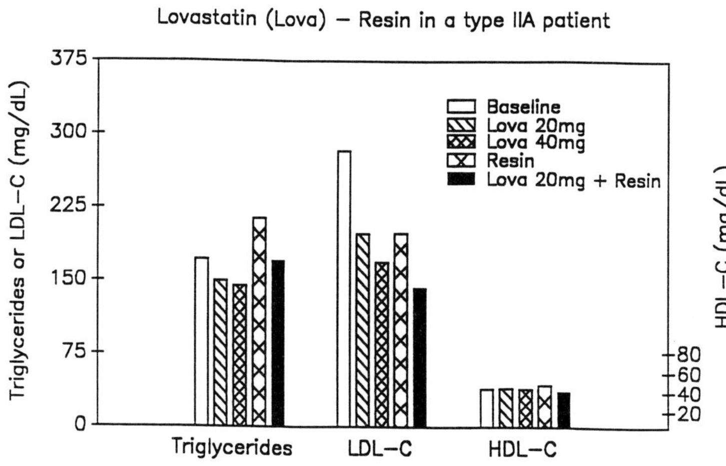

Figure 1. In this patient, Lova + Resin offered the greatest reduction in LDL-C levels. The combination was more effective than doubling the dose of lovastatin without resin.

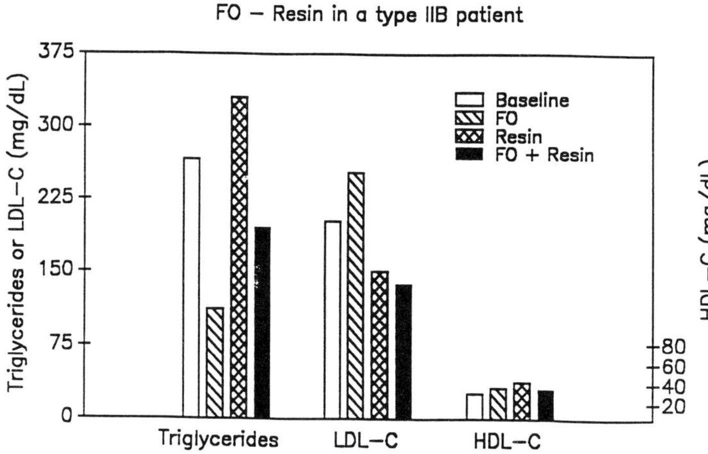

Figure 2. In this patient, FO + Resin provided the lowest LDL-C levels. The resin blunted the elevation of LDL-C levels seen with FO given singly. FO blunted the elevation of serum triglycerides seen when resin was given singly.

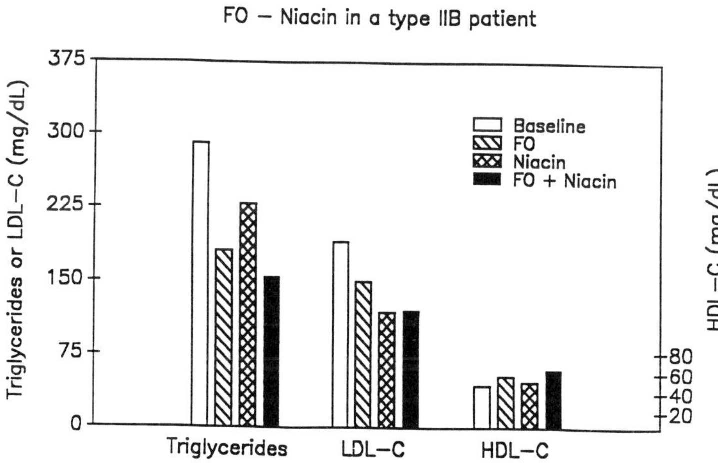

Figure 3. In this patient, FO + NA rendered effective control of LDL-C and triglyceride levels. Neither drug alone accomplished both objectives.

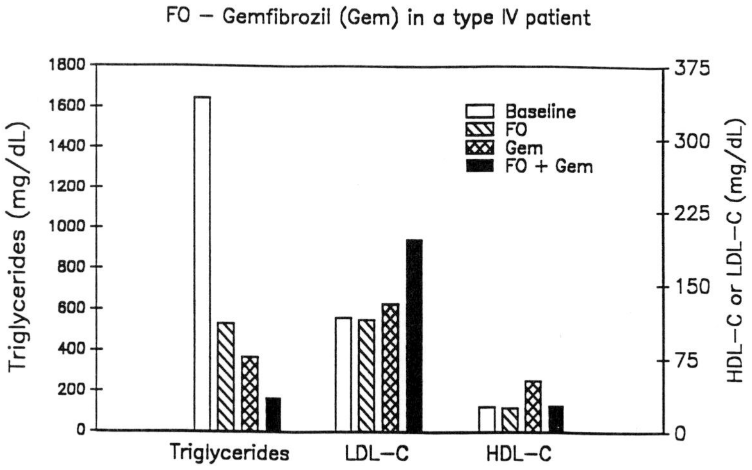

Figure 4. In this patient, serum triglyceride levels were reduced to normal only after FO + GEM treatment. The efficacy of the combination was judged to be equivocal because GEM alone provided the best effect on LDL-C/HDL-C rations while FO + GEM administration resulted in the highest LDL-C levels.

TABLE 4

COMBINED DRUG THERAPIES FOR DYSLIPIDEMIA

Combination	Advantages
Resins	
+ Niacin	Enhanced LDL-C reduction and HDL-C elevation. Blunting of hypertriglyceridemic effect of resins.
+ Probucol	Enhanced LDL-C reduction. Reduction of constipation due to resins.
+ Gemfibrozil	Enhanced LDL-C reduction and blunting of LDL-C elevation from gemfibrozil. Additional hypotriglyceridemic effect or blunting of hypertriglyceridemic effect of resins.
+ Lovastatin	Enhanced LDL-C reduction. Blunting of hypertriglyceridemic effect of resins.
+ Fish Oil	Prevention of LDL-C elevation from fish oils and of triglyceride elevation by resins in combined hyperlipidemia. Diarrhea and constipation from either agent may be ameliorated.
Lovastatin	
+ Gemfibrozil	Enhanced LDL-C reduction in isolated hypercholesterolemia or blunting of LDL-C elevation from gemfibrozil in combined hyperlipidemia. Enhanced hypotriglyceridemic effect. Enhanced HDL-C elevation.
+ Niacin	Enhanced LDL-C and triglyceride reduction in combined hyperlipidemia. Enhanced HDL elevation.
Niacin	
+ Fish Oil	Enhanced hypotriglyceridemic effect. Blunting of LDL-C elevation from fish oils in combined hyperlipidemia.
Gemfibrozil	
+ Niacin	Enhanced hypotriglyceridemic effect. Enhanced HDL-C elevation. Blunting of LDL-C elevation from gemfibrozil.
+ Fish Oil	Enhanced hypotriglyceridemic effect.

Adapted from Dujovne & Harris, 1989, Ann. Rev. Pharmacol. Toxicol., 29:265-268 (3).

Discussion

It is difficult, if not impossible, to predict the result of drug combination therapy in a given patient. Thus, it becomes necessary to perform a crossover type "clinical trial" in each individual patient to determine the best therapeutic combination.
The potential advantages of specific drug combinations are listed in Table 4. Any one of them may be indicated in a given patient and some were selected for the examples illustrated in the results section.
The major potential disadvantage of the use of drug combinations is the increased complexity of drug intake schedules. In some patients, combination drug therapy may decrease compliance and impair therapeutic efficacy. These factors are relevant when the treatment is a life-long undertaking such as in a large majority of hyperlipidemic patients. Nevertheless, the physician can carefully select the drugs and closely monitor laboratory results for efficacy and side effects to find drug combinations which will provide maximum benefit to the ever-growing number of patients requiring multiple drugs to effectively treat dyslipidemia-induced arteriosclerosis.

References

1. Harris, W.S., Dujovne, C.A., Zucker, M. and Johnson, B. (1988) 'Effects of a Low Saturated Fat, Low Cholesterol Fish Oil Supplement in Hypertriglyceridemic Patients: A Placebo-Controlled Trial', Ann Int Med 109(6), 465-470.

2. Jackson, B., Dujovne, C.A., DeCoursey, S., Beyer, P., Brown, E.F., and Hassanein, K. (1986) 'Method to Assess Dietary Compliance in Outpatient Clinical Trials', J Am Diet Assoc 86, 1531-1535.

3. Dujovne, C.A. and Harris, W.S. (1989) 'The Pharmacological Treatment of Dyslipidemia', Ann Rev Pharmacol and Toxicol 29, 265-288.

The authors wish to acknowledge the valuable contribution of Brenda Cannon, Beverly Fehner, Sherry Severson, and Sheryl Windsor during the performance of this research and the preparation of this manuscript.

*M. Sztern, M.D. is a recipient of the American Physicians' Fellowship Grant.

82
Hyperlipoproteinemia therapy: when to opt for drug combination?

F. DAIROU, J.L. DE GENNES, E. BRUCKERT and J. TRUFFERT

Hôpital de la Pitié, Service d'Endocrinologie-Métabolisme, 83 bv de l'Hôpital, Paris, 75013 France

ABSTRACT. Two or more hypolipidemic drugs can be used simultaneously in order to obtain an adequat level of LDL cholesterol (LDL C), triglycerides (TG), HDL cholesterol (HDL C), apolipoprotein B (Apo B), and apolipoprotein A1 (Apo A1) at which atherosclerosis is supposed to be stopped or even is regressing. Such a decision depends on the lipid levels but also on the type of hyperlipoproteinemia, age, side effects of drugs and clinical course of atherosclerosis. Drug combination remains a secondary decision after a dietetic period and a monotherapy period. We have studied several drug combinations in heterozygous forms of Familial Hypercholesterolemia (FH). Bile acid sequestrants (resin) associated to fenofibrate lower LDL C by 36%. A retrospective study with cholestyramin and ciprofibrate shows a sustained lowering action on LDL C. Hydroxymethyl coenzyme A reductase inhibitors (HMG I) associated with resin provides the same lowering action on LDL C. An association of HMG I and fibrate derivative must be specially cautious for adverse reactions : it decreases LDL C by 38%. In most cases of FH, one can reach a complete correction of LDL C modulating the posology of resin. In the remaining cases a third drug have to be added; it can be nicotinic acid or probucol.

INTRODUCTION

It has been clearly demonstrated from preventive trials, that cholesterol reduction must be drastic if we want to reach the main goal of treating dyslipoproteinemias : prevent or retard atherosclerotic complications. In severe forms of dyslipoproteinemia, complete lipid correction cannot be achieved by the means of diet alone or diet plus one single drug.

DECISION ACCORDING TO THE TYPE OF DYSLIPIDEMIA

1)Heterozygous Familial Hypercholesterolemia.
The most common situation requiring drug combination is represented by heterozygous FH. However, before any decision of drug combination, one have to appreciate individual response to treatment which can vary in a large proportion. Young adults and children, can be excellent responders to diet or monotherapy. Since in children, the risk of liver toxicity or unknown effects on growth, make all drugs but bile acids sequestrants, unsuitable, there is no possibility for drug combination in children. In adults such diet response must be appreciated after at least 6 weeks (in other types of dyslipidemia the diet period should be 2 or 3 months, especially in Combined Hyperlipidemia and in Hypertriglyceridemia) and the action of monotherapy evaluated after a minimum period of 4 months. Basal total cholesterol is not always a good indicator for drug response to treatment : individual variation can exist.

2)Homozygous FH.
Homozygous FH is an extreme state where response to medical treatment depends on the genetic defect. In children totally deficient in LDL receptor activity, so called negative receptor homozygotes, neither monotherapy nor multiple drug combination are able to lower consistantly LDL C. All classes of drug whose mechanism of action involves an enhanced synthesis of LDL receptor have a weak or nul lipid lowering effect. In defective receptor homozygotes, drug combination associated to LDL apheresis is useful to retard cholesterol rebond post apheresis and maybe, allows larger intervals between apheresis procedures. HMG I, resins and nicotinic acid or probucol are commonly used at the maximal tolerated posology.

3)Combined Hyperlipidemia.
In Combined Hyperlipidemia (CH), drug combination is rarely necessary, as long as diet is observed (1). First line drugs are fibrates derivatives which lead to a complete correction in most cases. In some resistant patients, fibrates and nicotinic acid have proven to be an effective combination, as demonstrated in the Stockholm Study. Up to now, efficacy of HMG I in CH is not clearly documented ; further studies are necessary to demonstrate the usefulness and tolerance of a combination of HMG I and fibrates in CH.

DECISION RELATED TO SIDE EFFECTS OF DRUGS

Poor compliance can be the consequence of drug side effects. Most side effects are dose related and can be blunted in reducing posology. The mean to limit adverse reactions and reach the same lipid lowering action as one single drug at full dosage, is to associate several drugs

whith different mechanism of action. Fibrates side effects have been extensively listed in the Coronary Drug Project (CDP) (2). Clofibrate was the drug used in CDP but most of clofibrate side effects can occur with fibrate derivatives. Muscle syndrome -myalgia and increased CPK-, liver toxicity, and maybe increased gallstone formation are dose dependant. While other complications like : skin rashes, gastro-intestinal pain, nausea, decreased libido or potentia, can be attributed to the type of molecule and can vary from one fibrate derivative to another. However tolerance of fibrates are generally acceptable if one avoid excessive posology, or respect contra-indications, such as renal failure, or liver disease, and establish a correct follow up of hepatic enzymes.
Resin intolerance makes the treatment uncomfortable in nearly 30% of cases. Such percentage can be reduced with progressive posology and usual advices in the use of resins. Side effects, abdominal pain, belching, bloating, constipation or diarrhea, gas, nausea, are quite dose related and a reduced dosage blunt them.

STUDIES IN HETEROZYGOUS FAMILIAL HYPERCHOLESTEROLEMIA.

European recommandations for optimal cholesterol level indicate dietary modifications for total cholesterol ranging from 200 to 250 mg/dl (3); LDL C is considered at risk above 170 mg/dl. This is the target one have to reach. If one consider the common basal level of total cholesterol in heterozygous FH between 350 and 400 mg/dl, the cholesterol lowering action one must achieve ranges between 20% and 50% with a mean value of 37%.

1)Resin-fenofibrate combination.

Combination of bile acid sequestrants and fibrates derivatives is a classical combination, used in France for nearly 15 years, since fenofibrate appeared in 1975. It has replaced the more classical combination of resin and clofibrate. Resin is generally used as first drug. This study involved 28 FH patients (7 females, 21 males), mean age was 46 years (range 18-62), familial history of FH, (all), xanthomatosis (22/28), premature coronary heart disease, (7/28). After a dietetic period of 2 months, and a wash out of any hypocholesterolemic drug, they were given cholestyramin alone at a daily dose of 16 g/day, during 4 months. At month 5, fenofibrate was added, 100mg thrice a day for two months. Colic disturbances was observed 8 times and 3 patients gave up. In five cases posology was reduced. No side effect was reported, due to fenofibrate use. Results are shown in table N° 1.

TABLE N° 1:CHOLESTYRAMIN (C) + FENOFIBRATE (F) (n=25)

MONTHS		0	1	2	3	4	5	6
TREATMENT			<..........	..C....	........>		<.....C+F	....>
LDL C	mg/dl	325	247	247	250	259	220	218
	%		**-24%**	**-24%**	**-23%**	**-20%**	**-32%**	**-33%**
APO B	mg/dl	209	174	171	175	182	152	144
	%		**-17%**	**-18%**	**-16%**	**-13%**	**-27%**	**-31%**
TG	mg/dl	125	124	126	138	143	100	100
	%		**-0,8%**	**+0,8%**	**+10%**	**+14%**	**-20%**	**-20%**
HDL C	mg/dl	45	49	49	51	50	52	55
	%		**+8%**	**+8%**	**+13%**	**+11%**	**+15%**	**+22%**
APOA1	mg/dl	138	153	150	157	157	155	161
	%		**+11%**	**+9%**	**+14%**	**+14%**	**+12%**	**+17%**

The number of patients whose LDL C fall under 170 mg/dl did not exceed 20%. Hypertriglyceridemic effect of resin is not only erased but reversed by fenofibrate addition. Increasing effect on HDL C and Apo A1 was surprising with resin alone but only significant for month 3. Later on, whith the increasing posology of cholestyramin, we observed an additionnal lowering action on LDL C and the number of patient with an LDL C under 170 mg/dl increased up to 55%.

2)Long term cholestyramine-ciprofibrate combination. This is a retrospective study, involving patients receiving cholestyramin and ciprofibrate for at least 3 years. They were 31 FH patients under a mean daily dose of cholestyramin of 12 g and ciprofibrate was given at a dose of 100 or 200 g/day. Results are given in table N° 2.

TABLE N° 2 : CHOLESTYRAMIN (C) + CIPROFIBRATE (CI) (n=31)

TREATMENT		Basal	C	C + CI
LDL C	mg/dl	280	244	212
	%		**-13%**	**-24%**
APO B	mg/dl	176	156	143
	%		**-11%**	**-19%**
TG	mg/dl	101	110	103
	%		**+8%**	**+1%**
HDL C	mg/dl	39	38	44
	%		**0**	**+12%**

The lowering action of this combination is less important explained by smaller posology of resin. Ciprofibrate is still able to erased the hypertriglyceridemic effect of resin after 3 years, however triglycerides are not lowered as they usually are in short term study with fenofibrate.

3)HMG I-resin combination.

Pravastatin is a new HMG I which is supposed to have a tissue selectivity of action with a higher hepatocytes impact. The number of patients was 44 (37 males and 7 females). Mean age was 44 (range 21-63), 37 patients had tendinous xanthomas, all had familial history of FH, 29 suffered for a previous coronary attack. Pravastatin was the first drug used alone during 4 months and resin was added at month 5 and 6. Posology was 40 mg/day for pravastatin and 16g/day for cholestyramin. Patients tolerated well HMG I despite slight increase of GGT and CPK, (in one case CPK went up 10 times normal level after physical activity) none patient dropped out. During combination, 21 patients complained of constipation or other colic disturbances. In five cases resin posology has to be reduced to 12 and even 8 g per day. None patient dropped out. Results are shown in table N° 3.

TABLE N° 3:PRAVASTATIN (P) + CHOLESTYRAMIN (C) (n=44)

MONTHS		0	1	2	3	4	5	6
TREATMENT			<.........	P.........	>	<.....	P+C	.......>
LDL C	mg/dl	347	258	256	248	252	223	221
	%		**-26%**	**-26%**	**-29%**	**-27%**	**-36%**	**-36%**
APO B	mg/dl	222	171	178	170	174	160	156
	%		**-17%**	**-18%**	**-16%**	**-13%**	**-27%**	**-31%**
TG	mg/dl	129	109	123	114	114	127	142
	%		**-16%**	**-5%**	**-12%**	**-12%**	**+2%**	**+10%**
HDL C	mg/dl	47	50	50	52	51	52	51
	%		**+6%**	**+6%**	**+1%**	**+11%**	**+15%**	**+22%**
APOA1	mg/dl	157	156	158	156	157	157	162
	%		**-1%**	**+1%**	**-1%**	**0**	**0**	**+3%**

With pravastatin alone, mean LDL decrease reached 27%, obtained as soon as the first month of treatment, and remained stable for 4 months. Combination of resin afforded an additionnal decrease of 9%. Patients whose LDL C reached 170 mg/dl represented 23% of population. Apo B results were comparable and additionnal decrease reached 7%. Triglyceride effect of pravastatin was small but nevertheless, significant on month 1, 3, and 4 when compared to basal level. It vanished on month 5 when cholestyramine was added and pravastatin was unable to avoid a 10% increase of TG at month 6. Prolongation with increased posology of resin, have shown the possibility to reach a lipid correction in 85% of patients. The effect of this combination on HDL class showed a slight increase in HDL C only detectable on month 3 and 4.

4)Combination of HMG I and fibrate.

It involved a small number of patients who entered the study of simvastatin in our group. They were 5 men and 6 women ; mean age was 41 years (range 28-54) , all 11 patients had FH with xanthomas. They received simvastatin alone, 40mg per day, in the evening, for at least 12 weeks. Previous and well documented intolerance to resin, lead us to decide an association of simvastatin and ciprofibrate. They were given ciprofibrate in the morning, once a day, 100 mg. Considering previous publications of muscle toxicity of such combination (4), a special attention was given to adverse reaction, with clinical and biological control monthly. We did not observe in these 11 cases any clinical and /or biological adverse reaction especially in muscular function. Results are shown in table N° 4.

TABLE N° 4:SIMVASTATIN-CIPROFIBRATE COMBINATION (n=11)

MONTHS		0	1	2	3	4
TREATMENT			<........S.......>		<........S+CI.......>	
LDL C	mg/dl	320	243	218	201	212
	%		**-24%**	**-32%**	**-37%**	**-34%**
APO B	mg/dl	212	172	157	140	148
	%		**-19%**	**-26%**	**-34%**	**-30%**
TG	mg/dl	124	105	117	94	90
	%		**-15%**	**-6%**	**-24%**	**-27%**
HDL C	mg/dl	36	40	33	40	36
	%		**+11%**	**-8%**	**+11%**	**0**
APOA1	mg/dl	127	138	131	150	151
	%		**+9%**	**+3%**	**+18%**	**+19%**

The monotherapy already allowed to lower LDL C by 28% and Apo B level by 25%. None patient had an LDL C under 180 mg/dl. Ciprofibrate provided an additional decrease of LDL C of 10%. 3 patients had a LDL C under 160mg/dl. Apo B level decrease by 12%, which represents a total decrease of 37% compared to basal level. Even in these normotriglyceridemic patients, ciprofibrate lowered TG by 17%. However we observed a discordant response on HDL parameters : HDL C increased only by 4% while Apo A1 increased by 11%.

5)Lp (a) change during drug combination.

As it has been already reported, none of these class of drug affected Lp (a) value alone or in combination (5). Since there was no significant change versus basal level of Lp (a) either for cholestyramine + fenofibrate or for pravastatin + cholestyramin.

TABLE N° 5:LP (a) CHANGE UNDER DRUG COMBINATION (n=21)

MONTHS	0	1	2	3	4	5	6
TREATMENT			<.........C.........>			<.....C+F.......>	
Lp (a) mg/dl	37	35	41	30	32	34	34
%		**-5%**	**+10%**	**-19%**	**-13%**	**-8%**	**-8%**
TREATMENT			<.........P.........>			<.....P+C.......>	
Lp (a) mg/dl	37	34	28	30	25	35	34
%		**-8%**	**-24%**	**-19%**	**-32%**	**-5%**	**-8%**

CONCLUSION

This four types of drug combination significantly reduces LDL C in FH and in some association increase HDL C. The main goal, prevent or retard the progression of atheroslerosis, have already been demonstrated with resin-nicotinic acid and resin-fibrate combinations. It remains to be demonstrated also for HMG I alone or in combination with other hypolipidemic drugs.

REFERENCES

1)Hyperlipidémies réfractaires à la correction thérapeutique ordinaire diététique et médicamenteuse.
JL DE GENNES, J LAMBROZO, J TRUFFERT.
2)The Coronary Drug Project Research Group. Clofibrate and niacin in coronary heart disease. JAMA, 1975, 231, 360.
3)Study Group : European Atherosclerosis Society. Strategies for the prevention of coronary heart disease : a policy statement of he European Atherosclerosis society. European Heart Journal, 8, 1987, 77-87.
4)C EAST, PA ALIVIZATOS, SM GRUNDY, PH JONES, JA FARMER. Rhabdomyolysis in patients receiving lovastatin after cardiac transplantation. N Engl J Med. 1988, 318, 46.
5)G KOSTNER. Lipoprotein Lp (a): Structural and functionnal aspects. in Atherosclerosis VII , NH FIDGE, PJ NESTEL ed. Elsevier, 1986, Amsterdam. 267.

83
Combined pharmacological treatment of heterozygous familial hypercholesterolemia

R. CARMENA

Department of Internal Medicine, Hospital Clinico Universitario, 46010 Valencia, Spain

ABSTRACT. Combined therapy of heterozygous familial hypercholesterolemia using a non-systemically acting drug (bile acid sequestrants) and a systemically acting one is frequently employed in clinical practice. A brief review of this topic is presented, with particular emphasis on the use of cholestyramine combined with pravastatin, a new HMG CoA reductase inhibitor.

Familial hypercholesterolemia (FH) is among the commonest of major genetic diseases, affecting-in the heterozygous form -one person in 500. The hypercholesterolemia is usually severe (above 300 mg/dl, 7.8 mmol/l) and is due to increased levels of LDL (above 190 mg/dl, 4.9 mmol/l) resulting from impaired function of LDL receptors (1).

Patients with FH constitute a unique group at high risk for premature coronary heart disease (CHD). Heterozygous men have a 8-10 fold greater risk of CHD than unaffected male subjects of comparable age. In some series, the risk of myocardial infarction among heterozygous men was 51 percent by age 50 and 85 percent by age 60 (1,2).

Dietary treatment alone for heterozygous FH patients is rarely adequate and cholesterol-lowering agents are commonly used. Inasmuch as these patients have one normal LDL receptor gene, the ideal agent would be one that caused an enhanced production of LDL receptors in the liver. One such class of drugs is made up of the bile acid-binding resins (cholestyramine and colestipol) wihich have been used extensively in the last two decades. These drugs bind bile acids in the intestinal lumen, increasing their fecal excretion. The interruption of the enterohepatic circulation of bile acids promotes a compensatory increase in the hepatic conversion of cholesterol to bile acids with a resultant depletion in the hepatic cholesterol pool. This, in turn, promotes a compensatory increase in hepatic cholesterol synthesis and an increased expression of LDL receptors on hepatocyte cells with a concurrent stimulation of LDL catabolism (3).

In general, treatment of heterozygous FH with resins results in a 25 percent lowering of LDL-cholesterol levels. The effectiveness of these agents is limited because of the compensatory increase in hepatic cholesterol biosynthesis as demoustrated by a 28% increase in urinary mevalonate excretion during cholestyramine treatment (4). Thus, bile acid sequestrants remain a cornerstone in the therapy of heterozygous FH patients but their efficacy can be enhanced when they are used in combination with a second drug.

There are two indications for introduction of a second drug in the treatment of heterozygous FH (5). The more common is failure to approach target cholesterol levels in an adequate trial of diet and a single drug. The other is marked and persistent hypertriglyceridemia occuring during resin therapy, despite attention to diet and to underlying causes of elevated triglycerides.

Mentioning resins specifically in the text underlines the fact that monotherapy with bile acid sequestrants has been widely used in the past two decades for treatment of heterozygous FH. Due to their mode of action and the therapeutic ceiling mentioned above, combined therapy using resins and other lipid lowering agent is not an uncommon treatment for FH patients at the present time. Among the drugs used in combination with the bile acid sequestrants, nicotinic acid, probucol, fibric acid derivatives and 3-hydroxy-3-methyl-glutaryl coenzyme A (HMG CoA) reductase inhibitors (lovastatin, simvastatin and pravastatin) have been used as recently reviewed by Illingworth (6).

Nicotinic acid was, until recently, the most widely prescribed second drug for use in combination with a bile acid sequestrant in the treatment of heterozygous FH patients inadequately controlled on monotherapy with a bile acid sequestrant. With such combination, the LDL cholesterol levels fell by 40-50 percent. However, the incidence of side effects with nicotinic acid is significant and few patients are able to tolerate the drug at the required dose.

Different combinations of resins and fibric acid derivatives have been used, resulting in an LDL-Cholesterol lowering between 12 and 42 percent (6). In our experience, the combination of cholestyramine and probucol, although safe from the point of view of toxicity and side effects, did not improve the hypolipidemic effect of cholestyramine alone (7).

The recent development of the HMG CoA reductase inhibitors constitutes a valuable new therapeutic approach for FH patients. This group of drugs act by decreasing the conversion of HMH CoA reductase to mevalonic acid and, ultimately, a reduction in de novo cholesterol biosynthesis. They reduce by 30-35% the 24-hour urinary excretion of mevalonic acid (4). Thus, the association of bile acid sequestrants and the new reductase inhibitors provide a logical approach to combined-drug therapy in patients with hypercholesterolemia that is inadequeately controlled on monotherapy with either agent.

Treatment of heterozygous FH with cholestyramine and pravastatin.

We have conducted a prospective, randomized, parallel, multicenter study using pravastatin, a HMG CoA reductase inhibitor, and comparing the efficacy of two combinations - cholestyramine and pravastatin or cholestyramine and bezafibrate - versus monotherapy with either cholestyramine or pravastatin in the treatment of heterozygous FH. A detailed description of the study's protocol with preliminary results at 6 months and an abstract with results at 12 mo. have been published (8,9).

A total of 110 heterozygous FH patients have now completed one year of therapy. According to the study's protocol, after a 3 month period of random assignation in double-blind fashion to either pravastatin (20 mg bid) or cholestyramine (8 g bid), the code was broken and the question of combined therapy was raised. If total cholesterol was below 300 mg/dl (7.7 mmol/l) monotherapy was continued at the same dose. In the patients with total cholesterol above such figure, combined therapy was began : patients on pravastatin added cholestyramine 8 g bid and those on monotherapy with cholestyramine added bezafibrate 400 mg qd HS. The study has been continued in open-label fashion; at the end of the first 9 months a total of 31 patients had received pravastatin, 24 pravastatin and cholestyramine, 21 cholestyramine and 22 bezafibrate and cholestyramine. There were 12 drop-outs, 8 in the cholestyramine group and 4 on pravastatin

The results at 12 months showed a total cholesterol decrease of 26.4% with pravastatin, 33.5% with pravastatin and cholestyramine, 25.0% with cholestyramine and 15% with bezafibrate and cholestyramine. The table below shows the LDL-Cholesterol changes observed during the 12 month period using the four different therapeutic regimens.

LDL-Cholesterol (mg/dl)

	Basal	3 mo.	12 mo.	% change
Pravastatin	257.7±45.3	181.7±31.8	175.0±37.2	-31.0 d
Cholestyramine	264.4±44.0	167.2±27.2	171.1±31.8	-33.4 b
Prava + Choles.	351.1±63.9	276.3±47.0	210.3±56.9	-40.0 bc
Bezaf.+ Choles.	329.6±95.9	294.3±114.2	267.9±119.8	-16.4

b= $p<0.05$ monotherapy vs the same monotherapy + other drug

c = p<0.05 combined therapy vs. combined therapy
d = p<0.05 monotherapy vs. the other monotherapy + other drug.

- - - - - - - - - - - - - - - - - - -

The HDL-Cholesterol rose in the four groups : 23.1% in patients on pravastatin, 13.7% with cholestyramine, 17.7% pravastatin and cholestyramine and 20.9% bezafibrate and cholestyramine. The Apo AI and AII increased in parallel with these figures. On the other hand, in the 4 mentioned groups the Apo B decreased by 9.5, 28.0, 23.6 and 9.5 percent respectively.

As far as total and LDL-Cholesterol changes, our results show no statistical difference between the two monotherapy groups. The combination of cholestyramine with pravastatin resulted in a significantly greater (p<0.05) reduction in total and LDL-Cholesterol than the one obtained using cholestyramine and bezafibrate or any form of monotherapy.

Thus, at the present time, use of a systemically acting drug such as pravastatin plus a non-systemically acting one (cholestyramine) is the preferred combination for treatment of heterozygous FH patients. However, in a small number of patients with severe heterozygous FH combinations of two drugs may fail to adequately control plasma cholesterol levels and a third drug coould be added under careful supervision. In Illingworth's recent review (6), three such triple combinations were discussed, using lovastatin (20-40 mg-qd) plus nicotinic acid (1-4.5 g qd) and either colestipol or cholestyramine (8-30 g qd). The decrease in the LDL-Cholesterol level ranged from 59 to 67 percent, together with a 10-20% increase in HDL-Cholesterol and a modest reduction in plasma triglycerides. Careful attention to adverse side effects should be given if this triple combinations are to be considered.

References.

1.- Goldstein,JL & Brown,MS. (1989) "Familial hypercholesterolemia". In: The Metabolic Basis of Inherited Disease, 6th Edition. Eds. C.R. Scriver, A.L. Beaudet, W.S. Sly & D. Valle. McGraw Hill, New York, pp 1215-1250

2.- Slack,J. (1969) "Risks of ischaemic heart-disease in familial hyperlipoproteinemic states". Lancet 2:1380-84

3.- Sheperd,J, Packard,CJ, Bicker,S, Lawrie,TDW & Morgan, HG. (1980) "Cholestyramine promotes receptor-mediated low-density lipoprotein catabolism. N Engl J Med, 302: 1219-1224

4.- Pappu,AS & Illingworth,DR. (1987) "Contrasting effects of lovastatin (mevinolin) and bile acid sequestrants on 24-hour urinary mavalonate in familial hypercholesterolemia (abstract). Arteriosclerosis, 7: 513A

5.- The recognition and management of hyperlipidaemia in adults: a policy statement of the European Atherosclerosis Society (1988). European Heart J. 9:571-600

6.- Illingworth,DR. (1989) "New horizons in combination drug therapy for hypercholesterolemia" Cardiology, 76 (suppl. 1): 83-100

7.- Carmena,R, Ascaso,JF, Serrano,S, Martínez-Valls,J & Soriano,P. (1984) "Treatment of heterozygous familial hypercholesterolemia with diet, cholestyramine and probucol". In: Treatment of Hyperlipoproteinemia. Eds.: L.A.Carlsson & A.G.Olsson. Raven Press, New York, pp 147-150.

8.- Carmena,R, de Oya,M, Franco,M, Martínez,ML, Mata,P, Gomez,JA, Serrano,S, Alvarez-Sala,L, Matesanz,J, Rubio, MJ & Gras,X. (1989) "Treatment of heterozygous familial hypercholesterolemia with pravastatin and/or cholestyramine. The Spanish Multicenter Pravastatin Study". Atherosclerosis VIII, Excerpta Medica, Amsterdam, pp 757-760

9.- Carmena,R, Serrano,S, Martinez,ML, de Oya,M, Alvarez-Sala,L, Franco,M, Gomez,JA, Mata,P, Rubio,MJ & Olivan, J. ((1989) "Combined therapy of heterozygous familial hypercholesterolemia with cholestyramine and pravastatin".(The Spanish Multicenter Pravastatin Study). Abstract Book, 7th Int.Meeting on Atherosclerosis and Cardiovascular Disease Univ. of Bologna, Italy.

HYPERTENSION AS A RISK FACTOR

84
Review of primary prevention trials of antihypertensive treatment

W.B. KANNEL

Boston University School of Medicine, Section of Preventive Medicine and Epidemiology, 720 Harrison Avenue, Suite 1105, Boston, MA 02118, USA

ABSTRACT. Epidemiologic studies of the role of hypertension in the evolution of cardiovascular disease stimulated large multicenter trials to evaluate the efficacy of antihypertensive treatment in the prevention of cardiovascular disease. These trials have convincingly demonstrated the efficacy of anti-hypertensive treatment in reducing overall mortality, stroke, cardiac failure and renal insufficiency. The evidence for coronary heart disease is weak and inconsistent despite two-thirds of trial endpoints due to CHD. Trials of mild hypertension lacked the power to detect a 50% reduction in CHD events. Even so, with fewer events they did show a clear benefit for stroke, left ventricular hypertrophy and hypertension progression. There is clear evidence that progression in severity of hypertension can be slowed by drug treatment. For any outcome treatment benefits for women and persons under age 50 were not demonstrated. A number of possible reasons for failure to show efficacy against CHD have been postulated. Trials may have been too short in duration to affect progression of atherosclerosis and started too late in life. Sample sizes were too small to detect even sizeable reductions in CHD. No attention was paid to whether the CHD risk profile was improved. The drugs used can adversely affect lipids, glucose tolerance and uric acid offsetting the benefits of the lowered blood pressure. Diuretics also may predispose to sudden death in susceptible persons. Trials suggest that for CHD prevention in hypertension, control of smoking and serum lipids are particularly important. The Gothenberg Trial demonstrates the importance of concomitant lowering of lipids. Existing trials suggest that we need to examine the efficacy of antihypertensive agents which do not adversely affect the CHD risk profile. Also, the efficacy of non-pharmacologic control of mild hypertension with obesity control, salt and alcohol restriction need to be tested.

Influence of Coronary Risk Profiles in Hypertension

Coronary heart disease (CHD) is now the commonest and most lethal of the cardiovascular sequelae of hypertension. All clinical manifestations of CHD occur in excess in hypertensive individuals. Risk increases in proportion to the degree of blood pressure elevation whether this is in the systolic or diastolic component, at any age, and in either sex. Even isolated systolic hypertension increases the risk. The significant adverse effect of raised blood pressure on two clearly atherosclerotic cardiovascular endpoints (CHD and intermittent claudication in the Framingham Study), is summarized in Figure 1.

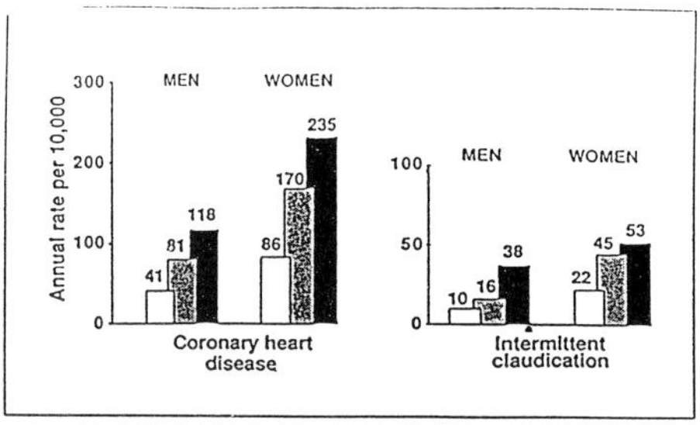

Figure 1. Age-adjusted risk of cardiovascular disease by hypertensive status at each biennial exam in subjects aged 35-84 (Framingham 26-year follow-up) P < 0.01 for all trends; □ normotensive (≤140/90 mmHg); ▣ mild; ■ definite (≥ 160/95 mmHg)

Risk factors associated with hypertension influence the coronary risk potential of hypertension more than the character of the blood pressure elevation. Although blood pressure independently contributes to CHD, the risk at any level of pressure elevation is markedly influenced by the coronary risk profile. For mild-to-moderate hypertensive persons in particular, the risk of CHD is concentrated in those who have an increased total/HDL-cholesterol ratio, impaired glucose tolerance, cigarette smokers, and those with ECG abnormalities. Figure 2 represents the effect of multiple risk factors on CHD incidence in hypertension in the Framingham Study.

RISK OF CHD OVER 8 YEARS IN MEN AGED 45 WITH SBPs OF 150 mm Hg AND 180 mm Hg BY INTENSITY OF OTHER RISK FACTORS (FRAMINGHAM 26 YR FOLLOW-UP)

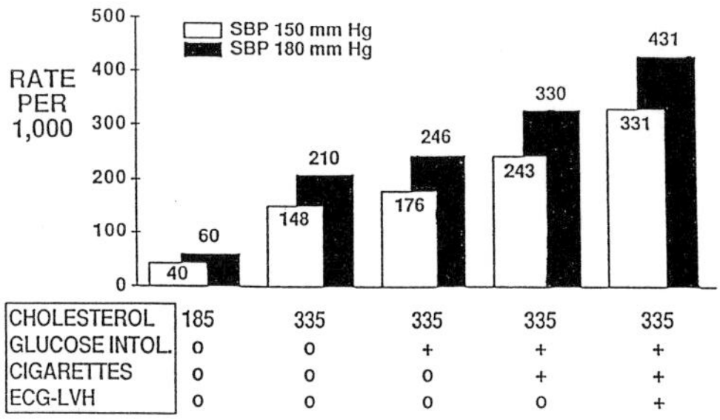

The presence of organ involvement signified by ECG-LVH proteinuria or impaired left ventricular function greatly augments the risk of CHD and generally indicates a compromised coronary circulation. Awaiting such evidence is dangerous since most myocardial infarctions and sudden deaths occur before such evidence appears.

Hypertension risk assessment requires consideration of the multivariate risk profile which provides a better basis for determining the nature and urgency of treatment required and a more sound basis for judging the efficacy of antihypertensive treatment. Optimal preventive management of hypertension for the prevention of CHD requires more than normalization of the blood pressure if the hazard of coronary events is to be reduced.

Hypertension is dangerous, whether systolic or diastolic, labile or fixed, at all ages and in both men and women. Adiposity, heart rate, alcohol intake, hematocrit, blood sugar, serum cholesterol and triglyceride are all related to occurrence of hypertension in one or both sexes (2). These also contribute to occurrence of the cardiovascular sequelae of hypertension. The influence of blood pressure on incidence of cardiovascular disease is independent of the other predisposing co-factors, but is greatly affected by them. Elevated pressures are often accompanied by hyperlipidemia, hyperglycemia, elevated fibrinogen and ECG abnormalities, all of which augment the risk (1,2). Coronary disease is now the commonest sequela of hypertension and the excess risk is concentrated in those with an increased LDL/HDL-cholesterol ratio, impaired glucose tolerance, ECG abnormalities and cigarette smokers. The beneficial effect of increasing levels of HDL-cholesterol against differing background concentrations of LDL-cholesterol is well illustrated in Figure 3.

RELATIVE RISK OF CHD BY HDL, LDL, AND SYSTOLIC BP IN MEN AGED 50-70 (FRAMINGHAM)

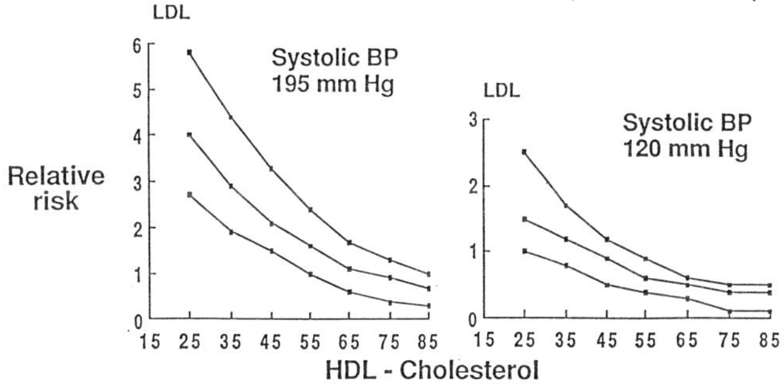

Hypertension is only a component of a multifactorial coronary risk profile which must be considered in implementing optimal therapy. Both the urgency for treatment and judgment of efficacy should be guided by the multivariate risk make-up.

Review of Major Primary Prevention Trials

Coronary heart disease, the main cause of death in developed countries, is now the chief cardiovascular sequela and lethal outcome of hypertension. It was hoped that control of hypertension, a powerful, independent contributer to CHD incidence, would reduce CHD morbidity and mortality in hypertensive persons. Occasional trials have given promising results, but there has been no consistent, convincing evidence that CHD morbidity and mortality is reduced by treatment of hypertension (3,4). Only vascular sequelae such as renal failure, stroke, aortic dissection, and cardiac failure have been reduced by antihypertensive therapy. However, results have not been consistent with regard to efficacy in hypertensive patients with and without target organ involvement, and in white women and subjects under age 50, benefits have been equivocal.

The bulk of mortality (60%) in hypertension occurs in those with mild to moderate elevations of blood pressure. The chief hazard is coronary disease. Although progression in severity of hypertension has been slowed with drug therapy, benefits for coronary outcome and mortality from all causes have been equivocal. Only a 10% reduction in CHD morbidity and mortality has been shown - improvements that are not only small, but not statistically significant (Table 1).

TABLE 1. Trials of Mild Hypertension

<u>9 Trials</u>: 43000 Subjects av. 5.6 Yrs. Duration

<u>Interventions</u>:

1. Thiazide Diuretics
2. Non-Selective B-Blockers
3. Av. 5.5 mmHg. Reduction in Diastolic Blood Pressure

<u>Outcomes</u>:

1. Fatal CHD and Non-Fatal MI Reduced: 8%
2. CHD Mortality Reduced: 8%
3. Fatal and Non-Fatal Stroke Reduced: 39%
4. Stroke Mortality: 38%
5. Total Mortality: 11%

In general, recent trials comparing B blockers with other antihypertensive drugs have not shown the expected promise implied by B-Blockers effectiveness following a myocardial infarction. However, two large trials suggest that they may be effective against CHD in male non-smokers (3,5). The MAPHY Study, in a subgroup analysis, on the other hand, suggests effectiveness of metoprolol only in smokers (6).

A number of possible reasons for the failure to show efficacy against CHD have been postulated (Table 2).

TABLE 2. Possible Reasons for Poor Results of Antihypertensive Rx for Coronary Disease

- -Presence of pre-existent C.A.D. and hard to regress
- -Treatment initiated too late in life
- -Too short a trial
- -Poor control of blood pressure - not enough contrast
- -Other risk factors not controlled
- -Adverse effects of anti-HBP Rx. on risk factors
- -Design limitations of trials

The trials may have been too short in duration to significantly affect atherosclerotic progression. Also, sample sizes were too small to detect even a sizable reduction in CHD events. Furthermore, no attention was paid to whether the CHD risk profiles was improved, as the drugs used are known to have adverse effects on blood lipids, glucose tolerance, and uric acid. There may also have been a predispositon to sudden death associated with antihypertensive therapy (7).

The trials suggest that for CHD prevention, control of smoking and serum lipids is particularly important in hypertensive persons and may be more effective than controlling the blood pressure alone. The Gothenburg Study results from their primary prevention trial suggests that serum cholesterol must be concomitantly reduced if antihypertensive treatment is to be effective against CHD (Table 3).

TABLE 3. Coronary Heart Disease Events by Change in Blood Pressure According to Serum Cholesterol Change: Gothenberg Primary Prevention Trial

Change in Systolic BP	Incidence of Coronary Heart Disease Change in Serum Cholesterol			
	>20%	-11 to 20%	-1 to 10%	<-1%
>-11%	2	6	10	1
2 to 11%	6	6	19	19
-2 to 7%	15	15	19	19
>+7%	25	25	25	33

(Samuelsson O., et al, JAMA 1987, 258:1768-1776.)

The trials suggest that we need continuing research to find optimal agents. Also, nonpharmacologic methods for management of mild hypertension, such as salt restriction, control of obesity, exercise, and reduced alcohol intake, would appear worthy of attention (2). Because a large number of persons with mild hypertension must be treated to benefit a few, drug treatment should be targeted at those with a poor cardiovascular risk profile where the bulk of events are concentrated. Also, the treatment must be harmless and free of side effects that adversely impact the quality of life. Trials in mild hypertension indicate that treatment must be multifactorial, because lowering of blood pressure alone is not enough. Also, the criterion for successful intervention against hypertension is improvement of the entire cardiovascular risk profile rather than the blood pressure alone.

Interdependence of Coronary Risk Factors

Major contributors to coronary heart disease identified through epidemiologic research fall into interdependent categories including: atherogenic traits, faulty living habits, signs of a compromised circulation and innate susceptibility (Table 4).

TABLE 4. Classes of Cardiovascular Risk Factors

Living Habits	Overeating; lack of exercise; cigarette smoking. Type A behavior?
Atherogenic Personal Attributes	High blood pressure; hyperglycemia; dyslipidemia; elevated fibrinogen
Indicators of Compromised Circulation	ECG abnormalities at rest; on exercise; on ambulatory monitoring; vascular bruits; echocardiographic abnormalities; myocardial perfusion deficits etc.
Host Susceptibility	In-born errors of metabolism; family history of premature cardiovascular disease

Modifiable atherogenic risk attributes include blood lipids, blood pressure, glucose tolerance and fibrinogen. Modifiable living habits include overeating, unrestrained weight gain, faulty diet, cigarette smoking and lack of exercise. Innate susceptibility is signified by premature vascular disease in close relatives.

The risk associated with each particular risk factor is markedly affected by coexistent others. At a given serum total cholesterol risk varies widely depending on the LDL/HDL-cholesterol ratio reflecting the net effect of the two-way traffic of cholesterol. Risk in diabetics varies widely depending on coexistent risk factors as does that associated with hypertension and dyslipidemia.

Preclinical indicators of a compromised coronary circulation including ECG-LVH, IV block, repolarization abnormality and abnormal exercise response also escalate the risk associated with modifiable risk factors.

Multifactorial Approach

Optimal risk predictions require a quantitative synthesis of risk factors into a composite profile expressing the multivariate risk. These have been facilitated by production of handbooks, calculators and P.C. software. Such risk assessment requires only ordinary office procedures and simple laboratory tests. Preventive management as well as risk estimation should be multifactorial if good results are to be acheived. Preventive strategies should include public health measures to shift the whole distribution of risk factors to a more favorable level, health education so people can protect their own health and preventive medicine for high risk candidates.

Agents used to correct blood pressure must be carefully selected so as not to use those that tend to worsen other elements of the cardiovascular risk profile such as the blood lipids, glucose tolerance and uric acid. Also, since hypertension is usually accompanied by higher than average lipid values these should be monitored and treated.

Cigarette smoking deserves a high priority in the hypertensive patient since all trials clearly indicate its pernicious effect. Weight control can minimize the need for drugs and improve all elements of the cardiovascular risk profile.

REFERENCES

[1] Kannel, W.B. (1989) 'Hypertension: Impact of risk factors', J Med Consultation 29,104-114.

[2] Kaplan, N. (1978) 'Factors affecting blood pressure', In, Clinical Hypertension, 2nd Edition, Williams & Wilking Co., Baltimore, MD, pp. 14-18.

[3] MacMahon, S.W., Cutler, J.A., Furberg, C.D., Payne, G H. (1986) 'The effects of drug treatment for hypertension on morbidity and mortality from cardiovascular disease: A review of randomized controlled trials', Prog CV Dis 24,(suppl),99-118.

[4] Thompson, S.G. (1985) 'An appraisal of the large-scale trials of antihypertensive treatment', In, Handbook of Hypertension, Epidemiology of Hypertension, Ed. C. J. Bulpitt, Elsevier Science Publishers, B.V., 6,331-343.

[5] MRC Trial of Treatment of Mild Hypertension. (1985) 'Principle Results', Brit Med J 291,97-104.

[6] Wikstrand, J., Warnold, I., Olsson, G., Tuomilehto, J., Elmfeldt, D., Berglund, G. (1988) 'Primary prevention with metropolol in patients with hypertension. Mortality results from the MAPHY Study', JAMA 259,13,1976-1982.

[7] Kannel, W.B., Cupples, L.A., D'Agostino, R.B., Stokes, J. III. (1988) 'Hypertension, antihypertensive treatment and sudden death: The Framingham Study', Hypertension 11,(suppl. II),II45-II50.

[8] Samuelsson, O., Wilhelmsen, L., Andersson, O.K., Pennert K., Berglund, G. (1987) 'Cardiovascular morbidity in relation to change in blood pressure and serum cholesterol in treated hypertension', JAMA 258,1768-1776.

85
Hypertension: why a risk factor for atheroscolerosis?

C. DAL PALU', P. PAULETTO and G. SCANNAPIECO
Clinica Medica I, Università di Padova, Italy

ABSTRACT

In spite of the extensive epidemiological, clinical and experimental studies, little is known about the pathophysiological links between hypertension and atherosclerosis. In the last years evidence has grown that both haemodynamic (i.e. shear stress, flow turbulence, etc.) and humoral (i.e. renin, catecholamines, etc.) factors present in hypertension exert their effects acting on vascular wall cells, in particular endothelial cells and smooth muscle cells (SMC). The same cellular elements play a major role in the development of atherosclerotic lesions when other risk factors are present, such as hypercholesterolemia. It has been recently shown that similarities do exsist between the effect of hypertension and of hypercholesterolemia on the arterial wall. In fact, in experimental hypertension increased endothelial permeability, accompanied by structural and/or functional endothelial changes, have been observed. Moreover,an increase of intimal SMC and an increased adhesion of monocytes to endothelium occur in hypertension. All these intimal changes present in hypertension are thought to represent the basis for the development of atherosclerosis in the presence of hypertension, as well as in the presence of hypercholesterolemia. In particular, a recent study from our group showed an incresed LDL binding to cultured SMC taken from hypertensive arteries as compared to cells taken from normotensive vessels. It therefore appears that several important pathophysiological mechanisms are common to hypertension and atherosclerosis: they could represent the link between these two important vascular diseases.

INTRODUCTION

Several epidemiological data are consistent with the relationship between hypertension as a major risk factor for atherosclerosis (1,2). Moreover, clinical and experimental studies do confirm the link between these vascular diseases (3,4,5). However, the sequence of events leading to atherogenesis in hypertension is not completely known. In the past, the haemodynamic factors have been thought to play the major atherogenic role through direct action on arterial wall. The view that some cellular and humoral factors associated with high blood pressure may play an independent and crucial role has grown today. In particular, data consistent with the hypotesis that the renin system and/or catecholamines may interact with

SMC and endothelium leading to vascular damage as observed in hypertension and in atherosclerosis will be summarized in this paper.

HAEMODYNAMIC FACTORS

Evidence that high blood pressure can damage vessels walls comes from both clinical and experimental observation. The haemodynamic blood flow pattern around vessel orifices, branches and at major curves in arteries appears to be linked to the appearance of early atherosclerotic lesions (6,7). Injury to the endothelium and the accumulation of platelets on altered or damaged surfaces is influenced by the patterns of blood flow rather than by pressure per se (7).Therefore, two different mechanisms are operating at the same time: 1) the increase in pressure leading to changes mainly at the arteriolar level and 2) the alteration of flow pattern, whose effects occur mainly at the large arteries level. Changes at the arteriolar level account for some clinical consequences of arterial hypertension, namely retinopathy, nephropathy, encephalopathy, and the appearance of cerebral microaneurysms of Charcot and Bouchard. Conversely, the alterations of arterial flow are involved in the development of diffuse intimal thickening, atherosclerotic plaques and aneurysms, and post-stenotic dilatations (8).

Both increased intraarterial pressure and flow turbulence play a role in increasing endothelial permeability (9,10) by causing endothelial denudation and/or functional alterations of the arterial endothelium, for instance, increased endothelial cell turnover. Increased pressure is associated with increased wall shear stress; however, the role of fluid shear stress in promoting endothelial injury and/or turnover is uncertain: both high and low stresses have been implicated. High shear stress is linked to alignment of endothelial cells, increased endothelial permeability and function (9,10). Paradoxically, however, there are regions of high laminar shear stress in vivo that are refractory to atherosclerosis and regions at low stress which are associated with wall injury (11,12,13).

Recent experiments demonstrate that, at least in vitro , endothelial cell turnover is considerably more sensitive to relatively low shear stresses in turbulent flow than to much higher shear stresses under conditions of laminar flow (9). Hence, turbulent or laminar flow conditions seem to represent the main determinants of endothelial cells turnover and consequent arterial wall damage through platelet deposition on deendothelialized areas. However, platelet attachment to areas with injured endothelium is quite limited (7). Conversely, on collagenous surfaces of severely damaged vessels platelets were seen to spread, degranulate, and attach to other platelets forming persistent layers (7).

HUMORAL AND CELLULAR FACTORS

According to the revised response-to injury hypothesis the above-mentioned events are liable to result in intimal proliferative lesions via the second pathway, as described by Ross (14). In the first one, observed in experimental hypercholesterolemia, injury to the endothelium induces continuous growth factors secretion which allows monocyte attachment.

Subendothelial migration of cholesterol-loaden macrophages leads to fatty streaks formation; subsequent release of growth factors by macrophages and/or endothelial cells may result in development of fibrous plaques. Macrophages may also injure the overlying endothelium with further platelet deposition and growth factors release. Growth factors induce migration from the media into the intima and intimal proliferation of SMC, which in turn secrete growth factors and produce collagen fibrils and proteoglycans. At this stage, a fully developed fibro-fatty plaque is present. In the alternative pathway the endothelium is injured and the endothelial cells turnover is accelerated. This may result in growth factors formation which stimulates migration and proliferation of medial SMC into the intima and additional growth factors release. This second pathway may be operative in hypertension-related atherosclerosis. As in the case with atherogenesis, SMC play a key role also in the development of medial hypertrophy in hypertension (15). This is accomplished through two main mechanisms, namely SMC hypertrophy and/or SMC hyperplasia (15). DNA synthesis by hypertensive SMC in large vessels consists of DNA duplication without either kariokinesis or cytokinesis (endoreplication). This results in hypertrophyc, polyploid cells that account for most of the increased mass of large vessels in hypertension (16). Conversely, in small vessels a true SMC hyperplasia (increased number of diploid SMC) has been described (15). However, in some experimental models of hypertension (i.e. aortic coarctation in the rat) SMC hyperplasia without SMC hypertrophy occurs (17). As in the case with atherosclerosis, mytogens like PDGF are thought to play a role which may be relevant expecially in inducing SMC proliferation at the microvascular level.

As for the atherogenic role of humoral factors specifically involved with hypertension, angiotensin II and catecholamines have been particularly investigated. The in vivo atherogenic role of norepinephrine has been evidentiated by Helin at al in a study carried out on rabbits kept on normal diet (18). Two weeks of norepinephrine i.v. injection (0.50 mg twice daily) resulted in significant increase of aortic sudanophilic lesions even in the absence of any persistent rise of blood pressure after noradrenaline injection. A similar result has been obtained by Kukreja et al (19) in monkeys kept on cholesterol-enriched diet and receiving a daily i.v. injection of adrenaline (50 µg/kg). Markedly advanced atherosclerosis and an increased aortic cholesterol content was observed in monkeys injected with adrenaline in comparison to controls. Although the rise in blood pressure following adrenaline injection was sharp, blood pressure levels recovered within 1 hour. Therefore, vascular damage consequent to catecholamines administration could be in at least in part independent from intraarterial pressure and related to a direct effect on the arterial wall. Studies on spontaneously hypertensive turkeys (20) are consistent with this view. In these animals atherosclerosis develops in the abdominal aorta in spite of having very high serum alpha-lipoproteins. As a consequence, hypertension and high catecholamines seem to be the main risk factors for atherosclerosis in these turkeys. By treating these animals soon after birth with a beta-blocker (oxprenolol) we could significantly reduce the development of atherosclerotic lesions even in the absence of any blood pressure reduction (20,21). A possible explanation could be that the development of atherosclerosis in turkeys is not only related to hypertension but more likely to their very high levels of catecholamines. Indeed, in vitro experiments demonstrate that catecholamines produce an increased growth rate of SMC in secondary culture (22). The effect is dependent upon the dose used, being more marked in the case with norepinephrine and epinephrine than with isoproterenol. Interestingly, this catecholamines-induced growth of cultured SMC was prevented in a dose-dependent manner by adding to the culture medium propranolol or, even more markedly, phentolamine. Catecholamines can also damage arterial wall independently from any action on vascular SMC by modifying metabolism and permeability of the arterial wall (23) and by reducing oxygen uptake by the media (24).

In hypertension, an atherogenic role independent from the haemodynamic modifications induced by high blood pressure could also be attributed to the renin-angiotensin system arousal. In fact, McGill et al (25) showed that hypertension was accompanied by increased incidence of atherosclerotic lesions in baboons fed a cholesterol-enriched diet for 13 months in comparison to baboons on cholesterol diet but with normal blood pressure. In this experiment two different models of renovascular hypertension were used, with high or low plasma renin activity. More severe atherosclerotic lesions were found in hypertensive animals with high plasma renin activity especially at the level of some districts, i.e. the carotid arteries. Angiotensin II and, to a lesser extent, vasopressin, have been reported to stimulate the growth of cultured SMC in a dose-dependent manner (26). Angiotensin-stimulated growth of SMC is quite limited in the absence of platelet-derived growth factors; by adding these factors to the culture medium, the angiotensin-induced growth of cultured SMC increases by about 6 folds (26). This in vitro experiment may clarify the mechanisms by which angiotensin could enhance atherogenesis in vivo: functional (angiotensin-induced) and/or structural (hypertension-induced) endothelial damage can lead to SMC exposure to the mitogenic activity of factors derived from platelets and/or macrophages, which in turn enhance the mitogenic activity attributed to angiotensin by itself.

On the whole, some humoral factors associated with high blood pressure, mainly catecholamines and angiotensin II, are thought to be atherogenic at least in part independently from any haemodynamic mechanism. These substances can in fact increase endothelial permeability and stimulate SMC growth. This latter may result either in medial hypertrophy and/or in intimal thickening depending on the presence of additional risk factors for atherosclerosis. Endothelin is another substance which is of potential interest for both vascular diseases; in fact endothelin induces a marked rise in blood pressure and, at the same time, has been proven to be an effective mitogenic factor for cultured SMC (27). However, in vivo evidences on a possible atherogenic effect of this polypeptide are still lacking.

LIPIDIC FACTORS AND HYPERTENSION

As discussed in the first section , an altered lipid metabolism may result in intimal thickening through interaction of cholesterol esters with different cell types of the arterial wall, mainly macrophages. However, in vitro studies carried out in our laboratory suggest that also vascular SMC may play a role in cholesterol metabolism of vascular wall. In particular, we have observed that SMC cultured from aorta of SHR bind larger amounts of LDL than SMC from the aorta of normotensive rats (28). This may represent an additional mechanism for lipid accumulation within the arterial wall and may contribute to explain why subjects with familial dyslipidemic hypertension are at high coronary risk, even more than patients with secondary dyslipidemias. This syndrome has been recently described in approximately 12% of patients with essential hypertension (29). It represents a clinical subtype of essential hypertension which has been described in siblings selected for early familial hypertension and found to have one or more of three fasting lipid abnormalities (high tiglycerides, low HDL, high LDL). Familial dyslipidemic hypertension consists of two subgroups; 1) familial combined hyperlipemia with high apolipoprotein B, small LDL particles, and high fasting plasma insulin levels; 2) subjects with upper central obesity, low HDL, high triglycerides and fasting plasma insulin (30). In these patients a common, unknown, pathophysiological link does probably exist among hypertension, abnormalities of lipid metabolism and hyperinsulinemia.

EFFECTS	HYPERTENSION	ATHEROSCLEROTIC PLAQUE
INTIMAL CHANGES		
(CELLULAR AND STRUCTURAL)		
-ENDOTHELIAL PROLIFERATION	+	+
-SMC PROLIFERATION	0	+++
-MONOCYTE INFILTRATION	?	++
-FOAM CELL FORMATION	0	++
-ENDOTHELIAL DENUDATION	0/+	++
-INCREASED THICKNESS	0	+++
(BIOCHEMICAL AND FUNCTIONAL)		
-LIPID ACCUMULATION	0	++
-COLLAGEN, ELASTIN AND GLYCOSAMINOGLYCAN ACCUMULATION	+	++
-INCREASED PERMEABILITY	+++	+++
MEDIAL CHANGES		
-SMC PROLIFERATION	0/+++	0
-SMC TETRAPLOIDY	+++/0	0
-INCREASED THICKNESS	+++	0/-

tab 1: Effects of hypertension and of atherosclerosis on the arterial wall.

	SMC FROM AP	SMC FROM HV
-MIGRATION FROM AORTIC EXPLANTS	+	+
-GROWTH RATE	+	+
-LDL BINDING AND/OR UPTAKE	+	+
-COLLAGEN PRODUCTION	+	?

tab 2: Main characteristics of SMC isolated from atherosclerotic plaques (AP) and from hypertensive vessels (HV).

CONCLUSIONS

Although the link between hypertension and atherosclerosis clearly emerge from several epidemiological, clinical and experimental studies only a few issues about the mechanisms have been elucidated as yet. Endothelial cells and, even more, SMC seem to play a central role in the development of both vascular diseases. Nevertheless, at the level of the arterial wall, besides structural and molecular similarities also important differences do exsist between the two diseases which are not fully understood (table 1). In particular, the role of vascular SMC need to be further investigated in view of the common modifications seen in this cells in both hypertension and atherosclerosis (table 2). On the other hand, it would be relevant to undertake clinical studies designed to clarify the impact of blood pressure lowering on the development of atherosclerotic lesions. In fact, at the present time we have only indirect evidences about the reduction of atherosclerotic lesions in hypertensive patients on antihypertensive treatment. These evidences mainly derive from the data concerning morbility and/or mortality due to ischemic heart disease not yet from a direct evaluation of the atherosclerotic lesions.

REFERENCES

1) Kannel WB, Wolf PA, McGee DL et al. J Am Med Assoc 1981; 245:1225.
2) Robertson WB and Strong JP. Lab Invest 1968;18:538.
3) Lusiani L, Visona' A, Castellani V et al. Int J Cardiol 1987; 17:51.
4) Sutton KC, Dai WS, Kuller LH. Stroke 1985:16:781.
5) Spence JD, Perkins DG, Kline RL et al. Atherosclerosis 1984; 50:325.
6) Roach MR, Scott M, Ferguson GC. Stroke 1982; 3:255.
7) Badimon L, Badimon JJ, Galvez A et al. Arteriosclerosis 1986;6:312.
8) Spence DJ. Canad J Neurol Sci 1976; 3:149.
9) Davies PF, Remuzzi A, Gordon EJ et al. Proc Natl Acad Sci 1986; 83: 2114.
10) Thibault LE and Fry DL. In "Haemodynamics and the arterial wall" Nerem RM & Guyton JR eds. (Univ. Houston Press, Houston,TX) 1980; 140.
11) Friedman MH, Hutchins GM, Bergeron CB et al. Atherosclerosis 1981; 39:425.
12) Zarins CK, Giddens DP, Bharadvaj BK et al. Circ Res 1983; 53:502.
13) Zand T, Nunnari J, Majno G et al. Fed Proc Fed Am Soc Exp Biol 1984; 43:712.
14) Ross R. N Engl J Med 1986; 314:488.
15) Schwartz SM, Campbell GR, Campbell JH. Circ Res 1986; 58:427.
16) Owens GK, Schwartz SM. Circ Res 1982; 51:280.
17) Owens GK, Reidy MA. Circ Res 1985; 57:695.
18) Helin P, Lorenzen I, Garbarsch C et al. Atherosclerosis 1970; 12:125.
19) Kukreja RS, Datta BN, Chakravarti RN. Atherosclerosis 1981; 40:291.
20) Pauletto P, Scannapieco G, Vescovo G et al. Meth and Find Exptl Clin Pharmacol 1988; 10:357.
21) Pauletto P, Pessina AC, Pagnan A et al. Artery 1983;12:220.
22) Blaes N, Boissel JP. J Cell Physiol 1983; 116:167.
23) Constantinides P, Robinson M. Arch Path 1969; 10:11.
24) Loss RJ, Minken SL, Samuelson P. J Atheroscl Res 1969; 88:89.
25) McGill HC, Carey KD, McMahan Ca et al. Arteriosclerosis 1985; 5:481.
26) Campbell-Boswell M, Lazzarini-Robertson A. Exp Med Path 1981; 35:265.
27) Grooms A, Mitchell A, Millar JA et al. 4th European Meeting on Hypertension 18th- 21th June 1989 (A-322).
28) Scannapieco G, Pauletto P, Pagnan A et al. J Hypert 1988; 6(suppl. 4):S269.
29) Williams RR, Hunt SC, Hopkins PN et al. JAMA 1988; 259:3579.
30) Hunt SC, Wu LL, Hopkins PN et al. Arteriosclerosis 1989; 9:335.

86
Hypertension in the elderly

G. ABATE, M. ZITO and M.A. CAVONI

Department of Gerontology and Geriatrics, via Nicolini 2, 66100 Chieti, Italy

ABSTRACT. The prevalence of hypertension and, particularly, of isolated systolic hypertension increases with aging.

On the physiopathological ground, senile hypertension is associated with a decreased compliance of aorta and large vessels, and with dysfunctions of the baroreceptorial reflexes and of some hormonal systems, causing an impaired homeostasis of the body fluids.

On the clinical ground, hypertension in the elderly is characterized by an increased pressor values variability, with a higher prevalence of hypertensive and hypotensive crises, which, in presence of blunted mechanisms of the peripheral blood flow regulation, can induce local ischemia symptoms.

On the therapeutical ground, caution must be due in the pharmacological treatment of elderly patients, also considering the specific complications of hypertension, the associated diseases and the higher incidence of the side effects of the drugs.

In this paper the above-mentioned topics are discussed underlining the opportunity of a careful and individual clinical evaluation.

1. EPIDEMIOLOGY

Epidemiological studies have reported that, in industrialized Western countries, both systolic (SBP) and diastolic (DBP) blood pressure show relevant age-associated changes. (1,2)

It is noteworth that, while the increase of SBP values is continuous throughout the decades, DBP increases only up to age 50-60 yrs and afterwards doesn't show any change or even decreases. (Figg. 1-2)

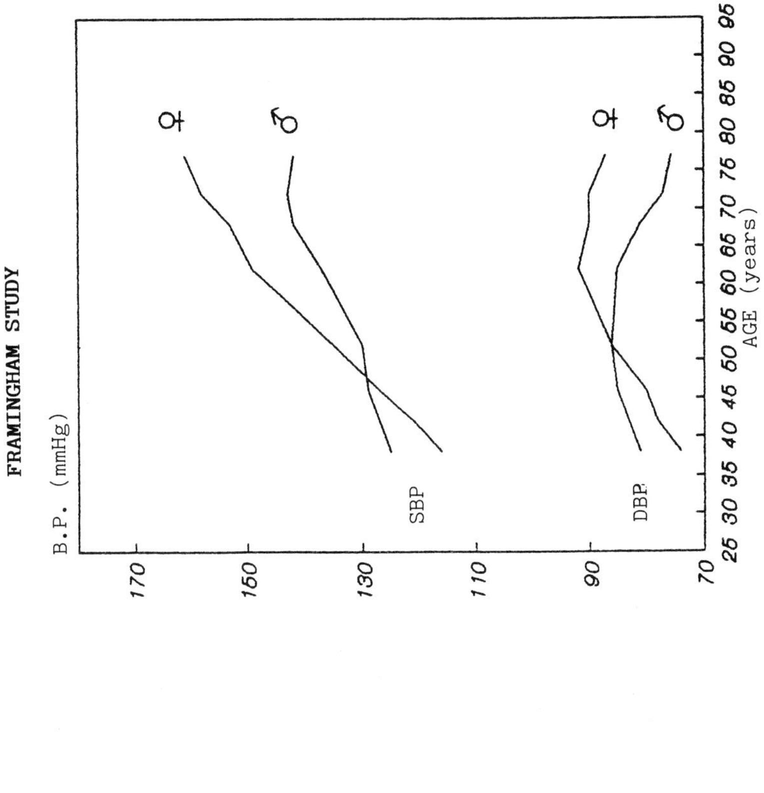

Fig. 1
Modified by Kannel W.B., 1978

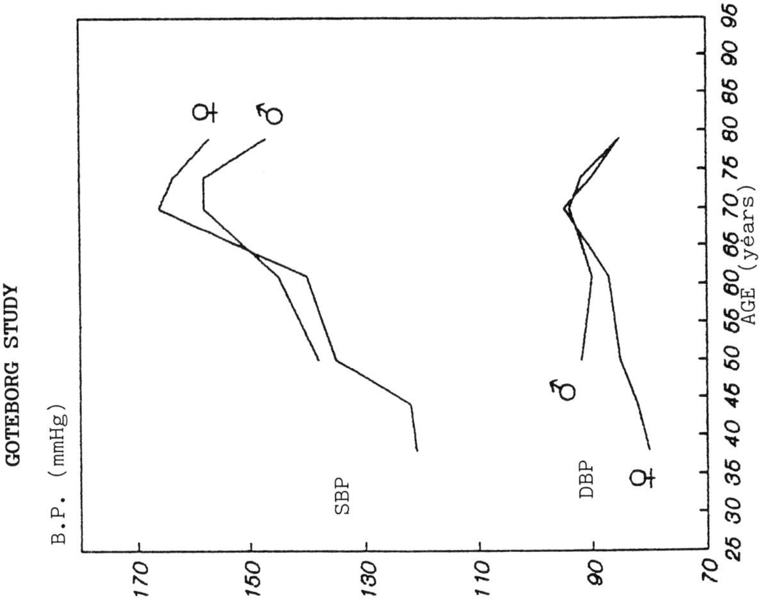

Fig. 2
Modified by Landhal S., 1986

In relation to this trend, in elderly subjects the prevalence of "isolated systolic hypertension" and of "mainly systolic hypertension", defined by the Koch-Weser formula (SBP > DBP - 15x2) is very high, varying from 20% to 50%. (3)
As different studies (Chicago Stroke Study, Framingham Study) have clearly shown, also in elderly subjects, hypertension is associated with an increased risk of cardiovascular diseases. (4,5)
However, it must be underlined that, according to several authors' opinion, in the very old, and particularly in istitutionalized subjects, the presence of an hypertensive status doesn't significantly influence the mortality ratio. (6)

2. PHYSIOPATHOLOGY

2.1. Vascular compliance

The decreased compliance of aorta and large vessels, due to subintimal thickening and medial sclerosis, is considered the main cause for systolic blood pressure increase in geriatric subjects.
Such a phenomenon leads to a reduction of the blood flow to peripheral organs during the diastolic phase; the increase in the arterial resistance, therefore, seems to be "concealed", so that DBP doesn't change and even decreases. (7)
For this reason the haemodynamic pattern of isolated SBP is quite different in relation to age: in young subjects, in fact, a hyperdynamic circulation, a high cardiac index, and a shortening in the rapid ventricular ejection time can be seen, while in elderly subjects the cardiac index is normal or reduced and the sphygmic wave velocity is increased. (8)

2.2. Baroreceptorial dysfunctions

A progressive deterioration of the baroreceptorial reflexes, with a decline of the heart rate responses relative to blood pressure changes, has been observed with increasing age. (9)
Recent studies have shown, both in humans and laboratory animals, age-related effects on baroreceptorial control of blood pressure, characterized by a decline of its dynamic component, while the long term modulation is preserved. (10)
Such dysfunctions are associated with an impaired sensitivity of cardiopulmonar baroreceptors , influenced by "low" pressor values. (11)
The clinical effects of the baroreceptorial impairment are an increase

of the sympathetic tone and a higher occurrence of hypotensive and hypertensive crises.

2.3. Hormonal changes

The renin secretion rate and, in a lesser degree, the plasmatic and urinary concentration of aldosterone decrease with age, both at baseline and during dynamic tests.

The reduced activity of this hormonal system, probably linked to an intrinsic defect or to a minor beta-adrenergic stimulation of juxtaglomerular apparatus (12), can explain the impaired effectiveness of homeostatic control of body fluids in the elderly and, therefore, the higher occurrence of water and salt depletion or overload.

On the other hand, an increase in the plasmatic levels of noradrenaline may be explained by a reduction of plasmatic clearance and mainly by a higher secretion rate of this hormone, due to the down-regulation of the baroreceptorial reflexes. (13)

Finally, beta-adrenergic stimulation decreases with age, both in relation to the decreased number of receptors and to their binding capacity, while alfa-adrenergic receptors show no functional alterations. (14)

3. CLINICAL FEATURES

3.1. Pressor variability

Monitoring studies, performed by invasive and non-invasive techniques, have reported that pressor variability, in elderly subjects, seems to be increased, above all in short term.

In other words, with the same mean pressor daily values, in the elderly compared with the young, a major incidence of hypotensive and hypertensive crises can be observed.

Hypertensive crises can occur in the course of many daily activities, such as static and dynamic exercise, sexual intercourse, smoking, etc.

Hypotensive crises are frequently observed in post-prandial period, during nocturnal hours, in postural changes, etc.; their clinical effects are more evident in elderly patients with local blood flow impaired homeostatic control.

The interaction of several factors can explain the increased blood pressure variability in the elderly; particularly the baroreceptorial dysfunctions, the senile changes of hydroelectrolitic homeostasis and the haemodynamic alterations linked to the aging of the cardiovascular

system. (Fig.3)

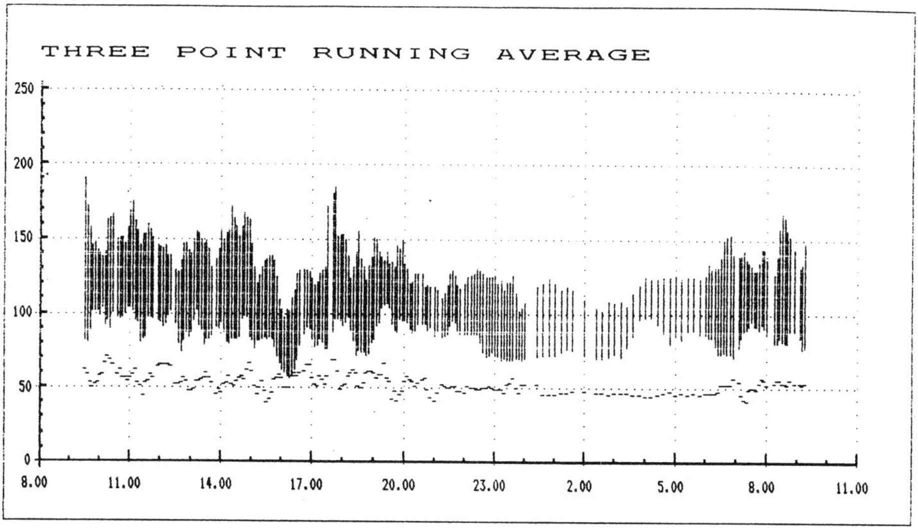

Fig. 3
24-h non-invasive recording of Blood Pressure in an elderly subject (77 yrs) with high pressor variability.

3.2. Specific complications

The specific complications of arterial hypertension are more frequent to be seen in the elderly as result of the interrelation, at vascular level, between the physiologic senile deterioration and the specific damage due to the hypertensive status.
Peculiar clinical aspects found in the elderly can be considered the following:
1) the association with coronary heart disease, which is often asymptomatic, but can worsen the prognosis, raising the incidence of complications, such as myocardial infarction, cardiac failure, life threatening arrithmias, etc.

2) the association with renal diseases (lithiasis, pyelonephritis, diabetic nephropathy, prostatic hypertrophy, etc.), which can allow a more rapid progression towards renal failure;
3) the frequent occurrence of small cerebral ischemic lesions (lacunae), which usually have no clinical relevance, but, sometimes, if repeated, could lead to a cognitive impairment, interrupting the nervous connections among the basal ganglia and different cortical areas.

3.3. Associated diseases

While in young subjects hypertension is usually found in otherwise healthy subjects, in the elderly it is commonly associated with other independent diseases which can interfere with the prognosis and the choice of drugs.
Among them, the cardiovascular, pulmonary, digestive, metabolic and, above all, the neurological diseases (mainly dementia), whose evaluation has a relevant importance in a wider clinical context, in order to establish the correct prognosis and treatment.

4. RATIONAL FOR THERAPY

The pharmacological treatment of senile hypertension is still controversial.
In the European Working Party on Hypertension in the Elderly study (EWPHE) (15) no significant reduction of the total mortality (-9%) was found; however, the cardiovascular mortality, mainly linked to decreased cardiac, but not cerebrovascular deaths, was significantly modified (-27%, p=0.037).
Severe cardiovascular events also decreased, while less severe cardiovascular complications, such as congestive heart failure, were more frequent among the treated group.
The study of subgroups, according to age, showed that the therapy was less effective in 75-79yrs group, while in ⩾80yrs group it was totally ineffective. (16)
The Hypertension in Elderly Patients in Primary Care study (HEP)(17) has reported that the treatment with antihypertensive drugs (atenolol, bendrofluazide or methyldopa) was associated with a decreased risk of stroke, fatal and non fatal (-42%), heart failure, and cardiac mortality incidence.
No data are yet available about the treatment of isolated systolic hypertension: a multicentric double-blind study (Systolic Hypertension

in the Elderly Program = SHEP) is at present in progress. (18)
On the basis of the collected data it can be stated that, in general terms, also in the elderly, the therapy of hypertension can reduce the incidence of cardiovascular complications.
Nevertheless, in some subgroups of patients (very old hypertensives or subjects with severe associated diseases), the treatment seems to be ineffective. In other subgroups the beneficial effect of therapy is still debated: for example, in patients with a high degree of variability, in which the risk of dangerous falls in blood pressure is foreseeable, or in patients with arterial stenosis, in which a critical reduction in regional blood flow can occur.
Conclusively, the following diagnostic and therapeutical approach to the elderly hypertensives can be proposed:
1) careful individual evaluation, with special regard to the age of the patients, the associated diseases and risk factors, and the results of non-invasive examinations (blood pressure monitoring, functional tests, hormones, echography, doppler ultrasonography, etc.);
2) non pharmacological therapeutical approach, based on physical exercise and dietary intake of calories and mineral salts;
3) rational pharmacological treatment, which must take into account:
a) the associated diseases, which can suggest the use of some drugs or represent a contraindication to others;
b) the occurrence of side effects, with a worsening of the quality of life.
Moreover, it can be underlined that, in the elderly, the usual dosage of antihypertensive drugs must be decreased, and that the blood pressure control must be achieved gradually in time, so that a progressive resetting of baroreceptorial mechanism can be restored.

BIBLIOGRAPHY

1) Kannel, W.B. (1978) "Hypertensive disease in the elderly: a consequence of arteriosclerosis or blood pressure?", Bull. N.Y. Acad. Med., 54,31.
2) Landhal, S., Bengtsson, C., Sicurdson, J.A., Svanborg, A., Svardsudd, K. (1986) "Age-related changes in blood pressure", Hypertension, 8, 1044.
3) Kannel, W.B., Dawber, T.R., McGee, D.L. (1980) "Perspective of systolic hypertension. The Framingham study", Circulation, 61, 1179.
4) Shekelle, R.B., Ostfeld, A.M. , Klawans, Jr.H.L. (1984) "Hypertension and risk of stroke in an elderly population", Stroke, 5, 71.

5) Kannel, W.B., Gordon, T. (1978) "Evaluation of cardiovascular risk in the elderly: the Framingham study", Bull. N.Y. Acad. Med., 54, 573.
6) Rajala, S., Haavisto, M., Heikinhelm, H. (1983) "Blood pressure and mortality in the very old", Lancet, i, 520.
7) Lakatta, E.G., Mitchell, J.H., Pomerance, A., Rowe, G.G. (1987) "Human aging: changes in structure and function", J. Am. Coll. Cardiol., 10 (suppl.A), 42.
8) Simon, A.C., Levenson, J.A., et al. (1985) "Haemodynamic mechanisms and therapeutic approach to systolic hypertension", J. Cardiovasc. Pharmacol., 7, S22.
9) Gribbin, P., Pickering, T.G., Sleight, P., Peto, R. (1971) "Effect of age and high blood pressure on baroreflex sensitivity in man", Circ. Res., 29, 424.
10) Mancia, G., Grassi, G., Bertinieri, G., Ferrari, A., Zanchetti, A. (1984) "Arterial baroreceptor control of blood pressure in man", J. Aut.Nerv.Syst., 11, 115.
11) Giannattasio,C., Cleroux, J., Serravalle, G., Valsecchi, M., Cuspidi, C., Sampieri, L., Bolla, G., Mazzola, C., Grassi, G., Mancia, G. (1988) "Riflessi cardiopolmonari e invecchiamento" (abstr.), Atti V Congr. Naz. Soc. Ital. Dell'ipertensione Arteriosa, Milano, p.32.
12) Yamada, T., Endo, T., Ito, K., Nagata, H., Izumiyama, T. (1979) "Age-related changes in endocrine and renal function in patients with essential hypertension", J. Am. Geriatr. Soc., 27, 398.
13) Veith, R.C., Featherstone, J.A., Linares, O.A., Halter, J.B. (1986) "Age differences in plasmonorepinephrine kinetics in humans", J. Hypertension, 41, 3, 319.
14) Davies, I.B., Sever, P.S. (1988) "Adrenoceptor function and ageing" in Bannister R. Autonomic failure. A textbook of clinical disorders of the autonomic nervous system, 2th edit. 357, Oxford, London.
15) Amery, A. et al. : Mortality and morbidity results from the European Working Party on high blood pressure in the elderly trial. Lancet, i, 1349, 1985.
16) Coope, J., Warrender, T.S. (1986) "Randomized trial of treatment of hypertension in elderly patients in primary care", Br. Med. J., 293, 1145.
17) Amery, A. et al. (1986) "Efficacy of antihypertensive drug treatment according to age, sex, blood pressure, and previous cardiovascular disease in patients over the age of 60", Lancet, ii, 589.
18) Hulley, S.B., Furberg, C.B., Gurland, B., McDonald, R., Perry, H.M., Shnaper, H.W., Schoenberger, J.A., Smith, W.M., Vogt, T.M. (1985) "Systolic Hypertension in the Elderly Program (SHEP): Antihypertensive efficacy of chlorthalidone", Am.J.Cardiol., 56, 916.

INVASIVE THERAPY OF CORONARY AND CEREBROVASCULAR DISEASES

87
Coronary and cerebral ischemia: surgery in one or two stages

A. PIERANGELI, G. MARINELLI, B. TURINETTO, M. CAZZATO, T. BOMBARDINI, F. ZACA' and D. ROVINETTI

Cardiac Surgery Department, Policlinico S. Orsola, via Massarenti 9, 40138 Bologna, Italy

ABSTRACT. At the Cardiac Surgery Dept. of the University of Bologna, 45 patients from 41 to 72 years have been treated for coronary and carotid atherosclerotic pathology. Among these patients, 31 have been operated in one stage (group A) and 14 in two stages (group B); in this late case the most serious damaged area was surgically approached primarily. The hospital mortality rate was 3.2% (1/31 pts.) in group A and 27.4% (5/14 pts.) in group B. This was due to myocardium infarction in group A and to cardiac or cerebral causes in group B. The average follow up was 43 months (3 min. - 120 max.): all patients were checked again both clinically and by carotid echo-Doppler examination. The late mortality rate was 6.4% (2/31 pts.) in group A due to probable myocardium infarction. In conclusion we obtained that the best approach in patients with coronary and carotid atherosclerosis lesions would be simoultaneous surgical treatment.

INTRODUCTION

Artheriosclerosis is a multivessel desease with a very high mortality when coronaries and carotids are involved.

At the Cardiosurgical Institute of the University of Bologna 45 patients underwent surgery between April 1979 and June 1989; 31 (group A) had a combined procedure and 14 (group B) a staged one.

The aim of this paper is to verify upon our experience whether the staged procedure is more effective than the combined one.

MATERIAL AND METHODS

Critical coronaries and carotideals lesions were present in 45 patients.

A lesion is considered critical when a narrowing of at least 50% in the carotid and 60% in the coronary is reached.

Patients in group A (31) had a combined procedure and in group B

(14) had a staged one; 41 were males and 4 females with a mean age of 63 ± 7.9 years (ranging from 41 to 72).

Mean follow up is 43 months (ranging from 3 to 120). Statistical evaluation was done with the χ square test.

According with table 1 data, there are not significant stathistical differences between the two groups as far as the type of angina, the ventricular score, the ejection fraction, the left ventricular endiastolic pressure, the number of involved vessels and performed grafts, the completeness of myocardial revascularization and the type of graft employed are concerned.

Table 1. CABG + ETC
(April 1979 - June 1989)
CLINICAL DATA

PATIENTS 45 — 31 combined procedure; 13 staged procedure (5*)

SEX: ♂ 41; ♀ 4 AGE: min. 41; max. 72 mean 63 ± 7.5

Mean follow up 43 months (3 - 120 months)

* 5 patients not completed surgery

		COMBINED PROC.	STAGED PROC.	P
ANGINA	stable	3 (9.7%)	3 (21.5%)	N.S.
	unstable	28 (90.3%)	11 (78.5%)	
VENTRICULAR SCORE	5-7	13 pt (42%)	5 (36%)	N.S.
	8-15	18 pt (58%)	9 (64%)	
EF mean		62.7 ± 11.2 (46% -> 81%)	58.2 ± 9.6 (41% -> 71%)	N.S.
EDVP mean		13.5 ± 8.9 (5 -> 30)	16.3 ± 11.2 (7 -> 30)	N.S.
VESSELS INVOLVED		*3.2 ± 1 (1->5) *12 LM (38.7%)	*3.4 ± 0.9 (1->4) *4 LM (28.5%)	N.S.
N.BYPASS		2.6 ± 0.9 (1 -> 5)	2.8 ± 0.7 (1 -> 4)	N.S.
COMPLETE REVASC.		22 (60.2%)	8 (66.7%)	N.S.
UNCOMPLETE REV.		9 (29.8%)	4 (33.3%)	
GRAFT		96.8% saph. 3.2% mamm.	100% saph.	N.S.

Interstingly most of the patients had a clinically unstable angina and more than 1/3 had left main trunk lesions.

In table 2 pre and intraoperative data regarding the carotids are shown and even in this case there are not statistically significant differences.

Table 2. CABG + ETC
(April 1979 - June 1989)
CLINICAL DATA

		COMBINED PROC.	STAGED PROC.	P
CAROTID	Monolat.	18 (59.1%)	7 (50%)(1 obs.)	N.S.
LESIONS	Bilat.	13 (40.9%)(2 obs.)	7 (50%)(1 obs.)	
CEREBRAL	YES	18 (58%)	10 (71.4%)	N.S.
SIGNS	NO	13 (42%)	4 (28.6%)	
PERIPHERAL	YES	8 (25.8%)	4 (28.5%)	N.S.
VASC.DISEASE	NO	23 (74.2%)	10 (71.5%)	
DIRECT SUTURE		9	/	
ETC + PATCH	20	19 (saph.vein)	10 (Sauvage)	
		1 (peric.)	1 (peric.)	
ETC + SCB		2	/	

It is important to emphasize that in more than 40% of the patients both carotids were involved but only in 71% (group B) and in 38% (group A) of the patients clinical signs of cerebral ischemia were present.

Moreover peripheral vasculopaty with claudicatio intermittens was also present in 29% of the patients: 3 of these patients, all in group A, have been later operated 2 for an abdominal aorta aneurysm and 1 for P.T.A. of the right iliac artery.

We now always use a patch to reconstruct the carotid after the E.T.C. whereas at the beginning of our experience we sutured directly the arteriotomy. In group A the patch was in saphenous vein and in group B in dacron Sauvage.

RESULTS

Hospital mortality was 3.2% (1/31) in group A and 35.7% (5/14) in group B. Death in group A was due to a perioperative infarction and the mortality rate is superimposable to that of isolated C.A.B.G.

In group B we first operated the most critical district: 6 in the coronaries and 8 in the carotids; 5 patients died: 3 for myocardial infarction and 2 for neurological coma.

Two patients died later in group A (6.4%) probably for myocardial infarction at 24 and 48 months postoperatively. Cardiac and cerebral mortality is 3.2% in group A and 7.1% in group B. These data are summarized in table 3 whereas in table 4 non letal late complications in still alive patients are reported.

Table 3. CABG + ETC (April 1979 - June 1989) RESULTS

Combined procedure *
(31 pt.)

HOSPITAL MORTALITY	LATE MORTALITY	CARDIAC MORBILITY	CEREBRAL MORBILITY
1 AMI (3.2%)	2 AMI ? (6.4%) 24-48 m.	1 AMI (3.2%)	1 Paresis (3.2%)°

* 12 left main
* 1 pt. aneurismectomy

° Cerebral morbility = 1.6%

Staged *
(14 pt.)

	HOSPITAL MORTALITY	LATE MORTALITY	CARDIAC MORBILITY	CEREBRAL MORBILITY
1° CABG (6 pt.)	3 (50%) 2 neur.coma 1 AMI	/	1 pt. (7.1%)	1 pt.(7.1%) emiparesis
1° ETC (8 pt.)	2 (25%) 2 AMI	/		

* 4 LM

Cerebral morbility = 1.6%

Table 4. CABG + ETC (April 1979 - June 1989) NO LETAL COMPLICATIONS

	COMBINED PROC.	STAGED PROC.
RISTENOSIS OR CAROTIDEAL OBSTR.	1 (3.5%)	2 (22.2%)
CAROTIDEAL STEN. CONTROLATERAL	1 (3.5%)	/
ANGINA	2 (7%)	1 (11.1%)
RENAL DIALISIS	1 (3.5%)	/

Interestingly in 1 patient a controlateral carotid stenosis, occured and 1 patient is now in chronic renal dyalisys.

DISCUSSION AND CONCLUSIONS

The problem of diagnosis and treating combined atherosclerotic coronary and carotid lesions is under discussion since almost 20 years and at the end of 1987 more than 1500 such patients are operated. A part from the diagnosis the surgical treatment can be combined as staged.

Upon our experience we are totally oriented towards combined surgery and our attitude is worldwide accepted. We perform a staged procedure only when there is a carotideal restenosis treating first the most involved district.

When the C.A.B.G. is first performed we keep the perfusion pressure during the E.C.C. at least of 70 mmHg and we don't low the hematocrit below 30% in order to achieve a better myocardial protection.

REFERENCES

1) Babu SC, Shaw PM, et al. (1985) "Coexisting carotid stenosis in patients undergoing cardiac surgery indications and guidelines for simultaneous operations" Am.J.Surg. 150, 207.
2) Thevenet A. (1985) "Traitement chirurgical des lésions associées aux sténoses carotidiennes avec AIT" In "Ateroma della carotide ed ischemia cerebrale reversibile" Editrice Compositori, Bologna.
3) Matar AF. (1986) "Concomitant coronary and cerebral revascularization under cardiopulmonary bypass" Am.Thor.Surg. 41,431.
4) Newmann DC, Hicks RG, Horton DA. (1987) "Coexistent carotid and coronary arterial disease" J.Cardiovasc.Surg., 28.
5) Hertzer NR, Young JR, Beven FG, et al. (1986) "Late results of coronary by-pass in patients with peripheral vascular disease" Clev.Clin., Q 52,2.
6) Pierangeli A, Marinelli G, Turinetto B. (1988) "Indicazioni chirurgiche nei pazienti con lesioni aterosclerotiche associate carotidee e coronariche" Atti Congr. Ischemia Cerebrale e cardiopatia. Il Pensiero Scientifico Ed.

88

Invasive monitoring of coronary blood flow in acute myocardial infarction: pathogenetic and therapeutic relevance

R. BUGIARDINI, A. POZZATI, G. MORGAGNI, A. BORGHI, F. OTTANI and P. PUDDU

Institute of Pathological Medicine and CCU, Policlinico S. Orsola, University of Bologna, Italy

ABSTRACT. The need to develop a reliable marker of reperfusion is important in view of the large number of pts in whom thrombolysis is now likely to be used. We measured coronary blood flow (CBF; thermodilution technique) in 12 pts presenting with acute myocardial infarction (AMI) and ST elevation in the anterior leads. After application of i.v. thrombolytic therapy (urokinase, 2 mil IU), CBF was measured every 30 min for 4 hrs and then every 4 hrs for 20 hrs. Coronary blood flow increased by more than 30% in 9 pts (G1) : from 86$\pm$24 to 126$\pm$46 ml/min; $p < 0.001$. No significant changes were seen in the remaining 3 pts (G2). Coronary angiography was performed in all pts and showed patency of the infarct-related artery in 8/9 G1 pts (89%) and occlusion in the remaining four pts. We conclude that measurement of CBF is a relatively simple technique that appears both sensitive and specific in detecting coronary reperfusion in anterior AMI.

Reocclusion of reperfused coronary arteries may limit the initial benefits obtained by thrombolysis in acute myocardial infarction (AMI). In-hospital transient or persistent reocclusion (i.e. post-infarction angina or reinfarction) following thrombolysis can be observed in 20 to 45% of patients diagnosed as being "successfully treated" (1). With this background, continuous monitoring of coronary patency with implied early detection of vessel reocclusion has to be considered a standard of primary importance for the understanding of both the pathophysiology and the therapeutic management of patients with AMI. Coronary revascularization can be indirectly assessed by the observation of the ST segment shifts during thrombolysis (2). Different patterns of variations suggests different modalities of reperfusion. These can be summarized as follows : (A) early and rapid normalization of ST elevation; (B) intermittent fluctuations of ST elevation with late

return to the baseline, or (C) with late persistence of this ECG abnormality; (D) no changes in ST elevation for many hours. Theoretically both changes in myocardial oxygen comsumption or variations in coronary blood flow (CBF) may account for the above mentioned patterns of ST changes. However, Hackett et al. (3) have recently demonstrated by angiography the existence of a subset of pts who develop reperfusion -reocclusion coronary cycles after successfull thrombolysis, thus indicating that a change in myocardial oxygen supply, rather than demand, is the real reason for the fluctuations of ST segment elevation observed during therapy.
Unfortunately, coronary angiography cannot be extensively performed in AMI, and procedure cannot be repeated when required by clinical or electrocardiographic observations.

1. Measurement of coronary blood flow

Keeping in mind these limitations, we looked for a simplified but sensitive method to assess coronary revascularization as many time as you need. Thus, we measured CBF by using the thermodilution technique (Wilton Webster Labs) after right heart catheterization and positioning of the catheter in the great cardiac vein, which drains blood from the anterior ventricular wall (4). We studied a series of pts with anterior AMI (chest pain $\leqslant$ 4 hrs, ST elevation in precordial leads) before and following i.v. urokinase (2 mil IU) (Fig. 1). Continuous monitoring of CBF, invasive arterial pressure, ST segment deviation, and CK plasma activity was performed for 24 hrs; this to obtain correlations between CBF and non invasive parameters of infarct-related artery patency. The data obtained confirm the existence of reocclusion cycles (Fig. 2) occurring in a subset of pts treated with thrombolysis.

CORONARY BLOOD FLOW DURING THROMBOLYSIS

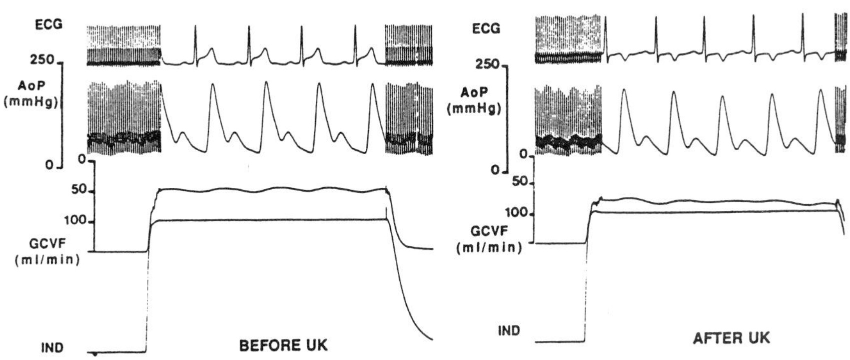

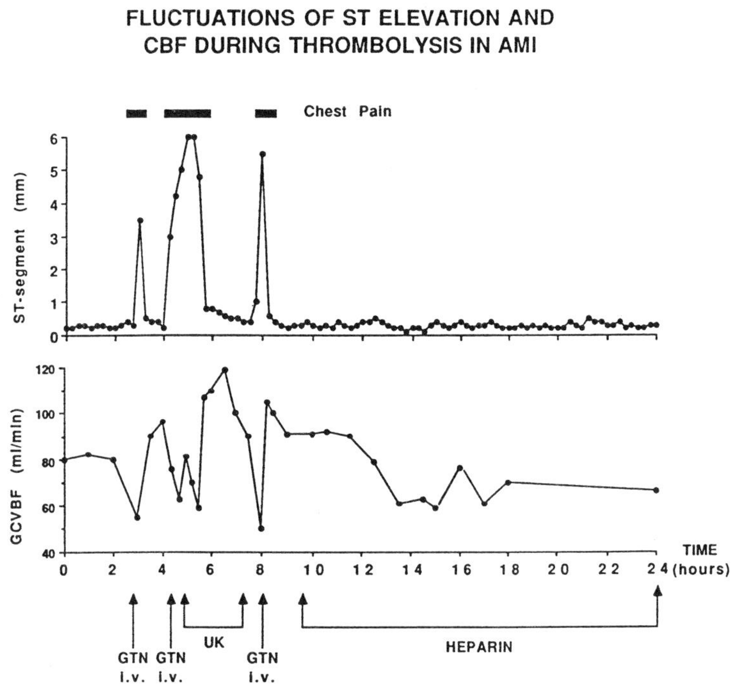

We observed an hyperemic response (increase > 30% of CBF) to coronary reperfusion in the majority of cases which is in agreement with other recent preliminary reports (5). Also, intermittency of CBF was observed in one third of pts; this usually occurs in the very early phase (6-12 hrs) of AMI, with a good correlation between CBF values and ST segment deviation. The evidence of these intermittent coronary occlusions has stimulated a number of therapeutic approaches to be done following thrombolysis. Efforts to prevent and/or resolve coronary reocclusion have been mainly directed towards antithrombotic drugs. Briefly, both repeated full doses or prolonged infusion of fibrinolytic agents, as well as continuous infusion of heparin and/or oral administration of aspirin have been suggested to be usefull in pts with AMI (6). Also, association between coronary dilators and thrombolytics have a rationale for their clinical application.

Indeed reocclusion is presumably due to rethrombosis and/or vasoconstriction in the infarct-related artery as suggested by several studies.

2. Paradoxic prothrombotic effect of thrombolysis

Fibrin generation is initiated by the thrombin induced cleavage of fibrinopeptide A (FPA) and B from the amino termini of fibrinogen chains. Thus FPA allows a monitoring of intravascular fibrin generation during AMI as well as thrombolysis. Rapold and al. (7) showed that FPA plasma levels are increased from the admission value in most pts under recombinant-tissue plasminogen activator (rtPA) infusion. Plasmin induced fibrinogenolytic peptides may elevate FPA levels, but their contribution is of minor importance during treatment with rtPA, which is a fibrin specific agent. Patients with clinical and ECGraphic evidence of recurrent coronary events after initial reperfusion had persistent high or reincreasing FPA plasma levels 30 min after completion of thrombolytic activity. This strongly suggests that post-reperfusion thrombin activity is due to enhanced fibrinogenesis, which in turn could be sustained by the reexposure of subendothelial collagen, or ischemia-related complicated lesions (8) through thrombolysis, or by procoagulant factors released from the same clot.

3. Role of vasoconstriction

A role for vasoconstriction is supported by the frequent prompt relief of reocclusion induced by nitrates during or following thrombolysis, and by the increase in the caliber of the residual stenosis that follows the intracoronary administration of nitrates (3). In addition, previous studies have clearly shown that spasm and stagnant flow resulting from it may enhance platelet aggregation (9), which may trigger thrombus formation at the site of the infarct-related coronary artery stenosis.

4. Clinical implications

The frequent intermittence of coronary blood flow observed following thrombolysis suggests that the majority of pts successfully treated are at high risk for early (within 24 hrs) recurrent coronary occlusion. Thus, strategies for intervention in AMI should not be based only on the achievement of coronary recanalization, but also on the prevention of the alternating cycles of reocclusion-reperfusion which may prelude up to recurrent coronary events.

Our preliminary data show that heparin infusion along with oral aspirin do not prevent the development of intermittent coronary occlusion nor the early (within 24 hrs) recurrence of AMI. Thus it seems conceivable to prolong (up to 24 hrs) the use of thrombolysis which can be complemented by high doses of powerful vasodilators such as i.v. nitroglycerin and/or calcium antagonists. These drugs should prevent vasoconstriction localized at the site of the infarct-related artery stenosis, which could result in a better delivery of thrombolytic agent along the thrombogenic coronary segment. This treatment can be used to "buy time" and prevent further myocardial damage while waiting for emergency revascularization.

References

(1) Barbash G.I., Hod H., Rath S., Miller H.I., Roth A., Har-Zahav Y., Modan M., Rotstein Z., Batler A., Zivelin A., Charnilass J., Kaplinsky E., Laniado S., Rabinowitz B., Seligsohn U. (1989) 'Intermittent, dose-related fluctuations of pain and ST elevation during infusion of recombinant tissue plasminogen activator during acute myocardial infarction', Am. J. Cardiol., 64, 225-228.

(2) Krucoff M.W., Green C.E., Satler L.F., Miller F.C., Pallas R.S., Kent K.M., Del Negro A.A., Pearle D.L., Fletcher R.D., Rackley C.E. (1986) 'Noninvasive detection of coronary artery patency using continuous ST-segment monitoring', Am. J. Cardiol., 57, 916-922.

(3) Hackett D., Davies G., Chierchia S., Maseri A. (1987) 'Intermittent coronary occlusion in acute myocardial infarction. Value of combined thrombolytic and vasodilator therapy', N. Engl. J. Med., 317, 1055-1059.

(4) Pepine C.J., Mehta J., Webster W.W., Nichols W.W. (1978) 'In vivo validation of a thermodilution method to determine regional left ventricular blood flow in patients with coronary disease', Circulation, 5, 795-802.

(5) Nicklas J.M., Diltz E.A., O'Neill W.W., Bourdillon P.D.V., Walton J.A. Jr., Pitt B. (1987) 'Quantitative measurement of coronary flow during medical revascularization (thrombolysis or angioplasty) in patients with acute infarction', J. Am. Coll. Cardiol., 10, 284-289.

(6) Fuster V., Stein B., Badimon L., Chesebro J.H. (1988) 'Antithrombotic therapy after myocardial reperfusion in acute myocardial infarction', J. Am. Coll. Cardiol., 12, 78A-84A.

(7) Rapold H.J., Kuemmerli H., Weiss M., Baur H., Haeberli A. (1989) 'Monitoring of fibrin generation during thrombolytic therapy of acute myocardial infarction with recombinant tissue-type plasminogen activator', Circulation, 79, 980-989.

(8) Ambrose J.A., Winters S.L., Arora R.R., Haft J.I., Goldstein J., Rentrop K.P., Gorlin R., Fuster V. (1985) 'coronary angiographic morphology in myocardial infarction : a link between the pathogenesis of unstable angina and myocardial infarction', J. Am. Coll. Cardiol., 6, 1233-1238.

(9) Bugiardini R., Chierchia S., Davies G., Crea F., Lenzi S., Maseri A., 1986) 'Differential transmyocardial platelet behavior in response to pacing and ergonovine-induced myocardial ischemia', Am. Heart J., 112, 255-262.

89
Prevention of stroke in bilateral carotid lesions

M. D'Addato

Department of Vascular Surgery, University of Bologna, via Massarenti 9, 40138 Bologna, Italy

The natural history of a carotid atherosclerotic lesion is well defined by many medical and surgical trials (7).

Monolateral stenoses greater than 70% or with gross ulcerations present a 5% average stroke-risk per year ().

Bilateral lesions are complicated by a greater incidence of stroke linked to the twin lesion and to a greater involvement of intracranial stenoses or occlusions (6). Even higher is the stroke rate in patients affected by a carotid stenosis associated with a contralateral occlusion (1). This event, moreover, is followed by a worse neurological symptomatology and by worse results, due to a lesser blood supply from the contralateral hemisphere.

The purpose of carotid endarterectomy (EA) is a reduction of the stroke-rate, a survival-rate improvement and, chiefly, a better quality of life.

The operative risk in patients with bilateral lesions increases progressively with the severity of the contralateral lesion. (6)

The aim of this study was to evaluate the indication and the surgical timing in these patients in order to obtain better results than with the conservative treatment.

Case evaluation

Between 1974 and 1983, 297 carotid EA were performed in 245 patients affected by bilateral carotid lesions, out of over 700 carotid reconstructive operations performed in the same time period.

Two hundred and seventeen EAs were performed in 165 patients affected by bilateral stenoses (BS), 120 males and 45 females, while 80 EAs were performed in patients with a stenosis associated with a contralateral internal carotid occlusion (S+O); 70 males and 10 females.

Preoperative symptomatology is reported in Tab. 1.

Tab. 1 : preoperative symptomatology

Neurological classification	B.S. (%)	S+O (%)
Asymptomatic	29.1	45.0
R.I.A.	46.5	35.0
mSTROKE-STROKE	11.3	6.2
Vertebro-bas;Borderline	13.1	13.8

The mean age of the first group (BS) was 62.6 years (38 - 78), while the mean age of the S+O group was 60 years.

The mean follow-up was respectively 21 and 15 months. All of the patients received antiplatelet treatment in the post-operative period; in the last 5 years this treatment began in the pre-operative period and continued in the follow-up. Before clamping 2.500 I.U. of heparin were injected i.v.

An intraluminal shunt was inserted when the back pressure was less than 50 mmHg, when a stroke was present in the history or when a cerebral damage in the contralateral hemisphere was present at the computed tomography. In the last 2 years, the need for shunt was decided when a 50% reduction of amplitude and a 20% lengthening of latency of the median nerve SEP component N. 20 was recorded.

Cumulative operative morbidity and mortality are reported in Fig. 1-3; the actuarial survival rate and stroke - free rate were calculated with the life - table analysis method and are reported in Fig. 1-3.

The patients with bilateral stenoses presented a lower operative stroke-rate than the patients with monolateral stenosis with no difference in the mortality rate. The patients with stenosis associated with a contralateral occlusion presented a higher operative stroke and mortality rate. In the follow-up, stroke-risk was less than 0.5% per year in both MS and BS group, while in the S+O group no late stroke was recorded, perhaps in relation to a shorter mean follow-up period.

Discussion

The surgical treatment of patients with bilateral carotid stenosis is followed, in many reports, by a higher complication-rate, the cause of which can be attributed to many factors, as a reduced collateral circulation, a reduced haemodynamic compense during surgery or an increased severity of intracranial and systemic vascular lesion. The operative timing, moreover, seems to be important also in determining the results.

Evaluating our results, an increase of the operative ipsilateral or contralateral stroke-risk cannot be confirmed, even if a reduced collateral circulation is confirmed by the need for an intraluminal shunt (Tab. 2).

Tab. 2 : need for shunt related to contralateral carotid

	%
Monolateral st.	7.7%
Bilateral st.	10.6%
Stenosis + occlusion	44.3%

The surgical timing in patients with bilateral stenoses is particularly important. The contemporaneous operation of both lesions is followed by a high incidence of complications due to: 1) "local nerve injury with following respiratory distress or problems with swallowing); 2) glomus nerve lesion (with hypertensive spikes); 3) hematoma or laryngeal edema; 4) uncontrollable ischemic complication after the 1st side EA in patients operated on in general anesthesia. For these reasons all but 5 patients with BS underwent a staged operation. In the 5 patients operated contemporarily on both sides, 2 deaths and 1 uncontrollable blood pressure were recorded.

In patients with bilateral lesion the carotid EA is indicated in symptomatic stenosis greater than 50% or in complicated plaques or in asymptomatic stenosis greater than 70%.

After a successful EA a patient with bilateral stenosis becomes a patient with a monolateral lesion; the indications for a 2nd EA are: a stenosis greater than 70% or an unstable plaque. Between the 2 operations, in consideration of the possible local nerve lesion, cranial nerve evaluation, cerebral CT scan and Duplex carotid evaluations are recommended and, in any case, a 15 day period between the 2 treatments is useful to obtain a stady state in the cerebral perfusion.

In the surgical timing in patients with BS, the more severe stenoses or, if similar, the symptomatic or the more unstable ones, were chosen for the 1st EA.

Following these patterns, carotid endarterectomy allowed us to obtain encouraging results even in high risk patients like those of the S+O group compared with a stroke-rate greater than 5% per year obtained with a non-operative treatment (4).

As the operative morbidity and mortality are prevalently due to myocardial infarction, cerebral haemorrhage and stroke, these results can be improved with a more accurate preoperative study, using SPECT to show brain ischemic areas at risk for stroke during clamping, and with a post-operative monitoring of patients with preoperative severe cerebral ischemia in which the autoregulation system may be non-functioning and who present, in the post-operative period, a cerebral hyperperfusion with high risk of cerebral haemorrhage. Patients with cardiac and respiratory deficits may be well operated under local anesthesia.

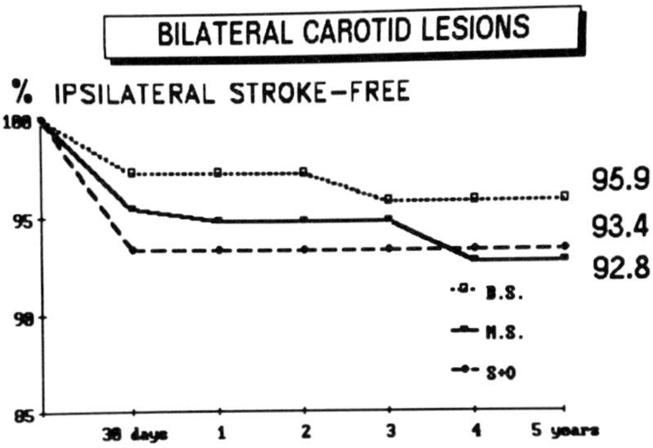

Fig. 1: Ipsilateral stroke-free rate in the follow-up in patients with monolateral stenosis (M.S.), bilateral stenosis (B.S.) and stenosis associated with a contralateral occlusion (S+O).

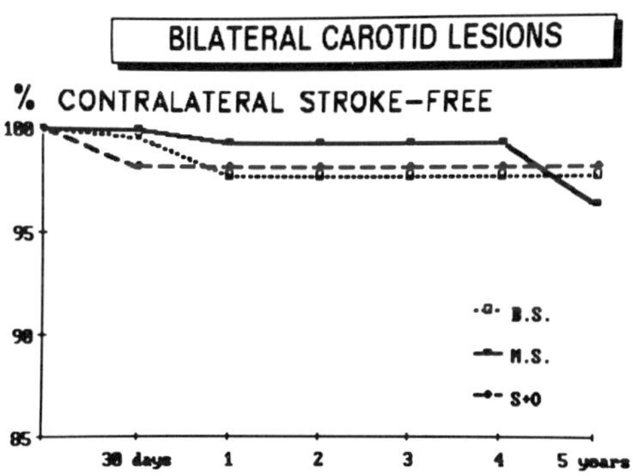

Fig. 2: Contralateral stroke-free rate in the follow-up, related to carotid lesion.

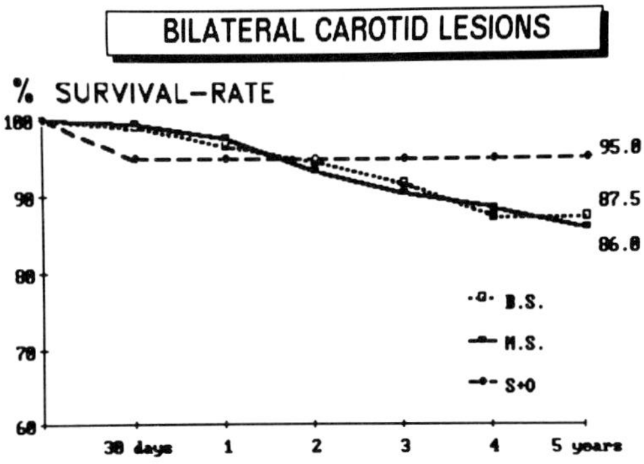

Fig. 3: Operative and follow-up survival-rate related to carotid lesion.

REFERENCES

1. BARNETT W.J.M.
   EC-IC By pass Study group. Failure of extracranial-intracranial arterial by pass to reduce the risk of ischemic stroke.
   N. Engl. J. Med. 313: 1191-1200, 1985.
2. BOUSSER M.G., ESCHWEGE E., HAGUENAU M., LE FAUCCONNIER J.M., THIBULT N., TOUBOUL D., TOUBOUL P.J.
   "AICLA" Controlled trial of aspirin and dipyridamole in the Secondary prevention of athero-thrombotic Cerebral Ischemia.
   Stroke 14 (1): 5-14, 1983.
3. FIELDS W.S., LEMAK N.A.
   Joint Study of extracranial arterial occlusion.
   X International carotid artery occlusion
   J.A.M.A. 235: 2734-8, 1976.
4. FRIEDMAN S.G., RILES T.S., LAMPARELLO P.J., IMPARATO A.M., SAKWA M.P.
   Surgical therapy for the patient with internal carotid artery occlusion and contralateral stenosis.
   J.V.S. 5: 856-61, 1987.

5. GENT M., BLAKELY J.A., EASTON J.D., ELLIS D.J., HACHINSKI V., HARBISON J.W., PANAK E., ROBERTS R.S., SICURELLA J., TURPIE A.G.G.
The canadian american ticlopidine study (Cats). in Thromboembolic stroke
the Lancet. 1217-20, 1989.
6. KIEFFER E., KOSKAS F., BAHNINI A., CORMIER F., GOUNY P., LESAGE R., PIQUOIS A., RUOTOLO C., SARFATTI P.O.
Résultats cliniques tardifs de la chirurgie carotidienne
In: Indications et résultats de la chirurgie carotidienne. Ed. AERCV, Paris, 1988. pp. 51-66.
7. THE AMERICAN CANADIAN CO-OPERATIVE STUDY GROUP
Persantine Aspirin Trial in cerebral ischemia - Part II: Endpoint results.
Stroke 16 (3): 406-15, 1985.

90 The role of percuraneous transluminal coronary angioplasty (PTCA) in the treatment of clinical syndromes of coronary atherosclerosis

A. BRANZI, G. PIOVACCARI, A. MARZOCCHI, G. MELANDRI, C. MARROZZINI, R. FATTORI and F. PRATI

Institute of Cardiovascular Diseases, University of Bologna, via Massarenti 9, Bologna, Italy

ABSTRACT. The treatment of ischemic heart disease has been strongly influenced over the last decade by the definitive acknowledgement that organic stenosis of coronary arteries and acute thrombotic occlusion on a preexisting stenosis are the two basic components of various clinical patterns of ischemic heart disease in the vast majority of cases.

Relevant therapeutic consequences are coronary bypass surgery and coronary angioplasty (PTCA) for the stenotic component and thrombolysis in acute infarction for the thrombotic component. Since the first successful operation in 1977, the use of PTCA has expanded dramatically. Whether it is applied or not frequently depends on organizational difficulties, due to the need for a surgical stand-by. But, in other circumstances, true scientific support for a very widespread diffusion is hard to imagine.

In our laboratory the percentage of PTCAs as compared to the number of coronary arteriographies performed between 1981 and 1988 was as follows: 0.3% (1981), 2.1% (1982), 5.9% (1983), 5% (1984), 9.5% (1985), 18.8% (1986), 21.2% (1987), 30.7% (1988). These data roughly indicate the percentage of PTCA candidates after diagnostic coronary arteriography today and thus the PTCA workload which must be considered when planning the activity of a catheterization laboratory.

The preliminary success rate in the initial series of 321 patients was 89%. In 38 of the patients in whom the procedure was unsuccessful, 18 had emergency and 13 elective bypass surgery, 6 were placed under medical treatment and one patient died suddenly one month after PTCA. Within the 1st year follow-up, 83 of 265 patients (31.3%) had further cardiac events: 3 acute myocardial infarction (AMI), 78 recurrence of angina and 2 died from cardiac-related causes. A second PTCA, carried out in 36 patients (46%) with recurrent angina, was successful in all cases with good long-term results in 27 (75%).

Probably one third or more of the patients with ischemic heart disease undergoing coronary arteriography are candidates for PTCA. It is envisaged that 20 to 25% of patients with a successful dilation will be re-examined with coronary arteriography within the first year and will need a second angioplasty in most cases. Apart from restenosis, a number of special clinical conditions will extend the indications and applications of PTCA: multivessel disease, stenosis of bypass grafts, total coronary occlusions, AMI with or without thrombolysis.

INTRODUCTION

Percutaneous transluminal coronary angioplasty (PTCA) has become a fundamental therapeutic tool in the treatment of the various clinical expressions of coronary atherosclerosis. Following its introduction in 1977, PTCA has met with an ever increasing number of indications, being applied in multiple coronary lesions, during AMI and in patients with previous aorto-coronary by-passes (1-8). The extension of the indications is basically due to the increased experience of the operators and a significant indications is basically due to the increased experience of the operators and a significant technological development in the materials used for the procedure (9). Due to these advances the percentage of successful PTCAs rose from the initial 67% to the present 90-95% (4-10). Thus the criteria for selecting eligible PTCA patients were progressively modified.

Original criteria

Between 1977 and 1982 the patients were carefully selected according to symptoms and anatomical pattern; they were all candidates for aorto-coronary by-pass with an arteriographic pattern typical of a normal left ventricular function, in the presence of a subtotal stenosis limited to a single main coronary vessel (4). Moreover, the patients had to have proximal, concentric, noncalcified stenoses, shorter than 10 mm and not affecting secondary branches (Tab.1). When these criteria were strictly applied, the PTCA candidates were found to be a very small minority, only 3.7% of the cases examined in the Coronary Artery Surgery Study (CASS) (11).

TABLE 1. Original selection criteria for PTCA candidates

Clinical
Angina pectoris Established myocardial ischemia Candidate for surgical revascularization
Angiographic
Single-vessel, proximal, concentric, subtotal, noncalcified lesions less than 10 mm long not involving secondary branches Well-preserved left ventricular function

Present criteria

The improvement in the results obtained have led to substantial changes in the selection criteria with extension of PTCA to patients with single and multi-vessel lesions, with eccentric, long, calcified stenoses and with total coronary occlusions. At present angioplasty is also carried out on patients with minimal symptoms but with clear atheromatous lesions of the main coronary vessels. The procedure is extended to highly symptomatic patients and those with non "ideal" arteriographic patterns: i.e. those cases which have already undergone aorto-coronary by-pass and have developed new stenoses in the native coronary vessels or reveal new pathologies obstructing the grafts (8) (Tab.2). At present the PTCA candidates are 25-30% of those patients undergoing diagnostic coronary arteriography (10).

PTCA in acute myocardial infarction

Since 1985, PTCA has been widely used to treat AMI (12-15). Mechanical dilation with a balloon offers two advantages as compared to thrombolysis: a more rapid reperfusion

80% of the cases in which thrombolytic therapy fails. PTCA can therefore be used alone or associated with thrombolysis to treat AMI (12).

TABLE 2. Present selection criteria for PTCA candidates

Clinical
Established myocardial ischemia with functional tests even in oligosymptomatic patients Acute Myocardial Infarction
Angiographic
"Simple" and "Complicated" single-vessel lesions (ulcerated, eccentric, calcified, long plaques) even at the coronary bifurcation Multivessel lesions, Total coronary occlusions Aorto-coronary grafts

A recent multicenter North American study (TAMI) has demonstrated that angioplasty carried out immediately after effective intravenous thrombolytic therapy does not lead to an improvement in the ventricular function and the prognosis in patients (16). Elective PTCA, 7-10 days after thrombolysis, is accompanied by a minor incidence of side-effects.

In the light of the results emerging from this study (16), PTCA is carried out in many cardiology centres under elective clinical conditions and, in particular, in cases with symptoms and/or evidence of residual myocardial ischemia. Immediate treatment of AMI with PTCA, with or without the association of thrombolytic therapy, would appear to be impossible on a large-scale due to the obvious organizational reasons. These therepeutic strategies may, however, be adopted in patients with myocardial infarction during hospitalization and particularly when diagnostic coronarography is carried out. During AMI with serious hemodynamic impairment, despite thrombolytic treatment, the use of PTCA may be justified in emergencies.

PTCA of multivessel lesions

The increase in the number of coronary angioplasties is mainly due to the extension of the procedure to patients with multi-vessel coronary disease. Following these indications, approximately 25-30% of the patients undergoing coronary arteriography have become candidates for PTCA (6-17-18).

There is still some dispute about the strategies to be followed in PTCA of multi-vessel lesions. In particular, it is not clear whether it is necessary to go ahead with a complete revascularization or if the procedure can be limited to the dilation of the stenosis in the vessel identified as being responsible for the ischemia or the symptoms (culprit lesion). The clinical results were better in the patients who had benefitted from complete revascularization, with a lower incidence of angina relapses and fewer aorto-coronary by-passes required.

PTCA after coronary surgery

Ten years after an aorto-coronary by-pass approximately 50% of vessel grafts reveal obstructive lesions with consequent recurrence of symptoms; moreover, there is a progressive expansion of the atheroscleroses in the native coronary vessels which contributes towards the clinical deterioration in these patients (19-20). A second operation involves higher mortality risks (between 2.3 and 16.7%) and worse clinical results over time (21).

Recently percutaneous coronary angioplasty was applied with success to graft and native coronary vessel stenoses. Considering the high number of patients undergoing aorto-coronary by-passes over the last decade, it is easy to understand the wide possibilities offered by PTCA both now and for the future. PTCA of venous by-passes has a greater incidence of failures, complications and new stenoses as compared to the treatment of native coronary lesions; therefore, where possible, combined dilation of the venous graft and the native coronary vessel appears to be beneficial.

Results and complications

The results of PTCA depend mainly on patient selection and the experience of the operators. At present the percentage of PTCA successes varies from 90-95%, in the cases with so-called "ideal" lesions (single, proximal, concentric and subocclusive), to 80-85% in the cases with multi-vessel diseases and after coronary surgery. In the cases with total coronary occlusion success is approximately 60% (10). Although there has been an improvement in the percentage success of immediate angiography, PTCA still shows a major number of complications which cannot be ignored (dissection and/or coronary thrombosis, myocardial infarction and death). The need to resort to an urgent aorto-coronary by-pass varies, according to the surveys, between 2 and 9%. Death during surgery oscillates between 0 and 14% and probably depends on the promptness of the operation once coronary occlusion has been established (Tab.3). Finally the overall mortality attributable to PTCA is approximately 1-1.5% (10).

TABLE 3. Incidence of CABG and perioperative complications after PTCA

Reference		Total no. of patients	Emergency CABG		Mortality		Perioperative AMI	
			No.	%	No.	%	No.	%
22 Cowley	1984	(3079)	202	6.6	13	6.4	90	45
23 Murphy	1984	(899)	32	3.7	0	0	21	66
24 Killen	1985	(3000)	115	3.8	13	11.3	50	43
25 Shiv	1985	(240)	14	5.8	2	14.3	5	36
26 Golding	1986	(1831)	81	4.4	2	2.5	37	46
27 Connor	1989	(996)	91	9.1	4	4.4	49	54
Card.Inst.BO.	1989	(606)	27	4.4	0	0	13	48

Follow-up

An important limit on PTCA is represented by coronary restenoses which occur in the first 6-8 months after the procedure.

In two surveys with average follow-ups of 12 and 72 months the reappearance of angina occurred in 13 and 33% (28-29). The percentage of patients with angina and other clinical signs of coronary insufficiency was much higher in those with multivessel lesions, especially if only partially treated (29).

Although there is the possibility of the atherosclerotic disease spreading to different coronary branches and segments from those dilated, it is obvious that restenosis is the fundamental cause of the reappearance of angina and therefore of the clinical failure of angioplasty over time. For a reliable assessment of the incidence of restenosis it is necessary to make a systematic arteriographic re-examination of the patients. A survey of 557 patients, re-examined in the NHLBI PTCA report, revealed restenosis in 33.6% (30). Other studies report restenosis percentages of between 29 and 40% (10, 31, 32) in patients treated mainly or exclusively for single-vessel lesions. The incidence of restenosis increases dramatically in patients treated for multivessel lesions, ranging from 46% to 56%, even if the percentage of restenoses referring to dilated lesions remains around 30% (10, 34). A total of 162 patients were studied at the Cardiology Institute in Bologna, with a total of 179 dilated lesions and a critical restenosis (≥70%) was found in 23.5% of the cases (33).

Medical therapy with calcium-antagonists, nitroderivates, anticoagulants and anti-platelet drugs do not appear to have a significant effect on the percentage of restenoses; therefore the best treatment of restenoses still remains the repetition of PTCA.

REFERENCES

1 Gruentzig, C.T. (1978) 'Transluminal dilatation of coronary-artery stenosis' (letter to the editor), Lancet 1, 263.

2 Levy, R.I., Mock, M.B., Willman, V.L., Passamani, E.R., Frommer, P.L. (1981) 'Percutaneous transluminal coronary angioplasty: a status report' (editorial). N. Engl. J. Med. 305, 399-400.

3 Mabin, T.A., Holmes, D.R. Jr., Smith, H.C., et al. (1985) 'Follow-up clinical results in patients undergoing percutaneous transluminal coronary angioplasty'. Circulation 71, 754-760.

4 Kent, K.M., Bentivoglio, L.G., Block, P.C., et al. (1982) 'Percutaneous transluminal coronary angioplasty: report from the registry of the National Heart, Lung and Blood Institutes'. Am. J. Cardiol. 49, 20111-2020.

5 Kent, K.M., Bentivoglio, L.G., Block, P.C., et al.. (1984) 'Long-term efficacy of percutaneous transluminal coronary angioplasty (PTCA): report from the National Heart, Lung and Blood Institute PTCA Registry'. Am. J. Cardiol. 53, 27C-31C.

6 Vlietstra, R.E., Holmes, D.R. Jr., Reeder, G.S., et al. (1983) 'Balloon angioplasty in multivessel coronary artery disease'. Mayo Clin. Proc. 58, 563-567.

7 Holmes, D.R. Jr., Vlietstra, R.E., Reeder, G.S., et al. (1984) 'Angioplasty in total coronary artery occlusion. J. Am. Coll. Cardiol. 3, 845-849.

8 Reeder, G.S., Bresnahan, J.F., Holmes, D.R. Jr., et al. (1986) 'Angioplasty for aortocoronary bypass graft stenosis'. Mayo Clin. Proc. 61, 14-19.

9 Kelsey, S.F., Mullin, S.M., Detre, K.M., et al. (1984) 'Effect of investigator experience on percutaneous transluminal coronary angioplasty'. Am. J. Cardiol. 53, 56C-64C.

10 Holmes, D.R. Jr., Vlietstra, R.E. (1986) 'Percutaneous Transluminal Corononary Angioplasty: Current Status and Future Trends'. Mayo Clin. Proc. 61, 865-876.
11 Holmes, D.R. Jr., Vlietstra, R.E., Fisher, L.D., et al. (1983) 'Follow-up of patients from the Coronary Artery Surgery Study (CASS) potentially suitable for percutaneous transluminal coronary angioplasty'. Am. Heart J. 106, 981-988.
12 Holmes, D.R., Smith, H.C., Vlietstra, R.E., et al. (1985) 'Percutaneous transluminal coronary angioplasty, alone or in combination with streptokinase therapy, during acute myocardial infarction'. Mayo Clin. Proc. 60, 449-456.
13 Papapietro, S.E., MacLean, W.A.H., Stanley, A.W.H. Jr., et al. (1985) 'Percutaneous transluminal coronary angioplasty after intracoronary streptokinase in evolving acute myocardial infarction'. Am. J. Cardiol. 55, 48-53.
14 O'Neill, W., Timmis, G.C., Bourdillon, P.D., et al. (1986) 'A prospective randomized clinical trial of intracoronary streptokinase versus coronary angioplasty for acute myocardial infarction'. N. Engl. J. Med. 314, 812-818.
15 Hartzler, G.O., Rutherford, B.D., McConahay, D.R., et al. (1983) 'Percutaneous transluminal coronary angioplasty with and without thrombolytic therapy for treatment of acute myocardial infarction'. Am. Heart J. 106, 965-973.
16 Topol, E.J., Califf, R.M., George, B.S., et al. (1987) 'A randomized trail of immediate versus delayed elective angioplasty after intravenous tissue plasminogen activator in acute myocardial infarction'. N. Engl. J. Med. 317, 581-8.
17 Cowley, M.J., Vetrovec, G.W., Di Sciascio, G., Lewis, S.A., Hirsh, P.D., Wolfgang, T.C. (1985) 'Coronary angioplasty of multiple vessels: short-term outcome and long-term results'. Circulation 72, 1314-1320.
18 Thomas, E.S., Most, A.S., Williams, D.O. (1988) 'Coronary angioplasty for patients with multivessel coronary artery disease: Follow-up clinical status'. Am. Heart J. 115, 8.
19 Ernst, S.M.P.G., van der Feltz, T.A., Ascoop, C.A.P.L., et al. (1987) 'Percutaneous transluminal coronary angioplasty in patients with prior coronary artery bypass grafting'. J. Throac. Cardiovasc. Surg. 93, 268-75.
20 Dorros, G., Lewin, R.F., Mathiak, L.M. (1988) 'Percutaneous transluminal coronary angioplasty in multivessel coronary disease patients: short- and long-term follow-up in single and multiple dilatations'. Clin. Cardiol. 11, 601-612.
21 Dorros, G., Ruben, Lewin, R.F., Mathiak, L.M., et al. (1988) 'Percutaneous transluminal coronary angioplasty in patients with two or more previous coronary artery bypass grafting operations'. Am. J. Cardiol. 61, 1243-1247.
22 Cowley, M.J., Dorros, G., Kelsey, S.F., et al. (1984) 'Emergency coronary bypass surgery after coronary angioplasty: The National Heart, Lung and Blood Institute's Percutaneous Transluminal Coronary Angioplasty Registry experience'. Am. J. Cardiol. 53 (Suppl. C), 22.
23 Murphy, D.A., Craver, J.M., Jones, E.L., et al. (1984) 'Surgical management of acute myocardial ischemia following percutaneous transluminal coronary angioplasty: Role of the intra-aortic balloon pump'. J. Thorac. Cardiovasc. Surg. 87, 332.
24 Killen, D.A., Hamaker, W.R., Reed, W.A. (1985) 'Coronary artery bypass following percutaneous transluminal coronary angioplasty'. Ann. Thorac. Surg. 40, 133.
25 Shiu, M.F., Silverton, N.P., Oakley, D. et al. (1985) 'Acute coronary occlusion during percutaneous transluminal coronary angioplasty'. Br. Heart J. 54, 129.
26 Golding, L.A.R., Loop, F.D., Hollman, J.L., et al. (1986) 'Early results of emergency surgery after coronary angioplasty'. Circulation 74 (Suppl.3), 26.

27 Connor, A.R., Vlietstra, R.E., Schaff, H.V., et al. (in press) 'Early and late results of coronary artery bypass after failed angioplasty: Actuarial analysis of late cardiac events and comparison with initially successful angioplasty'. J. Thorac. Cardiovasc. Surg.
28 Berger, E., Williams, D.O., Reinert, S., Most, A.S. (1986) 'Sustained efficacy of percutaneous transluminal coronary angioplasty'. Am. Heart J. 111, 233.
29 Gruentzig, A.R., King, S.B. III, Schlumpf, M., Siegenthaler, W. (1987) 'Long-term follow-up after percutaneous transluminal coronary angioplasty'. N. Engl. J. Med. 316, 1127.
30 Holmes, D.R., Vliestra, R.E., Smith, H.C., et al. (1984) 'Restenosis after percutaneous transluminal coronary angioplasty (PTCA): a report from the PTCA Registry of the National Heart, Lung and Blood Institute'. Am. J. Cardiol. 53, 77C.
31 Leimgruber, P.P., Roubin, G.S., Hollman J., et al. (1986) 'Restenosis after successful coronary angioplasty in patients with single-vessel disease'. Circulation 73, 710.
32 Henderson, R.A., Karani, S., Bucknall, C.A., Dritsas, A., Timmis, A.D., Sowton, E. (1989) 'Clinical Outcome of coronary angioplasty for single-vessel disease'. Lancet September 2, 546.
33 Marzocchi, A., Piovaccari, G., Marrozzini, C., Donti, A., Maresta, A., Magnani, B. (1988) 'Risultati a distanza dell'angioplastica coronarica: importanza della ristenosi'. Giorn. Ital. Cardiol. Vol. XVIII, 705-712.
34 Vandormael, M.G., Deligonul, U., Kern, M.J. (1987) 'Multilesion coronary angioplasty: clinical and angioplastic follow-up'. J. Am. Coll. Cardiol. 10, 246.

91
Invasive treatment of acute stroke

C. FIESCHI, D. TONI, M. SACCHETTI, P. PANTANO, E. MILLEFIORINI and M. FRONTONI

Department of Neurosciences, University of Rome, Viale dell'Università 30, 00185 Rome, Italy

Data pertaining the population of Rochester (Minnesota) in the early eighties [1] are consistent with the end of the decline of stroke which was recorded in that area from 1945 to 1974 [2]. However, the survival up to three days and the 30-day death of patients with cerebral infarction have never significantly decreased over the past four decades [3].

Therefore, stroke prevention, which appeared so effective until a few years ago, seems currently to have reached its limits, whereas available guidelines to treatment of acute brain ischemia are still needed now, as they were forty years ago.

Criticallly evaluating the failure of traditional trials of medical therapy, a few years ago Caplan and Stein [4] hypothesized that it could be basically related to an inhomogeneous grouping of patients. In fact, published studies had been always planned without considering the the peculiar and different pathophysiological problems underlying analogous clinical events.

In the same period, studies on animal models indicated the presence and limits of a possible therapeutic window: an early revascularization, within 4-8 hours from the experimental occlusion, was demonstrated as necessary to minimize the ischemic damage [5].

Functional studies on cerebral blood flow in cerebral ischemia, made possible on humans by PET and SPECT, have then showed the existence of an area of ischemic "penumbra", located around the infarcted area, in which an increased extraction of nutrients partially balances the decrease of blood supply [6; 7]. Over a limited period of time, neurons in that area would be maintained in a state of functional deficit liable to complete recovery if the blood flow is promptly restored [8].

Therefore, a counterpart of the experimentally demonstrated therapeutic window does exist, even if its limits are still to be clarly defined.

Considering the above mentioned criticisms on previous trials, together with the more recent experimental knowledge, one can come to the conclusion that a modern study on pharmacological treatment of acute ischemic stroke should be carried out on the basis of an early clinical observation and thorough evaluation, to take into account both the limits of the therapeutic window and the specific pathophysiological correlates which "functional" studies (PET and SPECT) can provide.

Furthermore, the perfusional state should be studied as soon as possible after the onset of cerebral ischemia, with neuroimaging techniques, and possibly monitored by means of noninvasive exams, possibly supported by angiography, since the role of collateral circulation is fundamental in the evolution of ischemic damage [9].

Indeed, when hypoperfusion lasts enough to cause ischemia, only if a "good" collateral circulation takes place very soon, the possibility reasonably exist to minimize tissue damage.

With these guidelines, a study in which all patients admitted to the Emergency Room were promptly examined by a neurologist, was undertaken [10].

When a diagnosis of probable focal cerebral ischemia was established, the patient was considered as eligible. Subjects older than 80 years of age, patients in coma or evaluated later than 4 hours from the onset of their signs or simptoms, and those with subtentorial clinical evidences, previous ischemic stroke, other invalidating diseases, or regression of symptoms within the recruitment period, were excluded.

Included patients had immediate brain CT scan to rule out any further cause of exclusion, like hemorrhages, tumors or other conditions mimicking stroke.

The enrolled ones underwent a complete evaluation including: neurological and cardiovascular hystory and exam; pertinent laboratory tests; 12-lead EKG; grading of neurological deficit by means of the Canadian Neurological Scale; transcranial and neck vessel Dopplersonography; Digital Subtraction Angiography of the cerebral arteries. An assessment of cerebral blood flow was also obtained in 32 patients, using Tc-99m-PAO as tracer and SPECT technique according to Holmes et al. [11].

Further exams were performed over the 30-day follow-up period, including repeated head CT scan and dayly monitoring of angiographically documented intracranial occlusions by Transcranial Doppler (TCD).

Patients with angiographically documented Internal or Middle Cerebral Artery occlusion were considered as having good collateral circulation only if the vessels distal to the occlusion were fully visualized within five seconds from the end of contrast injection.

Eighty out of 417 consecutively observed patients (19% of the eligibles) were included in the study and prospectively followed.

CT scan was performed, on average, within 3 hours, and angiography within 4 hours. from the onset of symptoms, with a maximum delay of 6 hours.

Eightyfour percent of patients had normal CT scan of the head on admission, 9% showed an early congruous hypodensity and 6% indirect signs of focal brain edema.

In 8 cases (10%) angiogram was normal and in 11 (14%) it showed an isolated plaque at the origin of tha ICA. The remaining 61 patients (76%) had complete occlusive arterial disease.

The patency of the intracranial arteries was monitored during follow-up with TCD in patients with MCA mainstem occlusion, 8 of whom had repeated angiography. An overall correlation between TCD and angiography was demonstrated in 90% of MCA mainstem occlusions (Zanette et al. 1988, personal communication).

Reperfusion occurred within 24 hours in 4 and within a week in 7 additional patients; none of these cases showed significant improvement following recanalization, and, remarkably, patients with documented intracranial occlusion nd poor or absent collateral filling at early angiography had the worst clinical outcome.

The presence of a good collateral supply was correlated to a lesser degree of both interemispheric and regional asymmetry index at SPECT. This neuroimaging technique could proven useful to differentiate subgroups of stroke patients according to the severity of both clinical and tissue damage evolution, being also able to demonstrate an early perfusional deficit while CT scan was still negative (Giubilei et al. 1989, in press).

Complete arterial occlusions in the symptomatic arteries, possibly embolic in nature, and spontaneously reversible were frequent (66%), confirming other results from studies on early angiography in cerebrovascular patients [12], and in contrast with previous data in less acute patients, indicating a strong prevalence of atherosclerotic extracranial carotid lesions in ischemic stroke [13].

The incidence of emboli reported in our series also exceeds the 40% of the Harvard Stroke Registry [14] and the 50% of an autopsy study [15].

The interval from the onset of stroke may provide an explanation for these differences: the shortest the latency, the hyghest seems to be the probability of detecting a complete occlusion.

If this is true, embolic cerebral ischemia is much more common than we believed in the past, and these data would strongly support the interest in studies with Kinases and r-TPA [16; 17] encouraged also by the results obtained with fibrinolytics in myocardial infarction [18].

In terms of therapeutic management, the administration of streptokinase and urokinase involves a significant risk of hemorrhagic complications because of their systemic anticoagulant action. Selective thrombolysis, due to higher affinity with fibrin-bound than with free plasminogen, may encourage the use of r-TPA or r-prourokinase in new trials.

Identifying the subgroup of strokes suitable for fibrinolytic treatment might just represent the right attempt to exploit a therapeutic window of still partially reversible ischemic damage, in order to achieve a timely regional perfusion optimized to good recovery.

Aimed to the same goal, vasodilating agents have been used.

Nimodipine, a calcium channel blocker, limited ischemic damage by improving CBF in animals after MCA occlusion [19] and gave interesting results in the clinical trial of Gelmers et al. [20]. Recently, CBF measurement by SPECT in patients treated with Nimodipine within 6 hours from onset, has evidentiated an increased flow at the periphery of the ischemic area [21].
Over the past few years, acquisition on the pathogenesis of irreversible ischemic brain damage have shown that an increase of intracellular calcium concentration may induce important metabolic disturbances. They involve Ca-dependent proteases and phospholipases activation with consequent release of toxic products, responsible for cytoscheletal disruption [22].

Calcium antagonists, with their properties of Ca-influx modulators, can therefore play a further role in protection against brain ischemia, additional to perfusional increase. Current research on animals is addressed to newer calcium entry blockers with peculiar charateristics, as Nilvadipine [23] and Emopamil [24] to be potentially evaluated in future clinical trials.
But the mainstream of brain protection takes also in account knowledge on the role of neuromodulators as glutamate, whose accumulation, in the ischemic area, is believed to be responsible for neurotoxicity [25]. A specific glutamatergic receptor, activated by N-methyl-D-aspartate (NMDA) is linked to an excessive Ca-influx, thus the blockade of that receptor, by means of competitive and non-competitive NMDA-antagonists should be attempted in experimental studies.
Membrane failure is also a major phenomenon characterizing irreversible ischemic injury [26]. Gangliosides, which interact with brain membranes by various metabolic effects [27], have been tested in animals, concerning possible protection in the acute phase [28].
Moreover, considering the recently demonstrated existence of growth factors stimulating CNS plasticity [29], gangliosides have been also considered in enhancement of neuronal "regeneration"[30].

On the basis of these data, an international multicenter study, involving six European countries and USA, on early treatment of ischemic stroke with monosialoganglioside (GM1) has been undertaken. Up to September 1989, the stroke registry has reported 7624 patients, 721 of whom were eligible (9.45%) and 698 randomly treated.

In conclusion, carefully planning a study on pharmacological treatment for acute ischemic stroke is a difficult task. It is necessary to be aware of logistical problems which can be solved only in higly qualified facilities; different services as Neuro Intensive Care Unit, Neuroradiology, Nuclear Medicine, Dopplersonography, have to work in a well organized cooperative system.
However, only well designed, protected and sufficiently extensive trials will provide clinically reliable and convincing evidence.

BIBLIOGRAPHY

1. Broderick JP, Phillips SJ, Whisnant JP, O'Fallon WM, Bergstral EJ. (1989) "Incidence rate of stroke in the eighties: the end of the decline of stroke?" Stroke 20, 577-588.

2. Garraway WM, Whisnant JP, Furlan AJ, Phillips LH, Kurland LT, O'Fallon WM. (1979) "The declining incidence of stroke", New Engl J Med 300, 499-452.

3. Garraway WM, Whisnant JP, Drury I. (1983) "The changing pattern of survival following stroke", Stroke 14, 699-702.

4. Caplan LR, Stein RW. (1986) "Stroke. A clinical approach", Butterworths publisher.

5. Weinstein PR, Anderson GG, Telles DA. (1980) "Neurological deficit and cerebral infarction after temporary middle cerebral artery occlusion in unanesthetized cats", Stroke 17, 318-324.

6. Lenzi GLL, Frackowiack RSJ, Jones T. (1982) "Cerebral oxygen metabolism and blood flow in human cerebral ischemic infarction", J Cereb Blood Flow Metab 2, 321-335.

7. Vorstrup S, Paulson OB, Lassen N. (1986) "Cerebral blood flow in acute and chronic ischemic stroke using Xenon-133 inhalation tomography", Acta Neurol Scand 74, 439-451.

8. Lenzi GLL, Frackowiack RSJ, Jones T, Heather JD, Lammertsma AA, Rhodes CG, Pozzilli C. (1981) "CMRO2 and CBF by Oxygen-15 inhalation technique: results in normal volunteers and cerebrovascular patients", Europ Neurol 20, 285-290.

9. Bozzao L, Fantozzi LM, Bastianello S, Bozzao A, Fieschi C. (1989) "Early collateral blood supply and late parenchymal brain damage in patients with middle cerebral artery occlusion", Stroke 20, 735-740.

10. Fieschi C, Argentino C, Lenzi GL, Sacchetti ML, Toni D, Bozzao L. (1989) "Clinical and instrumental evaluation of patients with ischemic stroke within the first six hours" J Neurol Sci 91, 311-322.

11. Holmes RA, Chaplin SB, Rayston FG et al. (1985) "Cerebral uptake and retention of Tc-99m hexamethilpropyleneamine oxime (Tc-99m HM-PAO)", Nucl Med Commun 6, 443-447.

12. Dalal PM. (1965) "Angiographic observation on spontaneous clot lysis", Lancet 1, 61-64.

13. Gurdjian ES, Lindner DW, Hardy WG, Thomas LM. (1961) "Completed stroke due to occlusive cerebrovascular disease. An analysis of 409 cases", Neurology (Minn.) 11, 724-733.

14. Mohr JP, Caplan LR, Melski JW, Goldstein RJ, Duncan GW, Kistler JP, Pessin MS, Blech HL. (1978) "The Harvard Cooperative Stroke Registry: a prospective registry", Neurology 28, 574-762.

15. Fisher M. (1954) "Occlusion of the carotid arteries. Further experiences", Arch Neurol Psychiat 72, 187-204.

16. Sloan MA. (1987) "Thrombolysis and stroke. Past and future", Arch Neurol 44, 748-768

17. The TPA-Acute Stroke Study Group. (1988) "An open multicenter study of the safety and efficacy of various doses of r-TPA in patients with acute stroke: preliminary results", Stroke 19, 9.

18. GISSI. (1987) "Long-term effects of intravenous thrombolysis in acute myocardial infarction: final report", Lancet 1, 871-874.

19. Mohamed AA, Gotoh O, Graham DI, Osborne KA, McCulloch J, Mendelow AD, Teasdale GM, Harper MH. (1985) "Effect of pretreament with the calcium antagonist nimodipine on local cerebral blood flow and histopathology after middle cerebral artery occlusion", Ann Neurol 18, 705-711.

20. Gelmers HJ, Gorter K, De Weerdt CJ, Wiezer HJA. (1988) "A controlled trial of nimodipine in acute ischemic stroke", N Engl J Med 318, 203-207.

21. Pozzilli C, Di Piero V, Pantano P, Rasura M, Lenzi GL. (1981) "Influence of nimodipine on cerebral blood flow in human cerebral ischaemia", J Neurol 236, 199-202.

22.Siesjo BK. (1981) "Cell damage in the brain. A speculative synthesis", J Cereb Blood Flow Metab 1, 155-185.

23. Kuwaki T, Satoh H, Ono T, Shibayama F, Yamashita T, Nishimura T. (1989) "Nilvadipine attenuates ischemic degration of gerbil brain cytoscheletal proteins", Stroke 20, 78-83.

24. Nakayama H, Ginsberg MD, Dietrich WD. (1988) "(S)-Emopamil, a novel calcium channel blocker and serotonin S2 antagonist, markedly reduces infarct size following middle cerebral artery occusion in the rat", Neurology 38, 1667-1673.

25. Rothmans SM, Olney JW. (1987) "Excitotoxicity and the NMDA receptor", TINS 10, 299-302.

26. Astrup J. (1982) "Energy-requiring cell functions in the ischemic brain", J Neurosurg 56, 482-497.

27. Davis CW, Daly JW. (1980) "Activation of rat cerebral cortical 3', 5'-cyclic nucleotide phosphodiesterase activity by gangliosides", Mol Pharmacol 17, 206-211.

28. Greenberg JH, Reivich M ,Urbanics R, Tanaka K, Dora E, Toffano G. (1986) "The effect of GM1 on cerebral metabolism, microcirculation and histology in focal ischemia", in Tettamanti G et al. (eds.), Gangliosides and neuronal plasticity, Liviana Press, Padova, pp. 397-405.

29. Freed WJ, De Medinaceli L, Wyatt RJ. (1985) "Promoting functional plasticity in the damaged nervous system", Science 227, 1544-1552.

30. Doherty P, Dickson JG, Flanigan TP, Walsh FS. (1985) "Ganglioside GM1 does not initiate, but enhances neurite regeneration of nerve growth factor-dependent sensory neurones", J Neurochem 44, 1259-1265.

Index